Practical Head and Neck Oncology

Practical Head and Neck Oncology

GUY J. PETRUZZELLI, MD, PhD, MBA, FACS

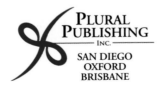

PLURAL PUBLISHING INC.

SAN DIEGO
OXFORD
BRISBANE

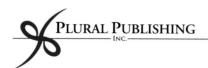

5521 Ruffin Road
San Diego, CA 92123

e-mail: info@pluralpublishing.com
Web site: http://www.pluralpublishing.com

49 Bath Street
Abingdon, Oxfordshire OX14 1EA
United Kingdom

Typeset in 10½/13 Garamond by Flanagan's Publishing Services, Inc.
Printed in Hong Kong by Paramount Printing

ISBN-13: 978-1-59756
ISBN-10: 1-59756-

Library of Congress Cataloging-in-Publication Data:
Practical head and neck oncology / [edited by] Guy J. Petruzzelli.
     p. ; cm.
  Includes bibliographical references and index.
  ISBN-13: 978-1-59756-113-6 (alk. paper)
  ISBN-10: 1-59756-113-4 (alk. paper)
  1. Head—Cancer. 2. Neck—Cancer. I. Petruzzelli, Guy J.
  [DNLM: 1. Head and Neck Neoplasms—diagnosis. 2. Head and Neck Neoplasms—surgery. 3. Head and Neck Neoplasms—therapy. WE 707 P8953 2008]
  RC280.H4P73 2008
  616.99'491—dc22

            2008014270

Contents

Preface

The care of patients with malignant neoplasms of the head and neck is an area of medial practice where superior outcomes are realized only through multispecialty collaboration. Each member of the health care team brings his or her own level of expertise, dedication, and sophistication to each patient encounter. The management of patients with head and neck cancer is constantly evolving. In *Practical Head and Neck Oncology* we have attempted to address some of the specific therapeutic challenges these patients present. Specifically, we included chapters on management of endocrine malignancies by Dr. Theodore Teknos, salivary gland malignancies by Dr. Daniel Deschler, surgery following chemoradiation therapy by Dr. Kerstin Stenson, and evaluation of the unknown primary cancer by Dr. Petruzzelli. Surgeons will find Dr. Urquharts's comprehensive chapter on lymphoreticular malignancies of the head and neck extremely useful to enhance their understanding of the complex group of neoplasms.

In addition to the surgical perspective we have included input from experts in other important disciplines involved in the management of patients with malignant tumors of the upper aerodigestive tract. Experts from the fields of radiation oncology (Dr. Emami), medical oncology (Dr. Clark), and oral and maxillofacial surgery (Drs. Beumer and Khan) have made important contributions in their respective fields.

The focus of the text is to provide clinicians useful information for the systematic and efficient evaluation, diagnosis, and treatment of patients with malignant head and neck tumors. General otolaryngologists-head and neck surgeons, plastic/reconstructive and oral/maxillofacial surgeons, radiation and medical oncologists, and other clinicians interested in caring for patients with tumors of the head and neck will find this text to be a concise resource providing critical and useful information for comprehensive treatment planning and monitoring therapy in their patients. By including chapters on the head and neck examination by Dr. Scianna and interpreting clinical studies by Dr. Pytinia, we hope students and residents will find this text an excellent reference for preparing to care for these challenging and fascinating patients.

The textbook is dedicated to the understanding, assessment, and comprehensive treatment of patients with malignant tumors of the head and neck and upper aerodigestive tract. It focuses on the practical evaluation of these patients with emphasis on sensible, efficient, and cost-effective evaluation.

Acknowledgments

I wish to acknowledge my mentors in the Department of Otolaryngology at the University of Pittsburgh Drs. Eugene Myers, Carl Snyderman, Riccardo Carrau, and in particular Dr. Jonas Johnson. From the beginning of my training these individuals stressed that superior patient outcomes are only possible through hard work, a commitment to excellence, and attention to every detail. They emphasized that improving patient care is only possible through continued self-examination, systematic data collection, and an unbiased critique of one's work.

The treatment of complex patients with rare diseases requires the dedication and commitment of many individuals and I been fortunate to have worked with outstanding clinicians in a variety of specialties. Many of whom were generous with their time and shared their expertise in this textbook. In particular I would like to thank Dr. Bahman Emami for his hours of instruction in the principles of radiation oncology and Dr. Thomas Origitano for his continued friendship forged over many hours in the operating room.

I also wish to thank Ms. Stephanie Meissner and Dr. Sadanand Singh at Plural Publishing for their support, patience, and commitment to this project.

Finally, I would like to recognize Ms. Kathy Rockford for her dedication and attention to detail throughout all phases of the preparation of this textbook. Her tenacity and professionalism were instrumental in completing this work.

Contributors

Amit Agrawal, MD
Assistant Professor
Department of Otolaryngology-Head and Neck
 Surgery
Arthur G. James Cancer Hospital and Richard J.
 Solove Research Institute
The Ohio State University
Columbus, Ohio
Chapter 18

Douglas Edwin Anderson, MD
Professor of Neurological Surgery
Loyola University Medical Center
Maywood, Illinois
Chapter 13

Amy Anstead, MD
Otolaryngology-Head and Neck Surgery
University of Illinois, Chicago
Chapter 24

William J. Benedict, Jr., MD
Assistant Professor of Neurosurgery
Emory University School of Medicine
The Emory Clinic
Atlanta, Georgia
Chapter 13

Michelle G. Bernstein, MA, CCC
Speech-Language Pathologist
Department of Otolaryngology
University of Miami Miller School of Medicine
Miami, Florida
Chapter 29

John Beumer, III, DDS, MS
Distinguished Professor and Chair

Division of Advanced Prosthodontics, Biomaterial
 and Hospital Dentistry,
University of California, Los Angeles
Los Angeles, California
Chapter 27

Brian B. Burkey, MD
Associate Professor
Vice-Chairman for Academic and Clinical Affairs
Director, Residency Program
Department of Otolaryngology-Head and Neck
 Surgery
Vanderbilt University Medical Center
Nashville, Tennessee
Chapter 28

Joseph I. Clark
Professor of Medicine
Loyola University Chicago
Cardinal Bernardin Cancer Center
Loyola University Medical Center
Maywood, Illinois
Staff Physician
Medical Service
Edward Hines, Jr VA Hospital
Hines, Illinois
Chapter 6

Cheryl M. Czerlanis, MD
Fellow, Division of Hematology and Oncology
Cardinal Bernardin Cancer Center
Loyola University Medical Center
Maywood, Illinois
Chapter 6

Daniel G. Deschler, MD, FACS
Director, Division of Head and Neck Surgery

Massachusetts Eye and Ear Infirmary
Massachusetts General Hospital
Associate Professor
Harvard Medical School
Boston, Massachusetts
Chapter 21

Stephanie Detterline, MD
Assistant Professor of Medicine
University of Cincinnati Medical Center
Cincinnati, Ohio
Chapter 2

Umamaheswar Duvvuri, MD, PhD
Chief Resident
Department of Otolaryngology
University of Pittsburgh Medical Center
Pittsburgh, Pennsylvania
Chapter 17

Steven B. Edelstein, MD
Professor and Vice-Chairman
Department of Anesthesiology
Loyola University Medical Center
Maywood, Illinois
Chapter 8

David W. Eisele, MD, FACS
Professor and Chairman
Department of Otolaryngology-Head and Neck
  Surgery
University of California, San Francisco
San Francisco, California
Chapter 19

Bahman Emami, MD, FACR, FASTRO
Professor and Chairman
Department of Radiation Oncology
Loyola University Medical Center
Maywood, Illinois
Chapter 5

Kevin S. Emerick, MD
Clinical Instructor
Department of Otology and Laryngology
Harvard Medical School
Department of Otolaryngology
Massachusetts Eye and Ear Infirmary
Boston, Massachusetts
Chapter 21

Allan G. Farman BDS, PhD, DSc
Professor of Radiology and Imaging Sciences
  Department of Surgical and Hospital
  Dentistry
University of Louisville
Louisville, Kentucky
Chapter 7

Tarik Y. Farrag, MD, MSc
Postdoctoral Fellow
Department of Otolaryngology-Head and Neck
  Surgery
Johns Hopkins Medical Institutions
Baltimore, Maryland
Chapter 16

Robert L. Ferris, MD, PhD, FACS
Associate Professor and Chief
Division of Head and Neck Surgery
Departments of Otolaryngology and of
  Immunology
Co-Leader, Cancer Immunology Program
University of Pittsburgh Cancer Institute
Pittsburgh, Pennsylvania
Chapter 17

Vivek V. Gurudutt, MD
Assistant Professor
Department of Otolaryngology-Head and Neck
  Surgery
Mount Sinai School of Medicine
New York, New York
Chapter 19

Ehab Hanna, MD
Professor of Surgery
Department of Head and Neck Surgery
University of Texas MD Anderson Cancer Center
Houston, Texas
Chapter 12

Sheng-Po Hao MD, FACS, FICS
Professor and Chairman
Department of Otolaryngology-Head and Neck
  Surgery
Chang Gung Memorial Hospital
Chang Gung University
Taiwan
Chapter 11

Timothy J. Hughes, MD
Department of Otolaryngology-Head and Neck
Surgery
Loyola University Medical Center
Maywood, Illinois
Chapter 8

Jason P. Hunt, MD
Assistant Professor
Division of Otolaryngology-Head and Neck Surgery
University of Utah Health Sciences Center
Salt Lake City, Utah
Chapter 28

Zafrulla Khan, DDS, MS, FACP
Diplomat, American Board of Prosthodontics,
Professor of Prosthodontics,
School of Dentistry
Adjunct Professor, Medical and Radiation
Oncology,
School of Medicine
Director, Maxillofacial/Oncologic Dentistry
James Graham Brown Cancer Center
University of Louisville,
Louisville, Kentucky
Chapter 7

Diane P. Kowalski, MD
Assistant Professor of Pathology and Surgery
(Division of Otolaryngology)
Director Head and Neck Division
Department of Pathology
Yale University School of Medicine
New Haven, Connecticut
Chapter 4

Michael E. Kupferman, MD
Assistant Professor of Surgery
Department of Head and Neck Surgery
University of Texas MD Anderson Cancer Center
Houston, Texas
Chapter 12

John P. Leonetti, MD
Professor and Vice-Chairman
Neurotology, Otology and Skull Base Surgery
Co-Director, Loyola Center for Cranial Base Surgery
Maywood, Illinois
Chapters 13 and 23

Donna S. Lundy, PhD
Associate Professor
Department of Otolaryngology
University of Miami Miller School of Medicine
Miami, Florida
Chapter 29

Daniel D. Lydiatt, DDS, MD, FACS
Professor
Division of Head and Neck Surgical Oncology
University of Nebraska Medical Center,
Medical Director
Methodist Estabrook Cancer Center
Omaha, Nebraska
Chapter 9

William M. Lydiatt, MD, FACS
Associate Professor
Division of Head and Neck Surgical Oncology
University of Nebraska Medical Center
Omaha, Nebraska
Chapter 9

John Maddalozzo, MD, FACS, FAAP
Associate Professor
Department of Otolaryngology-Head and Neck
Surgery
Feinberg School of Medicine
Northwestern University Medical School
Chicago, Illinois
Pediatric Otolaryngology-Head and Neck Surgery
Children's Memorial Hospital
Chicago, Illinois
Chapter 24

Sam J. Marzo, MD
Associate Professor
Residency Program Director
Department of Otolaryngology-Head and Neck
Surgery
Loyola University Health System
Maywood, Illinois
Chapter 23

Brett A. Miles, MD, DDS
Department of Otolaryngology-Head and Neck
Surgery
University of Texas Southwestern Medical Center
Dallas, Texas
Chapter 14

Brian A. Moore, MD, FACS
Chief, Otolaryngology-Head and Neck Surgery
Elgin AFB, Florida 32542
Clinical Assistant Professor
Tulane University Department of Otolaryngology
New Orleans, Louisiana
Chapter 10

Jeffrey S. Moyer, MD, FACS
Division of Facial Plastic and Reconstructive
    Surgery
Division of Head and Neck Surgery
Department of Otolaryngology-Head and Neck
    Surgery
University of Michigan Medical Center
Ann Arbor, Michigan
Chapter 22

Larry L. Myers, MD, FACS
Assistant Professor
Department of Otolaryngology-Head and Neck
    Surgery
University of Texas Southwestern Medical Center
Dallas, Texas
Chapter 14

Thomas C. Origitano, MD, PhD
Professor and Chair
Department of Neurological Surgery
Loyola Stritch School of Medicine
Loyola University Health System
Maywood, Illinois
Chapter 13

Guy J. Petruzzelli, MD, PhD, MBA, FACS
Professor and Senior Attending
Director Head, Neck & Skull Base Surgery
Department of Otolaryngology
Rush University Medical Center
Chicago, Illinois
Chapters 1, 13, 15, 20, and 23

Sheri Poznanovic, MD
Pediatric Otolaryngologist
Colorado Otolaryngology Associates
Colorado Springs, CO
Chapter 24

Kristen B. Pytynia, MD, MPH
Assistant Professor
University of Illinois

Chicago, Illinois
Chapter 30

Eleni D. Roumanas, DDS
Professor, Division of Advanced Prosthodontics,
    Biomaterials of Hospital Dentistry
Director, Graduate Prosthodontics
Co-Director, Maxillofacial Prosthetics
University of California-Los Angeles, School of
    Dentistry
Los Angeles, California
Chapter 27

Gail M. Santucci
Florida Radiology Consultants
Fort Myers, Florida
Chapter 3

Robert L. Schiff, MD
Clinical Associate Professor of Medicine
Loyola Stritch School of Medicine
Maywood, Illinois
Chapter 2

Joseph M. Scianna, MD
Northern Illinois ENT Specialist, Ltd
Clinical Assistant Professor
Sycamore, Illinois
Chapter 1

Ryan K. Sewell, MD, JD
Resident
Department of Otolaryngology-Head and Neck
    Surgery
University of Nebraska Medical Center
Omaha, Nebraska
Chapter 9

Edward M. Stafford, MD
Instructor
Department of Otolaryngology-Head and Neck
    Surgery
Johns Hopkins Medical Institutions
Baltimore, Maryland
Chapter 16

Kerstin M. Stenson, MD, FACS
Associate Professor of Surgery
Director of Head and Neck Program
University of Chicago Medical Center
Chicago, Illinois
Chapter 26

Paula A. Sullivan, MS, CCC-SLP, BRS-S
Speech-Language Pathologist
Malcom Randall VA Medical Center
North Florida/South Georgia Veterans Health
 System
Gainesville, Florida
Chapter 29

Theodoros N. Teknos, MD
Division Chief
Head and Neck Surgery
University of Michigan Health System
Ann Arbor, Michigan
Chapter 22

Ngan-Ming Tsang, MD, DSc
Associate Professor
Department of Radiation Oncology
Chang Gung Memorial Hospital
Chang Gung University
Taiwan
Chapter 11

Ralph P. Tufano, MD, FACS
Associate Professor
Division of Head and Neck Surgical Oncology
Department of Otolaryngology-Head and Neck
 Surgery
Johns Hopkins School of Medicine
Baltimore, Maryland
Chapter 16

Andrew C. Urquhart, MD
Department of Otolaryngology-Head and Neck
 Surgery
Marshfield Clinic
Marshfield, Wisconsin
Chapter 25

Mikhail Vaysberg, DO
Assistant Professor
Department of Otolaryngology
University of Florida, College of Medicine
Gainesville, Florida
Chapter 3

Joshua D. Waltonen, MD
Fellow, Head and Neck Oncology
Department of Otolaryngology-Head and Neck
 Surgery
The Ohio State University
Columbus, Ohio
Chapter 18

Steven J. Wang, MD
Assistant Professor
Chief of Otolaryngology, San Francisco Veterans
 Affairs Medical Center
Department of Otolaryngology-Head and Neck
 Surgery
University of California, San Francisco
San Francisco, California
Chapter 19

Randal S. Weber, MD
Professor and Chairman
Department of Head and Neck Surgery
University of Texas MD Anderson Cancer Center
Houston, Texas
Chapter 10

Chad A. Zender, MD
Director of Head and Neck Surgery
Department of Otolaryngology-Head and Neck
 Surgery
Loyola University Medical Center
Maywood, Illinois
Chapter 28

Lee A. Zimmer, MD, PhD
Assistant Professor
Department of Otolaryngology-Head and Neck
 Surgery
University of Cincinnati Medical Center
Cincinnati, Ohio
Chapter 3

To my daughter, Kara Celeste Petruzzelli, the source of all my joy and the light in my life.

To my wife, Patricia Graf, my companion and my compass.

To my parents, Jeanne and Vito Petruzzelli, for their sacrifices and the opportunities they provided.

To my patients and their families, for their trust and confidence. You have been my greatest teachers and inspiration; it is and will always be my privilege and honor to care for you.

Finally, to the memory of Fanchon Knight, RN, one of my heroes.

1

The Complete Head and Neck Examination

Joseph M. Scianna
Guy J. Petruzzelli

INTRODUCTION

"I will remember that there is art to medicine as well as science, and that warmth, sympathy, and understanding may outweigh the surgeon's knife or the chemist's drug."

from the modern version of the
Oath of Hippocrates[1]

From the days of Hippocrates and the birth of modern medicine our profession has been based on the physician-patient relationship. Although this relationship has evolved over many centuries, the basic premise of a patient with a problem and a story that presents to a treating clinician has remained the same. As a treating physician, one's duty and one's investigation begins from the moment the patient is met. Appearance, affect, attitude all are immediately impressed on one's mentis. The development of the history and the intimate details of progression are laid out, and then with impartial, adept hands, the act of the physical examination begins. Fine details of history and physicality are woven together to display a tapestry which will become a cohesive treatment plan.

THE HISTORY

The complete head and neck examination begins with a thorough medical history. The medical history begins with a chief complaint, which is frequently overlooked. All patients have an agenda for which they seek counsel. Although the patients' concerns might be misplaced in light of the findings of the physician, their complaint, the primary reason for which they have sought aid, should always be addressed. For the head and neck oncologist, significant insight into the stage and site of disease can be elucidated from the chief complaint. A complaint of pain with swallowing might draw attention to a potential hypopharynx malignancy, whereas a complaint of hearing loss might draw attention to a mass within the nasopharynx causing a secondary middle ear effusion. The chief complaint will provide a sturdy base on which the remainder of the history will be built.

For the head and neck oncologist, key historical points revolve on delineating a time line of events. The onset of pain, discomfort, dysfunction, or recognition of a lesion provides an invaluable clue to length of time that a lesion has existed. The progression of symptoms in number and severity demonstrates the magnitude of the problem. Specific questioning additionally should include discussions regarding exacerbating and alleviating factors, previous treatments that have had a negative or positive impact on the complaint, and associated symptoms.

A concise, systematic, and thorough questioning should include all major anatomic and physiologic areas of the head and neck. Otalgia, hearing loss, vertigo, otorrhea, and tinnitus represent common symptoms related to ear pathology. Dysphagia, odynaphagia, trismus, dysarthria, and hemoptysis can all be found in conjunction with oral cavity lesions. Lesions of the base of tongue, supraglottis, hypopharynx, or glottis may present with shortness of breath, hoarseness, chronic cough, vocal fold dysfunction, and/or hemoptysis. Nasopharyngeal, sinonasal, and anterior skull base malignancies can present with variable degrees of olfactory dysfunction, nasal obstruction, and epistaxis. Lesions in a variety of areas along the skull base can result in cranial nerve dysfunction causing vocal paralysis, dysarthria, double vision, blindness, numbness, tingling, or facial palsy. Lastly, constitutional symptoms of weight loss, fatigue, myalgia, headache, fevers, chills, and night sweats can all accompany a malignancy and have a significant impact on the patient's quality of life.

In addition to investigating the key components of the history of present illness, an understanding of important past medical and surgical historical events provides unparalleled contributory information as well as risk stratification. Previous medical and surgical interventions should be investigated and recorded. Previous adverse events related to surgery, anesthesia, or medications should be noted and a history of bleeding disorders, either individually or within the family, must be determined. In the head and neck oncologic population, a thorough discussion of tobacco use, alcohol use, and other exposures must be discussed. Exposure history should not only include a history of chemical exposure related to work or hobby, but should include discussions of sun exposure and/or radiation exposure as both have a significant malignant impact.

As scientific investigations proceed regarding the genetics of cancer, the family history can provide insight into the potential for malignant predisposition. Familial history, as previously discussed, can provide information regarding bleeding diatheses as well as potential complications related to use of anesthesia. Lastly, beyond familial history related to cancer, a thorough review of the patient's various organ systems should occur.

A review of systems can be extensive at times, but it provides for surgical risk stratification, and can also elucidate metastatic disease. A history of constitutional symptoms, if not previously addressed should be determined. The status of the patient's cardiopulmonary system should be questioned as cardiac output and pulmonary function not only have an impact on general anesthesia, but also can significantly influence surgical decision making. This is most important when discussing possible larynx conservation procedures, as FEV_1/FVC ratio of less than 50% predicted is contraindicative to a number of procedures.[2] Hepatic and renal function should also be questioned as dysfunction of either system will not only have an impact on anesthetic clearance but also on administration of adjunctive chemotherapeutic agents. Diseases or previous surgeries of the gastrointestinal tract may eliminate or complicate procedures like a gastric pull-up or jejunal free flap. The patient's neurologic status both centrally and peripherally should be investigated as metastatic or local disease extending intracranially can have a profound impact on prognosis, treatment, and outcome. Finally, the psychiatric status of the patient, if impaired or disordered, can have a complicating impact on treatment choices and strategies.

THE VITAL SIGNS

The first, most routine of portion of the physical exam requires a review of the vital signs. The vital signs traditionally consist of four different components: heart rate, blood pressure, respiratory rate, and temperature. As patient comfort has become a prime directive for quality assurance, the fifth vital sign of pain has been added. In addition, a sixth vital sign of oxygen saturation has inherent significance for the head and neck surgical oncologist.

Evaluation of the heart rate at its most basic level provides insight into the status of the cardiac system. With blood pressure measurement as an adjunct the two can accurately describe the overall hemodynamic status of the patient. A combination of an elevated heart rate and hypotension can signal volume depletion, anemia, or sepsis. A further adjunct to evaluation of the hemodynamic status can include the measurement of orthostatic blood pressure. In this procedure, heart rate and blood pressure are measured in supine, sitting, and standing positions. Approximately a 5-minute waiting period is included between measurements to allow for reactive compensation. A drop of at least 20 mm Hg diastolic pressure or 10 mm Hg systolic pressure is indicative of hypovolemic hypotension.[3] In addition to evaluation for hypovolemia or anemia that can be related to malnutrition, a slow or irregular heart rate can be indicative of a serious arrhythmia, or beta blockade. This irregularity can lead to difficulties with anesthesia, the necessity of perioperative prophylactic cardiac medication, and/or the need for further cardiac evaluation.

Although the presence of a fever may be indicative of an acute infective process, a hematopoetic malignancy, or other chronic inflammatory process, for the head and neck oncologist the respiratory rate, quality of respiration, and the oxygen saturation are of notable importance. As many patients with head and neck malignancy have the associated risk factors of alcohol and tobacco use, chronic obstructive pulmonary disease (COPD) is commonplace.[4] The sequela of COPD includes low resting oxygen saturation and increased respiratory rate and effort.[5] The laryngeal, supraglottic or base of tongue malignancy may result in airway obstruction leading to increased respiratory rate, increased respiratory effort, and in its late stages to decreased oxygen saturation.

As discussed in obtaining a complete history, evaluation of pain establishes the status of the patient. Pain can result in an elevated heart rate, elevated blood pressure, and elevated respiratory rate. Pain can be representative of the location of a malignancy and also the recurrence of a malignancy.[6] Pain can hamper obtaining an accurate history and performing a complete physical exam. Pain can negatively impact the discussions of treatment options, but can also highlight the necessity for treatment. It remains the physician's responsibility to investigate the issue of pain and pain management as part of the treatment outline.

THE CRANIAL NERVE EXAM

The anatomy of the head and neck houses the most complex association of nerves in the body. Twelve cranial nerves course throughout the skull base and neck and provide essential functions of movement, sensation, vision, taste, olfaction, and hearing. The anatomic course of these nerves along with there function can be delineated through a concise, but thorough clinical exam.

The first cranial nerve, the olfactory nerve, has its origin in the subcallosal portion of the hippocampal gyrus area of the uncus. The olfactory nerve is the shortest of all the cranial nerves and its sensory receptor neurons are located in the nasal mucosal of the anterior skull base and upper nasal cavity.[7] The sensory nerve fibers of the nasal mucosa extend through the cribriform plate of the anterior skull base to the olfactory bulb where synapses connect to the central nervous symptoms.

Olfactory dysfunction is often described by patients as a lack of the ability to smell strong odors, or a change in taste. The change in taste is related to the combination that aroma has with the basic sensations of salt, sweet, bitter, and sour.[8] Nasal obstruction remains the most common cause of anosmia, and patient history can provide adequate insight into the olfactory sense. However, multiple tests are available to assess olfactory function. These tests center on a "scratch and sniff" format in which a variety of well-known and well-described odors must be identified by the patient.[9] Although complex olfactory testing can provide a quantitative documentation of the first cranial nerve, it is largely unnecessary to evaluate the function to this extent.

The second cranial nerve, the optic nerve, is a special sensory nerve providing sight. A continuation of the axons of retina, the optic nerves travel posterior to form the optic chiasm which lies below and in front of the pituitary and behind the sphenoid sinus. At the optic chiasm, fibers from the temporal half of each visual field do not cross; the fibers from the nasal half of each visual field, however, do cross and extend toward the contra lateral visual cortex found within the occipital lobe. The ocular examination for the head and neck surgeon includes a basic examination of the eye and a visual field test.

Lesions located within the sphenoid, or along the pituitary sella may result in bilateral hemianopsia.[10] In addition an examination of the retina and optic disk may reveal papilledema. Papilledema may be present with intracranial extension of malignancy resulting in increased intracranial pressure.[11]

The pupillary reflex is based on light perception from the optic nerve as well as the interaction of the pupillary constrictors with the third cranial nerve, the oculomotor nerve producing a bilateral response. Light entering one pupil signals a pretectal pathway that stimulates the Edinger-Westphal nucleus of both eyes. Preganglionic, parasympathetic fibers from this nucleus exit the nucleus and arrive at the cilliary ganglion. From the cilliary ganglion, postganglionic parasympathetic fibers travel via the oculomotor nerve to the pupillary constrictors. Therefore, light presented to one eye, results in bilateral, parasympathetic stimulation, ultimately resulting in bilateral pupillary constriction.[12] This bilateral effect can be useful in determining the site of a skull base or intracranial lesion. Optic nerve dysfunction in one eye will impair the afferent limb of the reflex, but stimulus to the contralateral, intact optic nerve will result in bilateral constriction. Oculomotor nerve dysfunction in one eye will result in impairment of the efferent limb of the reflex. Stimulation will be transmitted to both cilliary ganglia, but only the eye with the intact or nonimpaired oculomotor nerve will constrict.

Further evaluation of the oculomotor nerve can be accomplished with evaluation of the muscles that are innervated by the nerve. The oculomotor nerve path begins in the midbrain at the level of the superior colliculus in the oculomotor nucleus. Nerve fibers originating here merge and extend through the tentorium cerebelli, continuing along the lateral aspect of the cavernous sinus as the third cranial nerve. The nerve divides into two major divisions as it passes through the superior orbital fissure. The superior division ultimately provides movement to the superior rectus and the levator palpebrae muscles; the inferior division provides innervation of the medial rectus, superior rectus, and the inferior rectus.[13]

A complete extraocular muscle evaluation includes examination of cranial nerves IV and VI (the trochlear nerve and abducens nerve, respectively). The trochlear nerve begins at the trochlear nucleus at the floor of the cerebellar aqueduct and passes through the lateral wall of the cavernous sinus, entering the orbit via the superior orbital fissure to innervate the superior oblique muscle.[14] The superior oblique muscle provides for inferior lateral movement of the orbit via its association with orbital trochlea. The abducens nerve begins in the abducens nucleus inferior to the facial colliculus, passes within the cavernous sinus, entering the orbit via the superior orbital fissure to innervate the lateral rectus. Impairment of the sixth cranial nerve will result in inability to gaze laterally.[15]

With the muscles and function of the eye having been examined, attention can now proceed to the evaluation of the fifth cranial nerve (the trigeminal nerve) and its three divisions. The trigeminal nerve, the largest of the cranial nerves, consists of a sensory root as well as a motor root. Originating from two nuclei, the fibers of the trigeminal nerve extend to the trigeminal ganglion at the petrous apex. The first division of the trigeminal nerve is an entirely sensory nerve that exits through the skull base via the superior orbital fissure. Sensation to the scalp, forehead, conjunctiva, cornea, nasal mucosa and frontal sinus are supplied via this ophthalmic division of the trigeminal nerve. Testing of this nerve can be accomplished via vibratory sensation over the forehead, or more clearly with the blink reflex.[16] With a cotton wisp, the cornea and/or conjunctiva can be stimulated to produce a protective blink response. Failure to respond is indicative of impairment.

The second division of the trigeminal nerve, the maxillary division, is found most distally exiting via the inferior orbital foramen. The maxillary division provides sensation to the middle one-third of the face as well as the lateral aspect of the nose. Testing of the maxillary division is centered on vibratory or light touch to this area, where failure of sensation is indicative of impairment.

The third division of the trigeminal nerve, the mandibular division, carries motor and sensory fibers. The motor fibers provide innervation to the muscles of mastication. Care must be taken when evaluating the muscles of mastication, as pain and direct extension of tumor into the pytergoid musculature may inhibit complete masticatory movement.[17] The sensory branch of the mandibular division of the trigeminal nerve can be evaluated at its distal exit from the mandible through the mental foramen. Vibratory or light touch can be evaluated over each hemimandible to establish impairment or dysfunction this nerve.[18]

The facial nerve (VII) is a mixed nerve that provides mimetic facial movement, taste to the anterior two-thirds of the tongue, and autonomic innervation of the submandibular gland. With fibers arising from the facial motor nucleus of the pons as well as the nervus intermedius, after an initial turn or genu, the facial nerve courses through the cerebellar pontine angle, entering the internal auditory canal (IAC), coursing in the superior, anterior quadrant of the IAC, and enters the temporal bone through the meatal foramen (the narrowest portion of the course of the facial nerve). The short labyrinthine segment of the facial nerve leads to the geniculate ganglion where a second turn or genu occurs. The nerve then courses through the middle ear, through the mastoid, and exits at the stylomastoid foramen. Extending anteriorly the nerve divides into two major divisions, further dividing into five distinct branches: the cervical branch, the mandibular branch, the buccal branch, the zygomatic branch, and the temporal branch. Each of these motor branches can be individually tested and noted. The most well-recognized and common grading of facial nerve function is the House-Brackman grade.[19] This grading system (Table 1–1) takes into account resting and kinetic function, as well as mass movement, other wise known as synkinesis.[20]

Further testing of the facial nerve is based on the autonomic and special sensory testing of the nerve. An inability to taste in the anterior two-thirds of one side of the tongue is indicative of dysfunction of the chorda tympani. With postganglionic fibers exiting the geniculate ganglion and extending to the lacrimal gland as the greater superficial petrosal nerve, tear production can be measured. Known as the Schirmer test, tear production in both eyes is measured on a reactive paper. Adequate tear production (greater than 5 mm of tear production in 5 minutes) is indicative of a functioning nerve from its nucleus to the geniculate ganglion.[21]

The vestibular-cochlear nerve (VIII) consists of two major components, an auditory component and a vestibular component. The auditory portion

Table 1–1. House-Brackman Facial Nerve Evaluation

Grade	Description
I	Normal function
II	Slight weakness on close inspection Normal tone and symmetry at rest Complete eye closure
III	Obvious asymmetry at rest Complete eye closure
IV	Obvious asymmetry at rest Gross asymmetry with movement Incomplete eye closure
V	Barely perceptible motion Gross asymmetry at rest and with movement
VI	Complete paralysis

of the nerve extends from spiral ganglia in the petrous portion of the temporal bone, through the cerebellar pontine angle into the IAC and eventually reaching the organ of Corti within the cochlea. Although audiometric testing can provide highly specific information regarding the auditory status, a basic tuning fork examination can accurately assess the function of the nerve in a short period of time. A Weber test is performed using a 512-Hz tuning fork. With the tuning fork vibrating, it is placed in the midline skull and the patient is asked in which ear the sound is louder. A normal response is that the sound appears to be midline. With a conductive loss, the sound will be heard louder in the side of the ear with the conductive loss. With a sensorineural loss, the sound will be heard in the only hearing ear, contra lateral to the ear with the hearing loss. A Rhinne test can be used to confirm the hearing loss. In this test the tuning fork is struck and the patient is asked to differentiate the strength of the sound with the tuning fork in front of the ear versus placement in contact with the mastoid behind the ear. A positive Rhinne, where air conduction is better heard than bone conduction, is considered a normal response. A negative Rhinne, where bone conduction is heard better than air conduction, confirms a minimal of a 30-dB conductive hearing loss.[22] Thus, an accurate picture of the status of the auditory portion of the eighth cranial nerve can be established with these two simple tests.

The testing of the vestibular portion of the eighth cranial nerve can be significantly more complex and not routinely performed in all patients with head and neck tumors.

Assessing for resting or spontaneous nystagmus can indicate a peripheral lesion. The direction, amplitude, and the ability of fixation to suppress the nystagmus should be noted. Additional tests that can be performed include head thrust and head shake tests to induce nystagmus as well as the Dix-Hall-Pike positioning test that is indicative of benign positional vertigo.[23] Observing gait, standing positional stability, and performing the Romberg test (standing, feet close together, eyes closed and evaluate sway) can all provide further quantification to the degree of vestibular dysfunction.

With fibers arising in the medulla and exiting the posterior skull base through the jugular foramen, the glossopharyngeal nerve (IX) provides sensation to the pharynx and tongue, innervates the stylopharyngeus muscle, and provides parasympathetic supply to the parotid gland via the lesser petrosal nerve and the otic ganglion. Glossopharyngeal dysfunction can result in a deviated palate or uvula as well as an absent gag reflex.[24]

The vagus nerve, or 10th cranial nerve, carries sensory, motor, and parasympathetic fibers, its course begins within medulla and exits the posterior skull base through the jugular foramen traveling through the neck, through the thoracic cavity and eventually providing innervation to a visceral structures within the abdominal cavity.[25] Contributing to sensation within the oropharynx, as well as providing muscular innervation of the palate, the vagal nerve can be assessed similarly to the glossopharyngeal nerve. A more specific test for evaluation of the vagal nerve is an evaluation of the vocal folds. Via the recurrent laryngeal nerve, all muscles of the larynx are innervated with the exception of the cricothyroid muscle which is innervated by the superior laryngeal branch of the vagus nerve. Evaluation of vocal fold motion can be established via mirror laryngoscopy or via flexible laryngoscopy which is discussed in more detail later.

The spinal accessory nerve, or cranial nerve XI, is the motor nerve that innervates the trapezius muscle as well as the sternocleiodomastoid (SCM) muscle. With fibers that originate in the upper spinal cord segments that join with cranial roots, it travels through the jugular foramen to provide its muscular innervation. Dysfunction of the spinal accessory nerve is manifested by a failure to be able to raise the outstretched arm beyond 90 degrees and impairment of a shoulder shrug. In addition, an impaired head turn may be seen; it is important to remember that the SCM muscle functions to turn the head toward the *contralateral* side. Therefore, dysfunction of the right spinal accessory nerve will result in impairment of the head turn to the left.[26]

The last of the 12 cranial nerves to evaluate is the hypoglossal nerve. Fibers of the 12th cranial nerve begin within the medulla and course out of the posterior skull base through the hypoglossal canal. The hypoglossal nerve functions to provide motor innervation of the extrinsic and intrinsic muscles of the tongue. Therefore, testing can be accomplished via examination of the resting tongue, extrusion of the tongue, and evaluation of lateral movement of the tongue. With hypoglossal dysfunction, hemiatrophy of the tongue may develop; in addition, extrusion of the tongue will result in characteristic deviation of the tongue toward the side of the impairment as well as limitation of lateral movement toward the impaired side.[27]

THE SKIN AND SCALP

The skin is the largest organ of the body.[28] A thorough evaluation of the skin and scalp can be accomplished in a short period of time. Evaluation should include notation of the Fitzpatrick skin type (Table 1–2) as this is directly relevant to the risk of having a skin malignancy such as melanoma, cutaneous squamous cell carcinoma, or basal cell carcinoma.[29,30] Evaluation of skin type, thickness, the presence or absence of rhytids, evaluation of the hairline, prediction of balding patterns, and previous surgical scars are all relevant for planning future operations and skin incisions. Skin lesions should be evaluated based on

Table 1–2. Fitzpatrick Scale of Skin Types

Grade	Description
1	Very white or freckled—Always burn
2	White—Usually burn
3	White to olive—Sometimes burn
4	Brown—Rarely burn
5	Dark brown—Very rarely burn
6	Black—Never burn

the four principles of size, color, symmetry, and border irregularity.[31] Potentially malignant lesion tend to be larger (>1 cm) and asymmetric, can present with a multitude of color abnormalities, may be ulcerative, and may have border irregularities especially the "cookie cutter" appearance.[31] Such lesions should be clearly noted and potentially biopsied (see discussion of skin biopsy).

THE EAR EXAM

Examination of the ear should include examination of the auricle, the conchal and tragal cartilage, the external auditory canal, and otoscopic examination of the tympanic membrane. Examination of the auricle requires evaluation for tenderness, erythema, and the presence of any lesions suggestive of an auricular skin cancer. The external auditory canal should be examined and any debris or cerumen should be removed to provide for clear evaluation of the tympanic membrane. Otoscopic examination can be done with either a hand-held otoscope or preferably with microscopic otoscopy. Microscopic otoscopy provides for binocular visualization as well as the ability to safely clean or palpate structures within the canal. Otoscopy should focus on evaluation of the tympanic membrane and identification of normal structures.

The status of the tympanic membrane should first be noted: intact or perforated, aerated or retracted. Perforations should be defined by central

or peripheral location as well as the size of the perforation in relation to the total surface area of the membrane. With an intact tympanic membrane, its pliability can be further assessed using pneumatic otoscopy. A hypermobile tympanic membrane may be indicative of ossicular discontinuity whereas a stiff tympanic membrane may be present in tympanosclerosis, otosclerosis, or with the presence of a mass or effusion within the middle ear.[32]

With an intact tympanic membrane, an effusion may be identified. A typical straw-colored effusion of serous otitis media should be differentiated from the dark effusion of acute infection or the hemotympanum associated with skull base fractures.[33] In addition, a clear effusion may be indicative of CSF leak within the middle ear.[34] Evaluation of the fluid can be accomplished via a diagnostic myringotomy; however, caution must be taken as a number of middle ear vascular abnormalities may be mistaken for an acute effusion or hemotympanum.

An aberrant carotid artery, a high-riding jugular bulb, glomus jugulare or glomus tympanicum may all present as a red to blue-hued mass behind the middle ear. An aberrant carotid artery is typically described as a red, pulsatile mass found behind the middle ear. The venous lesions of the glomus jugulare or tympanicum are generally described as being more purple to blue. Verification of a vascular lesion can be provided by gently palpating the lesion or with pneumatic otoscopy. A blanching of the lesion with increased pressure, a Brown sign, is indicative of a vascular lesion.[35] In addition, evaluation with a stethoscope placed over the mastoid or high in the neck may allow for identification of an audible bruit.[36]

ANTERIOR RHINOSCOPY

Evaluation of the nose includes examination of the external and internal nasal anatomy. Notation of external nasal deformity, nasal cartilage weakness, and nasal tip support may be important in reconstruction options for nasal skin cancers. Using a nasal speculum with proper illumination can provide excellent visualization of the structures of the nasal cavity. Nasal septal deviation may pose a potential obstacle for endoscopic evaluation, whereas a septal perforation may be related to intranasal drug use, chronic granulomatous disease, or secondary to an intranasal malignancy.[37] The septum can also be evaluated as a potential source of epistaxis. The anterior portion of the septum, Kiesselbach's plexus, is a frequent culprit in the routine nose bleed.[38]

In addition to evaluating the septum, the inferior turbinates and nasal cavity can be examined. Frequently mistaken for nasal polyps by primary care physicians, the inferior turbinates represent reactive mucosal structures functioning to heat, humidify, and filter the air as it passes through the nasal cavity.[39] A bluish hue of the middle turbinate may be indicative of otolaryngologic allergy. More importantly to the head and neck oncologist, however, a discoloration of the mucosa of the inferior turbinate may represent a mucosal melanoma. A mass protruding from beneath the inferior turbinate may represent a lacrimal duct or sac malignancy extending into the nasal cavity.

The list of masses of the nasal cavity is extensive (Table 1–3).[40,41] Masses within the nasal cavity can be divided into three major groups, benign, malignant, or vascular. The most common benign lesion is the nasal polyp.[42] With a typical pearl onion appearance and a boggy consistency, nasal polyps can generally be differentiated from other benign lesions. An important consideration when evaluating a benign nasal lesion is a consideration that a dehiscence of the skull base congenitally or secondarily may result in a formation of an encephalocele. Therefore, careful consideration should be taken when an intranasal office biopsy is considered.

The malignant lesions within the nasal cavity should be assessed thoroughly. Understanding that malignancies found within the nasal cavity may have originated from within a paranasal sinus, from the anterior skull base, projecting from the nasopharynx, or eroding through the maxilla from within the oral cavity is imperative. Palpation of the intranasal mass can provide valuable information regarding its consistency and friability. In addition, much like the Brown sign of the middle ear mass, palpation that demonstrates a blanching effect should warn the physician of the potential of a vascular lesion that may not be suitable for biopsy.[41]

Table 1–3. Nasal Masses

Benign
• Nasal polyp
• Osteoma
• Ossifying fibroma
• Meningioma
• Schwannoma
• Neurofibroma
• Juvenile angiofibroma
• Harmatoma
• Inverted papilloma
Malignant
• Squamous cell carcinoma
• Esthestioneuroblastoma
• Sinonasal neuroendocrine carcinoma
• Sinonasal undifferentiated carcinoma
• Adenoidcystic carcinoma
• Lymphoma
• Plasmacytoma
• Mucosal melanoma

THE ORAL CAVITY

The oral cavity houses multiple anatomic structures each of which must be assessed individually. The initial assessment begins with evaluating the patient's ability to open the mouth. Trismus, the incomplete opening of the mouth, may be present for a number of reasons. Invasion into the pterygoid musculature may inhibit the ability to open the mouth, whereas a retromolar trigone lesion may cause trismus secondary to pain. Trismus may also be secondary to previous therapy, radiation or otherwise, that has resulted in scarring or contracture. Measuring the degree of trismus, and understanding the underlying cause of the trismus impacts future examinations and obtaining an operative airway.[43]

The next crucial assessment of the oral cavity is an examination of the dentition and occlusion. Although the edentulous patient can be quite favorable for a transoral approach to the tongue base or larynx, reconstructing the mandible of an edentulous patient can be challenging. Assessment of the mandibular and maxillary alveolar ridges provides insight into the origin and potential invasion of a cancer into a tooth root.[44] The degree to which dentition is compromised can also affect the planning of radiation therapy as decayed or compromised teeth will need to be removed prior to initiation of therapy. Inspection of the mandibular and maxilla alveoli can be enhanced by the use of a dental mirror, providing visualization of the lingual surface of the alveolar gingiva and the palate.[44]

After careful inspection and palpation of the maxillary and mandibular alveolar ridges, one can proceed with inspection of the floor of the mouth, and the ventral aspect of the anterior tongue. In this area, bimanual palpation can be useful to determine if a lesion is arising from within a submandibular gland, or is separate from the gland. In addition, palpation and milking of the submandibular glands should induce salivary secretion through the submandibular ducts (Wharton's ducts) into the floor of mouth. On occasion, malignancy can result in duct obstruction and/or chronic sialadentitis. In this case saliva may not be expressed from the gland, or a foul, purulent discharge may be encountered. Lesions extending onto the ventral tongue can be palpated to help determine the depth of invasion. Careful assessment of the mobility of the ventral tongue can also be indicative of the degree of lingual invasion of a floor of mouth lesion.

As attention is turned toward the anterior, mobile tongue, palpation becomes essential. The anterior tongue is much more accessible to physical examination and an accurate prediction of the depth of invasion can be achieved.[45] Lesions originating on the dorsal tongue or lateral tongue must be assessed not only for length and depth, but also for extension into the floor of mouth. The malignant extension ventrally into the floor of the mouth or laterally into the lingual-gingival sulcus can alter surgical reconstructive plans as primary closure with this type of extension may result in tethering of the tongue.

With the anterior tongue, floor of mouth and alveolar ridges having been inspected, the buccal space and extension into the retromolar trigone should then be assessed. Involvement of a lesion of the buccal mucosa is more common in patients with a history of chewing tobacco and with patients having a history of use of betel nut.[46] The retromolar trigone represents the confluence of the buccal mucosa, the mandibular alveolar mucosa, and the mucosa covering the anterior tonsilar pillar.[47] With lesions in the retromolar trigone, one should assess the adherence of the lesion to the posterior mandible as this will provide insight into depth of invasion and impact treatment strategies.

Attention can then be turned to the hard and soft palate. As mentioned, lesions originating from the hard palate may erode into the nasal cavity. The converse is also true in that lesions originating from within the maxillary sinus or along the floor of the nasal cavity can erode into the oral cavity.[40] The hard and soft palate house numerous minor salivary glands. Lesions of these minor glands have a high likelihood for malignancy and therefore should be examined carefully with a low threshold for biopsy.[48] Lesions of the soft palate or uvula should be evaluated for extension into the tonsilar fossa. Delineation of the size and extent of the lesion again is an imperative component of a postsurgical reconstruction plan.

The tonsilar fossa can then be assessed. The tonsil lies within a fossa formed anteriorly by the mucosa covering the palatoglossus muscle and posteriorly by the mucosa covering the palatopharyngeus muscle. As part of Waldeyer's ring, the inferior tonsil communicates directly with the lymphoid tissue of the base of the tongue. The principles of inspection, palpation, and assessment of extent of invasion are employed when evaluating a tonsil. If a hyperactive gag reflex is present, then a topical anesthetic can be administered to allow for full assessment of the posterior oropharynx.

The posterior wall of the oropharynx can be inspected as well. Lesions arising from within the nasopharynx can extend inferiorly and be visible within the oropharynx. Lesions of the soft palate should be palpated to ensure separation between the lesion and the posterior oropharynx. Oropharyngeal fullness may represent a retropharyngeal fluid collection or spread of a malignancy to the retropharyngeal nodes. A submucosal lateral oropharyngeal or retropharyngeal mass should not be biopsied until contrast enhanced imaging has been obtained.

The last step in a complete oropharyngeal examination requires palpation of the base of the tongue. Although not easily visualized via transoral inspection, deep palpation of the base of the tongue can be accomplished with the cooperation of the patient. Again a hyperactive gag reflex can be suppressed with a topical anesthetic. Attempts should be made to differentiate between the normal lymphoid tissue of the base of the tongue and a submucosal mass.

THE NECK EXAM

Inspection of the neck is the first step in assessment. Obvious asymmetry or masses can be noted. The thickness and length of the neck can be estimated. The neck circumference as measured across the thyroid can be recorded. Swelling of the external jugular veins may be indicative of an internal jugular obstruction.

Palpation of the neck should proceed in a systematic manner. The lymphatic drainage of the neck is divided into six anatomic areas, each of which receives lymphatic drainage for a particular anatomic location within the aerodigestive tact (Fig 1–1).[49] Beginning with the parotid gland, palpation should extend into level IIB of the neck. Differentiating a

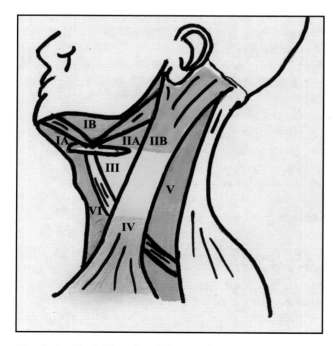

Fig 1–1. Nodal levels of the neck.

primary parotid tail lesion from lymphatic involvement in level IIB can be difficult, and bimanual palpation from within the oral cavity can be helpful.

Bimanual palpation also aids in differentiating the submandibular gland from other masses within I and IIA, likewise levels III, IV, and V are carefully palpated. When assessing a mass in any area of the neck a number of features should be noted. Particular attention is directed to the size of the mass, as this impacts the staging of the neck, and the mobility of the mass should be assessed.[49] A freely mobile mass is less worrisome than a fixed mass that cannot be separated from the SCM. In addition, a mass in level IIA that is mobile in the horizontal plane but not the vertical plain may be indicative of a vascular carotid body tumor. If a mass is pulsatile, and has a palpable thrill or an audible bruit, a vascular structure or mass should be considered.

Examination of the central compartment of the neck requires evaluation of the thyroid gland. With each lobe of the gland of the thyroid laying lateral to the trachea in the midline neck, the gland is centered at the second or third tracheal ring.[50] In the thin neck each lobe and occasionally the isthmus can be easily visualized. In most instances, however, palpation is necessary to adequately evaluate the gland. As each lobe of the gland is found deep to the strap musculature, having the patient initiate a swallow may help differentiate the borders of the gland. Whether the neck is examined from behind the patient or from an anterior approach the examiner should attempt to characterize the size of each lobe, the consistency of the lobe and the presence or absence of any nodularity.[51] Identification of a thyroid nodule that is obvious on physical examination lends itself to fine needle aspiration (FNA). In some instances ultrasonography is necessary for characterization of the thyroid as well as ultrasound-guided FNA.[52]

FLEXIBLE EXAMINATION OF THE LARYNX AND PHARYNX

The larynx and pharynx are evaluated following inspection and palpation of the mucosal surfaces of the head and neck. Mirror laryngoscopy should be attempted on all patients. The panoramic examination of the vallecula supraglottic and glottic larynx obtained with the mirror is an important initial step that, in some cases, may obviate the need for more costly fiberoptic endoscopy. Discomfort during the examination can be minimized by gentle retraction on the tongue and by avoiding contact between the soft palate and the posterior pharyngeal wall. Despite careful technique endoscopy may be necessary to obtain the necessary visualization for a complete head and neck examination.

Patient preparation begins with an explanation of the procedure and a discussion of topical anesthetic. A combination of a topical anesthetic agent and a vasoconstrictive agent is aerosolized and is applied in a short controlled burst transnasally.[53] Typically, the agent is expelled past the nasopharynx and the patient feels or tastes the agent in the oropharynx. The patient needs to be made aware of the anesthetic effect in that a globus sensation will likely develop.

In patients with a hyperactive gag reflex, topical anesthetic can be applied directly to the palate and/or base of tongue with a tongue blade. This is useful for transnasal esophagoscopy and for base of tongue biopsy in the office. For subglottic examination or vocal fold surgery (injection or biopsy) 4% plain lidocaine can be applied directly to the vocal fold transorally with a laryngeal cannula via a transcervical/transtracheal route.

After 10 minutes the flexible endoscopy can begin by inserting the scope into the nasal cavity. A severe septal deviation or a large intranasal mass may prevent insertion of the scope through one side of the nose. Beginning in the more open nasal cavity provides for an easier initial evaluation. Initially the size and the constriction of the mucosa of the inferior turbinates secondary to the vasoconstrictive agent should be assessed. Prominent vasculature of the nasal septum and the general shape and integrity of the septum should be recorded. Careful inspection of the middle turbinate and the middle meatus may identify neoplasm or an acute infection. The scope can be angle anteriorly to examine the area of the frontal recess and the anterior skull base and manipulation of the scope can provide visualization of the sphenoid os. The most direct route to visualize the sphenoid is accomplished medial to the middle turbinate and behind the superior turbinate.

In the nasopharynx size and character of the adenoid tissue should be noted. The area surrounding the eustachian tube orifice should also be inspected. Often a mass originating from one side of the nasopharynx is evident through examination of the contra lateral nasal passage. Masses of the nasopharynx should be assessed for pulsations, vascularity, friability, ulcerations, and potentially cystic nature.

As the flexible endoscope proceeds inferiorly, the posterior palate, the posterior aspect of the tonsils, and the posterior oropharynx can all be visualized. A large tonsil or tonsilar mass may produce an asymmetry in the lateral oropharyngeal wall.

Examination of the supraglottic larynx, glottis, subglottis, and hypopharynx should be accomplished in a manner similar to that of an operative direct laryngoscopy. The base of tongue can be examined with the vallecula accentuated by having the patient extrude the tongue. The area of the base of tongue should be characterized in relation to each inferior pole of the tonsil. In addition, obliteration of the vallecula or extension of a mass onto the lingual surface of the epiglottis is noted.

The tip of the laryngeal surface of the epiglottis can be examined. Each aryeptiglottic fold can be visualized and the laryngeal mucosal surface of each is inspected. The false vocal folds are assessed for symmetry and or fullness and the larynx and vocal processes should be in clear view.

The five vocal folds should be examined along their entire length. Careful attention should be paid to the anterior commisure. Lesions extending to the anterior commisure are noted to have a significant impact on therapeutic success.[54] The mobility of the vocal fold is characterized by having the patient vocalize. Videostroboscopy can be used to better characterize the mucosal wave, but is not essential for the initial exam. The resting position of the fold also should be noted, which when paralyzed may take a lateralized, paramedical, or medialized position.[55]

With satisfactory topical anesthesia the subglottis and trachea can be examined with the standard size fiberoptic scope. The patient should be directed to refrain from swallowing or speaking while the scope is between the vocal folds. Careful technique is necessary to prevent laryngospasm and caution should be exercised to avoid bleeding from friable tumors.

The hypopharyngeal mucosa (piriform sinus, posteriocoid, and posterium pharyngeal wall) is the final region to be evaluated hypopharynx. The piriform sinuses are inverted pyramids composed of medial mucosa extending from the aryepiglottic fold, lateral pharyngeal mucosa, and the posterior pharyngeal mucosa extending into the postcricoid area. At rest the redundant mucosa of this area is difficult to assess. To improve visualization the patient can be instructed to autosufflate their cheeks as if blowing up a balloon. This maneuver fills the piriform sinus with air dilating the region and allowing for characterization of the mucosa in this area.

The mucosa overlying the posterior cricoid lamina (posterocoid) can be visualized with autosufflation as well as placing the patient in the "sniffing position." A more complete hypopharyngeal examination, can be accomplished with a transnasal esophagoscope. Fitted with suction, biopsy port, and an insufflator, the TNE allows for complete office-based esophagoscopy.

Preparation for TNE is accomplished in a similar fashion as that of flexible laryngoscopy. The addition of the topical gel anesthetic that is allowed to migrate down the piriform sinus into the upper esophagus is helpful. By having the patient sit upright and lean forward, the postcricoid area can be insufflated. The patient can be instructed to swallow as well as this will permit entrance into the cervical esophagus. Using insufflation cervicothoracic esophagoscopy can be accomplished. With the various ports that are available for biopsy, the TNE can be used not only to sample suspicious lesions within the esophagus but also in the supraglottic larynx for biopsy.[56]

THE OFFICE BIOPSY

The office biopsy provides not only tissue for pathologic examination but also diagnostic clues based on consistency and, in some cases, can be therapeutic. Like all procedures the patient must be counseled on the risks and benefits of the procedure; informed consent should be documented. Consideration for patient safety, patient comfort, postbiopsy hemostasis, and potential complications is required.

In terms of patient safety and avoidance of potential complications, a few prudent measures can be taken. Reviewing patient medications specifically for aspirin-containing preparations or other anticoagulants will decrease the likelihood of difficult to control postbiopsy hemorrhage. Any previously obtained imaging should be reviewed. Consideration of the anatomic relationship of major neurovascular structures to the area being biopsied is paramount. Within the nasal cavity, the relationship of the skull base and the potential of encephalocele or other skull base defect should be realized. The proximity between the mass being biopsied and the airway should also be considered. A tenuous airway can be further compromised by postbiopsy hemorrhage, however minor, and may best be managed in an operative rather than office setting.

Topical and intralesional anesthesia can be provided in a number of ways. Topical mucosal anesthetics can be augmented by injection with local anesthetic with or without epinephrine.

Deciding where to biopsy and how to biopsy is dependent on the site. Cutaneous lesions, should be biopsied peripherally where the pathologist can compare normal tissue to abnormal tissue. Melanoma should be considered in the differential diagnosis of all cutaneous lesions. Because depth of invasion is an important element of melanoma staging, biopsies should be taken with a reasonable depth.[57] Other lesions should be biopsied to maximize the pathologic diagnosis, while minimizing the risks of hemorrhage. With lesions that are ulcerative, non-necrotic tissue should be obtained. With submucosal lesions, deeper biopsied material should be obtained.

In every instance, hemostasis must be obtained. Often with a small biopsy in an amenable area, tamponade for a short period of time can provide adequate hemostasis. Topical silver nitrate can also be employed to achieve local hemostasis. In some instances an electocautery unit is available and can be used; however, caution should be taken in patients with pacemakers or internal defibrillators who can be seriously harmed by improper use or grounding of the cautery machine.[58]

SUMMARY

The initial physical exam should be thorough and complete. The complete head and neck examination establishes the basis on which further diagnostic studies are obtained and therapeutic decisions are made. The history of present illness and key areas of the past medical history direct the emphasis of the physical exam. All areas of the head and neck are investigated. Tools such as the flexible laryngoscope and the TNE are employed to facilitate visualization of difficult to expose or evaluate areas. In addition, the office biopsy provides key information. Throughout all portions of the complete examination, communication between the patient and physician is paramount. Establishment of mutual respect and trust in this initial encounter will lay the foundation for the therapeutic relationship which may be needed to care for patient with malignant head and neck neoplasm.

REFERENCES

1. Louis Lasagna. Available from: http://www.pbs.org/wgbh/nova/doctors/oath_modern.html; Tufts University School of Medicine; 1964.
2. Beckhardt RN, Murray JG, Ford CN, et al. Factors influencing functional outcome in supraglottic laryngectomy. *Head Neck.* 1994;16(3):232-239.
3. Consensus statement on the definition of orthostatic hypotension, pure autonomic failure, and multiple system atrophy. The Consensus Committee of the American Autonomic Society and the American Academy of Neurology. *Clin Autonomic Research.* 1996;6(2):125-126.
4. Paleri V, Narayan R, Wight RG. Descriptive study of the type and severity of decompensation caused by comorbidity in a population of patients with laryngeal squamous cancer. *J Laryngol Otol.* 2004; 188(7):517-522.
5. Stenfors N. Physicain-diagnosed COPD global initiative for chronic obstructive lung disease stage IV in Ostersund, Sweden: patient characteristics and estimated prevalence. *Chest.* 2006;130(3):666-671.
6. Smit M, Balm AJ, Hilgers FJ, Tan IB. Pain as a sign of recurrent disease in head and neck squamous cell carcinoma. *Head Neck.* 2001;23(5):372-375.
7. Rombaux P, Mouraux A, Bertrand B, Nicolas G, Duprez T, Hummel T. Retronasal and orthonasal olfactory function in relation to olfactory bulb volume in patients with posttraumatic loss of smell. *Laryngoscope.* 2006;166(6):901-905.
8. de Araujo IE, Rolls ET, Kringelbach ML, McGlone G, Phillips N. Taste-olfactory convergence, and the representation of the pleasantness of flavour, in the human brain. *Eur J Neurosci.* 2003;18(7): 2059-2068.
9. Jackman AH, Doty RL. Utility of a three-item smell identification test in detecting olfactory dysfunction. *Laryngoscope.* 2005;115(12):2209-2212.
10. Fujimoto N, Saeki N, Miyauchi O, Adachi-Usami E. Criteria for early detection of temporal hemianopia in asymptomatic pituitary tumor. *Eye.* 2002;16(6): 731-738.
11. Whiting AS, Johnson LN. Papilledema: clinical clues and differential diagnosis. *Am Fam Physician.* 1992;45:1125-1134.
12. Yang LL, Niemann CU, Larson MD. Mechanism of pupillary reflex dilation in awake volunteers and in organ donors. *Anesthesiology.* 2003;99: 1281-1286.
13. Jacobson DM. A prospective evaluation of cholinergic supersensitivity of the iris sphincter in patients with oculomotor nerve palsies. *Am J Opthalmol.* 1994;118(3):377-383.
14. Sheik ZA. Trochlear nerve palsy. Retrieved August, 2005 from http://www.emedicine.com
15. Ehrenhaus MP. Abducens nerve palsy. Retrieved July, 2006 from http://www.emedicine.com
16. Cruccu G, Biasiotta A, Galeotti F, Iannetti GD, Truini A, Gronseth G. Diagnostic accuracy of trigeminal reflex testing in trigeminal neuralgia. *Neurology.* 2006;66:139-141.
17. Chong J, Som P, Silvers AR, Dalton JF. Extranodal non-Hodjkins lymphoma involving the muscles of mastication. *Am J Neuroradiol.* 1998;19: 1849-1851.
18. Jacobs R, Wu CH, Goossens K, Van Loven K, Van Hees J, Van Steenberghe D. Oral mucosal versus cutaneous sensory testing: a review of the literature. *J Oral Rehabil.* 2002;29(10):923.
19. House JW, Brackmann DE. Facial nerve grading system. *Otolaryngol Head Neck Surg.* 1985;93: 146-147.
20. Kang TS, Vrabec JT, Giddings N, Terris DJ. Facial nerve grading systems (1985-2002): beyond the House-Brackmann scale. *Otol Neurootol.* 2002; 23(5):767-771.

21. Nichols KK, Nichols JJ, Lynn Mitchell G. The relation between tear film tests in patients with dry eye disease. *Ophthalmic Physiol Opt.* 2003;23(6):553-560.

22. Emmett JR. Physical examination and clinical evaluation of the patient with otosclerosis. *Otolaryngol Clin North Am.* 1993;26:353-357.

23. Epley JM. The canalith repositioning procedure: for treatment of benign paroxysmal positional vertigo. *Otolaryngol Head Neck Surg.* 1992;107(3):399-404.

24. Shin JH, Lee HK, Kim SY, et al. Parapharyngeal second branchial cyst manifesting cranial nerve palsies: MR findings. *Am J Neuroradiol.* 2001;22:510-512.

25. Rielo D. Vagus nerve stimulation. Retrieved January 2006 from http://www.emedicine.com

26. Lunardi P, Mastronardi L, Farah JO, et al. Spinal accessory nerve palsy due to neurovascular compression. Report of a case diagnosed by magnetic resonance imaging and magnetic resonance angiography. *Neurosurgi Rev.* 1996;19(3):175-178.

27. Lo TS. Unilateral hypoglossal nerve palsy following the use of the laryngeal mask airway. *Can J Neurol Sci.* 2003;33(3):320-321.

28. Healy B. Skin deep. *US News and World Report.* Nov. 2005.

29. Zanetti R, Rosso S, Martinez C, et al. Comparison of risk patterns in carcinoma and melanoma of the skin in men: a multi-centre case-case-control study. *Br J Cancer.* 2006;94:743-751.

30. Fitzpatrick TB. The validity and practicality of sun-reactive skin types I through VI. *Arch Dermatol.* 1998;124(6):869-871.

31. Whited JD, Grichnick JM. Does this patient have a mole or melanoma? *JAMA.* 1998;279:696-701.

32. Jones WS, Kaleida PH. How helpful is pneumatic otoscopy? *Pediatrics.* 2003;112(3 pt 1):510-513.

33. Stiell IG, Clement CM, Rowe BH, et al. Comparison of the Canadian CT head rule and the New Orleans criteria in patients with minor head injury. *JAMA.* 2005;294:1511-1518.

34. Vukas D, Leonetti JP, Marzo SJ, et al. Spontaneous transtemporal CSF otorrhea: a report of 51 cases. *Ear Nose Throat J.* 2005; 84(11):700-706.

35. Santos VB, Polisar LA. Brown's sign: a tympanographic documentation. *Ear Nose Throat J.* 1966; 56(8):320-324.

36. Russell EJ, DeMichaelis BJ, Wiet R, Meyer J. Objective pulse synchronous "essential" tinnitus due to narrowing of the transverse dural venous sinus. *Int Tinnitus J.* 1995;1(2):127-137.

37. Farge D, Frances C, Vouldoukis I., et al. Chronic destructive ulcerative lesion of the midface and nasal cavity due to leishmaniasis contracted in Djibouti. *Clin Exper Dermatol.* 1987;12(3):211.

38. Doyle DE. Anterior epistaxis: a new nasal tampon for fast, effective control. *Laryngoscope.* 1985; 96(3):279-281.

39. Joniau S, Wong I, Rajapaksa S, Carney SA, Wormald PJ. Long term comparison between submucosal cauterization and powered reduction of the inferior turbinates. *Laryngoscope.* 2006;116(9):1612-1616.

40. Resto VA, Deschler DG. Sinonasal malignancies. *Otolaryngol Clin North Am.* 2004;37:473-487.

41. Melroy CT, Senior BA. Benign sinonasal neoplasms: a focus on inverted papilloma. *Otolaryngol Clin North Am.* 1005;39(3):601-617.

42. Bikhazi N. Contemporary management of nasal polyps. *Otolaryngol Clin North Am.* 2004;37(2):327-337.

43. Belleza WG, Kallman S. Otolaryngologic emergencies in the outpatient setting. *Otolaryngol Clin North Am.* 2006;90:329-353.

44. Miller EH. Dental considerations in the management of head and neck cancer patients. *Otolaryngol Clin North Am.* 2006;39(2):319-329.

45. Campana JP, Meyers AJ. Surgical management of oral cancer. *Otolaryngol Clin North Am.* 2006; 39(2):331-348.

46. Lin YS, Jen YM, Wang BB, Lee JC, Kange BH. Epidemiology of oral cavity cancer in Taiwan with emphasis on the role of betel nut chewing. *J Otorhinolaryngol.* 2005;67(4):230-236.

47. Robinson PN, Mickleson AR. Early diagnosis of oral cavity cancer. *Otolaryngol Clin North Am.* 2006; 39:295-306.

48. Toida M. Intraoral minor salivary gland tumors: a clinicopathological study of 82 cases. *Int J Oral Maxillofac Surg.* 2005;34(5):528-532.

49. Head and neck sites. In: American Joint Committee on Cancer. *AJCC Cancer Staging Manual.* 6th ed. New York, NY: Springer; 2002:17-88.

50. Miller FR. Surgical anatomy of the thyroid gland and parathyroid glands. *Otolaryngol Clin North Am.* 2003;36(1):1-7.

51. Sclabas GM, Staerkel GA, Shapiro SE. Fine-needle aspiration and correlation with histopathology in a contemporary series of 240 patients. *Am J Surg.* 2003;186:702-710.

52. Kim M, Lavertu P. Evaluation of a thyroid nodule. *Otolaryngol Clin North Am.* 2003;36(1):17-33.

53. Scianna JM, Chow JM, Hotaling AJ. Analysis of possible cross-contamination with the Venturi system atomizer. *Am J Rhinol.* 2005;19(5):503-507.

54. Steiner W. Impact of anterior commissure involvement on local control of early glottic cancer treated by laser microdissection. *Laryngoscope.* 2004;114(8):185-191.

55. Behrman A. Evidence-based treatment of paralytic dysphonia: making sense of outcomes and efficacy data. *Otolaryngol Clin North Am.* 2004;37(1): 75-104.

56. Price T. How we do it: The role of trans-nasal flexible laryngo-oesophagoscopy (TNFLO) in ENT: one year's experience in a head and neck orientated practice in the UK. *Clin Otolaryngol.* 2005;30(6): 551-556.

57. Fisher NM, Schaffer JV, Berwick M, Bolognia JL. Breslow depth of cutaneous melanoma: impact of factors related to surveillance of the skin, including prior skin biopsies and family history of melanoma. *J Am Acad Dermatol.* 2005;53(3):393-406.

58. Practice advisory for the perioperative management of patients with cardiac rhythm management devices: pacemakers and implantable cardioverter-defibrillators: a report by the American Society of Anesthesiologists Task Force on Perioperative Management of Patients with Cardiac Rhythm Management Devices. *Anesthesiology.* 2005;103(1): 186-198.

2

Preoperative Medical Evaluation of the Patient with Head and Neck Cancer

Robert L. Schiff
Stephanie A. Detterline

INTRODUCTION

Patients with head and neck cancer may first present to a primary care physician or to an otolaryngologist. When patients are newly diagnosed with head and neck cancer a complete history and physical exam should be done. That exam should evaluate if there is gross evidence of spread of the cancer, and ascertain if the patient has other medical problems. Many common medical problems may impact the management of the patient's cancer including conditions such as cardiovascular disease, chronic obstructive pulmonary disease, diabetes mellitus, and alcoholism.

Comorbid medical conditions are frequently present in patients with head and neck cancer. One series of 1,094 patients at a teaching hospital evaluated comorbid conditions in patients with head and neck cancer.[1] The mean age of the patients was 62.1 years and 83.2% were current or former smokers.[1] Pulmonary disease was present at the time of diagnosis of head and neck cancer in 17.9% of patients.[1] Other frequent comorbid conditions included diabetes mellitus (7.9%), prior myocardial infarction (6.7%), cerebrovascular disease (4.6%), and alcohol abuse (3.8%).[1]

Many patients with head and neck cancer will require surgery as part of their treatment. Patients should undergo a complete preoperative medical evaluation prior to any surgical procedure. The extent of the preoperative medical evaluation is determined by the type of surgery and by the patient's other medical problems. For example, whether the initial surgery is a minor procedure such as endoscopy or biopsy, or whether the patient is undergoing major surgery such as tumor resection or neck dissection will impact the extent of the preoperative medical evaluation. The surgical risk is affected by the type of surgery, the expected length of the procedure, and by other patient factors such as age and comorbid medical conditions.

One or more physicians may be involved in the preoperative medical evaluation of a patient with head and neck cancer. When a patient is undergoing a minor procedure the preoperative medical evaluation might be done just by the otolaryngologist. For some patients having minor procedures a preoperative medical evaluation will also be done by the patient's primary care physician or by a general internal medicine physician who is acting as a consultant. At many institutions when a major procedure is planned the patient's primary care physician or a consulting general internal medicine physician will be a part of the preoperative medical evaluation and risk stratification process, to evaluate the patient's surgical risk and what can be done to lessen the risk of surgery. The anesthesiologist also is usually involved in the preoperative evaluation for major surgery. Other physicians who also may be consulted in the preoperative evaluation include the fields of plastic surgery, medical oncology, radiation therapy, cardiology, and pulmonary medicine. Whether these or other specialists are involved will depend on the stage of the tumor, experience of the treatment team, and the wishes of the patient and their family.

Preoperative Testing

Preoperative laboratory tests that should be done prior to major surgery in all patients with head and neck cancer include a basic metabolic panel, complete blood count, and serum albumin. An electrocardiogram should also be done for all patients with a history of heart disease, for all male patients 40 years and older, and for all female patients 50 years and older.[2]

PREOPERATIVE CARDIAC EVALUATION

Two of the most frequent causes of postoperative morbidity and mortality for head and neck cancer patients are pulmonary and cardiac complications. All patients being considered for major surgery for head and neck cancer should be evaluated for pre-existing cardiovascular disease prior to surgery. That evaluation should include a complete cardiovascular history and physical exam and an ECG prior to major surgery for head and neck cancer.

Patients with particular medical comorbidities have an increased risk for perioperative cardiac complications. Many studies have evaluated which patients are at an increased risk for postoperative cardiac complications.[3,4] The American College of Cardiology/American Heart Association Task Force on Practice Guidelines updated their "Guidelines on Perioperative Cardiovascular Evaluation for Noncardiac Surgery" in 2007.[3] Medical problems that increase the risk for cardiac complications include: coronary artery disease, congestive heart failure, diabetes mellitus, chronic renal failure with a creati-

nine of greater than or equal to 2.0 mg per deciliter, severe valvular heart disease, and certain significant cardiac arrhythmias.[3] The most important cardiovascular complications of noncardiac surgery are myocardial infarction, congestive heart failure, and death. One study of 193 patients undergoing microvascular head and neck reconstruction for head and neck cancer found that 3.6% of patients had a perioperative myocardial infarction.[5] The identification of patients with an increased risk for perioperative myocardial infarction is particularly important because the mortality rate for a perioperative myocardial infarction is 30% to 50%.

One of the goals of the preoperative cardiac evaluation is to identify whether the patient has any of the risk factors for perioperative cardiac complications. If the patient is known or suspected to have one of those risk factors, then the patient should be evaluated prior to surgery by an internist or a cardiologist. The role of the internist or cardiologist will be to further delineate the cardiac risk for surgery, determine if other cardiac tests should be done prior to surgery, and to ascertain whether any measures can reduce the cardiac risk of surgery. The process of risk stratification and modification will depend on the cardiac problems identified, the status of those cardiac problems, and what type of oncologic surgery is planned.[3] The type of surgery that is planned affects the cardiac risk of noncardiac surgery. Surgical procedures have been grouped into high, intermediate, and low-risk procedures for cardiovascular complications.[3] Head and neck surgery is an intermediate-risk procedure.[3] Endoscopic procedures are classified as low-risk procedures.[3]

The status of a patient's coronary artery disease affects the perioperative cardiovascular risk. Unstable coronary syndromes such as acute or recent myocardial infarction, unstable angina, or severe angina are major clinical predictors of increased cardiovascular risk of surgery.[3] Decompensated congestive heart failure is also a major clinical predictor of increased cardiovascular risk of surgery.[3] Mild angina pectoris (Canadian Class I or II) or remote myocardial infarction are intermediate predictors of cardiovascular risk of surgery.[3] Compensated congestive heart failure is an intermediate predictor of cardiovascular risk of surgery.[3]

Preoperative Cardiac Testing

A question frequently asked is, should a patient undergo noninvasive cardiac testing prior to surgery for head and neck cancer? Whether a patient will benefit from preoperative noninvasive cardiac testing is a decision that should be made based on several factors. Those include: the type of surgery planned, the presence of any major or intermediate predictors of increased cardiovascular risk, whether or not the patient has had recent cardiac testing done, and the patient's functional capacity. A patient's functional capacity is determined by what daily activities they can perform such as dressing, walking, climbing stairs, exercise, or participation in sports. Perioperative cardiac risk is increased in patients who cannot do four METS (metabolic activity levels) of activities.[3] An activity level of four METS is typified by walking four blocks or by climbing a flight of stairs. The decision to perform noninvasive cardiac testing prior to surgery for head and neck cancer should be made by an internist or cardiologist. The majority of patients do not require noninvasive cardiac testing prior to head and neck surgery.

Perioperative Beta-Blockers

Once the patient has been scheduled for surgery are there any other measures that can reduce the risk for perioperative cardiac complications? Several prospective studies have shown that perioperative beta-blocker therapy may be beneficial for some patients undergoing noncardiac surgery.[6,7] Beta-blocker therapy may decrease the risk of perioperative cardiac complications for patients with major or intermediate predictors of increased cardiovascular risk (as described above), when major head and neck cancer surgery is done.[3,8] The goal of perioperative beta-blocker therapy is to reduce the risk of myocardial infarction, congestive heart failure, and death. Beta-blocker therapy should be started prior to surgery or on the morning of surgery. The ideal timing of and choice of perioperative beta-blocker therapy has not yet been determined; further clinical studies are examining these issues.[8] All patients who have known cardiovascular disease and/or hypertension should have their cardiac and antihypertensive medication continued up to and including the morning of surgery.

PREOPERATIVE PULMONARY EVALUATION

Evaluation of a patient's pulmonary status is an important aspect of the preoperative evaluation of the head and neck cancer patient. Postoperative pulmonary complications are a frequent cause of morbidity and mortality among surgical patients.[9] The patient with head and neck cancer frequently has risk factors that increase the risk of postoperative pulmonary complications including advanced age, cigarette smoking, and COPD.

Postoperative pulmonary complications occur in 16% of patients undergoing head and neck surgery.[9] A review by the American College of Physicians (ACP) reported that patients undergoing head and neck surgery had an increased risk for postoperative pulmonary complications (odds ratio 2.21, 95% CI 1.82–2.68).[10] Patients with head and neck cancer are at an increased risk for airway obstruction, particularly laryngeal obstruction, due to the mass effect of a tumor given the proximity of many head and neck cancers to the pharynx and respiratory tract.[11] The most frequent postoperative pulmonary complications include atelectasis, pneumonia, respiratory failure, exacerbation of COPD, and bronchospasm.[9]

A thorough history and physical exam to determine if the patient has significant risk factors for postoperative pulmonary complications is essential. The patient should also be evaluated for signs or symptoms of upper airway compromise such as stridor.[11] The most common patient-related risk factors for postoperative pulmonary complications are COPD (odds ratio 2.36), ASA class greater than or equal to 2 (odds ratio 4.87), poor exercise tolerance, albumin <35 g/L, CHF (odds ratio 2.93), ongoing cigarette use (odds ratio 1.36), and the presence of obstructive sleep apnea.[10] In addition, the risk of postoperative pulmonary complications increases with advancing age.

A large VA prospective cohort study evaluated cases to develop a risk index for predicting postoperative respiratory failure. The odds of developing postoperative respiratory failure increased with an albumin <30 g/L (odds ratio 2.16, 95% CI 1.86–2.51) as compared to a normal albumin (>40 g/L).[12] A preoperative BUN <8 mg/dL (odds ratio 1.47, 95% CI 1.26–1.72) or >30 mg/dL (odds ratio 1.41, 95% CI 1.22–1.64) were found to confer an increased risk of postoperative pneumonia.[13] The BUN and albumin are the only laboratory measures that have been shown to have predictive value for the development of pulmonary complications.

Pulmonary function testing is not routinely recommended prior to surgery for head and neck cancer. There is insufficient evidence to support routine spirometry as an independent predictor of postoperative pulmonary complications following noncardiothoracic surgery, even among patients with severe COPD. There is no clear cutoff level for FEV_1 and FVC below which the risk for surgery is unacceptable.[10] However, preoperative pulmonary function testing can be useful in the evaluation of patients with unexplained dyspnea or undiagnosed COPD.[9] Arterial blood gas analysis is not recommended for routine evaluation as it has not been shown to predict postoperative pulmonary complications.

Reducing the Risk of Pulmonary Complications

One of the most important roles of the physician performing the preoperative medical evaluation is to communicate their findings and recommendations to the anesthesiologist and the surgeon. There are several preoperative interventions that may reduce the risk of pulmonary complications. Smoking cessation in patients undergoing surgery for head and neck cancer should be recommended. The immediate benefit and ideal duration of smoking cessation prior to surgery to decrease postoperative pulmonary complications, however, is not clear. One multivariate study of 410 patients reported an adjusted odds ratio of 5.5 (CI 1.9–16.2) for the risk of postoperative pulmonary complications in smokers compared with nonsmokers.[14] Postoperative pulmonary complications can be decreased by delaying surgery to

treat an acute respiratory infection, and by optimizing airway management in patients with asthma or COPD. Postoperative maneuvers that have been shown to decrease the risk of pulmonary complications include lung-expansion techniques (deep breathing, incentive spirometry, or continuous positive airway pressure (CPAP)), and judicious use of NG intubation.[15]

NUTRITIONAL EVALUATION

Malnutrition may be a problem in the head and neck cancer patient because of impaired intake caused by the cancer, increased metabolic demand, or anorexia. Malnutrition is also a common and underrecognized problem in hospitalized patients, occurring in almost 40% of inpatients and documented in the medical record in only 20% of cases.[16] Malnutrition may contribute to an increased risk of poor wound healing, increased susceptibility to infection, overgrowth of bacteria, and increased frequency of decubitus ulcers. In a large study of hospitalized veterans undergoing surgery, those with malnutrition compared to a control group had an increased infection rate (42% vs 16%) and a higher rate of noninfectious complications (21% vs 9%).[17]

A thorough history is important to identify patient-related risk factors for malnutrition in patients with head and neck cancer. Patient related risk factors include a recent weight loss of greater than 10%, concurrent alcohol or drug use, advanced age, and chronic medical conditions such as chronic renal failure, liver disease, or lung disease.[18] In the head and neck cancer patient, it is important to elicit whether mechanical effects of the cancer are affecting the patient's ability to maintain nutrition. The physical exam should evaluate the patient for physical signs of malnutrition and a body mass index (BMI) should be calculated.

In head and neck cancer patients undergoing major surgery, the serum albumin level should be measured. In a large Veterans Administration (VA) study of 50,000 patients undergoing noncardiac surgery, serum albumin was the single strongest measure of 30-day morbidity and mortality.[19] If the albumin is found to be abnormal or there are other signs of malnutrition, optimizing nutrition before and after surgery is beneficial. Several small trials have demonstrated a benefit of preoperative enteral nutrition compared with no support, for the malnourished patient. The role of perioperative TPN is less clear. A VA trial demonstrated a significant reduction of postoperative complications in severely malnourished patients undergoing surgery who received TPN compared with the control group. However, the number of severely malnourished patients only represented 5% of the total number studied.[17]

HYPOTHYROIDISM IN THE HEAD AND NECK CANCER PATIENT

Hypothyroidism is a frequent complication in patients who have previously been treated for head and neck cancer. The preoperative evaluation of a patient who was previously treated for head and neck cancer should include screening for hypothyroidism with a TSH level. Patients who have had radiotherapy for head and neck cancer are at risk for developing hypothyroidism.[20-23] Patients who have had neck surgery and radiotherapy have the highest risk of developing hypothyroidism.[20-23] Patients who have had neck surgery without radiotherapy have a lower risk, but they may also develop hypothyroidism.[20-23]

The prevalence of hypothyroidism after treatment for head and neck cancer is estimated at 14.6% to more than 50%.[20-24] The wide range of estimates stems from the different methodologies used in studies which have evaluated the prevalence of hypothyroidism in these patients: different criteria have been used to define hypothyroidism, many of the studies are retrospective, and many have inadequate length of patient follow-up (2 years or less). The mean time to the development of hypothyroidism after treatment is from 8 to 24 months.[22,23,25]

Screening for hypothyroidism should also be part of a patient's care after they have had treatment for head and neck cancer.[20] Patients should be screened with a TSH level every 6 months for the first 5 years and every year after that.[20] If the TSH level is abnormal a free T3 and free T4 should be checked. Patients who develop hypothyroidism should be treated with levothyroxine.

SUMMARY

The general medical evaluation is a critical element in the comprehensive care of patients with tumors of the head and neck. Every attempt should be made to identify underlying medical conditions or diseases prior to the initiation of any therapies. This is particularly true in the cohort of patients with head and neck squamous cell carcinoma associated with the chronic abuse of tobacco and alcohol. Frequently, these patients forego routine physical examinations and do not have appropriate primary medical care.

Individuals presenting for the surgical treatment of malignant tumors of the head and neck represent a heterogeneous patient population ranging from healthy to those with multiple comorbidities. Some of the goals of the presurgical medical evaluation of these patients are to (1) identify acute potentially life-threatening medical problems requiring urgent intervention (ie, unrecognized severe coronary artery disease), (2) assess and stratify the overall risks to the patient of the potential stresses of the proposed oncologic surgery (ie, cardiopulmonary status), (3) recommend particular interventions to minimize preventable physiologic complications related to the stress of surgery (ie, beta-blocker protocol for postoperative MI), and finally (4) establish a relationship between the patient and a primary care provider for ongoing medical care (tobacco cessation, weight reduction). Establishing a Preoperative Assessment Clinic supervised by experienced internal medicine physicians is one way to provide this level of care. By creating the necessary infrastructure, presurgical consultations can be delivered in a systematic, efficient, cost-effective fashion maximizing the opportunity for appropriate testing and the timely and comprehensive evaluations needed for these frequently complex patients.

REFERENCES

1. Piccirillo JF, Lacy PD, Basu A, Spitznagel EL. Development of a new head and neck cancer-specific comorbidity index. *Arch Otolaryngol Head Neck Surg.* 2002;128:1172–1179.

2. Smetana GW, Macpherson DS. The case against routine preoperative laboratory testing. *Med Clin North Am.* 2003;84:7–12.

3. Fleisher LA, Beckman JA, Brown KA, et al. ACC/AHA 2007 guidelines on perioperative cardiovascular evaluation and care for noncardiac surgery: executive summary: a report of the American College of Cardiology/American Heart Association Task Force on Practice Guidelines. *Circulation.* 2007; 116:1–26.

4. Lee TH, Marcantonio ER, Mangione CM, et al. Derivation and prospective validation of a simple index for prediction of cardiac risk of major noncardiac surgery. *Circulation.* 1999;100:1043–1049.

5. Chiang S, Cohen B, Blackwell K. Myocardial infarction after microvascular head and neck reconstruction. *Laryngoscope.* 2002;112:1849–1852.

6. Mangano DT, Layug EL, Wallace A, Tateo I. Effect of atenolol on mortality and cardiovascular morbidity after noncardiac surgery: multicenter study of Perioperative Ischemia Research Group. *N Engl J Med.* 1996;335:1713–1720.

7. Poldermans D, Boersma E, Bax JJ, et al. The effect of bisoprolol on perioperative mortality and myocardial infarction in high-risk patients undergoing vascular surgery: Dutch Echocardiographic Cardiac Risk Evaluation Applying Stress Echocardiography Study Group. *N Engl J Med.* 1999;341: 1789–1794.

8. Fleisher LA, Beckman JA, Brown, KA, et al. ACC/AHA 2006 guideline update on perioperative cardiovascular evaluation for noncardiac surgery: focused update on perioperative beat-blocker therapy: a report of the American College of Cardiology/American Heart Association Task Force on Practice Guidelines. *J Am Coll Cardiol.* 2006;47:1–13.

9. Smetana GW, Conde MV. Pulmonary evaluation. In: Cohn SL, Smetana GW, Weed HG, eds. *Perioperative Medicine: Just the Facts.* New York, NY: McGraw-Hill; 2006:130–134.

10. Smetana GW, Lawrence VA, Cornell JE. Preoperative pulmonary risk stratification for noncardiothoracic surgery: systematic review for the American College of Physicians. *Ann Intern Med.* 2006;144: 581–595.

11. Online Web Site Up To Date. *Preoperative Management of Patients with Cancer.* Retrieved August 15, 2006 from www.uptodate.com

12. Arozullah AM, Daley J, Henderson WG, Khuri, SF. Multifactorial index for predicting postoperative respiratory failure in men after major noncardiac surgery. The National Veterans Administration Surgical Quality Improvement Program. *Ann Surg.* 2000;232:242–253.

13. Arozullah AM, Khuri SF, Henderson WG, Daley J. Development and validation of a multifactorial risk index for predicting postoperative pneumonia after major noncardiac surgery. *Ann Intern Med.* 2001;135:847–857.

14. Blumen LG, Mosca L, Newman N, Simon DG. Preoperative smoking habits and postoperative pulmonary complications. *Chest.* 1998;133:883–889.

15. Qaseem A, Snow V, Fitterman N, et al.. Risk assessment for and strategies to reduce perioperative pulmonary complications for patients undergoing noncardiothoracic surgery: a guideline from the American College of Physicians. *Ann Intern Med.* 2006;144:575–580.

16. Pirlich M, Schutz T, Kemps M, et al. Prevalence of malnutrition in hospitalized medical patients: impact of underlying disease. *Dig Dis.* 2003;21: 245–246.

17. The Veterans Affairs Total Parenteral Nutrition Cooperative Study Group. Perioperative total parenteral nutrition in surgical patients. *N Engl J Med* 1991;325:525–530.

18. Tess AV. Nutritional evaluation. In: Cohn SL, Smetana GW, Weed HG, eds. *Perioperative Medicine: Just the Facts.* New York, NY: McGraw-Hill; 2006:268–273.

19. Gibbs J, Cull W, Henderson W, et al. Preoperative serum albumin level as a predictor of operative mortality and morbidity: results from the National VA Surgical Risk Study. *Arch Surg.* 1999;134:36–42.

20. Smolarz K, Malke G, Voth E, et al. Hypothyroidism after therapy for larynx and pharynx carcinoma. *Thyroid.* 2000;10:425–429.

21. Gal RL, Gal TJ, Klotch DW, Cantor AB. Risk factors associated with hypothyroidism after laryngectomy. *Otolaryngol Head Neck Surg.* 200;123:211–217.

22. Tell R, Sjodin H, Lundell G, Lewin F, Lewensohn R. Hypothyroidism after external radiotherapy for head and neck cancer. *Int J Radiat Oncol Biol Phys.* 1997;39:303–308.

23. Sinard RJ, Tobin EJ, Mazzaferri EL, et al. Hypothyroidism after treatment for nonthyroid head and neck cancer. *Arch Otolarygol Head Neck Surg.* 2000;126:652–657.

24. Garcia-Serra A, Amdur RJ, Morris CG, Mazzaferri E, Mendenhall WM. Thyroid function should be monitored following radiotherapy to the low neck. *Am J Clin Oncol.* 2005;28:255–258.

25. Colevas AD, Read R, Thornhill J, et al. Hypothy-roidism incidence after multimodality treatment for stage III and IV squamous call carcinomas of the head and neck. *J Radiat Oncol Biol Phys.* 2001;51:599–604.

3

Radiographic Examination of the Head and Neck in Head and Neck Cancer

Lee A. Zimmer
Gail Santucci
Mikhail Vaysberg

INTRODUCTION

Cancer of the head and neck, and particularly squamous cell carcinoma (SCCa) is a challenge to health care providers. Before the advent of computed tomography (CT), practitioners relied on skilled physical examination to diagnose, stage, and manage patients with this disease. Often, though, persistent or recurrent disease would go undetected due to the inability of practitioners to see or feel disease in complex regions of the head and neck. This would lead to a delayed diagnosis with untoward outcomes for the patient.

The advent of CT, magnetic resonance (MR), positron emission tomography (PET), and the increased utilization of ultrasound in head and neck cancer imaging has improved the management of patients with SCCa of the head and neck. Imaging of the head and neck can improve surgical planning, aid in the localization of local regional and distant metastasis, and aid in the planning of radiation protocols (ie, Intensity Modulated Radiation Therapy [IMRT]).

The goal of the present chapter is to review current modalities for imaging head and neck cancer, in particular, SCCa. Emphasis is placed on matching imaging modalities with clinical situations.

PLAIN FILMS

With the advent of CT, MR, PET, and ultrasound (US) imaging techniques, plain film radiography has little role in providing practical information to the head and neck surgical oncologist. Historically, routine AP and lateral chest x-rays have been a practical screen for metastasis to the lungs. If a chest x-ray suggests metastatic disease, imaging of the chest with a CT scan is warranted. Patients with advanced stage head and neck cancer often undergo PET or combined PET-CT imaging. PET provides a thorough radiologic evaluation of the head, neck, lungs, and abdomen for metastatic disease (see PET section).

CT AND MRI CROSS-SECTIONAL IMAGING IN THE EVALUATION OF HEAD AND NECK CANCER STAGING AND SURVEILLANCE

Both primary and recurrent head and neck tumors are most accurately detected by panendoscopy; however, cross-sectional imaging plays an important role in staging.[1] It adds to the clinical evaluation of the primary tumor in assessing size, location, vascular invasion, bone invasion, and perineural spread of tumor.

Due to problems with inconsistency and a tendency to underestimate the size of small nodes when using palpation alone, cross-sectional imaging has become a primary tool in staging nodal disease.[2] CT and MRI will often demonstrate enlarged or morphologically abnormal lymph nodes in necks thought to be normal by palpation. Findings such as necrosis are much more specific for malignancy than enlargement alone (Figs 3–1 and 3–2).[3] Cross-sectional imaging plays a particularly important role in detecting retropharyngeal lymph nodes (Fig 3–3).

CT and MR have demonstrated similar accuracy in detecting nodal metastases. If additional evaluation of the primary tumor arising from the mucosal surface is desired, CT becomes the preferred technique.[4] A limitation of MR in this setting is motion artifact from breathing and swallowing. Motion artifact is related to significantly longer image acquisition times.

The presence of post-treatment changes including scar and edema complicate the cross-sectional evaluation of the neck. It has been suggested that the decision to use imaging should be based on clinical suspicion of recurrent disease, with no imaging study warranted for early stage disease with a low suspicion of recurrence. Cross-sectional imaging should be the initial study when there is a palpable mass or to restage after a biopsy-proved recurrence. PET can play an important role in patients with advanced disease with a low clinical suspicion of recurrence and in patients with nonspecific symptoms that could indicate recurrence.[5]

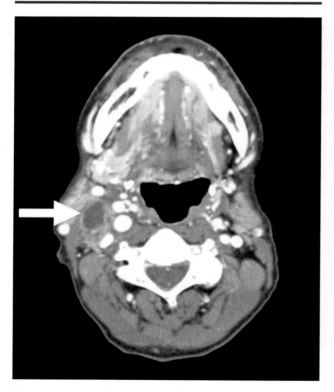

Fig 3–1. Axial CT image with contrast through the level of the mandible. Note lymph node (*arrow*) in right level II of the neck with area of central necrosis. FNA diagnosis revealed SCCa.

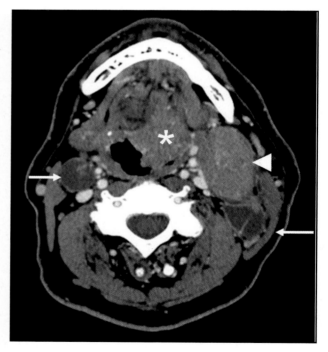

Fig 3–2. Axial CT image with contrast through the level of the mandible. Note large left-sided base of tongue SCCa with extension across the midline (*). Note multiple cystic lymph node metastases in level II (*arrows*) and single large solid metastasis in left level II of the neck (*arrowhead*).

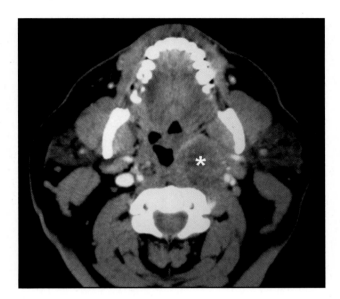

Fig 3–3. Axial CT image with contrast at the level of the angle of the mandible in a patient with a left-sided base of tongue squamous cell carcinoma (*not shown*). Note large, left-sided, solid metastatic lymph node in the retropharyngeal space (*).

IMAGING FEATURES OF MALIGNANCY

Evaluation of abnormal lymph nodes is based on size and morphology. The location of abnormal lymph nodes is usually described according to the anatomic classification by the American Joint Committee on Cancer Staging.[6] Use of a standard system facilitates communication between imagers and clinicians and produces more precise and reproducible nodal staging (Table 3–1).

Size is the first criterion used in evaluating cervical lymph nodes for metastatic disease. Lymph nodes at levels I and II are more frequently mildly enlarged by inflammatory processes and an upper limit of 1.5-cm maximal transverse dimension is used. Nodes at levels III to VII should be less than 1-cm maximal transverse dimension. There are no definite size criteria for retropharyngeal nodes, and they may be of concern even when considerably smaller than 1 cm in patients with pharyngeal cancer, papillary thyroid cancer, and ethesioneuroblastoma.[7]

Table 3–1. American Joint Committee on Cancer Classification of Cervical Lymph Nodes Based on Level and Location

Level I	
Ia	Submental
Ib	Submandibular
Level II	Anterior cervical lymph node chain. Lymph nodes in the internal jugular chain from the skull base to the level of the hyoid bone.
IIa	Nodes anterior, medial, or lateral to the internal jugular vein.
IIb	Nodes posterior to the internal jugular vein with a fat plane between the node and the vessel.
Level III	Nodes along the internal jugular chain between the hyoid bone and the cricoid cartilage.
Level IV	Nodes along the internal jugular chain between the cricoid cartilage and the clavicle.
Level V	Nodes along the spinal accessory chain, posterior to the sternocleidomastoid muscle.
Va	Level V nodes from the skull base to the lower border of the cricoid cartilage.
Vb	Level V nodes from lower border of cricoid cartilage to the clavicle.
Level VI	Nodes in the visceral compartment from the hyoid bone superiorly to the suprasternal notch inferiorly. On each side, the lateral border is formed by the medial border of the carotid sheath.
Level VII	Nodes in the superior mediastinum.

The finding of nodal necrosis is more indicative of nodal involvement by head and neck cancer than the finding of enlargement alone (see Figs 3–1 and 3–2). Even small necrotic nodes are usually malignant. CT and MRI are both accurate in correctly diagnosing nodal necrosis. A study by King et al[8] using pathologic analysis of surgical resection as the reference standard found a sensitivity of 91% and specificity of 93% for CT compared with a sensitivity of 93% and specificity of 89% for MR.

Extracapsular spread of nodal disease is an important prognostic indicator, as patients have a higher risk of recurrence and death when there is macroscopic extension of tumor beyond the capsule of the lymph node (Fig 3–4). Conversely, when tumor is confined to the lymph node or shows only microscopic invasion beyond the capsule there are no statistically significant differences in risk rates.[9] Imaging is less successful in making this distinction. CT is reported to have a sensitivity of 65% and a specificity of 93%, compared to a sensitivity of 78% and a specificity of 86% for MR.[10]

Calcified cervical lymph nodes are rare, seen in only 1% of 2,300 cases in one series.[11] Calcification is a finding with a limited differential diagnosis, including metastatic thyroid cancer, adenocarcinoma, and squamous carcinoma, in addition to tuberculosis and treated lymphoma. The pattern of calcification is not a predictor of benign or malignant disease.

Fixation of pharyngeal and laryngeal cancers to the prevertebral space can prevent surgical resection (see Fig 3–4). Concavity and abnormal enhancement of the prevertebral muscles adjacent to the mucosal space tumor on MR has been found to be sensitive (88%) but nonspecific (29%).[12] Preservation of the retropharyngeal fat plane between the tumor and the prevertebral compartment has been found to predict absence of fixation of tumor to the prevertebral fascia in 98% of cases.[13]

Invasion of the carotid arteries necessitates resection and reconstruction of the vessel if a complete resection is to be attempted. Yousem et al[14] using MR indicated that tumor should be considered to invade the artery when it involves greater than 270° of the vessel circumference (see Fig 3–4), whereas if involvement is 270° or less this is considered lack of vessel invasion. These criteria were demonstrated to have a sensitivity of 100% and a specificity of 88%. A study by Yoo et al[15] found clinical assessment of whether tumor could be dissected from the carotid artery without leaving residual tumor to be as predictive as CT (using more than 180° involvement) for vessel invasion.

Detection of bone invasion is important in tumor staging and surgical planning. Whereas CT has the advantage of improved resolution of bony architecture, MR can detect bone marrow abnormalities. The sensitivity and specificity reported for MR in the detection of mandibular invasion by oral cavity squamous cell carcinoma has ranged from 93 to 96% and 54 to 93%, respectively (Fig 3–5). CT has more consistently demonstrated high specificity of 87 to 88% with a similarly high sensitivity of 96 to 100%. False-positive cases on MR have been attributed to chemical shift artifact related to bone marrow fat.[16-18]

The prognostic significance of laryngeal cartilage abnormalities on imaging studies is controversial (Fig 3–6). Suspicion of cartilage invasion can preclude

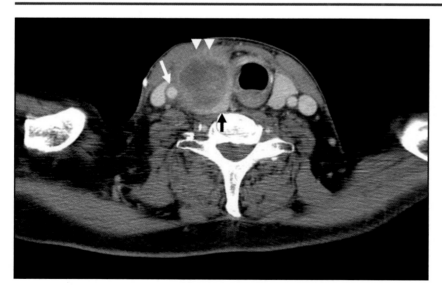

Fig 3–4. Axial CT with contrast at the level of the thyroid revealing a large metastatic lymph node in level IV of the neck. Note complete encasement of the right carotid artery (*white arrow*). Also note extracapsular extension of the involved lymph node (*arrowheads*) and involvement of the paraspinal muscles (*black arrow*).

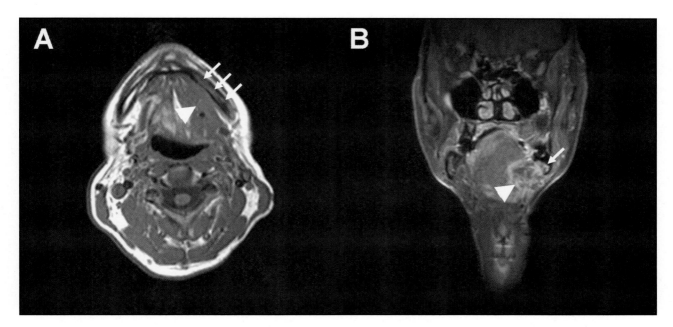

Fig 3–5. A. Axial T1-weighted MRI image without contrast through the level of the mandible. Note lesion along the left, lateral floor of mouth (*arrowhead*). Soft tissue is noted within the marrow space of the mandible on the left (*arrows*) consistent with mandibular invasion. **B**. Coronal T1-weighted MRI image with contrast through the level of the mandible in the same patient. Note lesion along the left, lateral floor of mouth (*arrowhead*) with invasion of the deep tongue musculature. Direct extension of tumor is identified invading the cortex and marrow space of the mandible (*arrow*).

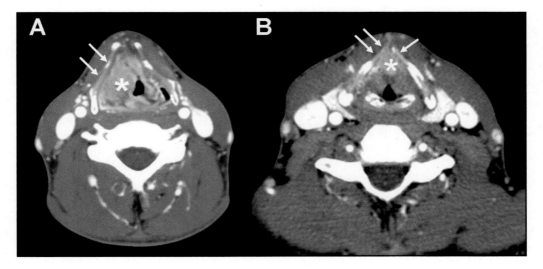

Fig 3–6. A. Axial CT scan with contrast through the level of the thyroid cartilage. Note mass on the right side of the glottis (*). The laryngeal mass has not invaded the thyroid cartilage (*arrows*). A clear plane is observed between the lesion and the thyroid cartilage. **B.** Axial CT scan with contrast through the level of the thyroid cartilage in another patient. Note mass involving the glottis and anterior commissure (*). Tumor is observed to be eroding and extending through the thyroid cartilage.

voice-sparing partial laryngectomy with radiation therapy, leaving total laryngectomy as the only option. A review of preoperative CT studies on a series of patients who underwent extended hemilaryngectomy demonstrated that cartilage abnormalities were not clearly associated with recurrence.[19] MR has demonstrated higher sensitivity than CT in detecting cartilage invasion by laryngeal and pyriform sinus cancer (89% vs 66%), but lower specificity (84% vs 94%). Inflammatory changes and fibrosis are indistinguishable from tumor on MR.[20]

Perineural spread of metastatic disease in the head and neck is seen most commonly in SCCa and adenoid cystic carcinoma. MR is generally the preferred method of imaging in this setting, demonstrating enlargement and abnormal signal and enhancement of involved nerves. MR also demonstrates changes from neuropathic atrophy and replacement of Meckel's cave with tumor (Fig 3–7). However, CT can play a complementary role by demonstrating foraminal enlargement or destruction and often demonstrates obliteration of fat planes at foraminal openings as well as on MR.[21,22]

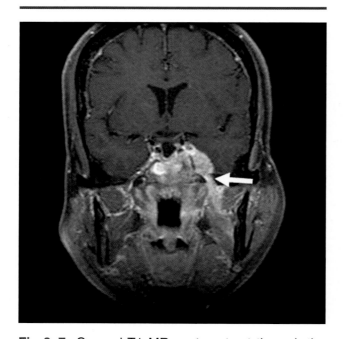

Fig 3–7. Coronal T1 MR post-contrast through the level of the pituitary gland. Note enhancement (*arrow*) with widening of the foramen ovale on the left. Note: extensive perineural spread of SCCa through the foramen ovale with intracranial spread.

IMAGING APPLICATIONS IN OTHER HEAD AND NECK TUMORS

Imaging in the management of thyroid cancer often involves several modalities, particularly when searching for sites of metastatic disease in the face of rising thyroglobulin levels. Contrast-enhanced CT is to be avoided when radioiodide therapy is planned. MR is often used to evaluate for recurrent tumor in the thyroid bed and metastatic lymph nodes. Enlarged nodes are suspicious for tumor involvement, as with other primary tumors. The use of size criteria generally results in a high sensitivity and low specificity.[23] Specificity for metastatic disease increases significantly when there are morphologic abnormalities such as cystic lymph nodes in metastatic papillary thyroid carcinoma.[24]

Paragangliomas demonstrate specific imaging features on MR. Internal flow voids are often particularly well-demonstrated on MRA (Fig 3–8). CT can be useful in demonstrating associated temporal bone destruction and catheter angiography is sometimes required for diagnosis in difficult cases. Angiography may also be performed prior to preoperative embolization.[25]

PET AND PET-CT IMAGING IN HEAD AND NECK CANCER

CT and MRI imaging has been the cornerstone in complementing the physical examination of the head and neck. The advent of PET and combined PET-CT may provide even more valuable information for the diagnosis and management of head and neck SCCa. The following section evaluates current data as to the utility of PET in the staging, treatment, and surveillance of head and neck cancer.

PET shows no advantage over traditional modalities for the identification and characterization of pri-

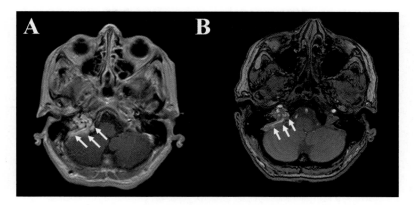

Fig 3–8. A. Axial MRA through the level of the cerebellar pontine angle (CPA). Note enhancing mass with flow voids in the right CPA (*arrows*) with internal flow voids consistent with a paraganglioma (glomus jugulare). **B.** Axial T1 MR postcontrast revealing an enhancing lesion in the right CPA consistent with a paraganglioma (glomus jugulare).

mary head and neck tumors.[26,27] PET imaging does not provide detailed anatomic information required for surgical or radiation planning. Combined imaging adds anatomic detail but information is lacking whether the addition of PET provides useful information when the primary treatment is surgical.

Patients with clinically staged N0 necks are particularly challenging as a number of these patients will harbor micrometastatic cancer in the cervical lymphatics. A number of studies evaluated the use of PET in the identification of nodal metastasis in patients with N0 necks on clinical examination.[26-29] Unfortunately, the specificity and sensitivity of PET in this patient population is similar to CT imaging alone. It is unclear whether combined imaging with PET-CT would improve the detection of neck metastasis not identified on traditional imaging modalities. It is unlikely that combined imaging will increase accuracy of nodal metastasis as PET does not detect occult nodal metastases less than 5 mm.

Patients with advanced stage (stage III and IV) SCCa of the head and neck have a high risk of distant metastasis. Several studies show a distinct advantage of PET in identifying synchronous lesions, particularly in the lung, compared to chest x-ray, CT, and bronchoscopy.[30,31] Teknos et al[32] evaluated

12 patients with stage III/IV SCCa of the head and neck with PET and CT. PET identified distant disease in 25% of patients whereas CT identified only 8% of distant lesions, suggesting that PET may be superior to other modalities for identifying distant disease.

UNKNOWN PRIMARY

Five to ten percent of patients with SCCa in the lymphatics of the neck have a primary tumor that cannot be identified by physical examination, panendoscopy, and conventional radiographic imaging.[33] PET may be a complementary study for patients with unknown primaries of the head and neck when conventional evaluation fails (Fig 3-9).[34,35] Kole and colleagues in 1998 evaluated 29 patients with unknown primaries of the head and neck and PET identified the primary lesion in 24% of the patients.[34] However, as PET changed the clinical management in only 10% of the patient population, the authors concluded that PET was not cost effective or beneficial to this patient population. Johansen and colleagues in 2002 evaluated 42 patients with unknown primaries of the head and neck with PET.[35] Discovery

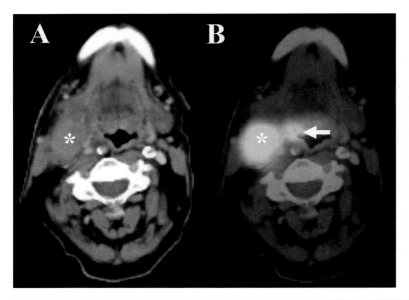

Fig 3–9. A. Axial CT image with contrast at the level of the mandible revealing a large right level II lymph node (*). FNA of the right lymph node revealed SCCa. No evidence of primary tumor on CT or physical examination. **B.** Axial PET/CT examination revealed evidence of increased uptake in the right base of tongue, inferior tonsil (*arrow*). Laryngoscopy with biopsy confirmed squamous cell carcinoma of the right base of tongue.

of the unknown primary altered treatment in 10 patients, allowing reductions in radiation protocols. The authors argued that PET in this setting may be beneficial to decrease the toxicity and associated morbidity of radiation therapy by avoiding wide-field radiation treatment.

Both PET and combined PET/CT are limited in identifying unknown primary cancers in the head and neck. First, as the resolution of PET and CT is limited to about 5 mm, small or superficial lesion may be undetected. Furthermore, basal uptake of radiotracer in the normal lymphoid tissues of Waldeyer's ring and the secretion of radiotracer from salivary glands may further obscure detection of small malignant primary lesions.

ORGAN-SPARING PROTOCOLS

A pretreatment PET would allow the medical and radiation oncologist to monitor the primary tumor's response to chemotherapy and/or radiotherapy. PET/CT can also be used to plan radiation fields for IMRT. The addition of PET to CT for IMRT planning allowed superior localization of the primary tumor compared to CT alone. Further studies are war-

ranted to evaluate whether this technology leads to more efficient treatment regimens and increased local and regional control.[36]

RESPONSE TO NONSURGICAL MODALITIES

Tumor response to chemotherapy can be monitored by PET by identifying changes in tumor metabolism (Fig 3–10).[37-39] Lowe evaluated the use of PET 2 and 10 months after chemotherapy and radiation in 30 patients presenting with stage III and IV head and neck cancer.[37] PET identified persistent tumor in all 16 treatment failures. However, Lonneux et al in 2000 demonstrated decreased specificity if PET images are obtained prior to 12 weeks postradiation due to the elevated uptake of glucose by inflammatory cells that are abundant in irradiated sites.[40] The data suggest that PET should be delayed until 8 weeks postchemotherapy and 12 weeks postradiation treatment. Another study evaluated the use of PET in patients participating in a neoadjuvant organ-preserving protocol.[38] In this setting, PET had 90% sensitivity and 83% specificity for accurately identifying persistent disease. The authors concluded that PET

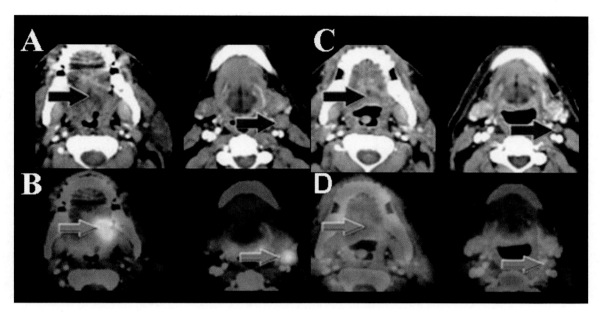

Fig 3–10. A. Axial CT image through the level of the mandible revealing normal anatomy in the left floor of mouth with adjacent, enlarged level I lymph node prior to treatment with chemotherapy and radiation (*arrows*). **B.** Corresponding PET/CT with FDG uptake in the left floor of mouth and level I lymph node. Subsequent biopsies revealed SCCa (*arrows*). **C.** Repeat axial CT image through the level of the mandible 12 weeks following the completion of chemoradiation. No evidence of tumor is present in the left floor of mouth or level I lymph nodes. **D.** Repeat axial PET/CT image through the level of the mandible 12 weeks following the completion of radiation. No evidence of FDG uptake present in the left floor of mouth or level I lymph nodes.

does play a role in the post-treatment surveillance of patients undergoing organ-sparing protocols for advance stage head and neck SCCa.

SURVEILLANCE OF ADVANCED TUMORS

Identification of recurrence by conventional imaging modalities is difficult secondary to tissue defects that develop secondary to surgery and the acute and chronic tissue effects of radiation (Fig 3–11). The specific uptake of FDG by aberrant glucose metabolism in malignancies offers a distinct advantage over traditional imaging techniques. Furthermore, combined PET/CT provides correlative anatomic imaging to guide diagnostic and therapeutic interventions.

The inability to reliably identify tumor recurrence leads to a delay in diagnosis and increases the number of nonsalvageable cases. Terharrd and colleagues[39] in 2001 demonstrated a delay of 26 months in the identification of recurrence in the larynx and hypopharynx using laryngoscopy. PET decreased this time interval from treatment to diagnosis to 14 months, and reduced the number of laryngoscopies and biopsies by 50%.

PET/CT shows a small but distinct advantage over PET alone for surveillance of head and neck cancer. In a recent study, 47 patients with suspected recurrent head and neck carcinoma and normal clinical examinations were evaluated with PET.[41] The average time from definitive treatment, including surgery and/or chemoradiation, to suspected recurrence on PET/CT was 22 months ±10 months. PET/CT identified recurrent disease in 70% of these patients.

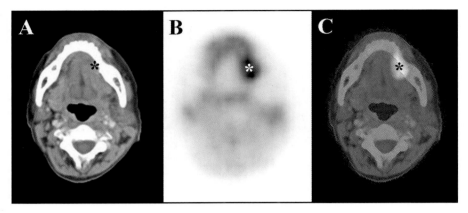

Fig 3–11. Axial CT (**A**), PET (**B**), and PET/CT (**C**) at the level of the mandible. Patient with a history of SCCa of the left floor of mouth resected 8 months prior. Physical examination revealed no evidence of tumor. CT scan revealed no abnormality. PET and PET/CT revealed presence of recurrent tumor (*).

The sensitivity of PET/CT was 100%, with a specificity of 60%. False positive exams were attributed to inflammation, infection, muscle activity, and high activity inherent in tissues of the head and neck. Another recent study examined 65 patients with suspected recurrent head and neck cancer with negative clinical exams. PET/CT increased the confidence of the radiologic interpretation of recurrence compared to PET and CT alone.[42] Routine surveillance with PET/CT provides advantages over PET and CT alone in the identification of head and neck recurrences.

ROLE OF PET IN THE POSTCHEMORADIATION NECK DISSECTION

Several studies have evaluated pathologic results in patients with a partial clinical response to chemoradiation.[26-28] Thirty-nine to 46% of patients with a partial clinical response to chemoradiation had residual disease in the neck. Thus, an incomplete response with palpable abnormalities in the neck is not an indicator of persistent, active disease. Furthermore, both CT and MRI fail to accurately predict the

pathologic status of residual lymph nodes following chemoradiation.[29-32]

The data above indicate that approximately 60% of individuals with N2-3 necks undergoing planned neck dissection following definitive concurrent chemoradiation did not need surgery. The true value may be higher as disease found on pathologic specimen may not be viable. This leads to increased hospital costs and the potential of increased surgical morbidity.

PET has been used extensively in head and neck cancer staging, assessment of treatment response, surveillance and detection of recurrence. PET and combined positron emission tomography with computed tomography (PET/CT) may further increase the detection of head and neck cancers.[33-35] Porceddu et al retrospectively evaluated the utility of PET for evaluating residual neck masses in patients treated with chemoradiation for mucosal head and neck SCCa.[43] PET had a negative predictive value and positive predictive value of 97 and 71%, respectively, with a mean follow-up of 34 months. Similar results have been reported in other retrospective studies.[37-39] The authors concluded that it is safe to follow patients with advanced neck disease with PET following chemoradiaton. Indeed, PET and PET/CT is considered standard of care for head and neck squamous cell carcinoma and not an experimental technology.

ULTRASONOGRAPHY IN HEAD AND NECK CANCER

Ultrasonography (US) has changed since the late 1960s. The evolution of computers, transducers, monitors and the progression from A to B-mode considerably improved the interpretability of US images. Current images from high-resolution US permit the identification of multiple types of head and neck lesions. US provides certain echogenic tissue characteristics suggestive of malignancy. Recent advances, including the use of contrast agents, tissue harmonic imaging, and 3-D multiplanar reconstruction, will enhance the resolution and interpretability of US images.[44] The most commonly performed US in head and neck SCCa is B-mode (gray-scale) using frequencies between 7.5 and 15 MHz. It is complemented by duplex and color flow analysis of tumor vascularity and surrounding vessels.[45]

High-resolution US is a noninvasive, cost-effective, and portable imaging method helpful in the management of patients with head and neck SCCA, especially for the diagnostic evaluation, surveillance, and treatment of cervical lymph nodes. Cervical ultrasonography distinguishes metastasis from other types of neck masses (prominent carotid sinus, laryngoceles, salivary glands, extension of primary tumor).[46] US can also assess cervical neck masses in high risk populations (ie, smokers, alcoholics, previously radiated patients), and assists in the detection of nonpalpable occult cervical metastatic foci. If residual disease is suspected, US permits metastatic surveillance of previously treated cervical areas despite extensive fibrosis. Furthermore, US aids in the surgical evaluation, including location of tumor, 3-dimensional size, remoteness from the skin surface, proximity to vital neighboring structures, and extracapsular spread. US also provides guidance for fine-needle aspiration biopsy (FNA) allowing for cytologic confirmation of metastatic disease (Fig 3–12).[47,48]

Assessment of cervical lymph nodes is essential for patients with head and neck carcinomas, as it helps to assess prognosis and select appropriate treatment. Gray scale and power-Doppler US is useful in predicting malignant characteristics of a neck mass based on visualized morphology, internal architecture, size and shape, extracapsular neoplastic infil-

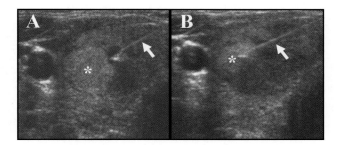

Fig 3–12. Axial ultrasound image of large mass adjacent to the left thyoid. **A.** FNA needle (*arrow*) approaching mass (*). **B.** FNA needle (*arrow*) within the tumor (*). FNA results confirmed SCCa.

tration, pattern of neovascularization, and vascular parameters. Features such as: round shape, absence of echogenic hilus, hyper/hypoechogenesity, intranodal cystic degeneration, absence of planes and sharp borders, and adjacent soft tissue edema are highly suggestive of malignancy.[49-52]

The advantages offered by US over CT or MRI include: volumetric 3D analysis of the lymph nodes achieved by manipulation of the transducer, absence of dental or fatty interferences, appreciation of calcifications, rapidness of FNA biopsy, lack of radiation and intravenous contrast hazards, decreased cost, and increased availability.[53] Furthermore, US can detect malignancies in lymph nodes less than 1 cm not detected by CT or MR.[46,54] CT and MR do have advantages over US: reproducibility that is not operator dependent: better evaluation of primary tumors, the ability to detect lymphadenopathy in the oropharynx, nasopharynx, retropharynx/esophagus, and below the sternum.[50,55] Thus, CT and/or MR must be considered in patients with tumors that have the tendency for metastatic spread to the above mentioned spaces.

The performance of US and US-guided FNAs in the management of head and neck cancer has a steep learning curve. In experienced hands, the average examination/procedure takes 10 minutes and the inadequate sample rate averages 5%.[56] Immediate fixation of the specimen is detrimental to its interpretability. On-site cytologic evaluation of the smears almost eliminates nondiagnostic aspirates. Factors limiting reproducibility of US-guided aspirates include node diameter less than 4 mm, patient compliance, needle size, resolution of the US image, criteria for cellularity of the biopsy specimen defined by the cytopathologist, the patients' neck anatomy (obese, stocky), and previous radiotherapy or surgery.[46] As a general rule, an US-guided FNA biopsy should be offered for any hypoechoic mass above 5 mm in size and should be performed on any lesion 1.0 cm or more with US characteristics suggesting malignancy. Due to the increased use of PET/CT technology, there have been a surge of positive radiologic findings with unknown relevance. US-guided FNA biopsy helps to determine the pathologic significance of these "hot" spots.

The rate of occult metastasis in head and neck SCCa depends on the tumor site, stage, degree of differentiation, and depth of invasion.[57] One may elect to observe the N0 neck with periodic US to monitor late cervical metastatic lymphadenopathy. Using US criteria mentioned above disease can be early and accurately identified.[58,59] The relapse rate and rates of neck metastasis have been equivocal due to strict follow-up and successful early salvage surgery. As a result of preoperative US evaluation and US-guided FNA biopsy, elective neck dissections can be avoided in a significant number of patients without negatively affecting their survival as the number of patients requiring any type of radical neck dissection has remained stable.[60]

US-guided FNA biopsy of sentinel lymph nodes for the detection of occult metastatic disease is still under investigation. The combination of lymphoscintigraphy and US-guided FNA biopsy of the sentinel lymph nodes is thought to be able to preselect N+ patients and to avoid the morbidity of open staging procedures. Although strong conceptually, this diagnostic alternative has not yet gained popularity due to conflicting reports of various false-negative results.[61-64] Achieving reduction of the risk of occult cervical metastasis to around 10% permits expectant management of the N0 neck, specifically when a patient can be followed with scheduled serial US-guided FNA biopsies.[50,65,66]

US can be utilized for examination of the efficacy of radiotherapy for patients with head and neck SCCa. Size reductions of primary tumors and the largest node before and during radiotherapy demonstrate the rate and extent of response to radiother-apy.[67] In a case where a lesion is operable, early identification of the tumor's radioresistance alters the course of therapy prior to upstaging the disease. Once primary radiochemotherapy is completed, the presence of a large amount of residual tumor volume and a high degree of lymph node vascularity on color Doppler sonography indicates a particularly bad prognosis for lesions of the aerodigestive tract.[68]

US image-guided laser therapy has been used for ablation of vascular and thyroid lesions.[69] It has also been applied for palliative management of recurrent head and neck cancer. For unresectable, hard to reach malignant cervical adenopathy, US-guided laser-induced thermal therapy is a minimally invasive outpatient procedure that offers limited morbidity. This type of palliation therapy has been found to reduce tumor-related pain and improve functional abilities.[70]

Head and neck carcinomas tend to metastasize to regional lymph nodes rather than to spread hematogenously. Clinical examination for the detection of metastases by palpation is unreliable. Furthermore, staging of the clinically negative neck in patients with head and neck SCCa continues to challenge the contemporary imaging techniques. Although their accuracy significantly supersedes the accuracy of clinical examination, neither US, CT scan, MRI, nor PET offer great sensitivity (50%–60%).[49,71,72] In addition, the combination of radiographic modalities is not complementary, which restricts the use of radiologic examination of the N0 neck to a single type. The choice of diagnostic cervical imaging largely depends on the tumor's site, morphology, thickness, T-stage, tumor behavior, and experience of the head and neck oncologist.[46,72] Absence of findings may not obviate the need for elective neck dissection, yet confirmation of metastatic disease certainly upstages the tumor and may alter the course and extent of therapy.

Comprehensive US examination of the head and neck with cytopathologic support from FNA biopsy is of great value. It is quick, safe, cost-effective, minimally invasive, and requires no intravenous contrast or ionizing irradiation. It improves care for head and neck oncology patients by offering improved pretreatment and post-treatment follow-up. In conjunction with ablative therapy, it improves quality of life in patients who have failed previous treatments.

It reduces the need for staging neck dissections and permits diagnosis of delayed cervical metastasis in observed patients without altering patients' survival. To avoid unpleasant surprises and negative consequences, one should be aware of the limitations of utilizing this technology. Visualization of certain anatomic structures can be limited, the malignant US features may not be apparent, and there is a size limitation for biopsy. In addition, it is operator-dependent; thus, the experience and skill of the ultrasonographer and cytopathologist are prerequisites for good results.

SUMMARY

CT imaging has been the workhorse in the characterization of the primary tumor and the localization of regional and distant metastasis of head and neck cancer. CT is superior to MR in determining bony invasion, particularly of the mandible. MR can be helpful in determining bone marrow and cartilage invasion and perineural spread. Both CT and MR are helpful in identifying carotid artery invasion. Neither CT nor MR is accurate at predicting extracapsular spread.

PET imaging offers an advantage over CT and MR for identifying SCCa in the head and neck. PET/CT adds detailed anatomy to increase confidence in the radiologist's interpretation of the images and assists in surgical planning. PET and PET/CT is advantageous for staging distant metastasis in stage III and IV disease, prospectively analyzing tumor response to chemotherapy and radiotherapy, determining the need for staged neck dissection in the nonoperative management of the N2 and N3 neck, and identifying recurrent disease. PET and PET/CT offers no advantage in staging the primary tumor or neck metastasis, or identifying the unknown primary tumor. Further studies are warranted to identify the appropriate timing of PET imaging following treatment of head and neck SCCa.

US is an exciting imaging modality for use in staging and surveillance of cervical metastasis. US also allows in office image guidance of fine needle aspiration. The accuracy of US-guided fine needle aspiration is greater than 95% in experienced hands. Hypoechoic lymph nodes greater than 5 mm and all lymph nodes greater than 1.5 cm should undergo US-guided fine needle aspiration if available. Further studies will establish the utility of this imaging modality readily available to the head and neck surgeon's office.

CONCLUSIONS

Imaging of patients with head and neck SCCa has advanced tremendously over the last 30 years. Exciting technology has increased the accuracy of identifying cancer in new and established head and neck cancer patients both in the office and the radiology suite. The future holds the promise of even more accurate, cancer-specific imaging modalities.

REFERENCES

1. Di Martino E, Nowak B, Hassan H, et al. Diagnosis and staging of head and neck cancer. *Arch Otolaryngol Head Neck Surg.* 2000;126:1457–1461.
2. Alderson DJ, Jones TM, White SJ, et al. Observer error in the assessment of nodal disease in head and neck cancer. *Head Neck.* 2001;23:739–743.
3. Atula TS, Varpula MJ, Kurki RJ, et al. Assessment of cervical lymph node status in head and neck cancer patients: palpation, computed tomography and low field magnetic resonance imaging compared with ultrasound-guided fine-needle aspiration cytology. *Eur J Radiol.* 1997;25:152–161.
4. Curtin HD, Ishwaran H, Mancuso AA, et al. Comparison of CT and MR imaging in staging of neck metastases. *Radiology.* 1998;207:123–130.
5. Mukherji SK, Wolf GT. Evaluation of head and neck squamous cell carcinoma after treatment. *AJNR.* 2003;24:1743–1746.
6. American Joint Committee on Cancer Staging. *American Joint Committee on Cancer Staging Manual.* 5th ed. Philadelphia, Pa: Lippincott Raven; 1997.
7. Som PM. Lymph nodes. In: Som PM, Curtin HD, eds. *Head and Neck Imaging.* 4th ed. St. Louis, Mo: Mosby; 2003. 1865–1934.
8. King AD, Tse GM, Ahuja AT, et al. Necrosis in metastatic neck nodes: diagnostic accuracy of CT, MR imaging, and US. *Radiology.* 2004;230:720–726.

9. Brasilino de Carvalho M. Quantitative analysis of the extent of extracapsular invasion and its prognostic significance: a prospective study of 170 cases of carcinoma of the larynx and hypopharynx. *Head Neck.* 1998;20:16–21.

10. King AD, Tse GMK, Yuen EHY, et al. Comparison of CT and MR imaging for the detection of extranodal neoplastic spread in metastatic neck nodes. *Eur J Radiol.* 2004; 52:264–270.

11. Eisenkraft BL, Som PM. The spectrum of benign and malignant etiologies of cervical node calcification. *AJR.* 1999;172:1433–1437.

12. Loevner LA, Ott IL, Yousem DM, et al. Neoplastic fixation to the prevertebral compartment by squamous cell carcinoma of the head and neck. *AJR Am J Roentgenol.* 1998;170:1389–1394.

13. Hsu WC, Loevner LA, Karpati R, et al. Accuracy of magnetic resonance imaging in predicting absence of fixation of head and neck cancer to the prevertebral space. *Head Neck.* 2005;27:95–100.

14. Yousem DM, Hatabu H, Hurst RW, et al. Carotid artery invasion by head and neck masses: prediction with MR imaging. *Radiology.* 1995;195: 715–720.

15. Yoo GH, Hocwald E, Korkmaz H, et al. Assessment of carotid artery invasion in patients with head and neck cancer. *Laryngoscope.* 2000;110(3 pt 1): 386–390.

16. Bolzoni A, Cappiello J, Piazza C, et al. Diagnostic accuracy of magnetic resonance imaging in the assessment of mandibular involvement in oral-oropharyngeal squamous cell carcinoma. *Arch Otolaryngol Head Neck Surg.* 2004;130:837–843.

17. Mukherji SK, Isaacs DL, Creager A, et al. CT detection of mandibular invasion by squamous cell carcinoma of the oral cavity. *AJR.* 2001;177:237–243.

18. Imaizumi A, Yoshino N, Yamada I, et al. A potential pitfall of MR imaging for assessing mandibular invasion of squamous cell carcinoma in the oral cavity. *AJNR Am J Neuroradiol.* 2006;27:114–122.

19. Thoeny HC, Delaere PR, Hermans R. Correlation of local outcome after partial laryngectomy with cartilage abnormalities on CT. *AJNR Am J Neuroradiol.* 2005;26:674–678.

20. Becker M, Zbären P, Laeg H, et al. Neoplastic invasion of the laryngeal cartilage: comparison of MR imaging and CT with histopathologic correlation. *Radiology.* 1995;194:661–669.

21. Ginsberg LE, DeMonte F. Imaging of perineural tumor spread from palatal carcinoma. *AJNR Am J Neuroradiol.*1998;19:1417–1422.

22. Caldemeyer KS, Mathews VP, Righi PD, Smith RR. Imaging features and clinical significance of perineural spread or extension of head and neck tumors. *RadioGraphics.* 1998;18:97–110.

23. Gross ND, Weissman JL, Talbot JM, et al. MRI detection of cervical metastasis from differentiated thyroid carcinoma. *Laryngoscope.* 2001;111:1905–1909.

24. Takashima S, Sone S, Takayama F, et al. Papillary thyroid carcinoma: MR diagnosis of lymph node metastasis. *AJNR Am J Neuroradiol.* 1998;19: 509–513.

25. Van den Berg R. Imaging and management of head and neck paragangliomas. *Eur J Radiol.* 2005;15: 1310–1318.

26. Wong WL, Chevretton EB, McGurk M, et al. A prospective study of PET FDG imaging for the assessment of head and neck squamous cell carcinoma. *Clin Otolaryngol Appl Sciences.* 1997;22: 209–214.

27. Laubenbacher C, Saumweber D, Wagner MC, et al. Comparison fluorine-18-fluorodeoxyglucose PET, MRI, and endoscopy for staging head and neck squamous cell carcinoms. *J Nucl Med.* 1995;36: 1747–1757.

28. Myers LL, Wax MK, Nabi H, Simpson GT, Lamonica D. Positron emission tomography in the evaluation of the N0 neck. *Laryngoscope.* 1998;108:232–236.

29. Stoekli SJ, Steinert H, Pfaltz M, Schmid S. Is there a role for positron emission tomography with 18F-fluorodeoxyglucose in the initial staging of nodal negative oral and oropharyngeal squamous cell carcinoma. *Head Neck.* 2002;24:345–349.

30. Stokkel MPM, Moons KGM, ten Broek F-W, van Rijk PP, Hordijk G-J. 18F-fluorodeoxyglucose dual-head positron emission tomography as a procedure for detecting simultaneous primary tumors in cases of head and neck cancer. *Cancer.* 1999;86: 2370–2377.

31. Wax MK, Myers LL, Gabalski EC, Husain S, Gona JM, Nabi H. Positron emission tomography in the evaluation of synchronous lung lesions in patients with untreated head and neck cancer. *Arch Otolaryngol Head Neck Surg.* 2002;128:703–707.

32. Teknos TN, Rosenthal EL, Lee D, Taylor R, MArn CS. Positron emission tomography in the evaluation of stage III and IV head and neck cancer. *Head Neck.* 2001;23:1056–1060.

33. Greco FA, Hainsworth JD. Cancer of unknown primary site. In: DeVita VT Jr, Hellman S, Rosenberg SA. *Cancer: Principles of Oncology.* 4th ed. Philadelphia, Pa: J.B. Lippincott; 1993:2072–2092.

34. Kole AC, Niewig OE, Pruim J, et al. Detection of occult primary tumors using positron emission tomography. *Cancer*. 1998;82:1160–1166.

35. Johansen J, Eigtved A, Buchwald C, Theilgaard SA, Hansen HS. Implication of 18F-fluoro-2-deoxy-D-glucose positron emission tomography on management of carcinoma of unknown primary in the head and neck: a Danish cohort study. *Laryngoscope*. 2002;112:2009–2014.

36. Heron DE, Andrade RS, Flickinger J, et al. Hybrid PET-CT simulation for radiation treatment planning in head and neck cancers: a brief technical report. *Int J Rad Oncol Biol Phys*. 2004;60:1419–1424.

37. Lowe VJ, Boyd JH, Dunphy FR, et al. Surveillance for recurrent head and neck cancer using positron emission tomography. *J Clin Oncol*. 2000;18:651–658.

38. Lowe VJ, Dunphy FR, Varvares M, et al. Evaluation of chemotherapy response in patients with advanced head and neck cancer using [F-18] fluorodeoxyglucose positron emission tomography. *Head Neck*. 1997;19:666–674.

39. Terhaard CH, Bongers V, van Rijk PP, Hordijk GJ. F-18-fluoro-deoxy-glucose positron emission tomography scanning in detection of local recurrence after radiotherapy for laryngeal/pharyngeal cancer. *Head Neck*. 2001;23:933–941.

40. Lonneux M, Lawson G, Ide C, Bausart R, Remacle M, Pauwels S. Positron emission tomography with flourodeoxyglucose for suspected head and neck tumor recurrence in the symptomatic patient. *Laryngoscope*. 2000;110:1493–1497.

41. Zimmer LA, Snyderman CH, Fukui MB, et al. Combined positron emission tomography/computed tomography imaging of recurrent head and neck cancer: the Pittsburgh experience. *ENT J*. 2005;84:104–110.

42. Branstetter BF, Blodgett TM, Zimmer LA, et al. Head and neck malignancy: is PET/CT more accurate than PET or CT alone? *Radiology*. 2005;235:580–586.

43. Porceddu SV, Jarmolowski E, Hicks RJ, et al. Utility of positron emission tomography for the detection of disease in residual neck nodes after (chemo) radiotherapy in head and neck cancer. *Head Neck*. 2005;27:175–181.

44. Lyshchik A, Drozd V, Reiners C. Accuracy of three-dimensional ultrasound for thyroid volume measurement in children and adolescents. *Thyroid*. 2004;14:113–120.

45. Ulrich JV. Ultrasound in dermatology. Part II. Ultrasound of regional lymph node basins and subcutaneous tumors. *Eur J Dermatol*. 2001;11:73–79.

46. Knappe M, Louw MM, Gregor RT. Ultrasonography-guided fine-needle aspiration for the assessment of cervical metastases. *Arch Otolaryngol Head Neck Surg*. 2000;126:1091–1096.

47. Hodder SC, Evans RM, Patton DW, Silvester KC. Ultrasound and fine needle aspiration cytology in the staging of neck lymph nodes in oral squamous cell carcinoma. *Bri J Oral Maxillofac Surg*. 2000; 38:430–436.

48. Kau RJ, Alexiou C, Stimmer H, Arnold W. Diagnostic procedures for detection of lymph node metastases in cancer of the larynx. *ORL; J Oto-Rhino-Laryngol Rel Spec*. 2000;62:199–203.

49. Takes RP, Righi P, Meeuwis CA, et al. The value of ultrasound with ultrasound-guided fine-needle aspiration biopsy compared to computed tomography in the detection of regional metastases in the clinically negative neck. *Int J Radiat Oncol Biol Phys*. 1998;40:1027–1032.

50. Ahuja A, Ying M. An overview of neck node sonography. *Invest Radiol*. 2002;37:333–342.

51. Sumi M, Ohki M, Nakamura T. Comparison of sonography and CT for differentiating benign from malignant cervical lymph nodes in patients with squamous cell carcinoma of the head and neck. *AJR*. 2001;176:1019–1024.

52. Steinkamp HJ, Beck A, Werk M, Rademaker J, Felix R. Extracapsular spread of cervical lymph node metastases: diagnostic relevance of ultrasound examinations. *Ultraschall in der Medizin*. 2003; 24:323–330.

53. Atula TS, Varpula MJ, Kurki TJ, Klemi PJ, Grenman R. Assessment of cervical lymph node status in head and neck cancer patients: palpation, computed tomography and low field magnetic resonance imaging compared with ultrasound-guided fine-needle aspiration cytology. *Eur J Radiol*. 1997;25:152–161.

54. Atula TS, Grenman R, Varpula MJ, Kurki TJ, Klemi PJ. Palpation, ultrasound, and ultrasound-guided fine-needle aspiration cytology in the assessment of cervical lymph node status in head and neck cancer patients. *Head Neck*. 1996;18:545–551.

55. Grotz KA, Krummenauer F, Al-Nawas B, et al. Does ultrasonographic-morphologic staging of lymph nodes in head and neck cancer lend itself to automation? *Ultraschall in der Medizin*. 2000;21:93–100.

56. Steward D, Danielson G, Afman C, Welge J. Parathyroid adenoma localization: surgeon-performed ultrasound versus sestamibi. *Laryngoscope*. 2006; 116:1380–1384.

57. Remmert S, Rottmann M, Reichenbach M, Sommer K, Friedrich H J. Lymph node metastasis in head-neck tumors. *Laryngo-Rhino-Otologie.* 2001;80: 27-35.

58. Yusa H, Yoshida H, Ueno E, et al. Follow-up ultrasonography for late neck metastases of head and neck cancer. *Ultrasound Med Biol.* 2002;28:725-730.

59. Yoshida H, Yusa H, Ueno E, Tohno E, Tsunoda-Shimizu H. Ultrasonographic evaluation of small cervical lymph nodes in head and neck cancer. *Ultrasound Med Biol.* 1998;24:621-629.

60. Wierzbicka M, Szyfter W, Kaczmarek J, Szmeja Z. Effect of ultrasonography on postoperative changes in treatment of neck lymph nodes and improvement of long-term results in patients with laryngeal neoplasms. *Otolaryngologia Polska.* 2002;56: 31-38.

61. Hoft S, Muhle C, Brenner W, Sprenger E, Maune S. Fine-needle aspiration cytology of the sentinel lymph node in head and neck cancer. *J Nucl Med.* 2002;43:1585-1590.

62. Pijpers DR, Castelijns HJ, van Diest JA, et al. Lymphoscintigraphy and ultrasound-guided fine needle aspiration cytology of sentinel lymph nodes in head and neck cancer patients. *Recent Results Canc Res.* 2000;157:206-217.

63. Werner JA, Dunne AA, Ramaswamy A, et al. Number and location of radiolabeled, intraoperatively identified sentinel nodes in 48 head and neck cancer patients with clinically staged N0 and N1 neck. *Eur Arch Oto-Rhino-Laryngol.* 2002;259:91-96.

64. Werner JA, Dunne AA, Ramaswamy A, et al. Sentinel node detection in N0 cancer of the pharynx and larynx. *Br J Canc.* 2002;87:711-715.

65. Cvorovic L, Milutinovic Z, Strbac M, et al. Significance of ultrasound and ultrasound-guided fine-needle aspiration for the detection of laryngeal occult metastases. *Vojnosanitetski Pregled.* 2005; 62:901-907.

66. van den Brekel MW, Stel HV, Castelijns JA, et al. Lymph node staging in patients with clinically negative neck examinations by ultrasound and ultrasound-guided aspiration cytology. *Am J Surg.* 1991;162:362-366.

67. Miyashita TT, Horiuchi JN, Sugizaki KK. Short-time ultrasound of head and neck squamous cell carcinoma under radiotherapy. *Ultrasound Med Biol.* 2001;27:13-19.

68. Dietz A, Delorme SR, Zuna IC, Vanselow B, Weidauer H. Prognostic assessment of sonography and tumor volumetry in advanced cancer of the head and neck by use of Doppler ultrasonography. *Otolaryngol Head Neck Surg.* 2000;122:596-601.

69. Dossing H. Bennedbaek FN. Hegedus L. Effect of ultrasound-guided interstitial laser photocoagulation on benign solitary solid cold thyroid nodules —a randomized study. *Eur J Endocrinol.* 2005; 152:341-345.

70. Bublik M, Sercarz JA, Lufkin RB, et al. Ultrasound-guided laser-induced thermal therapy of malignant cervical adenopathy. *Laryngoscope.* 2006;116: 1507-1511.

71. Stuckensen TK, Adams S, Baum RP. Staging of the neck in patients with oral cavity squamous cell carcinomas: a prospective comparison of PET, ultrasound, CT and MRI. *J Cranio-Maxillo-Fac Surg.* 2000;28(6):319-324.

72. Righi PD, Kopecky KK, Caldemeyer KS, et al. Comparison of ultrasound-fine needle aspiration and computed tomography in patients undergoing elective neck dissection. *Head Neck.* 1997;19(7): 604-610.

4

Principles of Head and Neck Pathology

Diane P. Kowalski

INTRODUCTION

The surgical pathologist, as a member of a multidisciplinary team caring for patients with head and neck cancer, serves a critical consultative role in the management of patients with malignancies of the head and neck. Historically, the pathologist provides diagnostic information, via the surgical pathology report, which will have both prognostic and therapeutic implications for the patient. Critical components of the pathology report may include the histologic classification and grade of the tumor, margin status, depth of invasion, angiolymphatic or perineural involvement, presence of lymph node metastasis, and extranodal extension. As our understanding of the molecular biology of head and neck cancer has increased, along with advancements in molecular techniques, the pathology report may also be used as the conduit for molecular test results.

This chapter begins with the classification of head and neck tumors from a histologic perspective. This is followed by a discussion on diagnostic methodology, including fine-needle aspiration biopsy, frozen section, histopathologic parameters, and molecular diagnostic trends. The latter part of the chapter reviews the natural progression of squamous cell carcinoma, with discussion of precursor lesions, early invasive carcinoma, and histologic parameters with prognostic significance. Finally, the common subtypes of squamous cell carcinoma are reviewed

for completeness. This chapter is not intended to be a comprehensive review of head and neck pathology. Due to space limitations, a detailed review of thyroid, salivary, and parathyroid pathology are not covered. Instead, the reader is referred to any of numerous texts on head and neck pathology to review these topics.

HISTOLOGIC CLASSIFICATION OF TUMORS

Tumors, or neoplasms, are abnormal growths of tissue. They can be benign or malignant. The histologic classification of any tumor is based on its cell of origin as evident by its lineage of differentiation. In the head and neck region, tumors may be divided into epithelial and nonepithelial origin. Malignancies with epithelial origin are called carcinomas (Table 4-1). The most common epithelial malignancy in the head and neck region is squamous cell carcinoma, which accounts for greater than 90% of head and neck malignancies. Squamous cell carcinoma arises from squamous epithelium lining the upper aerodigestive tract, or from cutaneous epithelium. Carcinomas can also arise from structures that are nonsquamous in origin, such as salivary glands, thyroid, parathyroid, and adnexal structures in skin. Epithelial malignancies with glandular differentiation, or with secretory properties, are called adenocarcinomas.

Table 4–1. Malignant Head and Neck Epithelial Tumors

Squamous Cell Carcinoma
    Verrucous carcinoma
    Papillary squamous cell carcinoma
    Basaloid squamous cell carcinoma
    Spindle cell carcinioma
    Adenosquamous carcinoma
    Acantholytic squamous cell carcinoma
    Carcinoma cuniculatum

Lymphoepithelial Carcinoma

Sinonasal Undifferentiated Carcinoma

Adenocarcinoma
    Intestinal-type adenocarcinoma
    Nonintestinal type adenocarcinoma

Neuroendocrine Tumors
    Typical carcinoid
    Atypical carcinoid
    Small cell carcinoma, neuroendocrine type

Nasopharyngeal Carcinoma
    Nonkeratinizing carcinoma
    Keratinizing squamous cell carcinoma

Nasopharyngeal Papillary Adenocarcinoma

Source: Adapted from World Health Organization Classification of Tumours, Pathology and Genetics Head and Neck Tumours (edited by Barnes et al, IARC Press, Lyon, 2005).

Nonepithelial tumors in the head and neck region may be mesenchymal or hematolymphoid in origin. Mesenchyme is tissue that derives from embryonic mesoderm. It develops into structures such as connective tissue, bone, cartilage, endothelial cells, and muscle. Malignancies with a mesenchymal origin are termed sarcomas. Primary head and neck sarcomas are rare, accounting for <1% of all tumors in the head and neck region.[1] Despite their overall rarity, one in three pediatric sarcomas occur in the head and neck.[2] Broadly speaking, sarcomas are classified by their lineage of differentiation, histologic grade, and anatomic location within the head and neck region. Histologic grade, a measure of how closely the tumor resembles normal tissue, carries independent prognostic significance.[3-5] See "Light Microscopy" section for detailed description of tumor grade. The most common sarcomas within the head and neck region include rhabdomyosarcoma, osteosarcoma, angiosarcoma, and malignant fibrous histiocytoma (Table 4-2). The incidence of many sarcomas varies greatly by age. Head and neck rhabdomyosarcoma is predominantly a pediatric disease with approximately 90% of these cases affecting children.[2,6] Adult rhabdomyosarcoma accounts for <1% of all neoplasms in this region.[2,6,7] Angiosarcoma is a rare vascular tumor with an exceedingly poor prognosis which typically occurs in elderly patients. Although uncommon, 50% of all cases occur in the head and neck area.[2,8] The majority of osteosarcomas involve the long bones of adolescent patients. Ten percent of osteosarcomas will occur in the head and neck region, most commonly involving the mandible or maxilla.[2,8,9] The average age of patients with head and neck osteosarcoma is approximately 10 to 15 years older than patients with osteosarcoma of the long bones, and typically occurs in patients in their 3rd to 4th decades.[2,10-12]

Tumors with hematolymphoid origin may also be primary in the head and neck (Table 4-3). Lymphomas are the second most common malig-

Table 4–2. Malignant Head and Neck Mesenchymal Tumors

Soft tissue tumors
- Fibrosarcoma
- Malignant fibrous histiocytoma
- Leiomyosarcoma
- Liposarcoma
- Rhabdomyosarcoma
- Angiosarcoma
- Kaposi sarcoma
- Malignant peripheral nerve sheath tumor
- Synovial sarcoma

Tumors of bone and cartilage
- Chondrosarcoma
- Mesenchymal chondrosarcoma
- Osteosarcoma
- Chordoma

Source: Adapted from World Health Organization Classification of Tumours, Pathology and Genetics Head and Neck Tumours (edited by Barnes et al, IARC Press, Lyon, 2005).

nancy in the head and neck region, and account for approximately 10% of patients with extranodal non-Hodgkin's lymphoma.[13,14] Greater than 60% of head and neck non-Hodgkin's lymphomas occur in

Table 4–3. Head and Neck Hematolymphoid Tumors

- Extranodal NK/T cell lymphoma
- Diffuse large B-cell lymphoma (DLBCL)
- Extramedullary plasmacytoma
- Extramedullary myeloid sarcoma
- Histiocytic sarcoma
- Langerhans cell histiocytosis
- Hodgkins lymphoma
- Follicular dendritic cell sarcoma/tumor
- Mantle cell lymphoma
- Follicular lymphoma
- Extranodal marginal zone B-cell lymphoma of MALT type
- Burkitt lymphoma
- T-cell lymphoma (including anaplastic large cell lymphoma)

Source: Adapted from World Health Organization Classification of Tumours, Pathology and Genetics Head and Neck Tumours (edited by Barnes et al, IARC Press, Lyon, 2005).

lymphoid tissue of Waldeyer's ring, with the most common site of involvement being the tonsil.[14,15] The most common extra nodal sites are paranasal sinus and nasal cavity.[13,14]

Finally, the head and neck region is replete with structures arising from neuroectoderm, which derives from neural crest cells. Representative components of neuroectoderm within the head and neck area include melanocytes, olfactory epithelium, Schwann cells, paraganglia, and neuroendocrine cells (APUD or diffuse neuroendocrine system).[16] Tumors that derive from these cells include malignant melanoma, olfactory neuroblastoma, schwannoma, paraganglioma, primitive neuroectodermal tumor (PNET)/Ewing sarcoma, malignant peripheral nerve sheath tumor (MPNST), and neuroendocrine carcinoma. Malignant melanoma is the most common tumor of neuroectodermal origin in the head and neck region. Approximately 90% of all malignant melanomas are cutaneous in origin.[17] The majority of the remaining cases, nearly 5%, are ocular in origin, whereas approximately 1% occur on mucosal surfaces.[17,18] Head and neck mucosal melanoma accounts for >50% of these cases, with the oral cavity being the most common location.[19-21] Olfactory neuroblastoma (esthesioneuroblastoma) is a malignant tumor of neuroectodermal origin which is thought to arise from the olfactory epithelium of the sinonasal tract (Fig 4–1). It is an uncommon

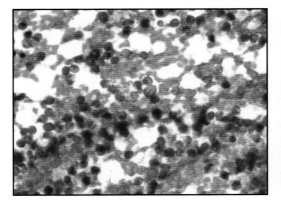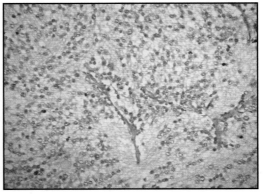

Fig 4–1. Olfactory neuroblastoma. *Left:* Fine-needle aspiration biopsy of recurrent olfactory neuroblastoma showing small round tumor cells with homogeneous, hyperchromatic nuclei and scant cytoplasm. *Right:* Similar cells as seen in the FNA but with abundant neurofibrillary stroma.

neoplasm accounting for approximately 3% of all tumors in the sinonasal region.[22] The upper nasal cavity in the region of the cribriform plate is the most common site of origin. It is thought to have a bimodal age distribution in the 2nd and 6th decades. Controversy exists surrounding this neoplasm due in part to the tumors variable biologic behavior, difficulty in histologic diagnosis, and lack of a universally accepted staging system. Several staging systems are currently used, each showing some correlation with prognosis. PNET/Ewing sarcoma represent a group of small round cell tumors with variable neuroecto-dermal differentiation and which primarily occur in children and adolescents. As many as 20% will occur in the head and neck region.[23-25]

DIAGNOSTIC METHODOLOGY

Light Microscopy

Light microscopy is the means by which a pathologist will evaluate the phenotypic characteristics of a tumor in order to determine its histogenesis. Tumor grade is a measure of differentiation, or the extent to which a neoplastic cell simulates its non-neoplastic counterpart. A well-differentiated tumor closely parallels the phenotypic characteristics of mature normal cells or tissues. Alternatively, poorly differentiated tumor cells look primitive and lack the structure and function of normal cells and tissues. With completely undifferentiated tumors, additional pathologic studies are often necessary to determine the histogenesis.

Immunohistochemistry

Immunohistochemistry refers to a technique of localizing cellular antigens using specific primary antibodies. The antigens may be nuclear, cytoplasmic, or on the cell surface. In the most common method, a labeled, species-specific secondary antibody then reacts with the primary antibody and can be visualized by a marker such as fluorescent dye, enzyme, or radioactive element. Formalin, the most common fixative used in pathology, preserves tissue

by cross-linking proteins. Although this is essential to inactivate enzymes that would otherwise degrade the tissue, cross-linking can alter the conformation or physically cover an antigenic site. This can effectively prevent an antibody from binding to its antigen. Retrieval of these masked antigens in formalin-fixed paraffin-embedded tissue can be enhanced by the application of techniques that use heat to help break the protein cross-links formed by formalin fixation. Antigen retrieval has been significantly enhanced by the application of microwave heat.[26] This has resulted in an expansion of specific antibodies developed against tumor antigen. The diagnostic utility of this technique is greatest in hematopoetic lesions and when a pathologist is faced with a poorly differentiated or undifferentiated tumor for which the histogenesis cannot be determined by light microscopy alone.

Frozen Section

Intraoperative frozen sections have long been accepted as a significant and integral component in the management and treatment of head and neck cancer patients.[27,28] Indications for frozen section examination include:

1. Adequacy of surgical margins
2. Confirmation of a histologic diagnosis immediately prior to a therapeutic surgical procedure
3. Evaluation of lymph nodes for metastatic disease
4. Assessment of the adequacy of tissue for diagnostic purposes and additional adjunctive testing
5. Diagnosis of an unknown pathologic process.

Arguably the most common indication for intraoperative frozen section consultation in head and neck cancer patients is evaluation of margins. Adequate surgical margins are an essential component of any oncologic surgery, particularly in the head and neck region, where patients with positive surgical margins have a significantly higher risk of local recurrence and a poorer prognosis.[29-32] In a study by Byers et al,[33] he observed a 12% local recurrence rate in oral cavity carcinomas with negative margins compared to 80% recurrence rate when margins were positive. Other factors which may be predictive of local control include anatomic location of the carcinoma and clinical T stage, both of which may influence the surgeon's ability to obtain clear margins.[30,32]

The accuracy of intraoperative frozen sections in head and neck patients with squamous cell carcinoma has been extensively reviewed with studies showing diagnostic accuracy rates between 96 and 99%.[34-37] These results compare favorably to similar studies in general surgery patients.[38,39] False positive and false negative rates in these same studies were <1% and <4%, respectively. Similar high rates of accuracy have been observed in salivary gland frozen sections with accuracy rates between 92% and 98.7%.[40-42] Despite this high degree of accuracy, discrepancies in frozen sections and errors will occur. Errors may be divided into two major groups: interpretive and sampling.[38,43] Interpretive errors are those where the pathologist fails to recognize and accurately diagnose a lesion that is present on the frozen section slide. Interpretive errors are most commonly seen in the setting of previously irradiated tissue, inflammation or necrosis where the morphology of the lesional tissue is obscured.[38,44] Knowledge of the clinical history and, if possible, review of preoperative biopsy material will help to minimize these errors. Sampling errors are defined as a lack of representative diagnostic material on the frozen section slide. Causes for this error include improper specimen orientation, inadequate gross examination of the specimen, and examination of tissue that is not representative of the pathologic process.[45] In all cases the pathologist is entirely dependent on well-preserved, representative tissue to make an accurate diagnosis. A cooperative and communicative relationship between pathologist and surgeon is imperative in light of the limitations of the technique and consequences of the frozen section diagnosis. Finally, contraindications and misuses of frozen section consultation include the following:

1. When the frozen diagnosis has no immediate impact and will not alter the surgical management of the patient
2. If a specimen is heavily calcified or ossified
3. If a specimen is small and no additional sampling is planned, where the frozen diagnosis could be equivocal and frozen artifact could impact final interpretation

4. For complex specimens which, under optimal conditions, would require extensive review (particularly lymphoproliferative disorders and melanocytic lesions).[16,46]

Fine-Needle Aspiration Biopsy

The technique of fine-needle aspiration (FNA) biopsy is widely accepted as a useful adjunct in the evaluation of head and neck lesions and is often used as the initial method of investigation.[47-50] FNA can be used on virtually any subcutaneous, palpable, discrete nodule. Sites in the head and neck region lending themselves to this procedure include thyroid, salivary glands, cervical lymph nodes, and orbit. Tumors in these locations are often superficial and easily accessible by fine-needle aspiration biopsy. Advantages of this technique include low cost, rapid and definitive diagnosis, few complications, and accuracy.[51-53]

The accuracy rates of FNA biopsy vary according to location within the head and neck region. Fine-needle aspiration biopsy of salivary gland lesions have reported accuracy rates between 89 and 92% (Fig 4–2).[50,54] In a retrospective review of 68 patients with preoperative FNA biopsies of salivary gland lesions, Tan et al was able to show a sensitivity and specificity of 100% (Fig 4–3) for identifying or excluding malignancy in adequate specimens.[54]

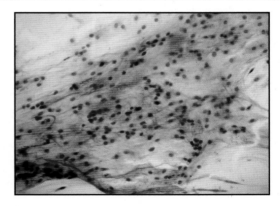

Fig 4–2. Pleomorphic adenoma. Fine-needle aspiration (FNA) biopsy of parotid. Fibromyxoid, fibrillar stromal material admixed with ovoid or spindled myoepithelial cells.

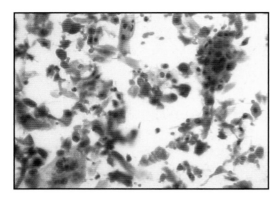

Fig 4–3. Metastatic squamous cell carcinoma. Fine-needle aspiration biopsy of cervical lymph node. Markedly atypical keratinized squamous epithelial cells.

Shaha et al demonstrated an overall accuracy rate of 96% in 136 aspiration biopsies of cervical adenopathy.[49] In that same study, accuracy rates for patients with a known squamous cell carcinoma approached 100%. The diagnostic accuracy rates of aspiration biopsy for non-Hodgkin's lymphoma in patients with adenopathy are variable, and range from 83 to 95%.[47,55] Some non-Hodgkin's lymphomas can be diagnosed and subclassified by fine needle aspiration when used in conjunction with flow cytometry.[47,56] A limitation of this technique in the clinical setting of suspected lymphoma is its inability to provide details on the architectural pattern of growth, which would preclude definitive subclassification of some lymphomas. In these cases, subsequent excisional biopsy would be necessary. Additionally, the differentiation of Hodgkin lymphoma subtypes is not possible with aspiration biopsy alone and requires tissue for diagnosis.[55] Finally, fine needle aspiration has utility in the staging workup of patients with lymphoma and in the diagnosis of recurrent disease.

MOLECULAR BIOLOGY AND MOLECULAR TECHNIQUES IN HEAD AND NECK CANCER

The emerging field of molecular diagnostics and its use in diagnosis and treatment of head and neck cancer patients is largely due to the surge in research over the past several years attempting to detail the understanding of the molecular basis of head and neck cancer. The term "field cancerization" was first described by Slaughter et al[57] to describe the observed increased incidence of second primary tumors in patients with head and neck cancer. Slaughter proposed that repeated exposure to carcinogenic insult in a region of tissue increased the risk of developing multiple independent premalignant foci. The persistence of abnormal tissue after surgery could explain second primary tumors and recurrences. More recent models have been proposed which suggest that a single premalignant stem cell develops into a clone of premalignant cells which migrate and colonize new remote foci.[58-62] Subsequent clonality studies provided evidence that the concept of "field cancerization" involves the migration and proliferation of clonally related cells that have undergone genetic alteration due to carcinogen exposure.[58-60] These cells undergo a series of accumulated genetic alterations resulting in varied phenotypic abnormalities ranging from premalignant lesions to invasive carcinoma.[63,64] In a study by Califano et al,[60] microsatellite analysis on 87 head and neck lesions showed that chromosomal loss progressively increased from benign hyperplasia through invasive carcinoma, and that many genetic alterations occur early in the disease process. In this study, Califano et al[60] propose a genetic progression model for head and neck cancer that shows the association between loss of genetic material and histopathologic progression.

Elucidation of key genetic alterations which occur in head and neck cancer has allowed the development, and in some cases, clinical implementation of molecular diagnostic tests which aid in early detection of disease, treatment or assessment of prognosis. The p53 tumor suppressor gene, located on chromosome 17p, has a significant role in the regulation of cell proliferation. Mutation of p53 is one of the most common and earliest of genetic alterations to occur in head and neck cancer and can result in p53 protein overexpression.[65-67] In a series of 58 squamous cell carcinomas of the larynx, Dolcetti et al[66] showed that 60% of the cases displayed overexpression of nuclear p53. Watling et al[65] had equally compelling results with 34 of 55 cases (62%) of head and neck squamous cancer showing p53 nuclear overexpression. Shin et al[67] conducted an imunohistochemical analysis of p53 overexpression in 33 patients with head and neck squamous cell carcinoma with tissue that included adjacent normal, hyperplastic, and dysplastic epithelium. Five of 24 (21%) samples of normal tissue adjacent to tumor, 7 of 24 (29%) samples of hyperplasia, and 9 of 20 (45%) samples of dysplasia showed p53 overexpression. Shin et al concluded that p53 expression can be altered in early phases of head and neck tumorigenesis and may be used as a marker for risk assessment. The knowledge of early p53 genetic alteration has been used as a marker in the molecular analysis of surgical margins.[68-70] Brennan et al[68] analyzed 25 cases of head and neck squamous cell carcinoma to determine if p53 mutation could be detected in histologically negative surgical margins. Using a PCR-based technique, Brennan's[68] analysis showed that 52% (13 of 25) of cases with histologically negative surgical margins were positive for p53 mutation. In 5 of these 13 patients (38%) tumor recurred locally, as compared to zero of 12 patients with p53 negative margins.[68] Boyle et al[71] analyzed the preoperative saliva of 7 head and neck cancer patients for mutations in the p53 gene using a PCR based technique. p53 alterations were identified in five of 7 (71%) patents.[71] Although these results are encouraging, application of these techniques to everyday clinical use has been limited.[70]

Microsatellite analysis of head and neck cancers looking for loss of heterozygosity (LOH) has helped elucidate areas of frequent allelic loss.[72-74] Studies have shown that one of the most frequent losses occur at chromosome 9p21,[73,74] site of p16, a tumor suppressor gene. p16 normally functions to inhibit cell cycle progression, leading to arrest of cell growth. Loss of this tumor suppressor gene results in unchecked cell division. Other areas with frequent allelic loss include chromosomes 3, 11q, 13q, and 17p.[72] Of interest is the fact that 17p is the site of the p53 tumor suppressor gene.

Another important mechanism for gene inactivation is hypermethylation at CpG islands within the promoter regions of important tumor suppressor genes. Sanchez-Cespedes et al[75] looked at gene promoter hypermethylation in tumors and serum of head and neck cancer patients. Fifty-five percent (52 of 95) of the primary tumors showed promoter hypermethylation in at least one of the four genes studied (p16, O-methylguanine-DNA-methyltrans-

ferase, glutathione S-trsnsferase, and DAP-kinase). A similar methylation pattern was detected in the corresponding serum of 21 of 50 (42%) patients.[75] This type of epigenetic alteration has been successfully used to detect aberrant methylated serum DNA in patients with non-small cell lung cancer.[76] These results indicate that detection of promoter hypermethylation in serum may be a useful marker for recurrent disease.

Protein overexpression is another mechanism associated with cancer progression. The epidermal growth factor receptor (EGFR) is a tyrosine kinase receptor which is overexpressed in many types of cancers.[77] Its significance lies in its association with cell proliferation, angiogenesis and cell motility, all of which enhance tumor progression.[77] Studies involving head and neck cancer have shown overexpression of EGFR to be associated with decreased relapse-free survival and poor prognosis.[78,79] In a study by Grandis et al,[80] EGFR protein levels were shown to increase with increasing stages of dysplasia in oropharyngeal lesions.

Molecular-based therapy for cancer patients is an emerging field that uses known genetic and protein alterations as molecular targets for possible therapeutic intervention. Therapeutic techniques targeted at inhibiting the action of EGFR, for example, are being developed and tested in clinical trials with hopeful results.[77,81] Other types of therapy with promise include gene therapy, immunotherapy and chemoprevention. An in-depth review of these topics is beyond the scope of this chapter. The reader is directed to listed references for further discussion.[77,82,83]

SQUAMOUS CELL CARCINOMA

Premalignant Lesions

The most commonly encountered lesions in the head and neck region are associated with alterations of the squamous mucosal surface and typically involve changes in cellular maturation and structure. The histologic changes associated with "premalignant" lesions in the head and neck region are broad and are accompanied by an equally broad collection of clinical and pathologic terms that are used to describe these changes.

Dysplasia, defined as an alteration in size, shape and organization of cells, is graded as mild, moderate, or severe (Fig 4-4). Dysplasia denotes not only abnormal cellular maturation, but cellular alterations including nuclear enlargement, hyperchromasia and mitoses. The greater the degree of dysplasia, the greater the likelihood of progression to invasive carcinoma.[84,85] The term carcinoma in situ implies full-thickness dysplasia of the mucosal surface without invasion through the basement membrane. In the upper aerodigestive tract, similar to the cervix, carcinoma in situ is generally considered to be synonymous with severe dysplasia (Fig 4-5). Carcinoma in situ is not, however, a prerequisite for the development of invasive carcinoma. In rare instances, an invasive carcinoma may arise from a minimally dysplastic basal layer without associated dysplasia of the remaining overlying squamous mucosa. Although the presence of keratinization implies some level of maturation of the surface mucosa, the risk of progression to invasive carcinoma in keratinizing lesions with mild, moderate, and severe dysplasia has been reported to be 5, 22, and 28%, respectively.[86]

Leukoplakia is a purely clinical term used to describe an abnormal patch of white tissue on the mucous membranes, often seen in the oral cavity, which cannot be attributed to any other disease process. The clinical term leukoplakia does not imply histologic dysplasia or atypia and is not necessarily suggestive of an underlying squamous cell carcinoma. Histologic changes associated with leukoplakia are variable and can range from simple hyperkeratosis to invasive cancer (Fig 4-6). Overall, the risk of progression to invasive carcinoma associated with leukoplakia is low. But a risk does exist and has been reported to be as high as approximately 10% when associated with dysplastic changes.[84,87] In contrast, erythroplakia is a clinical term used to describe bright red, "velvety" plaques seen on mucous membranes which are often indicative of an underlying dysplastic or malignant process.[88,89] In a study by Shafer et al[90] 91% of 58 cases from the oral cavity with a clinical diagnosis of erythroplakia were interpreted as either severe dysplasia, carcinoma in situ

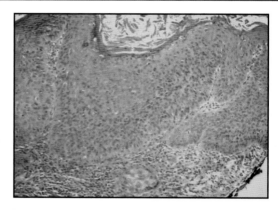

Fig 4–5. The squamous mucosa shows full-thickness squamous dysplasia (carcinoma in situ). A microscopic focus of invasive tumor is also present (*bottom center*).

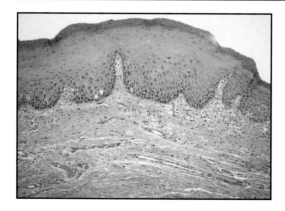

Fig 4–4. Parakeratotic squamous mucosa of the oral cavity with early bud-shaped rete ridges and cytologic changes at the basal layer suggestive of early mild dysplasia. This lesion was clinically identified as leukoplakia.

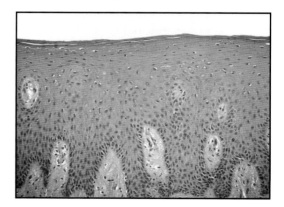

Fig 4–6. Hyperplastic squamous mucosa with parakeratosis. Clinically identified as leukoplakia.

or invasive carcinoma. Occasionally, when the clinical observation is made noting white patches interspersed with erythematous areas, the clinical term erythroleukoplakia or speckled leukoplakia may be used. Erythroleukoplakia has an increased likelihood of being associated with either squamous dysplasia or squamous carcinoma and should be treated as aggressively as erythroplakia.[84,87,91]

MICROINVASIVE SQUAMOUS CELL CARCINOMA

The term microinvasive carcinoma was initially used in the cervix to define a tumor with such limited invasion that the rate of metastasis was essentially zero. Application of the term to other anatomic sites has been problematic. The criteria for microinvasive carcinoma in the head and neck region is variable among expert pathologists. It is generally accepted that the term "microinvasive" implies extension of a malignant lesion through the basement membrane and into subepithelial stroma (Fig 4-7). The depth of invasion which defines microinvasive carcinoma is subjective. Reported acceptable depths, measured from the overlying epithelial basal lamina, range from 0.2 mm[92,93] to 0.5 mm,[86] without evidence of vascular or lymphatic invasion. The pattern of invasion as well as presence or absence of a stromal response provides additional histologic infor-

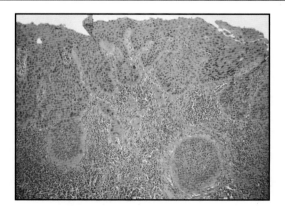

Fig 4–7. Full-thickness squamous dysplasia (carcinoma in situ) with microscopic invasion into subepithelial stroma.

mation in making the determination of invasion. The location of microinvasive carcinoma within the upper aerodigestive tract has prognostic significance. Microinvasive carcinoma of the laryngeal glottis is associated with a low risk of regional and distant metastatic disease due to the paucity of lymphatic spaces in this region.[92,94] These patients typically present earlier in the course of their disease due to voice changes which affords the opportunity of earlier and more conservative intervention. Patients with laryngeal glottic microinvasive carcinoma are at risk for local recurrence.[92,93] Where the concentration of lymphatic channels is greater, such as the hypopharynx, the risk of metastatic disease from microinvasive carcinoma increases. In general, microinvasive carcinoma consists primarily of in situ carcinoma with only minor foci representing the invasive component.

INVASIVE SQUAMOUS CELL CARCINOMA

Histologic Parameters

Numerous histologic parameters are evaluated and reported on by the surgical pathologist when the diagnosis of invasive squamous cell carcinoma is rendered. As previously discussed, margin status is one of the most significant parameters, with positive margins associated with increased risk of recurrence and decreased survival. Several additional parameters have independent prognostic significance, and are incorporated into the World Health Organization staging system (TNM system). This system uses both clinical and pathologic information to assess tumor size (T), regional nodal metastasis (N), and distant metastasis (M), that in turn is used to describe the anatomic extent of tumor, predict prognosis, and plan therapy. It has been well documented that the presence of nodal metastasis is associated with decreased patient survival and remains the most significant predictive factor for regional recurrence and survival (Fig 4-8).[95-99] The presence of extracapsular lymph node spread further prognostically subdivides patients with nodal metastasis, and has been found to be associated with a significant

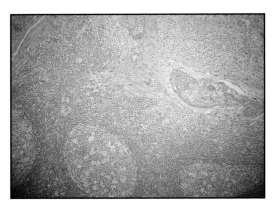

Fig 4–8. Metastatic squamous cell carcinoma to cervical lymph node (*middle right*) with reactive lymphoid follicles (*lower right and left*).

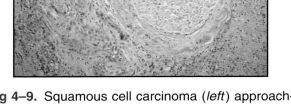

Fig 4–9. Squamous cell carcinoma (*left*) approaching and surrounding nerve (*center*).

reduction in survival when compared with patients with identical stage disease in whom metastasis is limited to the lymph node.[100-105] The size of the lymph nodes (>3 cm), total number with metastatic disease, lymph node level, and side relative to the primary tumor also carry prognostic significance.

Additional parameters which correlate closely with prognosis, and which supplement the TNM staging system, include tumor thickness, histologic grade, and perineural invasion. Some studies involving the oral cavity have shown a significant correlation between tumor thickness and regional lymph node metastasis and report that tumor thickness is a stronger predictor of nodal metastasis than maximum tumor size (T stage).[106-109] Although not standardized, maximal tumor thickness is accomplished by measuring vertically from the surface of the neoplasm, excluding surface keratin and inflammatory exudate, to the deepest area of tumor invasion. Breakpoints for tumor thickness that indicate increased risk for regional metastasis and prognosis have ranged from 1.5 mm to as much as 6 mm, depending on the primary location.

Studies addressing the significance of perineural invasion in head and neck cancer have been discordant. Several studies have found perineural spread to be a significant prognostic factor for locoregional recurrence and decreased survival and for an increased risk of concurrent nodal metastasis (Fig 4-9).[110-112] In contrast, Soo et al[112] showed no association between coexistent perineural invasion

and nodal metastasis in 141 composite resections. Likewise, Close et al[113] showed no statistical correlation between perineural invasion and regional lymph nodes in 43 patients with head and neck cancer of the oral cavity and oropharynx.

Other histopathologic parameters which have been shown in some studies to have prognostic significance in terms of overall survival include histologic grade[114,115] vascular invasion,[113,116,117] and pattern of invasion (Fig 4-10).[115] A study by Crissman et al[115] that looked at the prognostic value of multiple histologic parameters in 77 patients with oropharyngeal carcinoma, showed that the pattern of tumor invasion was the only statistically significant histologic parameter predictive of survival in T3 and T4 carcinomas. The authors conclude that neoplasms with invading thin, irregular cords and individual cells have a worse prognosis than invasive neoplasms with broad, pushing borders (Fig 4-11). It is likely that invasive tumors in the former category have greater access to vascular and lymphatic channels and would therefore be associated with increased risk of locoregional metastasis and lower overall survival (Fig 4-12).

Although some studies report histologic grade having prognostic significance, others have shown minimal survival differences between well and poorly differentiated tumors. The predictive value of histologic grade on patient survival was evaluated by Wiernik et al[114] with a retrospective review of 1,232 patients from two clinical trials between 1966 and

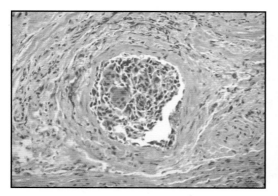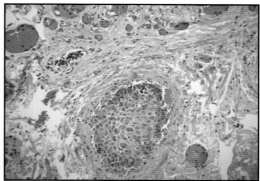

Fig 4–10. *Left and Right:* Squamous cell carcinoma showing vascular invasion. Endothelial cells lining vascular spaces may be difficult to identify with tumor invasion. Attachment of tumor to the endothelial lining is required to make this interpretation.

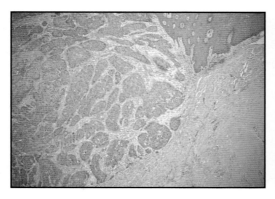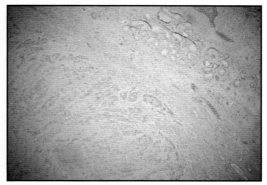

Fig 4–11. *Left and Right:* Laryngeal (glottic) invasive squamous cell carcinoma. The advancing edge of the tumors (*left and middle in both images*) shows a well-defined "pushing" border and cohesive nests of tumor. This pattern of tumor growth is associated with a more favorable prognosis.

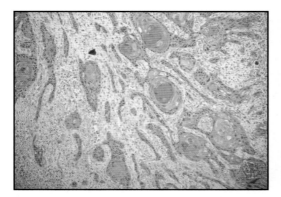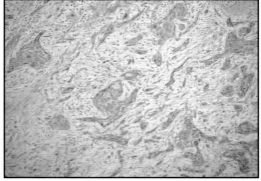

Fig 4–12. *Left and Right:* Laryngal (glottic) invasive squamous cell carcinoma. The pattern of invasion at the advancing edge of the tumor (*bottom of both images*) is described as infiltrating single cells and irregular cords. This pattern has been associated with increased locoregional and distant metastasis, and decreased survival.

1985 with carcinoma of the larynx and hypopharynx. The authors conclude that there were highly significant differences in survival and tumor-free intervals between those patients with well-differentiated tumors and those with anaplastic tumors. The authors state that the differences in prognosis may in part be due the more favorable distribution of site and stage in patients with well-differentiated tumors, as a statistically greater number of well-differentiated tumors were primary laryngeal tumors. In contrast, Roland et al[118] reported only a minimal difference in survival between well-differentiated and poorly differentiated squamous cancers of the head and neck in nearly 2,000 patients, and concluded that tumor grade does not have significant prognostic significance. Contributing to these inconsistent results may be variable degrees of differentiation within a given tumor as well as differing histologic criteria used to access differentiation, which may interject an element of subjectiveness and inter observer variability when determining histologic grade.[86] Other parameters reported to correlate with locoregional recurrence and survival include lymphatic invasion and depth of invasion.[119-121]

In all cases of conventional invasive squamous cell carcinoma of the head and neck region, the pathologist recognizes abnormal growth of abnormal squamous epithelium with deep invasion into submucosal stromal tissue, commonly involving deep muscle or cartilage (Fig 4–13). The invasion is beyond that which is acceptable for the classification of either microinvasive carcinoma, as previously defined,

or superficially extending invasive carcinoma. Superficially extending invasive carcinoma is defined as squamous cell carcinoma with invasion into and through the lamina propria, without involvement of deep muscle, regardless of angiolymphatic invasion.[86] The prognostic significance of this type of invasive carcinoma is unclear.

VARIANTS OF SQUAMOUS CELL CARCINOMA

Verrucous Carcinoma

Verrucous carcinoma is a well-differentiated form of squamous cell carcinoma which typically occurs in an older population, more commonly in males with a history of tobacco use. Human papillomavirus has also been investigated and shown to have an etiologic role in the development of verrucous carcinoma.[122,123] The oral cavity, particularly the bucal mucosa, accounts for he majority of all cases of verrucous carcinoma of the head and neck. The laryngeal glottic region is another common site, with rare cases reported in the nasopharynx and sinonasal cavity.[124,125] Verrucous carcinoma is a low-grade malignant tumor which can be locally aggressive but which typically does not metastasize. The clinical characteristics include an exophytic, papillary, or warty lesion with variable coloration ranging from tan to red to white. The lesion is often broad

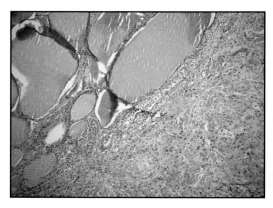 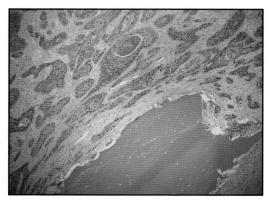

Fig 4–13. *Left:* Squamous cell carcinoma of the larynx with deep invasion into thyroid tissue (*upper left*). *Right:* Squamous cell carcinoma of the mandible with invasion into bone.

based, nonulcerated, and usually keratinizing. Specific histopathologic features must be identified for a tumor to qualify as a verrucous carcinoma. Characteristics that define verrucous carcinoma include well-differentiated, benign-appearing squamous epithelium with marked keratinization and blunt, pushing, deep epithelial invaginations (Fig 4-14). The dysplastic features and mitoses typically seen in squamous cell carcinoma are lacking in verrucous carcinoma. The stroma immediately adjacent to tumor exhibits a chronic inflammatory response comprised of lymphocytes and plasma cells. Superficial biopsies will not show diagnostic features of malignancy. Only a biopsy deep enough to show the tumor-stromal interface may be diagnostic.

With complete excision, the overall prognosis of verrucous carcinoma is excellent. Lesions may recur if incompletely excised, but local metastasis in uncommon. Distant metastases do not occur. Surgery is the usual and most effective treatment for local control. Radiotherapy may also be used in selective cases despite early reports suggesting that radiotherapy treatment alone was associated with an increased risk of anaplastic transformation. Later studies demonstrated that anaplastic transformation of verrucous carcinoma may occur in a subset of patients treated with either surgery or radiotherapy alone with equal frequency.[126] The differential diagnosis of verrucous carcinoma includes hyperplastic processes, benign neoplasms, as well as conventional squamous cell carcinoma with a verrucoid growth pattern. The most challenging of these is the distinction between

a benign reactive hyperplastic process and verrucous carcinoma. As both lesions lack cytologic atypia, this distinction is often based in part on the appearance of the underlying epithelial invaginations. In verrucous carcinoma the epithelial invaginations are described as broad and pushing, whereas in hyperplasia, particularly pseudoepitheliomatous hyperplasia, they are often described as elongated, thin and frequently attached to each other (Fig 4-15). Both lesions may be accompanied by a brisk chronic inflammatory infiltrate, and in general, lack mitoses.

Brief mention of two lesions termed verrucous hyperplasia and proliferative verrucous leukoplakia is in order as these lesions often occur in the oral cavity and have been shown to have the propensity to progress to verrucous carcinoma or conventional squamous cell carcinoma.[127] These lesions have been described as a spectrum or continuum of irreversible proliferative mucosal changes which may evolve into lesions with variably keratinized exophytic growth with verrucous processes lacking the pushing invasion seen in verrucous carcinoma.[127,128] Proliferative verrucous leukoplakia is often associated with a history of long-standing flat leukoplakia which undergoes rapid proliferation and development of an exophytic or papillary appearance (Fig 4-16). Verrucous hyperplasia may be encountered in sites other than the oral cavity, such as the larynx and sinonasal tract.[127] These lesions represent a spectrum of verrucoid lesions which have the capacity to recur and the potential to progress to carcinoma.[16] Shear et al[128] described a series of 68 cases with oral verrucous hyperplasia. Verrucus carcinoma was seen in 20 cases (29%), epithelial dysplasia in 45 (68%), and leukoplakia in 36 (53%). Treatment is complete surgical excision where possible, with close follow-up as these lesions frequently recur and have the potential to rapidly progress.[129]

PAPILLARY SQUAMOUS CELL CARCINOMA

Papillary squamous cell carcinoma is recognized as a distinct variant of conventional squamous cell carcinoma which occurs more frequently in males in the 6th to 7th decades.[130,131] Etiologic factors associ-

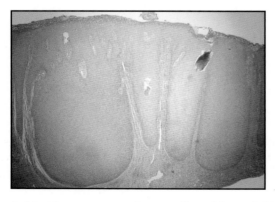

Fig 4–14. Verrucous carcinoma: Broad-based, blunt epithelial invaginations with pushing borders which lack cytologic features of malignancy.

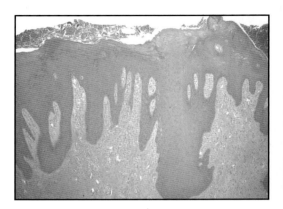 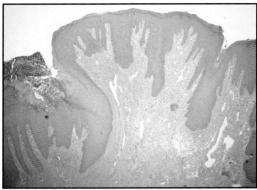

Fig 4–15. *Left and Right:* Pseudoepitheliomatous hyperplasia of the oral cavity is represented by a thickening or hyperplasia of the squamous mucosa with extreme elongation or downward growth of the squamous pegs but without cytologic evidence of malignancy. The surface is often keratinized. Tangential sections can be mistaken for invasive squamous cell carcinoma.

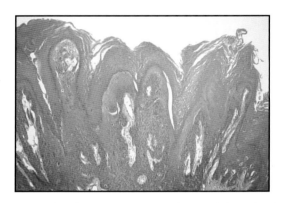

Fig 4–16. Proliferative verrucous leukoplakia with dysplastic progression. Exophytic, papillary squamous mucosa of the oral cavity with extensive keratinization and cytologic dysplasia. This lesion was associated with adjacent flat leukoplakia and represents an irreversible proliferative mucosal process with evolution to severe dysplasia.

ated with papillary squamous cell carcinoma include alcohol and tobacco use.[131] Evidence of a direct etiologic role for HPV has not been elucidated, although HPV types 6, 11, 16, and 18 have been detected by PCR and in situ hybridization in some cases of papillary squamous cell carcinoma with minimal surface keratinization.[132] Although the larynx is the most common site of involvement, other sites include the sinonasal tract, oralpharynx, hypopharynx, and naso-

pharynx.[131,132] Papillary squamous cell carcinoma often arises as a solitary lesion but may arise in association with multiple papillary lesions or in patients with a previous history of a papilloma at that same site.[130,132]

The clinical appearance of papillary squamous cell carcinoma is that of an exophytic, friable papillary to polypoid lesion arising from a variably thickened stalk which may appear thin or broad-based and which can measure as much as 6 cm.[130] The histologic features are characterized by an exophytic lesion with papillary fibrovascular cores and obviously dysplastic overlying squamous epithelium (Fig 4–17). The morphologic features of the fibrovascular cores may vary and can range from thin and elongated to broad-based and blunt. The malignant nature of the squamous epithelium distinguishes this entity from the more common benign papilloma. Minimal surface keratinization is seen. Invasion into adjacent stroma can be difficult to identify and may require thorough sectioning. Clusters of tumor cells at, or deep to, the mucosal-stromal interface, in association with a chronic lymphoplasmacytic response will help in this determination

The recommended treatment for either in situ or invasive papillary squamous cell carcinoma is surgery. Adjuvant therapy may be used for invasive tumors in accordance with guidelines for conventional squamous cell carcinoma. The prognosis for patients with papillary squamous cell carcinoma is

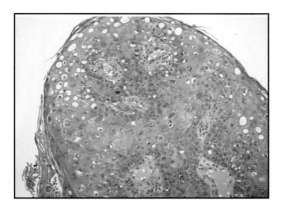

Fig 4–17. Papillary squamous cell carcinoma of the larynx with exophytic papillary growth, minimal surface keratinization, cytologically malignant epithelium, and delicate fibrovascular cores.

generally considered to be somewhat improved over conventional squamous cell carcinoma.[131] This may be due in part to the fact that these tumors are predominantly exophytic, and often of lower clinical stage. Patients presenting with more advanced disease and higher clinical stage have a prognosis similar to conventional squamous cell carcinoma when matched stage for stage.[132]

SPINDLE CELL CARCINOMA

Spindle cell carcinoma, also known as sarcomatoid carcinoma and carcinosarcoma, is a variant of squamous cell carcinoma with biphasic (epithelial and spindled) or monophasic (spindled) morphology that has been the focus of histogenetic controversy. Spindle cell carcinoma, as with conventional squamous cell carcinoma, occurs more commonly in males in their 6th to 7th decades, and has been associated with alcohol and tobacco use. Radiation therapy also has an etiologic role. Some studies have reported 30% of patients with spindle cell carcinoma have a history of radiation therapy for conventional squamous cell carcinoma.[133] The most common site of occurrence is the larynx, specifically the glottic region, followed by the oral cavity, hypopharynx, and rarely, the sinonasal region.[133-136] Depending on the location of the primary tumor, patients may pre-

sent with variable symptoms, including hoarseness and dysphagia.[133] On gross examination, the tumors often appear exophytic, polypoid, and ulcerated.

The diagnosis of spindle cell carcinoma may be elusive in small biopsy specimens where the epithelial component is commonly absent. Sampling of the epithelial component may require multiple biopsies targeting the base of the lesion, nonulcerated areas, and the margins, where the squamous component is most consistently identified (Fig 4–18). In the common scenario of absent squamous epithelium due to extensive ulceration, the differential diagnosis is much more problematic and may include other malignancies such as spindle cell melanoma, high-grade sarcoma, or a postradiation reactive process. Treatment for spindle cell carcinoma is similar to conventional squamous cell carcinoma of similar stage. Surgery is the primary treatment modality. Radiotherapy and chemotherapy may be used as adjuvant therapy. The prognosis is poor and is similar to conventional squamous cell carcinoma when tumors are matched stage for stage.

It is the spindle cell component of this tumor that has led to various theories on histogenesis, which in turn resulted in the various synonyms for this neoplasm. Extensive immunohistochemical and ultrastructural evidence has been reported which supports epithelial origin for both the squamous and mesenchymal components.[133-136] Cytokeratin immunoreactivity and ultrastructural evidence of tonofilaments and desmosomes in the epithelial and spindle cell components suggests an epithelial derivation.[133,135,137,138] Despite this, a lack of keratin immunoreactivity in the spindle cell component of a proportion of cases has been consistently reported in studies.[133,135,136]

Ansari-Lari et al[139] performed p53 immunohistochemical analysis on 23 spindle cell carcinomas, in part, to clarify the clonal relationship between the epithelial and sarcomatoid components of the tumors. Eighteen of 23 (78%) tumors showed p53 positivity. In 20 tumors with biphasic histology, the paired epithelial and mesenchymal components of each tumor consistently showed concordant p53 expression for intensity and distribution.[139] A clonal relationship between the two components was further confirmed at the genetic level through DNA sequence analysis of three biphasic tumors which

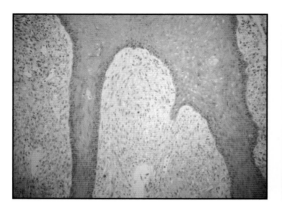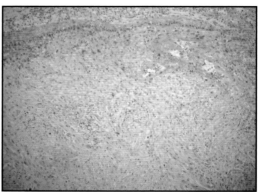

Fig 4–18. Spindle cell (sarcomatoid) carcinoma of the hypopharynx. *Left:* At the time of presentation, this lesion clinically appeared ulcerated and fungating. A spindle cell proliferation is seen extending to the squamous mucosal surface which is focally ulcerated (*top right*). The patient had a history of radiation therapy for a previous head and neck squamous carcinoma. *Right:* Spindle cell proliferation immediately adjacent to nonulcrated squamous mucosa.

showed identical base pair substitutions in p53 mutations in the conventional and spindle components.[139] Choi et al[140] provided further evidence for clonal origin by reporting 58 of 74 tumors (79.5%) with identical results in matching squamous and spindled components for LOH and retention of heterozygosity. A growing body of evidence suggests that this tumor arises from a common progenitor cell with the capacity for variable differentiation and phenotypic expression.

BASALOID SQUAMOUS CELL CARCINOMA

Basaloid squamous cell carcinoma is an aggressive variant of squamous cell carcinoma which was first described by Wain et al in 1986.[141] As with conventional squamous cell carcinoma, basaloid squamous cell carcinoma occurs most commonly in males, in the 6th to 7th decades, and has a strong association with alcohol and tobacco use.[142-147] The tumor has a tendency to originate in the oropharynx and hypopharynx, specifically the base of tongue and piriform sinus, as well as the supraglottic larynx and palantine tonsil.[142,145,147] Less commonly, the tumor may arise in the sinonasal tract.[143] Common present-

ing complaints often include dysphagia, pain, neck mass, hoarseness, and weight loss. The natural biologic behavior of this variant of squamous cancer is that of a high-grade, aggressive tumor which is often multifocal and deeply infiltrative, and which frequently presents with local regional and distant metastasis, and advanced stage.[143,145,146]

Basaloid squamous cell carcinoma is a biphasic epithelial malignancy with histologic characteristics of conventional squamous cell carcinoma, invasive or in situ, and a more prominent basaloid component (Fig 4–19). The basaloid cells are typically small, with scant cytoplasm, hyperchromasia, and inconspicuous nucleoli. There is often an abrupt transition between the squamous and basaloid components, with the basaloid component often closely opposed to the mucosal surface. The pattern of tumor growth is variable and may be solid nests, cribriform trabecular, or pseudoglandular. Other notable histologic features include frequent mitoses, comedo necrosis, peripheral palisading of basaloid cells, microcyst formation, and less commonly, a spindle cell component.[145-147] Immunohistochemical analysis is consistently positive for epithelial markers, such as cytokeratin AE1/AE3, CAM 5.2, and EMA. Vimentin and S-100 show variable expression. Rare neuroendocrine expression for synaptophysin has also been reported.[144] The differential diagnoses of basaloid

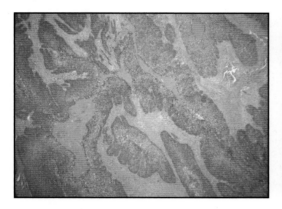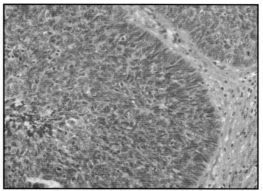

Fig 4–19. Basaloid squamous carcinoma of the base of tongue. *Left:* Infiltrative basaloid tumor in lobular configuration with central lobular necrosis and focal squamous differentiation (*bottom right*). *Right:* High-power view showing small, crowded hyperchromatic cells with scant cytoplasm and peripheral nuclear palisading.

squamous cell carcinoma includes adenoid cystic carcinoma and small cell neuroendocrine carcinoma. Although adenoid cystic carcinoma typically consists of small basaloid cells, a malignant squamous component is not a characteristic finding. Unlike basaloid squamous cell carcinoma, small cell neuroendocrine carcinoma should demonstrate unequivocal immunoreactivity with neuroendocrine markers, such as chromogranin and synaptophysin.

Basaloid squamous cell carcinoma is a rapidly fatal disease which typically is treated with aggressive surgery, including radical neck dissection, and adjuvant chemoradiaton. It has been reported by some to be more aggressive and carry a poorer prognosis than conventional squamous cell carcinoma.[141,142,145]

ADENOSQUAMOUS CARCINOMA

The World Health Organization defines adenosquamous carcinoma as a rare aggressive neoplasm which originates from surface epithelium and with histologic features of conventional squamous cell carcinoma and adenocarcinoma.[148] The tumor has a predilection for males in their 7th decade with a history of smoking and alcohol consumption. Adenosquamous carcinoma may originate in the larynx, tongue, floor of mouth, tonsillar pillars, and maxillary alveolus.[149-152]

The existence of this tumor as a distinct entity has been debated because of the histologic features it shares with mucoepidermoid carcinoma of salivary origin (Table 4–4). The WHO now recognizes adenosquamous carcinoma as a variant of squamous cell carcinoma due to the consistent aggressive nature of this tumor, which is in contradistinction to the biologic behavior of most cases of mucoepidermoid carcinoma. In a study by Keelawat et al[149] which examined 12 cases of adenosquamous carcinoma, 70% experienced local recurrence, 75% had regional metastasis, and 20% developed distant metastasis. Forty percent (40%) of patients were dead of disease at a mean follow-up of 40 months. Keelawat et al[149] combined these 12 cases with those in the literature for a total of 58 cases which revealed similar findings. Nearly 43% of patients were dead of disease at a mean follow-up of approximately 25 months.[149]

By definition, histologic features must include both a squamous and glandular component. The squamous component, in situ or invasive, originates from the mucosal surface and is typically localized to the superficial part of the tumor. The second component, adenocarcinoma, tends to occur deeper in the tumor, and has nonspecific histologic features which do not resemble any specific salivary neoplasm. True ductal lumina are present as is intracytoplasmic and intraluminal mucin.[149] Treatment includes

Table 4–4. Benign and Malignant Salivary Gland Tumors

Malignant Epithelial Tumors	Benign Epithelial Tumors
Acinic cell carcinoma	Pleomorphic adenoma
Mucoepidermoid carcinoma	Myoepithelioma
Adenoid cystic carcinoma	Basal cell adenoma
Polymorphous low-grade adenocarcinoma	Warthin tumor
Epithelial-myoepithelial carcinoma	Oncocytoma
Clear cell carcinoma, not otherwise specified	Canalicular adenoma
Basal cell adenocarcinoma	Sebaceous adenoma
Sebaceous carcinoma	Lymphadenoma
Sebaceous lymphadenocarcinoma	Sebaceous
Cystadenocarcinoma	Nonsebaceous
Low-grade cribriform cystadenocarcinoma	Ductal papillomas
Mucinous adenocarcinoma	Inverted ductal papilloma
Adenocarcinoma, not otherwise specified	Intraductal papilloma
Myoepithelial carcinoma	Sialadenoma papilliferum
Carcinoma ex pleomorphic adenoma	Cystadenoma
Carcinosarcoma	
Metastasizing pleomorphic adenoma	
Squamous cell carcinoma	
Small cell carcinoma	
Large cell carcinoma	
Lymphoepithelial carcinoma	
Sialoblastoma	

Source: Adapted from World Health Organization Classification of Tumours, Pathology and Genetics Head and Neck Tumours (edited by Barnes et al, IARC Press, Lyon, 2005).

surgical resection of tumor and regional lymph nodes. Adjuvant radiation therapy and chemotherapy may also be indicated.

NASOPHARYNGEAL CARCINOMA/ LYMPHOEPITHELIAL CARCINOMA

Nasopharyngeal carcinoma (NPC) is a variant of squamous cell carcinoma with light microscopic, immunohistochemical, or ultrastructural evidence of squamous differentiation.[24] Synonyms used for nasopharyngeal carcinoma have included lymphoepithelioma, undifferentiated carcinoma of nasopharyngeal type, and lymphoepithelioma-like carcinoma. The World Health Organization (WHO) classifies nasopharyngeal carcinoma into keratinizing and nonkeratinizing types.[148] The nonkeratinizing types are further subdivided into differentiated and undifferentiated types. Globally, nasopharyngeal carcinoma is an uncommon tumor, accounting for <1% of all cancers worldwide.[24] However, geographic regions with a markedly increased incidence include southern China, Southeast Asia, and the Arctic region. In Hong Kong, a region with one of the highest reported incidences world wide, >20 males per 100,000 will develop nasopharyngeal carcinoma, as opposed to <1 among Caucasian males in Western countries.[153] Suggested etiologic factors include environmental, dietary, and most notably, Epstein-Barr virus (EBV) infection. Nearly invariable association of EBV with nasopharyngeal carcinoma, specifically the nonkeratinizing types, along with elevated titers of anti-EBV antibody, evidence of clonal proliferation of viral DNA, and evidence of viral DNA genes in precursor-type dysplastic lesions, suggest an oncogenic role for EBV.[154]

Subclassification of nonkeratinizing carcinoma into differentiated and undifferentiated is done by convention, but their distinction has no significant clinical or prognostic significance. A bimodal age distribution exists for undifferentiated carcinoma with peaks in the second and sixth decades. The keratinizing and nonkeratinizing differentiated types typically occur in adults. Unlike nonkeratinizing carcinoma, keratinizing nasopharyngeal carcinoma is less often associated with regional nodal metastasis, is less responsive to radiation therapy and has been associated with tobacco use.[155-157]

The histopathology of the keratinizing type is that of an invasive carcinoma with obvious keratinization and intercellular bridges, similar to conventional squamous cell carcinoma. The tumor grows in irregular nests and islands and is associated with a prominent desmoplastic stromal response and mixed inflammatory infiltrate (Fig 4–20). Involvement of the surface mucosa may also be identified, representing squamous cell carcinoma in situ. These findings are in contrast to the nonkeratinizing differentiated subtype which presents with malignant cells showing moderately well-defined cell borders, eosinophilic cytoplasm, and occasional intercellular bridges. Rare keratinization may also be noted. Undifferentiated carcinoma consists of syncytial aggregates of large cells with indistinct cell borders, vesicular nuclei, prominent nucleoli, and scant cytoplasm. The Regaud pattern of undifferentiated carcinoma is described as tumor cells forming defined nests surrounded by a dense lymphoplasmacytic infiltrate. In contrast, the Schmincke pattern consists of single malignant cells or loose aggregates of cells which blend with a reactive lymphocytic infiltrate.

Nasopharyngeal carcinoma, specifically the nonkeratinizing types, is highly radiosensitive, making radiation therapy the primary treatment modality. Surgery and chemotherapy may be used in select cases. Negative prognostic factors include older age, keratinizing histology, cervical lymph node metastasis, and cranial nerve involvement.[158,159] Survival rates are variable and are dependent on the extent of disease. Clinical stage has been reported to have the greatest prognostic significance.[160]

Undifferentiated carcinoma arising in head and neck sites other than the nasopharynx has been reported, and is termed lymphoepithelial carcinoma. Lymphoepithelial carcinoma is a poorly differentiated malignant tumor that is histologically indistinguishable from undifferentiated nasopharyngeal carcinoma. Histologic characteristics include undifferentiated epithelial cells, most often in sheets or single cells, surrounded by a prominent, reactive lymphoplasmacytic infiltrate. This variant of squamous cell carcinoma has been described in the larynx, hypopharynx, oropharynx, and salivary glands.[161-165] Unlike its counterpart in the nasopharynx, lymphoepithelial carcinoma is uncommonly associated with EBV infection. It is a potentially aggressive tumor with a propensity for early cervical lymph node metastasis and mortality in approximately one third of patients.[163,164]

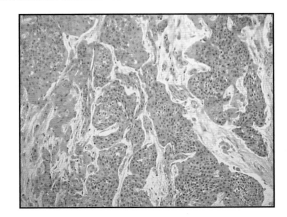

Fig 4–20. Keratinizing squamous cell carcinoma of the nasopharynx.

SUMMARY

In conclusion, there is a realistic expectation that as our knowledge of the biology of head and neck cancer continues to expand, promising new therapeutic options will continue to be developed with the goal of earlier detection, improved local control, and increased survival. Well-developed clinical trials continue to provide valuable information regarding the natural biology of head and neck cancer which, for example, can be integrated to develop molecularly targeted therapies or to optimize treatment modalities. The role of the pathologist is unique in this setting by naturally bridging the disciplines of investigative medicine and clinical medicine. The pathologist is poised to continue to play a significant role as a member of a multidisciplinary team that participates in the care and management of head and neck cancer patients.

REFERENCES

1. Kraus DH, Dubner S, Harrison LB, et al. Prognostic factors for recurrence and survival in head and neck soft tissue sarcomas. *Cancer.* 1994:74;697-702.
2. Sturgis E, Potter B. Sarcomas of the head and neck region. *Curr Opin Oncol.* 2003:15:239-252.
3. Mendenhall WM, Mendenhall CM, Werning JW, et al. Adult head and neck soft tissue sarcomas. *Head Neck.* 2005;27:916-922.
4. Coindre JM. Grading of soft tissue sarcomas: review and update. *Arch Pathol Lab Med.* 2006; 130:1448-1453.
5. Kilpatrick SE. Histologic prognostication in soft tissue sarcomas: grading versus subtyping or both? A comprehensive review of the literature with proposed practical guidelines. *Ann Diagn Pathol.* 1999;3:48-61.
6. Callender TA, Weber RS, Janjan N, et al. Rhabdomyosarcoma of the nose and paranasal sinuses in adults and children. *Otolaryngol Head Neck Surg.* 1995:112;252-257.
7. Simon JH, Paulino AC, Smith RB, et al. Prognostic factors in head and neck rhabdomyosarcoma. *Head Neck.* 2002;24:468-473.
8. Holden CA, Jones EW. Angiosarcoma of the face and scalp. *J Royal Soc Med.* 1985:78;30-31.
9. Delgado R, Maafs E, Alfeiran A, et al. Osteosarcoma of the jaw. *Head Neck.* 1994;16:246-252.
10. Ha PK, Eisele DW, Frassica FJ, Zahurak ML, Edward F. Osteosarcoma of the head and neck: a review of the Johns Hopkins experience. *Laryngoscope.* 1999:109;964-969.
11. Mark RJ, Sercarz JA, Tran L, et al Osteogenic sarcoma of the head and neck. The UCLA experience. *Arch Otolaryngol Head Neck Surg.* 1991:117; 761-766.
12. Oda D, Bavisotto LM, Schmidt RA, et al. Head and neck osteosarcoma at the University of Washington. *Head Neck.* 1997;19:513-523.
13. Yuen A, Jacobs C. Lymphomas of the head and neck. *Semin Oncol.* 1999:26;338-345.
14. Jacobs C, Weiss L, Hoppe R. The management of extranodal head and neck lymphomas. *Arch Otolaryngol Head Neck Surg.* 1986;112:654-658.
15. Jacobs C, Hoppe R. Non-Hodgkin's lymphomas of head and neck extranodal sites. *Int J Radiat Oncol Biol Phys.* 1985:11:357-364.
16. Wenig BM, Cohen J-M. General principles of head and neck pathology. In: Harrison LB, Sessions RB, Hong WK, eds. *Head and Neck Cancer: A Multidisciplinary Approach.* 2nd ed. New York, NY: Lippincott, Williams, and Wilkins; 2004: 11-48.
17. Chang AE, Karnell LH, Menck HR. The National Cancer Data Base report on cutaneous and noncutaneous melanoma: a summary of 84,836 cases from the past decade. The American College of Surgeons Commission on Cancer and the American Cancer Society. *Cancer.* 1998;83:1664-1678.
18. Tomicic J, Wanebo HJ. Mucosal melanomas. *Surg Clin North Am.* 2003;83:237-252.
19. Hicks MJ, Flaitz CM. Oral mucosal melanoma: epidemiology and pathobiology. *Oral Oncol.* 2000: 36;152-169.
20. Doval DC, Rao CR, Saitha KS, et al. Malignant melanoma of the oral cavity: report of 14 cases from a regional cancer center. *Eur J Surg Oncol.* 1996;22:245-249.
21. Patel SG, Prasad ML, Escrig M, et al. Primary mucosal malignant melanoma of the head and neck. *Head Neck.* 2002;24:247-257.
22. Diaz EM, Johnigan RH, Pero C, et al. Olfactory neuroblastoma: the 22-year experience at one comprehensive cancer center. *Head Neck.* 2005; 27:138-149.
23. Wanebo HJ, Koness RJ, MacFarlane JK, et al. Head and neck sarcoma: report of the Head and Neck Sarcoma Registry. Society of Head and Neck Sur-

geons Committee on Research. *Head Neck.* 1992; 14:1-7.

24. World Health Organization Classification of Tumours. Pathology and Genetics. In: Nasopharynx. Barnes L, Eveson JW, Reichart P, Sidransky D, eds. *Head and Neck Tumours.* Geneva, Switzerland: WHO; 2005:chap 2.

25. Raney RB, Asmar L, Newton WA, et al. Ewing's sarcoma of soft tissues in childhood: a report from the intergroup rhabdomyosarcoma study, 1972 to 1991. *J Clin Oncol.* 1997:15;574-582.

26. Shi S-R, Key ME, Kalra KL. Antigen retrieval in formalin fixed, paraffin-embedded tissues: an enhancement method for immunohistochemical staining based on microwave oven heating of tissue sections. *J Histochem Cytochem.* 1991; 39:741-748.

27. Nakazawa H, Rosen P, Lane N, Lattes R. Frozen section experience in 3000 cases. Accuracy, limitations, and value in residency training. *Am J Clin Pathol.* 1968;49:41-51.

28. Ackerman LV, Ramirez GA. The indications for and limitations of frozen section diagnosis; a review of 1269 consecutive frozen section diagnoses. *Br J Surg.* 1959;46:336-350.

29. Loree T, Strong E. Significance of positive margins in oral cavity squamous carcinoma. *Am J Surg.* 1990;160:410-414.

30. Jacobs J, Ahmad K, Casiano R, et al. Implications of positive surgical margins. *Laryngoscope.* 1993;103:64-68.

31. Batsakis J. Pathology consultation. Surgical margins in squamous cell carcinomas. *Ann Otol Rhinol Laryngol.* 1988;97:213-214.

32. Johnson R, Sigman J, Funk G, Robinson R, Hoffman H. Quantification of surgical margin shrinkage in the oral cavity. *Head Neck.* 1997;19:281-286.

33. Byers R, Bland K, Borlase B, Luna M. The prognostic and therapeuticl value of frozen section determinations in the surgical treatment of squamous carcinoma of the head and neck. *Am J Surg.* 1978;136:525-528.

34. Remsen K, Lucente F, Biller H. Reliability of frozen section diagnosis in head and neck neoplasms. *Laryngoscope.* 1984;94:519-524.

35. Gandour-Edwards R, Donald P, Wiese D. Accuracy of intraoperative frozen section diagnosis in head and neck surgery: experience at a university medical center. *Head Neck.* 1993;15:33-38.

36. Ord R, Aisner S. Accuracy of frozen sections in assessing margins in oral cancer resection. *J Oral Maxillofac Surg.* 1997;55:663-669.

37. Cooley M, Hoffman H, Robinson R. Discrepancies in frozen section mucosal margin tissue in laryngeal squamous cell carcinoma. *Head Neck.* 2002;24:262-267.

38. Holaday W, Assor D. Ten thousand consective frozen sections. A retrospective study focusing on accurancy and quality control. *Am J Clin Pathol.* 1974;61:769-777.

39. Ferreiro J, Myers J, Bostwick D. Accuracy of frozen section diagnosis in surgical pathology: review of a 1-year experience with 24,880 cases at Mayo Clinic Rochester. *Mayo Clinic Proc.* 1995;70; 1137-1141.

40. Granick M, Erickson R, Hanna D. Accuracy of frozen-section diagnosis in salivary gland lesions. *Head Neck Surg.* 1985;7:465-467.

41. Rigual N, Milley P, Lore J, Kaufman S. Accuracy of frozen-section diagnosis in salivary gland neoplasms. *Head Neck Surg.* 1986;8:442-446.

42. Gnepp D, Rader W, Cramer S, Cook L, Sciubba J. Accuracy of frozen section diagnosis of the salivary gland. *Otolaryngol Head Neck Surg.* 1987;96:325-330.

43. Zarbo RJ, Hoffman GG, Howanitz PJ. Interinstitutional comparison of frozen-section consultation. A College of American Pathologists Q-Probe study of 79,647 consultations in 297 North American institutions. *Arch Pathol Lab Med.* 1991;115: 1187-1194.

44. Gandour-Edwards R, Donald P, Lie J. Clinical utility of intraoperative frozen section diagnosis in head and neck surgery: a quality assurance perspective. *Head Neck.* 1993;15:373-376.

45. Barney P. Histopathologic problems and frozen section diagnosis in diseases of the larynx. *Otolaryngol Clin North Am.* 1970;3:493-515.

46. Luna MA. Uses, abuses, and pitfalls of frozen section diagnoses of diseases of the head and neck. In: Barnes L ed. *Surgical Pathology of the Head and Neck.* 2nd ed. Vol 1. New York, NY: Marcel Dekker Inc; 2001:1-12.

47. Ramzy I, Rone R, Schultenover S, Buhaug J. Lymph node aspiration biopsy—diagnostic reliability and limitations—an analysis of 350 cases. *Diagn Cytopath.* 1985;1:39-45.

48. Schultenover S, Ramzy I, Page C, LeFebre S, Cruz A. Needle aspiration biopsy: role and limitations in surgical decision making. *Am J Clin Pathol.* 1984;82:405-410.

49. Shaha A, Webber C, Marti J. Fine-needle aspiration in the diagnosis of cervical lymphadenopathy. *Am J Surg.* 1986;152:420-423.

50. Layfield L, Tan P, Glasgow J. Fine-needle aspiration of salivary gland lesions. Comparison with frozen sections and histologic findings. *Arch Pathol Lab Med*. 1987;111:346–353.

51. Amedee RG, Dhurandhar NR. Fine-needle aspiration biopsy. *Laryngoscope*. 2001;111:1551–1557.

52. Fulciniti F, Califano L, Zupi A, et al. Accuracy of fine needle aspiration biopsy in head and neck tumors. *Oral Maxillofac Surg*. 1997;55:1094–1097.

53. Schelkun PM, Grundy WG. Fine-needle aspiration biopsy of head and neck lesions. *J Oral Maxillofac Surg*. 1991;49:262–267.

54. Tan LGL, Khoo MLC. Accuracy of fine needle aspiration cytology and frozen section histopathology for lesions of the major salivary glands. *Ann Acad Med Singapore*. 2006;35:242–248.

55. Qizilbash A, Elavathil L, Chen V, Young J, Archibald S. Aspiration biopsy cytology of lymph nodes in malignant lymphoma. *Diagn Cytopath*. 1985;1:18–22.

56. Young N, Al-Saleem T. Diagnosis of lymphoma by fine-needle aspiration cytology using the revised European-American classification of lymphoid neoplasms. *Cancer*. 1999;87:325–345.

57. Slaughter D, Southwick H, Smejkal W. Field cancerization in oral stratified squamous epithelium. *Cancer*. 1953;6:963–968.

58. Worsham M, Wolman S, Carey T, et al. Common clonal origin of synchronous primary head and neck squamous cell carcinomas: analysis by tumor karyotypes and fluorescence in situ hybridization. *Hum Pathol*. 1995;26:251–261.

59. Bedi G, Westra W, Gabrielson E, Koch W, Sidransky D. Multiple head and neck tumors: evidence for a common clonal origin. *Cancer Res*. 1996;56:2484–2487.

60. Califano J, Van der Riet P, Westra W, et al. Genetic progression model for head and neck cancer: implications for field cancerization. *Cancer Res*. 1996;56:2488–2492.

61. Braakhuis BJM, Tabor MP, Kummer JA, et al. A genetic explanation of Slaughter's concept of field cancerization: evidence and clinical implications. *Cancer Res*. 2003;63:1727–1730.

62. Braakhuis BJM, Tabor MP, Leemans CR, et al. Second primary tumors and field cancerization in oral and oropharyngeal cancer: molecular techniques provide new insights and definitions. *Head Neck*. 2002;24:198–206.

63. Califano J, Westra W, Meininger G, et al. Genetic progression and clonal relationship of recurrent premalignant head and neck lesions. *Clin Cancer Res*. 2000;6:347–352.

64. Partridge M, Pateromichelakis S, Phillips E, Emilion G, Langdon J. Profiling clonality and progression in multiple premalignant and malignant oral lesions identified a subgroup of cases with a distinct presentation of squamous cell carcinoma. *Clin Cancer Res*. 2001;7:1860–1866.

65. Watling D, Gown A, Coltrera M. Overexpression of p53 in head and neck cancer. *Head Neck*. 1992;14:437–444.

66. Dolcetti R, Doglioni C, Maestro R, et al. p53 overexpresson is an early event in the development of human squamous cell cacinoma of the larynx: genetic and prognostic implications. *Int J Cancer*. 1992;52:178–182.

67. Shin DM, Kim J, Ro JY, et al. Activation of p53 gene expression in premalignant lesions during head and neck tumorigenesis. *Cancer Res*. 1994;54:321–326.

68. Brennan J, Mao L, Hruban R, et al. Molecular assessment of histopathologic staging in squamous-cell carcinoma of the head and neck. *N Engl J Med*. 1995;332:429–435.

69. Nathan C-A, Amirghahri N, Rice C, Abreo F, Shi R, Stucker F. Molecular analysis of surgical margins in head and neck squamous cell carcinoma patients. *Laryngoscope*. 2002;112:2129–2140.

70. Ball V, Righi P, Tejada E, et al. P53 immunostaining of surgical margins as a predictor of local recurrence in squamous cell carcinoma of the oral cavity and oropharynx. *Ear Nose Throat*. 1997;76:818.

71. Boyle JO, Mao L, Brennan JA, et al. Gene mutations in saliva as molecular markers for head and neck squamous cell carcinomas. *Am J Surg*. 1994;168:429–432.

72. Nawroz H, van der Riet P, Hruban R, Koch W, Ruppert M, Sidransky D. Allelotype of head and neck squamous cell carcinoma. *Cancer Res*. 1994;54:1152–1155.

73. van der Riet P, Nawroz H, Hruban R, et al. Frequent loss of chromosome 9p21-22 early in head and neck cancer progression. *Cancer Res*. 1994;54:1156–1158.

74. Cairns P, Polascik T, Eby Y, et al. Frequency of homozygous deletion oat p16/CDKN2 in primary human tumours. *Nature Genet*. 1995;11:210–212.

75. Sanchez-Cespedes M, Esteller M, Wu L, et al. Gene promoter hypermethylation in tumors and serum of head and neck cancer patients. *Cancer Res*. 2000;60:892–895.

76. Esteller M, Sanchez-Cespedes M, Rosell R, et al. Detection of aberrant promoter hypermethylation

of tumor suppressor genes in serum DNA from non-small cell lung cancer patients. *Cancer Res.* 1999;59:67-70.

77. Woodburn J. The epidermal growth factor receptor and its inhibition in cancer therapy. *Pharmacol Ther.* 1999;82:241-250.

78. Dassonville O, Formento J, Francoual M, et al. Expression of epidermal growth factor receptor and survival in upper aerodigenstive tract cancer. *J Clin Oncol.* 1993;11:1873-1878.

79. Maurizi M, Almadori G, Ferrandina G, et al. Prognostic significance of epidermal growth factor receptor in laryngeal squamous cell carcinoma. *Br J Cancer.* 1996;74:1253-1257.

80. Grandis J, Tweardy D, Melhem M. Asynchronous modulation of transforming growth factor a and epidermal growth factor receptor protein expression in progression of premalignant lesions to head and neck squamous cell carcinoma. *Clin Cancer Res.* 1998;4:13-20.

81. Barker A, Gibson K, Grundy W, et al. Studies leading to the identificationi of ZD1839 (IressaTM): an orally active, selective epidermal growth factor receptor tyrosine kinase inhibitor targeted to the treatment of cancer. *Bioorg Med Chem Ltt.* 2001;11:1911-1914.

82. Hoffmann TK, Dworachi G, Tsukihiro T, et al. Spontaneous apoptosis of circulating T lymphocytes in patients with head and neck cancer and its clinical importance. *Clin Cancer Res.* 2002;8:2553-2562.

83. Barrera JL, Verastegui E, Meneses A, et al. Combination immunotherapy of squamous cell carcinoma of the head and neck. *Arch Otolaryngol Head Neck Surg.* 2000;126:345-351.

84. Silverman S, Gorsky M, Lozada F. Oral leukoplakia and malignant transformation. A follow-up study of 257 patients. *Cancer.* 1984;53:563-568.

85. Blackwell K, Fu Y-S, Calcaterra T. Laryngeal dysplasia. *Cancer.* 1995;75:457-463.

86. Barnes L. Diseases of the larynx, hypopharynx, and esophagus (chapter 5). In: Barnes L, ed. *Surgical Pathology of the Head and Neck.* 2nd ed. Vol 1. New York, NY: Marcel Dekker Inc; 2001:157.

87. Mashberg A, Samit A. Early diagnosis of asymptomatic oral and oropharyngeal squamous cancers. *CA Cancer J Clin.* 1995;45:328-351.

88. Mashberg A, Feldman L. Clinical criteria for identifying early oral and oropharyngeal carcinoma: erythroplasia revisited. *Am J Surg.* 1988;156:273-275.

89. Bouquot J, Gnepp D. Laryngeal precancer: a review of the literature, commentary, and comparison with oral leukoplakia. *Head Neck.* 1991;13:488-497.

90. Shafer WG, Waldron CA. Erythroplakia of the oral cavity. *Cancer.* 1975;36(3):1021-1028.

91. Mashberg A. Erythroplasia: the earliest sign of asymptomatic oral cancer. *J Am Dent Assoc.* 1978;96:615-620.

92. Crissman JD, Zarbo RJ, Drozdowicz S, Jacobs J, Ahmad K, Weaver A. Carcinoma in situ and microinvasive squamous carcinoma of the laryngeal glottis. *Arch Otolaryngol Head Neck Surg.* 1988;114:299-307.

93. Gillis T, Incze J, Strong S, Vaughan C, Simpson G. Natural history and management of keratosis, atypia, carcinoma in situ, and microinvasive cancer of the larynx. *Am J Surg.* 1983;146:512-516.

94. Crissman JD, Zarbo RJ. Dysplasia, in situ carcinoma, and progression to invasive squamous cell carcinoma of the upper aerodigestive tract. *Am J Surg Pathol.* 1989;13(suppl 1):5-16.

95. Kalnins I, Leonard A, Sako K, Razack M, Shedd D. Correlation between prognosis and degree of lymph node involvement in carcinoma of the oral cavity. *Am J Surg.* 1977;134:450-454.

96. Leemans C, Tiwari R, Nauta J, van der Waal I, Snow G. Regional lymph node involvement and its significance in the development of distant metastases in head and neck carcinoma. *Cancer.* 1993;71:452-456.

97. Leemans C, Tiwari R, Nauta J, van der Waal I, Snow G. Recurrence at the primary site in head and neck cancer and the significance of neck lymph node metastases as a prognostic factor. *Cancer.* 1994;73:187-190.

98. Schuller D, McGuirt W, McCabe B, Young D. The prognostic significance of metastatic cervical lymph nodes. *Laryngoscope.* 1980;90:557-570.

99. Mamelle G, Papurik, Luboinski B, et al. Lymph node prognostic factors in head and neck squamous cell carcinomas. *Am J Surg.* 1994;168:494-498.

100. Johnson J, Myers E, Bedetti C, et al. Cervical lymph node metastases. Incidence and implications of extracapsular carcinoma. *Arch Otolaryngol.* 1985;111:534-537.

101. Snyderman N, Johnson J, Schramm V, et al. Extracapsular spread of carcinoma in cervical lymph nodes. Impact upon survival in patients with carcinoma of the supraglottic larynx. *Cancer.* 1985;56:1597-1599.

102. Richard J, Garnier H, Michaeu C, Saravane D, Cachin Y. Prognostic factors in cervical lymph node metastasis in upper respiratory and digestive tract carcinomas: study of 1,713 cases during a 15-year period. *Laryngoscope.* 1987;97:97-101.

103. Hirabayashi H. Koshii K, Uno K, et al. Extracapsular spread of squamous cell carcinoma in neck lymph nodes: prognostic factor of laryngeal cancer. *Laryngoscope.* 1991;101:502-506.

104. Myers J, Greenberg J, Mo V, Roberts D. Extracapsular spread. A significant predictor of treatment failure in patients with squamous cell carcinoma of the tongue. *Cancer.* 2001;92:3030-3036.

105. Johnson J, Barnes E, Myers E, et al. The extracapsular spread of tumors in cervical node metastasis. *Arch Otolaryngol.* 1981;107:725-729.

106. Spiro R, Huvos A, Wong G, et al. Predictive value of tumor thickness in squamous carcinoma confined to the tongue and floor of the mouth. *Am J Surg.* 1986;152:345-353.

107. Mohit-Tabatabai M, Sobel H, Rush B, Mashberg A. Relation of thickness of floor of mouth stage I and II cancers to regional metastasis. *Am J Surg.* 1986;152:351-353.

108. Frierson H, Cooper P. Prognostic factors in squamous cell carcinoma of the lower lip. *Hum Pathol.* 1986;17:346-354.

109. Baredes S, Leeman D, Chen T, Mohit-Tabatabai M. Significance of tumor thickness in soft palate carcinoma. *Laryngoscope.* 1993;103:389-393.

110. Byers R, O'Brien J, Waxler J. The therapeutic and prognostic implications of nerve invasion in cancer of the lower lip. *Int J Rad Oncol Biol Phys.* 1978;4:215-217.

111. Goepfert H,. Dichtel W, Medina J, Lindberg R, Luna M. Perineural invasion in squamous cell skin carcinoma of the head and neck. *Am J Surg.* 1984;148:542-547.

112. Soo K-C, Carter R, O'Brien C, et al. Prognostic implications of perineural spread in squamous carcinomas of the head and neck. *Laryngoscope.* 1986;96:1145-1148.

113. Close L, Burns D, Reisch J, Schaefer S. Microvascular invasion in cancer of the oral cavity and oropharynx. *Arch Otolaryngol Head Neck Surg.* 1987;113:1191-1195.

114. Wiernik G, Millard P, Haybittle JL. The predictive value of histological classification into degrees of differentiation of squamous cell carcinoma of the larynx and hypopharynx compared with the survival of patients. *Histopathology.* 1991;19; 411-417

115. Crissman J, Liu W, Gluckman J, Cummings G. Prognostic value of histopathologic parameters in squamous cell carcinoma of the oropharynx. *Cancer.* 1984;54:2995-3001.

116. Close L, Brown P, Vuitch M, Reisch J, Schaefer S. Microvascular invasion and survival in cancer of the oral cavity and oropharynx. *Arch Otolaryngol Head Neck Surg.* 1989;115: 1304-1309.

117. Poleksic S, Kalwaic HJ. Prognostic value of vascular invasion in squamous cell carcinoma of the head and neck. *Plast Reconstr Surg.* 1978:61; 234-240.

118. Roland NJ, Caslin AW, Nash J, Stell PM. Value of grading squamous cell carcinoma of the head and neck. *Head Neck.* 1992;14(3):224-229.

119. Ravasz L, Hordijk G, Slootweg P, Smit F, Tweel I. Uni- and multivariate analysis of eight indications for post-operative radiotherapy and their significance for local-regional cure in advanced head and neck cancer. *J Laryngol Otol.* 1993;107: 437-440.

120. Moore C, Kuhns J, Greenberg R. Thickness as prognostic aid in upper aerodigestive tract cancer. *Arch Surg.* 1986;121:1410-1414.

121. Olsen K, Caruso M, Foote R, et al. Primary head and neck cancer. Histopathologic predictors of recurrence after neck dissection in patients with lymph node invovement. *Arch Otolaryngol Head Neck Surg.* 1994;120:1370-1374.

122. Brandsma JL, Steinberg BM, Abramson AL, Winkler B. Presence of human papillomavirus type 16 related sequences in verrucous carcinoma of the larynx. *Cancer Res.* 1986;46:2185-2188.

123. Abramson AL, Brandsma J, Steinberg B, Winkler B. Verrucous carcinoma of the larynx. Possible human papillomavirus etiology. *Arch Otolaryngol Head Neck Surg.* 1985;111(11):709-715.

124. Medina JE, Dichtel W, Luna M. Verrucous-squamous carcinomas of the oral cavity. A clinicopatholgic study of 104 cases. *Arch Otolaryngol.* 1984;110:437-440.

125. Batsakis J, Hybels R, Crossman J, Rice D. The pathology of head and neck tumors: verrucous carcinoma, part 15. *Head Neck Surg.* 1982;5: 29-38.

126. McDonald JS, Crissman JD, Gluckman JL. Verrucous carcinoma of the oral cavity. *Head Neck Surg.* 1982;5(1):22-28.

127. Murrah V, Batsakis J. Proliferative verrucous leukoplakia and verrucous hyperplasia. *Ann Otol Rhinol Laryngol.* 1994;103:660-663.

128. Shear M, Pindborg J, Odont D. Verrucous hyperplasia of the oral mucosa. *Cancer.* 1980;46: 1855-1862.

129. Crossman J, Gnepp D, Goodman M, Hellquist G, Johns M. Preinvasive lesions of the upper aerodigestive tract: histologic definitions and clinical limitations (a symposium). *Pathol Ann.* 1987;22: 311-352.

130. Crissman J, Kessis T, Shah K, et al. Squamous papillary neoplasia of the adult upper aerodigestive tract. *Hum Pathol.* 1988;19:1387-1396.

131. Thompson LDR, Wenig BM, Heffner DK, Gnepp DR. Exophytic and papillary squamous cell carcinomas of the larynx: a clinicopathologic series of 104 cases. *Otolaryngology.* 1999;120(5):718-724.

132. Suarez P, Adler-Storthz K, Luna M, et al. Papillary squamous cell carcinomas of the upper aerodigestive tract: a clinicopathologic and molecular study. *Head Neck.* 2000;22:360-368.

133. Lewis J, Olsen K, Sebo T. Spindle cell carcinoma of the larynx: review of 26 cases including DNA content and immunohistochemistry. *Hum Pathol.* 1997;28:664.

134. Berthelet E, Shenouda G, Black M, Picariello M, Rochon L. Sarcomatoid carcinoma of the head and neck. *Am J Surg.* 1994;168:455-458.

135. Zarbo R, Crissman J, Venkat H, Weiss M. Spindle-cell carcinoma of the upper aerodigestive tract mucosa. An immunohistologic and ultrastructural study of 18 biphasic tumors and comparison with seven monophasic spindle-cell tumors. *Am J Surg Pathol.* 1986;10:741-753.

136. Ellis G, Langloss J, Heffner D, Hyams V. Spindle-cell carcinoma of the aerodigestive tract. An immunohistochemical analysis of 21 cases. *Am J Surg Pathol.* 1987;11:335-342.

137. Takata T, Ito H, Ogawa I, et al. Spindle cell squamous carcinoma of the oral region. An immunohistochemical and ultrastructural study on the histogenesis and differential diagnosis with a clinicopathological analysis of six cases. *Virchows Arch A Pathol Anat Histopathol.* 1991;419:177-182.

138. Meijer JW, Ramaekers FC, Manni JJ, et al. Intermediate filament proteins in spindle cell carcinoma of the larynx and tongue. *Acta Otolaryngol.* 1988;106:306-313.

139. Ansari-Lari, Hoque MO, Califano J, et al. Immunohistochemical p53 expression patterns in sarcomatoid carcinomas of the upper respiratory tract. *Am J Surg Pathol.* 2002;26:1024-1031.

140. Choi H-R, Sturgis EM, Rosenthal DI, et al. Sarcomatoid carcinoma of the head and neck. Molecular evidence for evolution and progression from conventional squamous cell carcinomas. *Am J Surg Pathol.* 2003;27:1216-1220.

141. Wain SL, Kier R, Vollmer RT, et al. Basaloid-squamous carcinoma of the tongue, hypopharynx, and larynx: report of 10 cases. *Hum Pathol.* 1986;17:1158-1166.

142. Banks E, Frierson H, Mills S, et al. Basaloid squamous cell carcinoma of the head and neck. A clinicopathologic and immunohistochemical study of 40 cases. *Am J Surg Pathol.* 1992;16: 939-946.

143. Wieneke J, Thompson L, Wenig B. Basaloid squamous cell carcinoma of the sinonasal tract. *Cancer.* 1999;85:841-854.

144. Morice W, Ferreiro J. Distinction of basaloid squamous cell carcinoma from adenoid cystic and small cell undifferentiated carcinoma by immunohistochemistry. *Hum Pathol.* 1998;29:609-612.

145. Barnes L, Ferlito A, Altavilla G, et al.Basaloid squamous cell carcinoma of the head and neck: clinicopathological features and differential diagnosis. *Ann Otol Rhinol Laryngol.* 1996;105:75-82.

146. Luna MA, el Naggar A, Parichatikanond P, et al. Basaloid squamous carcinoma of the upper aerodigestive tract. Clinicopathologic and DNA flow cytometric analysis. *Cancer.* 1009;66:537-542.

147. Muller S, Barnes L. Basaloid squamous cell carcinoma of the head and neck with a spindle cell component. An unusual histologic variant. *Arch Pathol Lab Med.* 1995;119:181-182.

148. World Health Organization Classification of Tumours. Pathology and Genetics. Salivary gland. In: Barnes L, Eveson JW, Reichart P, Sidransky D, eds. *Head and Neck Tumours.* Geneva, Switzerland: WHO;2005:chap 5.

149. Keelawat S, Liu CZ, Roehm PC, et al. Adenosquamous carcinoma of the upper aerodigestive tract: a clinicopathologic study of 12 cases and review of the literature. *Am J Otolaryngol.* 2002;23: 160-168.

150. Napier SS, Gormley JS, Newlands C, et al. Adenosquamous carcinoma. A rare neoplasm with aggressive course. *Oral Surg Oral Med Oral Pathol Oral Radiol Endod.* 1995;79:607-611.

151. Scully C, Porter SR, Speight PM, et al. Adenosquamous carcinoma of the mouth: a rare variant of squamous cell carcinoma. *Int J Oral Maxillofac Surg.* 1999;28:125-128.

152. Ellis G, Auclair P, Gnepp D. *Surgical Pathology of the Salivary Glands. Major Problems in Pathology.* Vol. 25. Philadelphia,Pa: Saunders, 1991.

153. Lee AWM, Foo W, Mang O, et al. Changing epidemiology of nasopharyngeal carcinoma in Hong Kong over a 20-year period (1980-99): an encouraging reduction in both incidence and mortality. *Int J Cancer.* 2003;103:680-685.

154. Raab-Traub N. Epstein-Barr virus in the pathogenesis of NPC. *Cancer Biol.* 2002;12:431-441.

155. Evitkovic E, Bachouchi M, Armand JP. Nasopharyngeal carcinoma. Biology, natural history and therapeutic implications. *Hematol Oncol Clin North Am.* 1991;5:821-838.

156. Fandi A, Cvitkovic E. Biology and treatment of nasopharyngeal cancer. *Curr Opin Oncol.* 1995; 7:255-263.

157. Zhu K, Levine RS, Brann EA, et al. A population-based case-control study of the relationship between cigarette smoking and nasopharyngeal cancer (United States). *Cancer Causes Control.* 1995;6:507-512.

158. Barnes L, Kapadia SB. The biology and pathology of selected skull base tumors. *Neurooncol.* 1994; 20:213-240.

159. Richardson MS. Pathology of skull base tumors. *Otolaryngol Clin North Am.* 2001;34:1025-1042.

160. Baker SR, Wolfe RA. Prognostic factors in nasopharyngeal malignancy. *Cancer.* 1982;49: 163-169.

161. Coskun BU, Cina U, Sener BM, et al. Lymphoepithelial carcinoma of the larynx. *Auris Nasus Larynx.* 2005;32:189-193.

162. Marioni G, Mariuzzi L, Gaio E, et al. Lymphoepithelial carcinoma of the larynx. *Acta Otolaryngol.* 2002;122:429-434.

163. Ferlito A, Weiss LM, Rinaldo A, et al. Clinicopathological consultation. Lymphoepithelial carcinoma of the larynx, hypopharynx, and trachea. *Ann Otol Rhinol Laryngol.* 1997;106:437-444.

164. MacMillan C, Kapadia SB, Finkelstein SD, et al. Lymphoepithelial carcinoma of the larynx and hypopharynx: study of eight cases with relationship to Epstein-Barr virus and p53 gene alterations, and review of the literature. *Hum Pathol.* 1996;27:1172-1179.

165. Easton JM, Levine PH, Hyams VJ. Nasopharyngeal carcinoma in the United States. A pathologic study of 177 US and 30 foreign cases. *Arch Otolaryngol.* 1980;106:88-91.

5

Basic Principles of Radiation Therapy in Head and Neck Cancers

Bahman Emami

INTRODUCTION

Radiation oncology is a medical discipline, which addresses the causes, prevention, and treatment of human cancers with special emphasis on the role of ionizing radiation. One of the most significant progresses in the last two decades has been the creation of a multidisciplinary approach for management of head and neck cancers. Radiation oncology along with surgery and medical oncology, pathology, and radiology are the integral components of this multidisciplinary approach. Approximately 60% of all cancer patients receive radiation therapy as a component of their treatment. This chapter attempts to review the role of radiation in management of head and neck cancers.

PHYSICAL ASPECTS OF RADIATION THERAPY

Ionizing radiation is part of the spectrum of electromagnetic energy that produces physical and biochemical events when they interact with the atoms of irradiated material. The absorption of energy from radiation and biological material leads to excitation or to ionization. The rising of an electron in an atom or a molecule to a higher energy level without actual rejection of the electron is called excitation. If the radiation has sufficient energy to eject one or more orbital electrons from the atom or the molecule, the process is called ionization and that radiation is said to be ionizing radiation. For convenience it is usual to classify ionizing radiation as electromagnetic or particulate. Gamma rays are nonparticle radiation beams emitted by naturally occurring radioactive isotopes. X-rays are nonparticle radiation beams produced by manmade sources, such as linear accelerators. Particle radiation beams most commonly used in radiation therapy include electrons, protons (charged particles), and neutrons (uncharged particles).

During the process of radiation when a beam of ionizing radiation interacts with material, it ejects an electron from an atom. These high-speed electrons transfer their energy to the material by producing ionization and excitations of atoms along their pathways. The absorbed energy per mass unit of material is radiation-absorbed dose.

Units of Radiation

Radiation dose absorbed in tissue is measured in Gray (Gy), defined as energy deposited per kg of mass. Older unit RAD (radiation absorbed dose) equals 0.01 Gy. One cGy equals 1 RAD. Roentgen (R) is a unit of radiation exposure in air. Activity of a radioactive isotope is measured in curies, which is a number of disintegrations per second undergone by 1 g of radium.

Nomenclature

The International Commission of Radiation Units and Measurements (ICRU) has recommended definitions of important concepts in treatment planning in radiation therapy (International Commission of Radiation Units and Measurements Report 50 [ICRU-50]).[1]

Gross tumor volume (GTV) is defined as all known gross tumor that is seen on imaging, palpable, or determined in any other way.

Clinical target volume (CTV) is defined as areas suspected of harboring microscopic cancer cells. In head and neck cancer, it generally includes microscopic extension of the primary tumor into the surrounding apparently normal tissue and/or clinically normal lymph nodes suspected of bearing microscopic disease.

Planning target volume (PTV) is a margin of normal tissue surrounding the previously described volumes that are included in radiation volume to account for organ movement and inaccuracies of daily setup. Inaccuracies in daily setup can be minimized by using proper immobilization technology.

Equipment Used in Clinical Radiation Therapy

High-energy x-rays produced by linear accelerators are by far the most commonly used beams for head and neck radiation therapy in the United States. Linear accelerators produce high-energy x-rays by bombarding a heavy-metal target with fast electrons. Low-energy x-rays such as produced by orthovoltage or superficial machines have poor tissue penetration characteristics and deposit excessive dose in superficial tissues; thus, they are suitable for treatment of superficial skin lesions.

Cobalt teletherapy units house isotope Co60 that emits gamma rays. Cobalt-60 machines have been extensively used for radiation therapy in the past but now are largely replaced by linear accelerators. However, they are still the most common radiotherapy machines in the rest of the world.

BIOLOGICAL EFFECTS OF IONIZING RADIATIONS AND BIOLOGICAL BASIS OF RADIATION THERAPY

The critical target in cell death is in the nucleus and it is probably DNA. Ionizing radiation damages DNA in at least four different ways: double-helix strand breaks, single-strand breaks, base damage, and damage to cross-links in which both DNA-DNA and DNA-protein cross-links are involved (Fig 5–1).

These physical and biochemical phenomena take place in fractions of a second at the time of the radiation exposure. Various nuclear and cytoplasmic molecular changes then follow, leading to loss of reproductive ability, cell cycle delays, somatic transformation, and mutations, among others.

Chromosomes may be damaged by ionizing radiation. Classically, the damage is not detected in interphase and only appears as the cells go through cell division. Kaplan has reported that the frequency of mutations produced by the single- or double-strand breaks on the DNA molecule depends on not only the number of initial breaks but also the adequacy of the repair mechanisms.[2]

Carcinogenesis

Ionizing radiation has the potential to induce cancer in any organ. The adult thyroid gland may tolerate as much as 40.0 cGy without significant changes, but in children who received between 2.0 and 8.0 cGy to the neck for thymic enlargement, the development many years later of thyroid carcinoma, usually of the papillary type, has been reported.

Cell Kill by Ionizing Radiation

When a cell is hit by an ionizing particle, different kinds of damage may take place. Lethal damage occurs when the cell loses its ability for unlimited proliferation. After radiation exposure, the cell and its progeny die, although as many as five to six cell divisions may occur. Potentially lethal damage consists of less severe impairment of the proliferative ability of the cell from which it may recover, but any

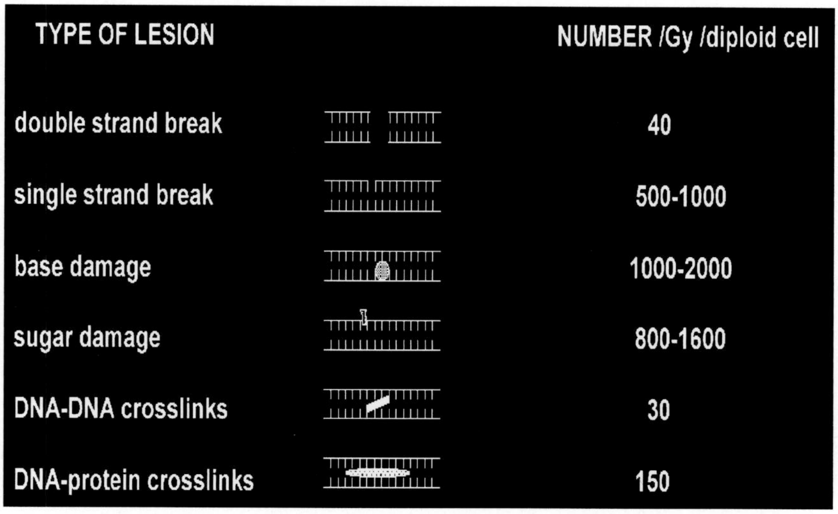

TYPE OF LESION		NUMBER /Gy /diploid cell
double strand break		40
single strand break		500-1000
base damage		1000-2000
sugar damage		800-1600
DNA-DNA crosslinks		30
DNA-protein crosslinks		150

Fig 5–1. Types of DNA damage to irradiation.

modification in its environment interferes with repair and causes the cell to die.

Sublethal damage occurs when the injury induced by the ionizing radiation can be repaired by the cell. After exposure to ionizing radiation, the cells exhibit changes in their growth rate, including prolongation of the generation time and mitotic delay.

FACTORS AFFECTING THE BIOLOGICAL EFFECTS OF IONIZING RADIATION

Cell Sensitivity to Radiation

In cell cultures and experimental animals the sensitivity of cells to ionizing radiation and to most chemotherapeutic agents varies according to the phase of the cell cycle in which exposure of the cell to the physical or chemical event occurs.[3] In cell culture tumor cells are most sensitive in M phase and more resistant in S phase of the cell cycles.

In clinical practice, a distinction must be made between cell sensitivity to radiation, tumor response, and curability. Some tumors, such as lymphomas, and small cell undifferentiated carcinomas, are sensitive

to radiation and may disappear after low or moderated doses, but the patient may not necessarily be cured and eventually dies of disseminated disease.

Oxygen Enhancement Effect (Reoxygenation)

With sparsely ionizing radiation, such as x-rays or gamma rays, a given biological effect produced by a given dose is two to three times greater in the presence of oxygen than if it is absent. This augmentation is called the *oxygen enhancement ratio (OER)*. Oxygen must be present during the radiation exposure. The oxygen enhancement effect is lessened or absent in high linear energy transfer (LET) radiations, such as alpha particles, fast neutrons, and pimesons. Although increasing concentrations of oxygen result in more sensitization to radiation, Gray reported that no significant gain is observed when the oxygen pressure is over 30 mm Hg.[4] Suit and Shalek[5] suggested that the hypoxic cell population determines the response of a tumor to and probability of control of a tumor by radiation. Fractionated radiation causes a decrease in the size of the tumor and the initial number of cells, as well as new blood vessel proliferation and reoxygenation. Kallman[6] noted that these changes result in a transfer of hypoxic tumor cells to a more oxygenated compartment, and this transfer in turn eventually leads to complete sterilization of the tumor without significant injury to the surrounding normal tissues. The lack of oxygen enhancement effect in the biological events induced by high LET particles has resulted in renewed interest in the clinical applications of these radiations.

Linear Energy Transfer (LET)

LET represents the energy transferred by an ionizing particle per unit length of pathway. Because most ionizing particles are not energetic, the LET that results from a beam of energy is an average of all the particles or photons in the beam. In addition, at the molecular level, the energy per unit length of track varies. So the LET of an ionizing particle depends in a complex way on the energy and charge of the particle: The greater the charge and the smaller the velocity, the higher the LET.

Because of these varying amounts of energy released in an absorber, equal doses of various types of radiation do not produce the same biological effects on the absorber, or patient. The term *relative biological effect* (RBE) was established to compare the biological effectiveness of a given ionizing radiation with a certain standard, which are 250-kV x-rays. For instance, cobalt 60 has a relative biological effect of approximately 0.95, and neutrons have a relative biological effect of between 2.0 and 2.5, depending on their energy.

REPAIR OF RADIATION DAMAGE (DOSE FRACTIONATION)

Radiation therapy is given in daily fractions four or five per week, on the presumption that normal cells generally have a greater and faster capacity to repair sublethal damage and cell repopulation between fractions. This time-dose relation depends on individual sensitivity of the cells and their repair ability, size of the radiation fractions, total dose given, time between fractions and of overall treatment, initial hypoxic subpopulation and reoxygenation that takes place throughout the fractionated therapy, and the type of ionizing radiation used.

In prescribing the treatment of the patient, the specifications should include not only the volume of tissue treated and the total dose given but also the number of fractions and the overall period of time in which they are administered.

DOSE FRACTIONATION IN RADIATION THERAPY OF HEAD AND NECK CANCER

In the United States, conventional dose fractionation used in head and neck cancers treatment is 1.8 to 2.0 Gy per fraction, delivered as one fraction per day, for overall treatment duration of around 6 to 7 weeks. In an effort to increase therapeutic efficacy, different fractionation schedules are explored, generally aimed to increase the number of daily fractions and decrease the overall treatment duration. The stated rationale for such approach are several. If the cells are most sensitive in G2/M phase of mitotic cycle, increasing the number of fractions should theoretically increase the probability of strike in the most sensitive phase. Furthermore, as the number of surviving cells is reduced by the initial part of therapy, the remaining cells proliferate more rapidly —a phenomenon known as accelerated repopulation. More frequent radiation treatments should in theory counteract rapid proliferation. Finally, by splitting the daily radiation dose into 2 smaller fractions, the late effects are thought to be reduced owing to difference in radiation sensitivity between rapidly cycling cells such as tumor and quiescent cells such as normal tissue. Due to a phenomenon known as "shoulder" on a cellular survival curve, rapidly proliferating cells sustain relatively more damage by smaller doses of radiation compared to noncycling cells. By repeating frequent administrations of smaller than usual fractions, the therapeutic window of radiation is increased allowing for higher radiation dose. To enumerate possible permutations of the design of altered fractionations, two main schemas, namely, hyperfractionation and accelerated fractionation, have been tested extensively in advanced head and neck cancers. Hyperfractionation exploits the difference in fractionation sensitivity between tumors and normal tissues manifesting late morbidity. The clinical trial of European Organization for Research for treatment of cancer (EORTC) showed a moderate (10–15%) improvement in local control of oropharyngeal carcinomas.[7] Incidence of acute toxicities was significantly higher and the late morbidities were within the range observed in conventional fractionation schedules. In contract, in accelerated fractionations it is thought that tumor proliferation is a major cause of radiotherapy failures. Therefore, by reducing the overall time without decreasing the total dose, an attempt has been made to circumvent the above problem. The excessive mucosal toxicities have not allowed more than 2 weeks reduction in overall treatment time in most of the trials. One version of accelerated fractionated regimen by the Danish Head and Neck Study Group (DAHNCA7)[8] delivered six fractions per week. In this randomized trial a total of 1485 patients were accrued. The incidence of acute severe mucositis and dysplasia was significantly higher in the experimental group receiving six fractions per week. The 5-year actuarial local regional control was 70% and 60% for accelerated versus conventional fractionated regiment, respectively ($p = 0.0005$). Another hybrid variant of concomitant boost was pursued by the Radiation Therapy Oncology Group (RTOG).[9] In this trial (RTOG 9003) three altered fractionation regimens were compared with standard fractionation of 70 Gy in 35 fractions over 7 weeks.[10] The experimental arms were hyperfractionation, split course-accelerated fractionation, and concomitant boost regimen. A recent analysis of over 1000 patients from this study revealed that the concomitant boost and hyperfractionation regimen showed modest improvement of 10 to 15% in local regional control. Acute mucosal reactions were significantly higher in altered fractionations but there were no difference in the late complication rate at one and two years (Table 5–1).

MODES OF RADIATION THERAPY

Primary Radiotherapy: External Beam Radiotherapy

Primary radiotherapy is generally delivered through external beam radiation with various energies of x-rays or electron beams. Cobalt gamma rays are in

Table 5–1. Altered Fractionation—2-Year Outcomes From the Radiation Therapy Oncology Group 90-03 Trial

	Fractionation Schedule			
Parameter	Conventional (70 Gy/35 Fx/7 wk)	Hyperfractionation (81.6 Gy/68 Fx/7 wk)	Accelerated Split Course (67.2 Gy/42 Fx/6 wk)	Accelerated Concomitant Boost (72Gy/42 Fx/6 wk)
No. of patients	268	263	274	268
Local-regional control	46%	54% ($p = .045$)	48% ($p = .55$)	55% ($p = .050$)
Disease-free survival	32%	38% ($p = .067$)	33% ($p = .026$)	39% ($p = .054$)
Overall survival	46%	55% ($p = .13$)	46% ($p = .86$)	51% ($p = .40$)
Grade 3 + acute toxicity	35%	55% ($p = .0001$)	51% ($p = .0002$)	59% ($p = .0001$)
Grade 3 + late toxicity	28%	28% (NS)	28% (NS)	38% ($p = .011$)
Grade 3 + late toxicity at 2 years	6%	13% (NS)	8% (NS)	8% (NS)

p-values reflect comparison of the experimental arms with standard fractionation.

Data from Fu et al. *Int J Radiat Oncol Biol Phys.* 2000;48:7-16 (ref 9).

NS = nonsignificant; Fx = fractions.

Source: Reprinted with permission from ref 10 Mendenhall et al. Altered fractionation. *Laryngoscope*, 2003: 113.

declining use in the United States but still are the most frequently used modes in the rest of the world. The choice of type and beam energy depends on the location and the geometric parameters of the area to be treated. Occasionally, kilovoltage x-rays are also used for very superficial skin lesions. In most centers, using conventional radiation regimens (1.80–2.00 Gy per day, 5 treatments per week), the gross tumor is radiated to 66 to 70 Gy and potential microscopic extensions of the tumor to 46 to 50 Gy. During the last two decades, some radiation oncologists who believe that modest improvement in local regional control of 10% to 15% justifies significant increase in acute toxicities, have utilized either hyper- or accelerated fractionations. However, when combining radiation with other modalities such as chemotherapy and/or surgery, the conventional fractionation is still common practice and use of altered fractionation with surgery and/or chemotherapy is still considered experimental.

Brachytherapy

Brachytherapy is the delivery of radiation through interstitial implants, intracavitary applications, and/or molds. Brachytherapy is usually combined with external beam radiation therapy as a boost to the gross tumor volume. The rational for using brachytherapy is delivery of higher doses of radiation to the gross tumor while minimizing dose to normal tissues. It should be noted that process of brachytherapy is highly operator dependent and many training programs do not have adequate training for this technique. Examples of brachytherapy are use of interstitial implants as a boost in carcinoma of base of tongue (Fig 5–2) or in treatment of recurrent oral cavity cancers and examples of intracavitary brachytherapy are in treatment of recurrent nasopharyngeal cancers.

Combination of Surgery and Radiation Therapy

Intermediate advanced carcinomas of head and neck, when medically operable, is usually treated with surgery followed by postoperative radiation therapy.

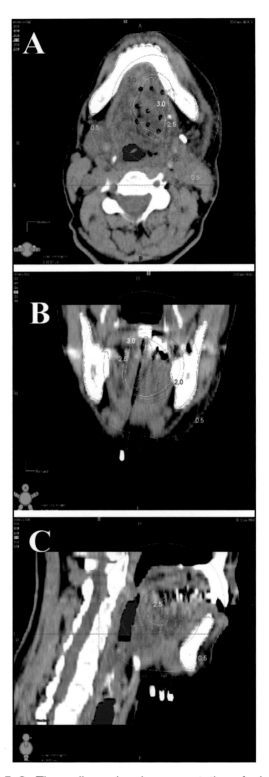

Fig 5–2. Three-dimensional representation of a base of tongue implant. **A.** Cross-section. **B.** Coronal view. **C.** Sagittal view.

The general indication for postoperative radiation therapy include close or positive surgical margins, perineural spread, lymph/vascular invasion, tumor extension into bone or neck soft tissues, presence of multiple metastatic nodes in the neck, and extracapsular extension (ECE) of nodal disease. In general, the entire operative bed is included in the postoperative target volume. Donor sites of skin graphs or flaps usually are not considered part of the operative bed. The usual dose is 58 to 60 Gy in conventional fractionation. In case of extracapsular extension and/or surgical positive margins the dose is increased to 64 to 66 Gy. Again, as a general rule, postoperative radiation therapy should start on complete healing of the surgical wound. This is usually 4 to 6 weeks after surgery. Extending the interwall from surgery to initiation of radiation beyond 8 weeks is not considered an optimal course of treatment.

In certain clinical situations use of preoperative radiotherapy can be considered. These include when cancer is marginally resectable. Use of preop radiation therapy is an uncommon event because of surgeons' desires to operate in nonradiated tissues. In primary radiotherapy treatment of patients who present with large cervical nodes, a regimen of preoperative radiation followed by planned neck dissection is still a common practice. In most preoperative treatments, the delivered dose is 50 Gy in 25 fractions, which is required for utilization of subclinical disease. The timing of neck dissection is usually 4 to 6 weeks after completion of radiation.

Combination of Radiotherapy with Systemic Treatments

Although this subject is discussed in detail in other chapters, a brief overview is indicated here. Systemic chemotherapy can be given prior to (neoadjuvant) and concurrent with and subsequent to (adjuvant) to local radiation therapy. Several metaanalysis of large number of patients have confirmed that most effective mode of combination of systemic treatment and radiotherapy is the use of concurrent form.[11,12] Neoadjuvant as well as adjuvant radiotherapy with the currently used cisplatin-based regimen has little or no therapeutic benefits. Concurrent radiation has resulted in significant improved cure rate in certain subsites such as nasopharynx[12] and only modest improvement in treatment of other advanced head and neck cancers.[11]

PROCESS OF RADIATION THERAPY

The process of radiation therapy is initiated with evaluation and staging of the patient, both anatomically and pathologically. Comprehensive evaluations of the physiologic and functional status of the normal tissues are an essential part of this evaluation. After the decision is made on the regimen to be used (eg, conventional fractionation, hyperfraction, radiation-chemotherapy), the technical process of administering radiation therapy initiates with simulation. In the past this planning process was with a single radiograph, called *simulator film* (Fig 5–3). On obtaining the simulation film, which is usually in anteroposterior or lateral projection, a portal would be outlined by the radiation oncologist that presumably contained the area of gross tumor as well as areas of subclinical disease. After appropriate measurements of the dimensions of this area of the film and the separation of the patient, calculations would have been carried out and the delivery of treatment would commence. This technique is labeled *1D radiation therapy*.

Introduction of CT scanning in the practice of radiation oncology in the 1970s was an important step, not only for evaluation of the patients but also for planning purposes as reported.[13] This technique of planning, which is currently used in many radiation therapy departments around the world, is labeled *2D treatment planning* as described below. Nevertheless, even after two decades of use of using 2D technology, serious limitations exist with this technique.

TECHNOLOGIC ADVANCES IN RADIATION THERAPY

Two-dimensional planning has been practiced in radiation therapy for decades. The entrance path of radiation beam is drawn on a plain radiograph, shaped around the tumor and subclinically involved

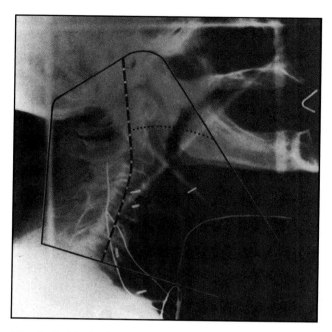

Fig 5–3. Typical postoperative simulation film of a patient with advanced-stage cancer of the laryngopharynx. *Dashed line*, initial field reduction (after 50 Gy, to shield spinal cord; *dotted line*, final reduction (after 60 Gy). Wires mark surgical scars and stoma. Slanting line used on lower borders reduces length of the spinal cord treated by the primary field, allows better caudal coverage of mucosal surfaces while simultaneously bypassing shoulders, and facilitates matching with low-neck field. Reproduced with permission from Amdur RJ et al. *Int J Radiat Oncol Biol Phys.* 1989; 16:25–36.

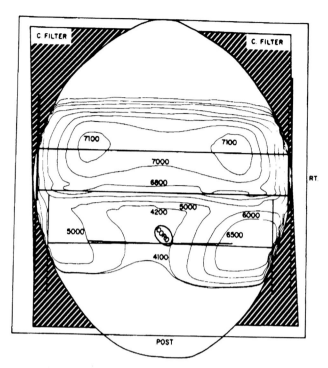

Fig 5–4. Two-dimensional radiotherapy: isodose curves of a set of beam arrangements in a head and neck cancer patient.

areas (see Fig 5–3). Dose distribution is then calculated on one or few slices of the CT scan. The plan is judged to be adequate if the desired isodose curve encompasses the desired target volume on the single CT slice (Fig 5–4). There are a number of problems with that kind of planning. The gross tumor on a plain radiograph frequently is not seen or delineated and cervical lymph nodes are obscured. Soft tissue anatomy is poorly seen on plain radiographs. One single CT slice is hardly representative of the entire head and neck volume. Even if isodose distribution is obtained on multiple CT slices, there is no algorithm to calculate dose distribution over the entire organ of interest. These shortcomings are thought to be at least partially responsible for poor

results obtained with radiation therapy in treatment of head and neck cancers.

In the 1990s the advent of computer technology led to development of three-dimensional conformal radiation therapy (3D-CRT),[14] which has replaced older, 2D technology in many academic, and nonacademic centers during the past decade.

Three-dimensional conformal radiotherapy is not just an add-on to the 2D radiation oncology planning process. Rather, it represents a radical change in practice, particularly for radiation oncologists. The 2D treatment planning approach emphasizes the use of conventional simulator for designing beam portals based on standardized beam arrangement techniques and bony landmarks visualized on planner radiographs. Three-dimensional treatment planning emphasizes a volumetric image-based virtual simulation approach for defining tumor and organs at risk volumes for the individual patients. A review of various stages and procedures involved in 3D-CRT is shown in Table 5–2.

Table 5–2. The Process of 3D Radiation Therapy Planning and Conformal Radiotherapy

I. Delineation of target volumes
- Evaluation of patient, tumor (staging), and normal tissue/organs
- Patient immobilization
- Computed tomographic scanning
- Contouring of target volumes and normal organs
- Volumetric computed tomography data transfer to radiation treatment system

II. Planning and Optimization
- Virtual simulation: design of portals and initial beam arrangement
- Three-dimensional dose calculations and display (dose-volume histogram, dose surface, dose statistics)
- Plan evaluation-optimization of three-dimensional beam arrangement

III. Predelivery preparation
- Digitally reconstructed radiograph (DRR)
- Block template
- Verification of portals
- Marking of patient
- Radiographic verification
- Block making (Cerrobend) and block check
- Multileaf collimation

IV. Treatment delivery

V. Treatment verification and documentation
- Portal films
- On-line imaging
- Record and verifying system

INTENSITY MODULATED RADIOTHERAPY (IMRT)

As mentioned above, progress in computerized treatment planning and delivery of radiation therapy has made it possible to conform the dose of radiation precisely to the predetermined target volumes and therefore reduce the radiation dose to the critical normal tissue structures resulting in reduction of morbidity. Such precision radiotherapy usually is accomplished by use of series of x-ray beams individually shaped to conform to the target, thus the creation of three-dimensional conformal radiotherapy. Technologic advances have also made possible to modify the intensity of individual beams/beamlets across the radiation field and thus enhancement of capability of conforming dose distribution in three-dimensions. This form of radiation therapy is called Intensity Modulated Radio Therapy (IMRT).[15] Published experiences from single institutions are suggestive of reduction in radiation-induced complications such as xerostomia. Long-term results of the use of IMRT in clinical settings are not available (Table 5–3).

It should be noted that by treating head and neck patients with IMRT technique, large volumes of unintended normal tissues would receive low doses of radiation. Potential of increase radiation-induced second malignancies in these areas is of major concern.[22]

SITE-SPECIFIC CLINICAL RESULTS

Oral Cavity

Lip

Small cancers of the lip (less than 2 cm) that do not involve the oral commissure are treated equally well with surgery or radiation therapy with excellent cosmetic and functional results. Radiation therapy is the preferred option for lesions larger than 2 cm or those involving the commissure, in which surgical resection results in microstomia or oral incontinence. Radiotherapy can be delivered by external beam, brachytherapy, or often a combination of both. Postoperative radiotherapy is also recommended for positive margins or lesions with perineural invasion. Results of treatment in carcinoma of the lip are shown in Table 5–4.

Oral Tongue and Floor of Mouth

Surgical resection is generally preferred in medically operable patients. Depending on risk factors a modified neck dissection may also be included. Postoperative radiation therapy is recommended for large

Table 5–3. Locoregional Control After IMRT for Head and Neck Cancer

| Study (ref) | No of Pts. | Primary Site | RT | | FU-Months | | Control | | |
			Definitive	Postop	Median	Range	Local (%)	Regional (%)	Interval (yrs)
Chao et al[16]	126	Various	52	74	26	12–55	85		2
Lee et al[17]	67	NPX	67	0	31	7–72	98		4
Chao et al[18]	74	OPX	31	43	33	9–60	87		4
Eisbruch et al*[19]	133	Various, non-NPX	60	73	32	6–107	82		3
Kam et al[20]	63	NPX	63	0	29	8–45	92	98	3
Kwong et al[21]	33	NPX	33	0	29	11–42	100	92	3

Abbreviations: IMRT, intensity-modulated radiotherapy; RT, radiotherapy, NPX, nasopharynx; OPX oropharynx.
*Patients treated from 1994 to 2002; three-dimensional conformal radiotherapy was used before 1996, and IMRT thereafter.

Table 5–4. Carcinoma of the Lip: Results of Treatment

Author	No. of Pts.	Tx	Local Control	5-year Cause-Specific Survival
MacKey and Seller[23]	2854	XRT	<2 cm 97%	65%
Baker and Krause[24]	279	XRT	≤3 cm 90%*	94%
		Surgery	>3 cm 80%	71%
Mohs and Snow[25]	1119	Mohs Surgery	<2 cm 97%	
			>2 cm 60%	

XRT: External radiation therapy.
*No difference between surgery or external radiation therapy in lesions ≤3 cm.

primary tumors, close or positive surgical margins, presence of perineural or vascular invasion, and multiple positive nodes with or without extracapsular extension. Recently for patients with positive surgical margins and/or positive nodes with extracapsular extension postoperative concurrent chemoradiotherapy is considered standard of care.[26] Small lesions (T1–T2) can equally be cured by radiation alone (Tables 5-5 and 5-6). However surgical approach is preferred. Advanced lesions with deep muscle invasion, which are often associated with cervical lymph node metastasis, are unlikely to be cured by radiation alone (see Tables 5-5 and 5-6). They are best managed by planned combined surgery and postop-

erative radiation therapy and/or radiochemotherapy (Tables 5-7 and 5-8).

It is important to note that initial oncologically negative surgical margins is one of the most important prognostic factors as compared to close margins or initially positive and re-section negative margins (Table 5-9).

Nasopharynx

Carcinomas of the nasopharynx are characterized by high incidence of cervical lymph node metastasis and relative high incidence of distant metastasis.

Table 5–5. T1 T2 Carcinoma of the Oral Tongue: Results of Treatment with Radiotherapy

Author (ref)	No. of Pts	XRT Tx	Local Control T$_1$	Local Control T$_2$	Cause-Specific Survival T$_1$	Cause-Specific Survival T$_2$
Lefebvre et al[27]	299	I ± E	98*	89*	57	46
Shibuya et al[28]	226	I ± E	92	82	84	76
Wendt et al[29]	103	I ± E	81	67	—	—
Horiuchi et al[30]	117	I + E	94	77	76	63
Decroix[31]	382	E ± I	86	78	80	56
Mezeron et al[32]	155	I	87	54	90	71

*Minimum follow-up for local control was 2 months.
XRT: Radiotherapy; I: Interstitial radiotherapy; E: external beam radiotherapy.

Table 5–6. T1 and T2 Carcinoma of the Floor of the Mouth: Results of Treatment

Author	Therapy	No. of Patients	Local Control (%) T1	Local Control (%) T2	5-yr Cause-Specific Survival Rate (%) T1	5-yr Cause-Specific Survival Rate (%) T2
Rodgers et al[33]	XRT	73	86	69	96	70
	S + XRT	8	1/1	7/7	—	—
	S	22	90	75	4/6	5/6
Mazeron et al[34]	XRT + ND	116	93.5	74.5H	94	61.5H
Matsumoto et al[35]	XRT	90	89	76H	95	79H
					—	54I
Nason et al[36]	S (ND)	114	—	—	69	64

Abbreviations: XRT, External radiation therapy; S, Surgery; ND, nodal dissection.

Table 5–7. Results of Radiotherapy in Cancers of Oral Tongue (556 patients)

	% LC	% LRC	% DSS (5-yr)	% OS (5-yr)
Stage I	95	82	82	71
Stage II	65	56	48	43
Stage III	54	44	33	33
Stage IV	36	20	19	23

LC: Local Control; LRC: Local Regional Control; DSS: Disease-Specific Survival; OS: Overall Survival.
Modified from ref 37.

Table 5–8. Results of Radiotherapy in Cancers of Floor of Mouth (207 Patients)

	% LC	% LRC	% DSS (5-yr)	% OS (5-yr)
Stage I	97	86	91	74
Stage II	73	67	48	46
Stage III	64	58	47	39
Stage IV	0	0	0	0

LC: Local Control; LRC: Local Regional Control; DSS: Disease-Specific Survival; OS: Overall Survival.
Modified from ref 37.

Based on current evidence from clinical trials the standard treatment for stage I to II nasopharynx cancer is radiotherapy. The standard for stage III to IV nasopharyngeal cancer is combination of radiation therapy and chemotherapy.[38] In intergroup phase III trial, the primary regimen was concurrent chemotherapy and radiotherapy.[39] Although the course of adjuvant chemotherapy was part of the intergroup protocol, significant number of patients did not receive full prescribed adjuvant chemotherapy according to protocol.[39] There is no analysis of the detrimental effect on this group of patients. The value of adjuvant chemotherapy in this setting still is not clear. Neck dissection is indicated in a very small number of patients who have residual neck disease 2 to 3 months after completion of combined chemoradiotherapy.

Several prospectively controlled phase III randomized trials have shown the superiority of combination of chemotherapy and radiotherapy over radiotherapy alone (Table 5–10). The results of recent meta-analysis are shown in Table 5–11. Several meta-

Table 5–9. Oral Cavity Cancers Treated with Surgery and Postoperative Irradiation: Influence of Margin Status on Local Control (Literature Review)

Margin Status	Oral Tongue No. Controlled/Total (%)		Floor of Mouth No. Controlled/Total (%)	
	MSKCC	U of FL[a]	MSKCC	U of FL[a]
Negative	7/9 (78%)	9/12 (75%)	9/9 (100%)	10/13 (77%)
Close	10/16 (62%)	7/11 (64%)[b]	6/8 (75%)	8/9 (89%)[b]
Positive	2/4 (50%)	1/4 (25%)	4/5 (80%)	8/13 (62%)
Total	19/29 (66%)	17/27 (63%)	19/22 (86%)	26/35 (74%)

MSKCC, Memorial Sloan-Kettering Cancer Center (Zelefsky MJ, Harrison LB, Fass DE, et al. 1993): University of Florida (Parsons JT, Mendenhall WM, Springer Sp, et al, 1997).

[a]Local-regional control

[b]Includes close and initially positive

Source: Reproduced with permission from Ang KK, Garden AS, eds. Lippincott Williams & Wilkins; 2006: 60.

Table 5–10. Results of Concurrent Chemo-Radiotherapy ± Adjuvant Chemotherapy in Stage III/IV Nasopharyngeal Carcinoma

Author (yr)	No of Patients	% OS	p	% DFS	p	Median Follow-up
Al-Sarraf et al (IG-0099) (2001)[39]	RT = 69 RT + C = 78	37 67	0.001	28 58	<0.001	>60 mo
Chan, et al (2005)[40]	RT = 174 RT + C = 176	59 70	0.065	54 60	0.16	66 mo
Lin, et al (2003)[41]	RT = 143 RT + C = 141	53 72	0.002	54 72	0.001	65 mo
Wee, et al (2005)[42]	RT = 110 RT + C = 111	46 65	0.01	45 55	0.04	60 mo

Abbreviations: RT: radiotherapy, C: chemotherapy.

analysis from a large number of patients treated in clinical trials have established the current standard of chemoradiotherapy for advanced nasopharyngeal cancer (see Table 5–11). Modern radiotherapy tech-niques such as three-dimensional conformal radiotherapy and/or intensity-modulated radiotherapy (IMRT) (Fig 5–5) have significantly contributed to the improvement of the results of treatment of patients

Table 5–11. Results of Meta-Analysis of the MAC-NPC Collaborative Group According to Sequence of Chemo-RT

Chemotherapy Schedule	No of Patients	Hazard Ratio (95% CI)	Risk Reduction
Neoadjuvant	RT = 415 C–RT = 415	0.99 (0.80–1.21)	1%
Concurrent	RT = 381 RT + C = 384	0.60 (0.48–0.76)	40%
Adjuvant	RT = 189 RT–C = 191	0.97 (0.69–1.38)	3%
Total	RT = 985 RT–C = 990	0.82 (0.71–0.94)	18%

Abbreviations: RT: radiotherapy, C: chemotherapy.
Data from ref 12.

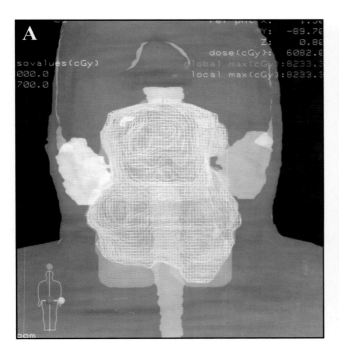
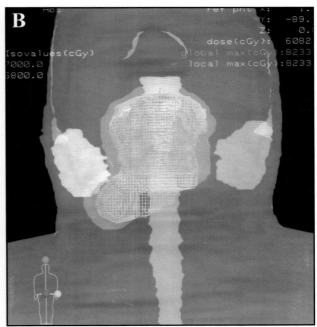

Fig 5–5. Three-dimensional representation of tumor volumes and radiation dose in a patient with T3N1 nasopharyngeal carcinoma. **A**. 5700 cGy to CTV$_1$; **B**. 7000 cGy to the gross tumor volume and node. *Note:* sparing parotid glands and prevention of xerostomia.

with carcinoma of the nasopharynx (Table 5–12). The progress in this area is both in control of the tumor as well as significant reduction in side effects in radiotherapy such as xerostomia and hearing loss. The results of one such study from our own institution is shown in Table 5–13.

Oropharynx

Palatine Arch (Soft Palate and Tonsils)

Primary radiotherapy is treatment of choice for T1, T2, N0 to N1 carcinomas. Small group of patients, who have residual nodal disease 6 weeks after completion of radiotherapy, can be considered for neck dissection.

Combination of radiation with chemotherapy is treatment of choice for infiltrative T3 and selected T4 or N2 to N3 carcinomas. Tumor dose of 70 Gy

Table 5–12. Results of IMRT in the Treatment of Nasopharyngeal Carcinoma

Author (yr)	No of Patients	% LC	Median F.U. (mo)
Lee et al (2002)[17]	67	97 (4 yr)	31
Kam et al (2004)[20]	63	92 (3 yr)	29
Kwong et al (2004)[21]	33	100 (3 yr)	33
Emami et al (2007)[43]	21	100 (2 yr)	31

Abbreviations: LC; local control.

with conventional fractionation plus concurrent cisplatin-based chemotherapy is standard of care. T4 tumors with bone invasion or extensive normal tissue destruction, anatomic deformation, or functional dysfunction can be considered for surgery and postoperative chemoradiotherapy. Due to excellent clinical results and very low morbidity using modern techniques of radiotherapy, surgical intervention should be discouraged in this group of patients to avoid risk of anesthesia and other surgical complications. Results of modern radiotherapy in carcinomas of oropharynx as shown in Table 5–14.

Base of Tongue

Early primary tumors of T1, T2, and early T3, N0 to N1 can be treated equally well with primary radiation therapy and/or intraoral laser resection of primary, selective neck dissection and postoperative radiation therapy. Infiltrative T3 and selected T4 or N2 to N3 tumors are best treated with combined modality therapy of surgery followed by chemoradiotherapy. In general, when treated with nonsurgical treatment of chemoradiotherapy, neck dissection is indicated in patients who have residual neck mass (clinically or radiographically) 6 weeks after completion of therapy. Routine neck dissection after concurrent chemoradiotherapy should be discouraged.[48] Over 85% of patients with post-treatment negative neck will have no disease in the neck.[49] As other primary tumors of the oropharynx, T4 tumors with extensive normal tissue destruction with anatomic or physiologic dysfunction should be treated with surgery and postoperative chemoradiotherapy.

Table 5–13. Squamous Cell Carcinoma of the Nasopharynx (Loyola)

Treatment	2 Year	
	Progression-Free Survival	Overall Survival
2D XRT Alone (59 pts)	49%	60%
3D CRT/IMRT + Chemo (21 pts)	75%	90%

Abbreviations: XRT; external radiation therapy.
Source: Emami et al. Presented at 5th International Conference on Head and Neck Cancer. San Francisco, Calif; 2000 (ref 43).

For cancers of pharyngeal wall, although small tumors can be successfully treated with radiation alone, most lesions of T2 to T4 are best treated with surgery followed by postoperative radiation therapy. As for neck metastasis, N0 patients are successfully treated with radiation therapy without any surgical intervention. Patients with clinically or radiographically positive cervical nodal metastasis should be treated with ipsilateral surgery followed by postop-

erative radiation therapy and or chemoradiotherapy in high-risk patients. Results of radiotherapy treatment of patients with base of tongue and pharyngeal wall are shown in Tables 5-15 and 5-16.

Hypopharynx

The best management for hypopharyngeal carcinomas is that which achieves the highest local regional

Table 5–14. Treatment Results of Primary Radiotherapy in Cancers of Oropharynx

Study	No of Patients	OS	LC	LRC	RFS	Median FU (mo)
Chao et al[18]	74	87%	NR	87%	81%	33
Garden et al[44]	80	NR	NR	94%	NR	17
Haung et al[45]	41	89%	94%	89%	91%	14
DeArruda et al[46]	50	98%	98%	86%	NR	18
Mendenhall et al[47]	64	83%	94%	91%	86%	36

Abbreviations: OS: overall survival; LC: local control; LRC: local-regional control; RFS: relapse-free survival.

Table 5–15. Results of Treatment in Carcinomas of Base of the Tongue

Investigator	No of Patients	Nodal Involvement	Laryngectomy	Operative/ Treatment Mortality	5-yr Survival	5-yr Loco-Regional Control
Surgery						
Foote 1993[50]	55	51%	16%	4%	55%	48%
Kraus 1993[51]	100 (+ RT in 63)	62%	20%	0%	55% 65%	72%
Radiation Therapy						
Mak 1995[52]	54 (+ ND in 20)	83%	0%	0%	59% 65%	76%
Hinerman 1994[53]	107 (+ ND in 58)	82%	1%	0%	44% 64%	71%
Surgery plus Irradiation						
Riley 1983[54]	28	—	—	—	25%	78%
Thawley 1983[55]	101	74%	2% total 33% partial	—	45%	60%

Abbreviations: RT: radiotherapy; ND: nodal dissection.

Table 5–16. Pharyngeal Wall Cancer: Treatment Results

Author	# Pts	Therapy	Local Control (%)				
			T1	T2	T3	T4	Overall
Moez-Mendez[56]	164	RT	91	73	61	37	60
	25	S+RT		5/5		75	45
Mendenhall[57]	49	RT qd ± implant		50		31	39
	13	RT (bid)		5/5		5/8	77
Emami[58]	62	RT					47
	41	RT + S					66
	24	S + RT					66

RT, radiation therapy; S, surgery; qd, daily; bid, twice daily.
81% of patients had tumor >4 cm.

control and least functional damage in terms of respiration, deglutition, and phonation. In general, most T1 N0 and selected T2 N0 lesions can be treated equally well with curative radiation therapy and/or conservation surgery. Invasion of larynx by piriform sinus cancer with vocal fold fixation predicts a poor outcome to curative radiation therapy. Larger lesions, especially with the ones with cervical nodal metastasis are best treated with combined surgical resection and adjuvant radiotherapy and/or radiochemotherapy in high-risk patients. Due to the fact that most of these patients have advanced disease at presentation, often with associated cervical nodal metastasis and also because most lesions are understaged at presentation, the general approach has been to use combined surgery followed by postoperative radiation therapy and/or chemoradiotherapy. Results of treatment of cancers of piriform cancer are depicted in Table 5-17.

Larynx

Glottic Carcinomas

Patients with T_{is}, T1 to T2 N0 carcinoma of the glottic larynx can be treated equally with transoral laser resection, open partial laryngectomy, or radiotherapy. The goals of treatments are cure and laryngeal

preservation with good quality voice. Additional goals are minimized risk of serious complications and minimizing cost. There is no randomized trial comparing any of the above options. Therefore, the decision will be made based on nonrandomized trials, which have their own known pitfalls. Although a small percentage of patients with very small vocal fold lesions can be treated with laser surgery, primary radiotherapy is preferred modality for T1 to T2 tumors. This approach results in excellent local control, superior voice quality (as compared with any kind of surgery) and more cost effective. The results of treatment of early glottic larynx with radiation therapy are shown in Tables 5-18, 5-19, and 5-20. In a recent prospective randomized trial of altered fractionation versus conventional fractionation radiotherapy of early glottic cancer (T1a–T1b) by Yamazaki et al,[69] the 5-year local control was 92% for 2.25 Gy/day compared to 77% for 2.00 Gy/day ($p = 0.004$). The corresponding 5-year cause specific survival rates were 100% and 97%. Patient with the T2 lesion (especially bulky T2 lesions) should preferably be treated with hyperfractionation. A recently completed RTOG study has shown superiority of hyperfractionation over conventional fractionation.[70] The results are shown in Table 5-20. Patients with advanced stage lesions are mostly treated with concurrent radiation and chemotherapy as a preferred larynx preservation treatment. The results of recent published

Table 5–17. Piriform Sinus Cancer: Treatment Results

Author	No. of Patients	Therapy	Local Tumor Control			5-yr survival		
			T1-T2	T3-T4	Overall	T1-T2	T3-T4	All Patients
Bataini[59]	434	RT	67%	33%	47%	26%	17%	19%*
Mendenhall[60]	50	RT + ND	74%	26%	49%	60%†	23%†	49%†
	53	S + RT	4/6	72%	25%	43%†	24%†	25%†
	8	RT (bid)	3/4	1/4				
Dubois[61]	209	RT	73%	34%	25%	11%	3%	5%
	154	S + RT	43%§	33%§	35%§	37%§	30%§	33%§
El-Badawi[62]	48	RT	—	—	75%			
	125	S + RT	—	—	89%			47%
Vandenbrouck[63]	152	RT	77‡	49‡	45%	—	—	(3 yr) 25%
	198	S + RT			80%	—	—	3%
Marks[64]	137	RT + S	—	—	72%	—	—	→43%
Samant[65]	23	Chemo + RT**			92%***			23%
Garden[66]	82	RT + RND	79%			52%		
Chevalier[67]	49#	CS + RT	98%			47%		

RT, radiation therapy; S, surgery; ND, neck dissection; qd, daily; bid, twice daily.

*Determinate 5-year survival: 41%.

†Determinate survival.

§Locoregional.

‡Evaluation at last follow-up: 91 of 153 had complete response; subsequently, 22 had recurrences with eventual local control of 69 of 152 (45%).

**Intra-arterial chemotherapy.

***Reported endpoint is clinical complete response (not 5-year local control).

#Early lateral margin tumors.

Table 5–18. Early Laryngeal Cancer

T_{is} Glottic Treatment: XRT (31% have had ≥1 stripping)

No. of Patients	5-year Local Control
67	98%

Source: Data from ref 68 Spayne et al. IJROBP 49(5):1235, 2001.

larynx preservation trials are shown in Table 5–20. Subgroup of patients with glottic T3 tumors who are clinically and radiographically N0 at presentation and whose surgical alternate would have been total laryngectomy, are treated with hyperfractionation radiation therapy at our institution with minimum 2-year follow-up; 17 of 19 patients are alive, NED with preserved larynx, and excellent voice quality.[71]

Supraglottic Larynx

Primary management of supraglottic laryngeal cancers are highly individualized based on the epicenter of the primary tumor, stage of the primary tumor,

Table 5–19. T1 T2 Cancer of Glottic Larynx: Results of Radiotherapy

Author (yr)	No of Patients	Stage	% Ultimate % LC	LC	% CSS	% OS	Median FU
Mendenhall et al	230	T_{1a}	94	98	98	82	9.9 yr
	61	T_{1b}	93	98	98	79	9.9 yr
	146	T_{2a}	80	96	95	77	9.9 yr
	82	T_{2b}	72	96	90	77	9.9 yr
Garden et al	114	T_{2a}	74	—	—	—	6.8 yr
	116	T_{2b}	70	—	—	—	6.8 yr
	230	T_2	72	91	92	73	6.8 yr

Abbreviations: LC: local control; CSS: cause-specific survival; OS: overall survival; FU: follow-up.
Source: Modified from Mendenhall et al (ref 72). *Cancer.* 2004; 100(9):1766–1792.

Table 5–20. A Randomized Trial of Hyperfractionation Versus Standard Fractionation in T2 Squamous Cell Carcinoma of the Vocal Fold

Five-year Rates	SFX	HFX	*p*-value
Endpoint	% (95% CI)	% (95% CI)	
Local control	70 (62, 79)	79 (71, 87)	0.11
Disease-free survival	37 (27, 46)	51 (41,61)	0.07
Overall survival	62 (52, 72)	73 (64, 82)	0.19

Abbreviations: SFX: Standard fractionation; HFX: hyperfraction.
Source: Data from Trotti et al (ref 70).

presence or absence of cervical nodes, and status of pulmonary functions. Small epiglottic cancers can be treated with surgery alone (provided clean surgical margins). Otherwise radiation therapy is the preferred mode of therapy for T1 tumors of supraglottic larynx. In patients with good pulmonary functions who present with T2 to T3 supraglottic laryngeal cancers and normal vocal fold mobility, supraglottic laryngectomy followed by postoperative radiation therapy is the treatment of choice. In patients with medically inoperable, radiation therapy alone or concurrent chemoradiotherapy should be considered. For advanced laryngeal lesions with fixed vocal fold, concurrent chemoradiotherapy is the treatment of choice (Table 5-21).

The standard treatment for T4 tumors is total laryngectomy with postoperative radiation treatment. Management of nodes are dependent on clinically/radiographically determined presence of cervical nodal metastasis. For N0 patients, radiotherapy can achieve excellent control. Patients with clinically positive nodes should be treated with neck dissection followed by postoperative radiation therapy and/or radiochemotherapy in high-risk groups, such as patients with extranodal extension.

Paranasal Sinuses

Although surgery alone may be adequate for very uncommon T1 tumors, combination of surgery followed by postoperative radiation therapy is the standard treatment for T2 to T4 tumors (Table 5–22). Due to the complex anatomy of this region and var- ied pattern of local extensions to the base of skull, orbital structures, and so forth, intensity modulated radiotherapy (IMRT) is essential for radiotherapeutic

Table 5–21. RTOG Larynx Preservation Trial

Treatment Arm	No of Patients	Local control (%)	% Loco-Regional Control	5-yr* OFS	% Larynx 5-yr* OS	Preservation Rate
I-Radiation alone (QD fractionation)	173	101 (58)	56	27	56	70
II-Induction chemo followed by radiation	173	112 (64)	61	38	55	72
III-Concurrent chemoradiation	172	137 (80)	78	36	54	88

*Estimate

DFS = Disease-free survival; OS = Overall survival.

Note: Median follow-up 3.8 years.

Source: Data from Chen AM, et al (ref 73). *Int J Radiat Oncol Biol Phys.* 2006;66:1044–1050.

Table 5–22. Results of Treatment in Carcinoma of Paranasal Sinuses

Author (ref)	No of Patients	Primary Site	Treatment	% LC	% 5-yr CSS	% 5-yr OS
Katz et al[74]	78	Mixed	RT	49	56	50
			S + RT	79		
Jiang et al[75]	34	Ethmoid	RT	64	63	55
			S + RT	74		
Waldron et al[76]	29	Ethmoid	RT	41	58	39
Jiang et al[77]	73	Maxillary	S + RT	78	64	48
Paulino et al[78]	48	Maxillary	RT	23	42	47
			S + RT	59		
Bristol et al[81]	146	Maxillary	S + RT	70	57	51
			S + RT*	82	76	62
Hawkins et al[79]	62	Nasal cavity	RT	49	47	52
			S + RT	85		
Ang et al[80]	45	Nasal cavity	RT **	85	83	75
			S + RT**			

*After improved dosimetry.

**27 patients S + RT and 18 patients RT alone.

RT: radiotherapy; S: Surgery; LC: local control; CSS: cause specific survival; OS: overall survival.

management of this group of patients (Fig 5-6 and Table 5-23). Although IMRT for paranasal malignancies does not appear to significantly improve disease control, the complication rates in all three reports ore significantly lower than reports from 2D radiotherapy techniques.

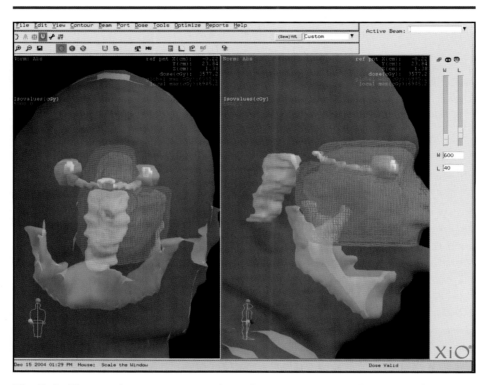

Fig 5–6. Dose volume representation of postoperative radiotherapy (IMRT) in a patient with paranasal cancer. *Note:* complete sparing of both optic nerves and chiasm.

Table 5–23. Results of IMRT in Treatment of Cancers of Paranasal Sinuses

Author (ref)	No of Patients	Tx	% LC (5 yr)	CSS (5 yr)	OS (5 yr)
Daly[82]	36	S + RT	58	55	45
Duthoy et al[83]	39	S + RT	68*	—	59*
Nagda et al[85]	54†	S + RT	75**		75**
	13pt‡	S + RT	92***	64***	90***

*4 year results.

**2 year results.

***3 year results.

†All histologies.

‡Adenoid cystic.

Abbreviations: LC: Local control; CSS: cause-specific survival; OS; overall survival; S: surgery; RT: radiotherapy.

Salivary Gland

Malignant tumors of salivary glands are best treated with surgery followed by postoperative radiation therapy. In a recent report by Tehaard et al[84] on 565 patients with salivary gland carcinomas the 10-year local control with surgery and surgery with postoperative radiotherapy was 76% and 90%, respectively ($p = 0.0005$). Postoperative radiation therapy even in the case of a negative prognostic factors has resulted in increased long-term local regional control. In another reanalysis of the report by Tehaard et al,[84] the significant improvement with postoperative radiotherapy was for both positive and close surgical margins.[84] Although surgery alone is considered adequate therapy for completely resected pleomorphic adenomas, management of recurrences of this pathology is still controversial. General surgical consensus is that repeated surgeries in this group of patients are justified, whereas most radiation oncologists recommend postoperative radiation therapy after first recurrence. In cases inoperable or unresectable salivary gland tumors, it has been postulated that these tumors are radioresistant. Review of literature reveals the fallacy of this perception. Tehaard et al[84] reported on 44 such patients treated with radiation therapy alone. With doses of over 66 Gy, 50% local regional control was achieved. Chen et al[73] achieved 70% 5-year local regional control in 44 patients treated with radiation therapy alone.

In summary, patients with head and neck cancer should be evaluated and treated with a multidisciplinary team of surgeons, radiation oncologists, and medical oncologists who are specialized in head and neck oncology. Although published clinical results can be used as a general guide, individualization of treatment strategy play an important role in management of these patients.

REFERENCES

1. *ICUR-50 Prescribing, Recording, and Reporting Photon Beam Therapy*. Bethesda, Md: International Commission on Radiation Units and Measurements; 1993.

2. Kaplan HS. Biochemical basis of reproductive death in irradiated cells. *AJR Am J Roentgenol*. 1963;90: 907–916.

3. Terasima T, Tolmach LJ. Variations in several responses of Hela cells to x-irradiation during division cycle. *Biophysical J*. 1963;3:11–33.

4. Gray LH. Radiobiologic basis of oxygen as modifying factor in radiation therapy. *AJR Am J Roentgenol*. 1961;85:803–815.

5. Suit HD, Shalek RJ. Response of anoxic C3H mouse mammary carcinoma isotransplants (1-25 MM3) to x-irradiation. *J Natl Cancer Inst*. 1963;31:479–493.

6. Kallman RF. The phenomenon of reoxygenation and its implications for fractionated radiation therapy. *Radiology*. 1972;105:135–142.

7. Horiot JC, Lefur RN, Guyen T, et al. Hyperfractionation versus conventional fractionation in oropharyngeal carcinoma: final analysis of a randomized trial of the EORTC cooperative group of radiotherapy. *Radiother Oncol*. 1992;25:231–241.

8. Overgaard J, Hansen HS, Specht L, et al. Five compared with six fractions per week of conventional radiotherapy of squamous-cell carcinoma of head and neck: DAHANCA 6 and 7 randomized controlled trial. *Lancet*. 2003;362:933–940.

9. Fu KK, Pajak TF, Trotti A, et al. A radiation therapy oncology group (RTOG) phase III randomized study to compare hyperfractionation and two variants of accelerated fractionation to standard fractionation radiotherapy for head and neck squamous cell carcinomas: first report of RTOG 9003. *Int J Radiat Oncol Biol Phys*. 2000;48:7–16.

10. Mendenhall WM, Riggs CE, et al. Altered fractionation and/or adjuvant chemotherapy in definitive irradiation of squamous cell carcinoma of the head and neck. *Laryngoscope*. 2003;113:546–551.

11. Pignon JP, Bourhis J, Domenge C, Deisgne L, on behalf of the MACH-NC Collaborative Group. Chemotherapy added to locoregional treatment for head and neck squamous-cell carcinoma: three meta-analyses of updated individual data. *Lancet*. 2000;255:949–955.

12. Baujat B, Audry H, Bourhis J, et al. Chemotherapy in locally advanced nasopharyngeal carcinoma: an individual patient data meta-analysis of eight randomized trials and 1753 patients. *Int J Radiat Oncol Biol Phys*. 2006;64:47–56.

13. Emami B, Melo A, Carter BL, Munzenrider JE, Piro AJ. Value of computed tomography in radiotherapy of lung cancer. *Am J Roentgenol*. 1978;131:63–67.

14. Purdy JA, Emami B. 3D *Radiation Treatment Planning and Conformal Therapy: Internal Sympo-*

sium Proceedings. Madison, Wisc: Medical Physics Publishing; 1993.

15. Chao KSC, Ozyigit G, eds. *Intensity Modulated Radiation Therapy for Head and Neck Cancer.* Philadelphia, Pa: Lippincott Williams & Wilkins; 2003.

16. Chao KSC, Low DA, Perez CA, et al. Intensity-modulated radiation therapy in head and neck cancers: the Mallinckrodt experience. *Int J Cancer.* 2000; 90:92–103.

17. Lee N, Xia P, Quivey JM, et al. Intensity-modulated radiotherapy in the treatment of nasopharyngeal carcinoma: an update of the UCSF experience. *Int J Radiat Oncol Biol Phys.* 2002;53:12.

18. Chao KS, Ozyigit G, Blanco AI, et al. Intensity-modulated radiation therapy for oropharyngeal carcinoma: impact of tumor volume. *Int J Radiat Oncol Biol Phys.* 2004;59:43.

19. Eisbruch A. Intensity-modulated radiation therapy in the treatment of head and neck cancer. *Nature Clin Pract Oncol.* 2005;2(1):34–39.

20. Kam MK, Teo PM, Chau RM, et al. Treatment of nasopharyngeal carcinoma with intensity-modulated radiotherapy: the Hong Kong experience. *Int J Radiat Oncol Biol Phys.* 2004; 60:1440.

21. Kwong DL, Pow EH, Sham JS, et al. Intensity-modulated radiotherapy for early-stage nasopharyngeal carcinoma: a prospective study on disease control and preservation of salivary function. *Cancer.* 2004;101:1584.

22. Hall EJ, Wuu CS. Radiation-induced second cancers: the impact of 3D-CRT and IMRT. *Int J Radiat Oncol.* 2003;56(1);83–88.

23. MacKay E, Sellers A. A statistical review of carcinoma of the lip. *CMAJ.* 1964;90:670–672.

24. Baker S, Kraus C. Carcinoma of the lip. *Laryngoscope.* 1980;90:19–27.

25. Mohs F, Snow S. Microscopically controlled surgical treatment for squamous cell carcinoma of the lower lip. *Surg Gynecol Obstet.* 1985;160:37–41.

26. Cooper JS, Pajak TF, Forastiere AA, et al. Postoperative concurrent radiotherapy and chemotherapy for high-risk squamous-cell carcinoma of the head and neck. *N Engl J Med.* 2004;350:1937–1944.

27. Lefebvre J, Coche-Dequeant B, Castelain B, et al. Interstitial brachytherapy and early tongue squamous cell carcinoma management. *Head Neck.* 1990;12:232–236.

28. Shibuya H, Hoshina M, Takeda M, et al. Brachytherapy for stage I and II oral tongue cancer: an analysis of past cases focusing on control and complications. *Int J Radiat Oncol Biol Phys.* 1993;26:51–58.

29. Wendt C, Peters L, Delclos L, et al. Primary radiotherapy in the treatment of stage I and II oral tongue cancers; importance of the proportion of therapy delivered with interstitial therapy. *Int J Radiat Oncol Biol Phys.* 1990;18:1287–1292.

30. Horiuchi J. Okuyana T. Shibuya H, et al. Results of brachytherapy for cancer of the tongue with special emphasis on local prognosis. *Int J Radiat Oncol Biol Phys.* 1982;8:829–835.

31. Decroix Y, Ghossein N. Experience of the Curie Institute in treatment of cancer of the mobile tongue: I. Treatment policies and results. *Cancer.* 1981;47:496.

32. Mazeron J, Crook J, Benck V, et al. Iridium 192 implantation of T1 and T2 carcinomas of the mobile tongue. *Int J Radiat Oncol Biol Phys.* 1990;19:1369–1376.

33. Rodgers LJ, Stringer S, Mendenhall W, et al. Management of squamous cell carcinoma of the floor of mouth. *Head Neck.* 1993;15:16–19.

34. Mazeron J, Grimard L, Raynal M, et al. Iridium-192 curietherapy for T1 and T2 Epidermoid carcinomas of the floor of mouth. *Int J Radiat Oncol Biol Phys.* 1990;18:1299–1306.

35. Matsumoto S, Takeda M, Shibuya H, et al. T1 and T2 squamous cell carcinoma of the floor of the mouth: results of brachytherapy mainly using 198Au grains. *Int J Radiat Oncol Biol Phys.* 1996;34:833–841.

36. Nason R, Sako K, Beecroft W, et al. Surgical management of squamous cell carcinoma of the floor of mouth. *Am J Surg.* 1989;158:292–296.

37. Pernot M, Luporsi E, Hoffstetter S, et al. Complications following definitive irradiation for cancers of the oral cavity and the oropharynx (in a series of 1134 patients). *Int J Radiat Oncol Biol Phys.* 1997;37:577–585.

38. Ang KK, Garden AS, eds. *Radiotherapy for Head and Neck Cancers, Indications and Techniques.* 3rd ed. Philadelphia, Pa: Lippincott Williams & Wilkins; 2006.

39. Al-Sarraf M, LeBlanc M, Giri PG, et al. Chemotherapy versus radiotherapy in patients with advanced nasopharyngeal cancer: phase II randomized intergroup study 0099. *J Clin Oncol.* 1998;16:1310.

40. Chan ATC, Teo PM, Leung TW, et al. Overall survival after concurrent cisplatin-radiotherapy compared with radiotherapy alone in locoregional advanced nasopharyngeal carcinoma. *J Natl Cancer Inst.* 2005;97:536–539.

41. Lin JC, Jan JS, Hsu CY, et al. Phase III study of concurrent chemoradiotherapy alone for advanced nasopharyngeal carcinoma: positive effect on

overall and progression-free survival. *J Clin Oncol.* 2003;21:631–637.

42. Wee J, Eng HT, Tai BC, et al. Randomized trial of radiotherapy versus concurrent chemoradiotherapy followed adjuvant chemotherapy in patients with American Joint Committee on Cancer/International Union Against Cancer Stage III and IV Nasopharyngeal Cancer of the Endemic Variety. *J Clin Oncol.* 2005;23(27), 6730–6738.

43. Emami B, Clark J, Mirkovic N, Crossan P, Petruzzelli G. Modern management of advanced squamous cell cancer of nasopharynx: preliminary results. 5th International Conference on Head and Neck Cancer. San Francisco, Calif; 2000.

44. Garden AS, Asper JA, Morrison WH, et al. Is concurrent chemoradiation the treatment of choice for all patients with stage III or IV head and neck carcinoma? *Cancer.* 2004;100:1171.

45. Haung K, Le N, Xia P. Intensity-modulated radiotherapy in the treatment of oropharyngeal carcinoma: a single institutional experience. *Int J Radiat Oncol Biol Phys.* 2003;57:S302.

46. DeArruda FF, Puri DR, Zhung J, et al. Intensity-modulated radiation therapy for the treatment of oropharyngeal carcinoma: the Memorial Sloan-Kettering Cancer Center Experience. *Int J Radiat Oncol Biol Phys.* 2006;64(2);363–373.

47. Mendenhall WM, Amdur RJ, Stringer SP, et al. Radiation therapy for squamous cell carcinoma of the tonsillar region: a preferred alternative to surgery? *J Clin Oncol.* 2000;18:2219.

48. Bernier J, Cooper JS, Pajak TF. Defining risk levels in locally advanced head and neck cancers: a comparative analysis of concurrent postoperative radiation plus chemotherapy trials of the EORTC (#22931) and RTOG (#9501). *Head Neck.* 2005; 27:843–850.

49. Rengan R, Pfister DG, Lee NY, Kraus D, et al. *Long-term neck control rates after complete response to chemoradiation in patients with advanced head and neck cancer.* 2007 Multidisciplinary Head and Neck Cancer Symposium; Rancho Mirage, Calif; 2007.

50. Foote RL, Olsen KD, Davis DL, et al. Base of tongue carcinoma: patterns of failure and predictors of recurrence after surgery alone. *Head Neck.* 1993; 15:300–307.

51. Kraus DH, Vastola P, Huvos AG, et al. Surgical management of squamous cell carcinoma of the base of the tongue. *Am J Surg.* 1993;166:384.

52. Mak AC, Morrison WH, Garden AS, et al. Base of tongue carcinoma: treatment results using concomitant boost radiotherapy. *Int J Radiat Oncol Biol Phys.* 1995;33(2):289–296.

53. Hinerman RW, Parsons JT, Mendenhall WM, et al. External beam irradiation alone or combined with neck dissection for base of tongue carcinoma: an alternative to primary surgery. *Laryngoscope.* 1994;104:1466.

54. Riley RW, Lee WE, Goffinet D, et al. Squamous cell carcinoma of the base of the tongue. *Arch Otolaryngol Head Neck Surg.* 1983;91:143.

55. Thawley SE, Simpson JR, Perez CA, et al. Preoperative irradiation and surgery for carcinoma of the base of the tongue. *Ann Otol Rhinol Laryngol.* 1983;92:485.

56. Moez-Mendez RT, Fletcher GH, Guillamondeque OM. Analysis of the results of irradiation in the treatment of squamous cell carcinoma of the pharyngeal wall. *Int J Radiat Oncol Biol Phys.* 1978; 4:579.

57. Mendenhall WM, Parsons JT, Mancuso AA, et al. Squamous cell carcinoma of the pharyngeal wall treated with irradiation. *Radiother Oncol.* 1988; 11:205–212.

58. Emami B, Marks JE, Senunus L, et al. Carcinoma of the pharyngeal wall. *Proceedings of the Second World Congress on Laryngeal Cancer*, Amsterdam, The Netherlands; 1994.

59. Bataini P, Brugere J. Berniere J. Results of radical radiotherapeutic treatment of carcinoma of the pyriform sinus. *Int J Radiat Oncol Biol Phys.* 1982;8:1277.

60. Mendenhall WM, Parsons JT, Stringer SP, et al. Radiotherapy alone or combined with neck dissection for T1–T2 carcinoma of the pyriform sinus: an alternative to conservation surgery. *Int J Radiat Oncol Biol Phys.* 1993;27:1017–1027.

61. Dubois JB, Guerrier B, DiRuggeriero JM, et al. Cancer of the piriform sinus: treatment by radiation therapy alone and after surgery. *Radiology.* 1986; 160:831.

62. El-Badawi SA, Goepfert H, Fletcher GH. Squamous cell carcinoma of the piriform sinus. *Laryngoscope.* 1982;92:357.

63. Vandenbrouck C, Eschwege F, DeLa Rochefordiere A. Squamous cell carcinoma of the pyriform sinus: Retrospective study of 351 cases treated at the Institute Gustave-Roussy. *Head Neck Surg.* 1987; 10:4.

64. Marks JE, Spector JG. Hypopharynx. In: Perez CA, Brady LW, eds. *Principles and Practice of Radiation Oncology.* 2nd ed. Philadelphia, Pa: JB Lippincott; 1992.

65. Samant S, Kumar P, Wan J, et al. Concomitant radiation therapy and targeted cisplatin chemotherapy for the treatment of advanced pyriform sinus carcinoma: disease control and preservation of organ function. *Head Neck.* 1999;21:595–601.

66. Garden AS, Morrison WH, Clayman GL, et al. Early squamous cell carcinoma of the hypopharynx: outcomes of treatment with radiation alone to the primary disease. *Head Neck.* 1996;18:317–322.

67. Chevalier D. Supraglottic hemilaryngopharyngectomy plus radiation for treatment of early lateral margin and piriform sinus carcinoma. *Head Neck.* 1997;19:1–5.

68. Spayne JA, Warde P, O'Sullivan B, Payne D, et al. Carcinoma-in-situ of the glottic larynx: results of treatment with radiation therapy. *Int J Radiat Oncol Biol Phys.* 2001;49(5):1235–1238.

69. Yamazaki H, Nishiyama K, Tanaka E, et al. Radiotherapy for early glottic carcinoma (T1N0M0): results of prospective randomized study of radiation fraction size and overall treatment time. *Int J Radiat Oncol Biol Phys.* 2006;64(1):77–82.

70. Trotti A, Pajak T, Emami B, et al. A randomized trial of hyperfractionation versus standard fractionation in T2N0 carcinoma of the vocal cord. *Int J Radiat Oncol Biol Phys.* 2006;66(3):S15.

71. Garza R, Emami B, Petruzzelli G. Hyperfractionated radiation therapy of T3 laryngeal carcinoma: single institution experience. Submitted for publication.

72. Mendenhall WM, Wering JW, Hinerman RW, et al. Management of T1–T2 glottic carcinomas. *Cancer.* 2004;100:1786–1792.

73. Chen AM, Bucci MK, Quivey JM, et al. Long-term outcomes of patients treated by radiation therapy alone for salivary gland carcinomas. *Int J Radiat Oncol Biol Phys.* 2006;66:1044–1050.

74. Katz TS, Mendehnall WM, Morris CG, et al. Malignant tumors of the nasal cavity and paranasal sinuses. *Head Neck.* 2002;24:821–829.

75. Jiang GI, Morrison WH, Garden AS, et al. Ethmoid sinus carcinomas: natural history and treatment results. *Radiother Oncol.* 1998;49:21–27.

76. Waldron JN, O'Sullivan B, Warde P, et al. Ethmoid sinus cancer: twenty-nine cases managed with primary radiation therapy. *Int J Radiat Oncol Biol Phys.* 1998;41:361–369.

77. Jiang GL, Ang KK, Peters LJ, et al. Maxillary sinus carcinomas: natural history and results of postoperative radiotherapy. *Radiother Oncol.* 1991;21: 193–200.

78. Paulino AC, Fisher SG, Marks JE. Is prophylactic neck irradiation indicated in patients with squamous cell carcinoma of the maxillary sinus? *Int J Radiat Oncol Biol Phys.* 1997;39:283–289.

79. Hawkins RB, Wynstra JH, Pilepich MV, et al. Carcinoma of the nasal cavity—results of primary and adjuvant radiotherapy. *Int J Radiat Oncol Biol Phys.* 1988;15:1129–1133.

80. Ang KK, Jiang GL, Frankenthaler RA, et al. Carcinomas of the nasal cavity. *Radiother Oncol.* 1992; 24:163–168.

81. Bristol IJ, Ahamad A, Garden AS, et al. Postoperative radiotherapy for maxillary sinus cancer: long-term outcomes and toxicities of treatment. *Int J Radiat Oncol Biol Phys.* 2007;68:719–730.

82. Daly ME, Chen AM, Bucci K, et al. Intensity-modulated radiation therapy for malignancies of the nasal cavity and paranasal sinuses. *Int J Radiat Oncol Biol Phys.* 2007;67:151–157.

83. Duthoy W, Boterbert T, Claus F, et al. Postoperative intensity-modulated radiotherapy in sinonasal carcinoma. Clinical results in 39 patients. *Cancer.* 2005;104:71–82.

84. Terhaard CHJ. *Postoperative and primary radiotherapy for salivary gland carcinomas: indications, techniques and results.* 2007 Multidisciplinary Head and Neck Cancer Symposium. Rancho Mirage, Calif; 2007.

85. Nagda SN, Emami B, Pederson A, et al. Target volume delineation and conformal radiation therapy in the management of adenoid cystic carcinoma of the paranasal sinuses. [Abstract]. Fourth International Symposium on Malignancies of the Chest and Head and Neck. *J Thorac Oncol.* 2006;1:915.

6

Principles of Chemotherapy in Head and Neck Oncology

Cheryl Czerlanis
Joseph I. Clark

SYSTEMIC CHEMOTHERAPY FOR HEAD AND NECK MALIGNANCIES

Chemotherapy has emerged as a vital element of the multimodality approach to the treatment of squamous cell cancers of the head and neck (SCCHN). The role of chemotherapy varies according to the disease stage. For patients with potentially curable locoregionally advanced SCCHN, chemotherapy is used as an adjunct to other treatment modalities. Chemotherapeutic approaches that have been investigated include induction, or neoadjuvant chemotherapy, concurrent chemoradiotherapy, adjuvant systemic therapy, or a combined approach. In patients with metastatic or advanced, recurrent locoregional disease that is otherwise incurable, chemotherapy is utilized with palliative intent. This chapter reviews the role of systemic cytotoxic chemotherapy and targeted agents in the treatment of SCCHN.

LOCOREGIONALLY ADVANCED DISEASE

The majority of patients present with locally or regionally advanced disease.[1] The historic treatment for patients with stage III or IV disease involved a combination of surgery and postoperative radiation therapy if tumor resection was feasible, versus radiation therapy alone. Despite improvements in local treatments, the overall prognosis was poor due to low rates of locoregional control.[2] In an attempt to improve outcomes, strategies to integrate chemotherapy into the multimodality approach for the treatment of locally advanced disease were introduced.

NEOADJUVANT (INDUCTION) CHEMOTHERAPY

The sensitivity of SCCHN to chemotherapy in recurrent and metastatic tumors led investigators to study single-agent and combination chemotherapy agents earlier in the disease course as part of the multimodality approach. The rationale for induction, or neoadjuvant, chemotherapy, was to achieve the following theoretical benefits: gain the ability to increase locoregional control by diminishing the disease burden prior to the definitive intervention; decrease the development of distant metastatic disease; improve organ preservation rates; and perhaps lead to a survival benefit.[3]

Some chemotherapy regimens have been associated with complete response rates of 30% and overall response rates of 90% in untreated patients.[4]

However, responses are transient and definitive surgery and/or radiation therapy is needed for locoregional control. The combination of 5-fluorouracil (5-FU) and cisplatin in the neoadjuvant setting in locally advanced head and neck cancer, showed disease activity, but the majority of the trials did not yield a definitive survival benefit.[5-9] Two phase III trials that showed a survival benefit from induction chemotherapy are discussed below.

A phase III study by the Gruppo di Studio sui Tumori della Testa e del Collo (GSTTC) randomized patients to receive either induction chemotherapy (cisplatin and infusional 5-FU) followed by locoregional treatment or locoregional treatment alone.[10] Local therapy included surgery and subsequent radiotherapy for patients with resectable disease or radiotherapy alone for those with unresectable disease. In a subset of patients with *unresectable* and inoperable disease only, there was a benefit in terms of disease-free survival and overall survival attributed to chemotherapy. The group who received chemotherapy had an improvement in the time to distant metastases regardless of operability. In this arm, there was a reduction in the 3-year estimate of distant metastases from 38% to 14% (*p* = .002). Other studies suggest that that there is a decrease in distant metastases related to induction chemotherapy,[6,11] and locoregional relapse represents the pattern of disease failure in this population.

The Groupe d'Etude des Tumeurs de la Tete Et du Cou (GETTEC) conducted a randomized phase III trial that enrolled a total of 318 patients with squamous cell oropharyngeal cancer between 1986 and 1992.[12] Patients were randomized to neoadjuvant cisplatin and infusional 5-FU followed by locoregional treatment versus the same locoregional treatment without chemotherapy. Overall survival was significantly better in the neoadjuvant chemotherapy arm than in the control group, with a median survival of 5.1 years versus 3.3 years (*p* = .03).

Despite these results and the fact that phase II trials showed high response rates, a number of phase III trials failed to show a survival benefit for neoadjuvant chemotherapy.[11,13,14] The benefit of adding chemotherapy to local treatment strategies in patients with advanced SCCHN has been determined by meta-analyses. Multiple meta-analyses have not shown a survival benefit specifically for neoadjuvant chemotherapy,[15,19] although a benefit for chemoradiotherapy was supported. The Meta-Analysis of Chemotherapy on Head and Neck Cancer (MACH-NC) trial performed a pooled analysis of 10,741 patients from 63 trials that were reported from 1965 to 1993.[16] Chemotherapy was associated with an improvement in survival (4% at 5 years) in nonmetastatic SCCHN treated by locoregional treatment, although there was no significant benefit associated specifically with neoadjuvant chemotherapy. A higher benefit (8%) was attributed to concomitant chemoradiotherapy. The updated data presented as ASCO in 2004 added new studies done from 1994 to 2000, to include an additional 24 trials with a combined total of 16,000 patients.[19] The newer trials focused mainly on concomitant chemoradiotherapy approaches. The updated pooled analysis validated a survival benefit of 8% at 5 years in the concomitant chemoradiotherapy trials (*p* ≤ .0001). An evaluation of the types of chemotherapy found that the magnitude of benefit for platinum-based chemotherapy was associated with an overall lower risk for death compared to other chemotherapy regimens (hazard ratio [HR] for death 0.88, 95% CI, 0.79–0.97). There was no benefit for multidrug regimens versus single-agent chemotherapy.

Whether the addition of taxanes to current cisplatin and 5-FU-containing regimens will improve the outlook for neoadjuvant therapy remains under investigation. The clinical activity of single-agent docetaxel and paclitaxel was established in several phase II trials done in patients with advanced or recurrent head and neck cancer,[20-24] with response rates ranging from 21 to 42%. The most common grade 3 or 4 toxicity was neutropenia.

The EORTC trial 24971 enrolled patients with unresectable stage III or IV SCCHN and randomized 358 patients to receive PF (cisplatin 100 mg/m^2 on day 1, and continuous infusion (CI) 5-FU 1000 mg/m^2 daily on days 1 to 5) or TPF (docetaxel 75 mg/m^2 on day 1, cisplatin 75 mg/m^2 on day 1, and CI 5-FU 750 mg/m^2 daily on days 1 to 5) every 21 days.[25] The treatment protocol included four cycles of chemotherapy, unless disease progression or unacceptable toxicity occurred during the treatment period. The induction chemotherapy was followed by a protocol-defined radiotherapy regimen in all patients who did not have evidence of disease progression during the study period. With a median follow-up of 32 months, progression-free survival was significantly improved with TPF versus PF (median 8.2 versus 11.0 months, HR 0.72; p = .0071). At a median follow-up of 51 months, there was also a significant improvement in median overall survival in the TPF group (median 14.2 versus 18.6 months, HR 0.71; p = .0052). Three-year overall survival rates were estimated at 23.9% (95% CI 17.9–30.5) for the PF arm and 36.5% (95% CI 29.3–43.6) for the TPF arm. The rate of grade 3 and 4 leucopenia and neutropenia was higher with TPF and severe thrombocytopenia was more common in the PF arm.

In the TAX-324 trial, patients with oral cavity, oropharynx, larynx, or hypopharynx cancer were randomized to receive either standard PF (cisplatin 100 mg/m-2 and CI 5-FU 1000 mg/m^2/day for 5 days) or TPF (docetaxel 75 mg/m^2, cisplatin 100 mg/m^2, and 5-FU 1000 mg/m^2 daily for 4 days) every 3 weeks for up to three cycles.[26] The neoadjuvant chemotherapy was followed by radiation therapy concurrent with weekly carboplatin (AUC 1.5). Three-year survival data indicate that there was a significant survival advantage in favor of TPF over PF (62% vs 48%, HR 0.70; p = .058). The absolute toxicities were comparable in both arms. Stomatitis, the dose-limiting toxicity, was less common in the docetaxel-containing arm.

An additional phase III trial included patients (n = 382) with previously untreated stage III or IV locally advanced SCCHN. Patients were randomized to receive PCF (paclitaxel 175 mg/m^2 on day 1, cisplatin 100 mg/m^2 on day 2, and CI 5-FU 500 mg/m^2 on days 2 through 6) versus CF (cisplatin 100 mg/m^2 on day 1, CI 5-FU 1,000 mg/m^2 on days 1 to 5).[27] Patients who achieved a complete response or a partial response of 80% of the initial tumor burden went on to receive chemoradiotherapy in both arms. The complete response rate was higher in the PCF group (33% vs 14%) and there was a nonsignificant trend toward an overall survival benefit. In patients with unresectable disease, overall survival was significantly improved (36 months versus 26 months, p = .04). Mucositis was more common in the CF arm.

NEOADJUVANT CHEMOTHERAPY— THE ROLE IN ORGAN PRESERVATION

Two large, randomized trials showed a benefit with respect to organ preservation with PF induction chemotherapy. The Veterans Affairs Laryngeal Cancer Study randomized 332 patients with previously untreated advanced (stage III or IV) laryngeal cancer to receive either induction chemotherapy (cisplatin and 5-FU) followed by definitive radiation versus conventional laryngectomy followed by postoperative radiation.[6] In the chemotherapy arm, there were more local recurrences (p = .0005) and fewer distant metastases (p = .016). Laryngeal preservation was achieved in 64% of the patients in the induction chemotherapy arm. The median survival was not altered between the treatment strategies.

An additional phase III prospective, randomized trial by the EORTC compared a larynx-preserving treatment to include induction chemotherapy plus definitive radiation therapy versus conventional therapy (total laryngectomy with partial pharyngectomy, radical neck dissection, and postoperative radiation) in patients with previously untreated cancers of the hypopharynx.[28] The chemotherapy arm received cisplatin and 5-FU for two cycles, after which partial or complete responders received a third cycle. Patients with a complete response after the second or third cycle were treated via irradiation (70 Gy), whereas nonresponders underwent conventional surgical resection with postoperative radiation (50–70 Gy). The induction chemotherapy arm led to preservation of the larynx in 42% of the patients and a decrease in failure rates at distant sites without a change in the overall survival.

CONCOMITANT CHEMORADIOTHERAPY FOR SCCHN

Chemoradiotherapy has been studied mainly as an alternative to radiation alone in advanced, unresectable SCCHN. Concomitant chemoradiotherapy has the potential advantage of eradication of the locoregional tumor burden with a synergistic radiosensitizer effect.

In addition, systemic chemotherapy can decrease micrometastatic disease. Chemotherapy also offers a survival advantage when given concomitantly or alternating with radiation therapy, regardless of tumor resectability, when compared with radiation alone.[7]

Multiple chemotherapeutic agents that have shown activity in SCCHN have been investigated in combination with radiation therapy, including methotrexate,[29,30] bleomycin,[31] mitomycin C,[31,31] 5-FU,[33-35] carboplatin, and cisplatin,[36] Randomized trials investigating single-agent cisplatin in concert with radiation have shown a benefit in terms of survival[37,38] and organ preservation.[36] Some of the phase III randomized trials that involve platinum-based agents, both as single and combination therapies in concurrent chemoradiation trials are summarized in Table 6-1.

The Intergroup RTOG 91-11 trial was a three-arm randomized trial that compared induction chemotherapy with cisplatin/5-FU followed by radiation therapy in patients who achieved a response, versus concomitant radiotherapy with single-agent cisplatin on days 1, 22, and 43, versus irradiation alone.[36] The trial enrolled 547 patients with stage III or IV

Table 6–1. Selected Phase III Randomized Trials with Concurrent Platinum-Based Chemoradiotherapy

	Resectable Disease (%)	Number of Patients	Concurrent Chemotherapy Regimen	Radiation regimen	3-year PFS (%)	3-year OS (%)
Wendt et al[64]	0	140	Arm A: None	H 70.2 Gy total dose— 1.8 Gy BID	NR	24
		130	Arm B: PF/LV	H 70.2 Gy total dose— 1.8 Gy BID		49 (p <.0003)
Brizel et al[65]	47	60	Arm A: None	H 75 Gy total dose— 1.25 Gy BID	41	34
		56	Arm B: PF	H 70 Gy total dose— 1.25 Gy BID	61 (p = .08)	55 (p = .07)
Adelstein et al[66]	100	50	Arm A: None	C 66-72 Gy total dose— 1.8–2 Gy daily	51 (5 yr)	48 (655 yr)
		50	Arm B: PF	C 66-72 Gy total dose— 1.8–2 Gy daily	62 (p = .04)	50 (p = .55) *NS
Jeremic et al[37]	NR	65	Arm A: None	H 77 Gy total dose— 1.1 Gy BID	25 (5 yr)	25 (5 yr)
		65	Arm B: P	H 77 Gy total dose— 1.1 Gy BID	46 (p =. 0068)	46 (p = .0075)
Al-Sarraf et al[38]	NR	69	Arm A: None	C 70 Gy total dose— 1.8–2 Gy daily	24	46
		78	Arm B: P	C 70 Gy total dose— 1.8–2 Gy daily	69 (p <.001)	76 (p <.001)
Calais et al[67]	NR	113	Arm A: None	C 70 Gy total dose— 2 Gy daily	20	31
		109	Arm B: CP/F	C 70 Gy total dose— 2 Gy daily	42 (p = .04)	51 (p = .02)

Abbreviations: NR, not recorded; P, cisplatin; F, 5-fluorouracil, CP, carboplatin; LV, leucovorin; PFS, progression-free survival; OS, overall survival; *NS, not significant.

resectable laryngeal cancer with a primary endpoint of larynx preservation. The laryngeal preservation rate favored the concomitant chemoradiotherapy arm, with laryngeal preservation in 84% of patients in the concomitant group versus 71% of patients in the induction chemotherapy arm and 66% in the radiation alone arm. Overall survival was similar in the three arms. There was no statistically significant benefit associated with induction chemotherapy plus RT over RT alone ($p = .27$). The authors concluded that concomitant chemoradiotherapy provided a benefit over a sequential chemoradiotherapy regimen and radiotherapy alone with regard to the primary trial endpoint, laryngeal preservation.

The value of a concurrent chemoradiotherapy regimen has been evaluated in several meta-analyses. As previously discussed, the updated MACH-NC collaborative meta-analysis showed a 19% reduction in the risk of death and an overall 8% improvement in 5-year survival with concurrent chemoradiotherapy compared with RT alone.[19] There was no advantage to multidrug over single-drug regimens. In addition, Browman et al. conducted a systematic analysis for the use of concomitant chemoradiotherapy in patients with locally advanced SCCHN.[39] A total of 18 randomized controlled trials involving 3,192 patients were evaluated in the pooled analysis; there was a reduction in mortality for concomitant therapy compared to RT alone (odds ratio [OR], 0.62; 95% CI 0.52–0.74; relative risk, 0.83; risk reduction, 11%; $p <.00001$). The magnitude of the benefit was higher for platinum-based chemotherapy regimens.

A third meta-analysis investigated concurrent chemotherapy with various radiotherapy regimens in a pooled analysis of 10,225 patients with unresectable locally advanced SCCHN.[40] Trials comparing RT alone with concurrent or alternating chemoradiation (5-FU, cisplatin, carboplatin, mitomycin C) were analyzed according to the radiation schedule (conventionally fractionated RT vs hyperfractionated RT vs accelerated RT) and the chemotherapy regimen. An overall survival benefit of 12.0 months was attributed to the addition of chemotherapy to radiation therapy of any type or schedule ($p< 0.001$). Radiation therapy combined with simultaneous 5-FU, cisplatin, carboplatin, and mitomycin C as a single drug or 5-FU-based chemotherapy multiagent regimens resulted in a survival advantage irrespective of the employed radiation schedule.

Further randomized studies are needed to determine the optimal combination or single-agent chemotherapeutic regimens, as well as the dose and schedule for concurrent chemoradiation approaches. In addition, the highly effective locoregional control achieved with concomitant chemoradiotherapy has led to an interest in whether the addition of induction chemotherapy in a sequential fashion would decrease distant metastases and improve survival.[41] Large, phase III multicenter trials are ongoing to investigate the role of induction chemotherapy prior to chemoradiotherapy.

ADJUVANT THERAPY IN PATIENTS WITH RESECTED HIGH-RISK DISEASE

Systemic chemotherapy after definitive locoregional control is designed to decrease both the occurrence of distant metastases and microscopic residual disease. In patients with pathologically high-risk locally or regionally advanced head and neck cancers that have been resected, adjuvant therapy has historically involved radiotherapy. Chemotherapy has been tested alone and in the context of adjuvant chemoradiotherapy in this setting. Early studies revealed that adjuvant chemotherapy alone was associated with a decrease in distant metastases, but no definite benefit in overall survival.[13,42] In the Intergroup study 0034,[42] eligible patients ($n = 442$) had completely resected tumors of the oral cavity, oropharynx, hypopharynx, or larynx. After surgical resection, they were randomized to receive either three cycles of cisplatin and 5-FU chemotherapy followed by postoperative radiotherapy (CT/RT) or postoperative radiotherapy alone (RT). There was a significant decrease in the overall incidence of distant metastases (23% on the RT arm vs 15% on the CT/RT arm; $p = .03$). However, there was no overall survival benefit, improvement in disease-free survival, or decrease in locoregional failure. A subgroup of high-risk patients was identified who showed a greater benefit in local control and survival; these patients had at least two positive neck lymph nodes, positive resection margins, and/or extracapsular extension.

Although there was no overall survival benefit, this trial had implications for the design of subsequent clinical trials.

Additional randomized trials have investigated the role of adjuvant chemoradiotherapy in high-risk patients. The EORTC phase III trial 22931 compared concomitant cisplatin and irradiation with radiotherapy alone as adjuvant treatment in patients with stage III or IV head and neck cancer.[43] Poor-risk characteristics were classified as oral cavity or oropharyngeal tumors with positive nodes at level IV or V, extracapsular extension, vascular embolism, and perineural involvement. Randomization occurred after patients underwent surgery with curative intent; 167 patients were randomized to receive radiotherapy alone (total dose of 66 Gy in conventionally fractionated doses of 2 Gy each over 6.5 weeks) and 167 to receive the same radiation regimen along with cisplatin 100 mg/m-2 on days 1, 22, and 43 of the radiation schedule. The primary endpoint of the trial was progression-free survival. After a median follow-up of 60 months, the rate of progression-free survival and overall survival showed a benefit in favor of the combined modality group. The estimated 5-year disease-free survival was 47% in the concomitant chemoradiotherapy group versus 36% in the radiotherapy alone group ($p = .04$). Grade 3 or higher adverse events were higher in the combined modality group (41% versus 21%; $p = .001$); however, the late toxicities were similar between the two arms. The incidence of local or regional relapses was lower in the chemoradiotherapy group ($p = .007$), but the addition of chemotherapy did not significantly affect the development of distant metastases.

An RTOG trial defined high-risk pathologic disease as two or more positive nodes, extracapsular extension, and insufficient (<5 mm) or positive resection margins.[44] The study design was similar to the EORTC trial; the chemotherapy regimens were identical and the radiation was delivered in a conventionally fractionated fashion, with a total dose of 60 to 66 Gy in 30 to 33 fractions over a period of 6 to 6.6 weeks. With a median follow-up of 45.9 months, the rate of local and regional control was significantly higher in the combined modality group compared to radiation therapy alone (HR for disease or death, 0.78; 95% CI 0.61 to 0.99; $p = .04$). The overall survival and rate of distant metastases were not significantly affected. The incidence of grade 3 or 4 adverse effects was 36% in the radiotherapy group and 77% in the combined modality group, including four deaths that were related to treatment. However, the presence of severe late toxicities was not increased by the addition of chemotherapy. In a joint analysis that combined the data from the EORTC and RTOG trials, risk factors for which there was an increased benefit to the addition of chemotherapy to radiation included nodal extracapsular extension and microscopically involved survival margins.[45]

In the postoperative setting, the management of high-risk patients needs to be further investigated with regard to the optimal regimen for both chemotherapy and radiation. The data suggest that there is better locoregional control with the postoperative chemoradiotherapy versus radiotherapy alone in high-risk patients; however, only the EORTC trial demonstrated a benefit in overall survival. In addition, the incidence of severe early adverse effects, namely, mucosal and hematologic events, was increased due to the addition of the chemotherapy. Due to the inherent increase in toxicity, it is important to optimize the delivery of the chemoradiotherapy and to identify the appropriate subgroup of patients in which to use this intervention. Further clinical trials are needed to determine the role of adjuvant chemotherapy in patients with SCCHN.

CHEMOTHERAPY FOR METASTATIC OR RECURRENT DISEASE

Despite advances in the multimodality treatment of patients with SCCHN, many patients present with or develop metastatic disease or incurable recurrent, advanced disease.[46] Many of the patients who develop disease recurrence will not be appropriate candidates for local therapy such as surgical salvage or radiation therapy. In this patient population, chemotherapy is utilized for palliation. Various cytotoxic chemotherapy drugs have activity in advanced head and neck cancer, including cisplatin, carboplatin, 5-FU, methotrexate, paclitaxel, and docetaxel. Several randomized trials have shown activity in a variety of chemotherapeutic drugs in this setting; however, there has been no sustainable survival benefit (Table 6–2).

Table 6–2. Selected Phase III Randomized Trials of Chemotherapy in Recurrent or Metastatic Squamous Cell Cancer of the Head and Neck

	Number of Patients	Chemotherapy Regimen	Overall Response Rate (%)	P value	Overall Survival (%)
Clavel et al[48]	382	Arm A: CABO	34	$p < .001$ over P	NS
		Arm B: PF	31	$p = .003$ over P	
		Arm C: P	15		
Forastiere et al[49]	277	Arm A: CF	32	$p < .001$ over MTX	NS
		Arm B: CP/F	21	$p = 0.05$ over MTX	
		Arm C: MTX	10		
Jacobs et al[68]	249	Arm A: PF	32		NS
		Arm B: P	17		
		Arm C: F	13		
Liverpool[47]	200	Arm A: P	14		NS
		Arm B: MTX	6		
		Arm C: PF	11		
		Arm D: P/MTX	12		

Abbreviations: CABO, cisplatin/methotrexate/bleomycin/vincristine; P, cisplatin; F, 5-fluorouracil, CP, carboplatin; MTX, methotrexate; NS, not significant.

Table 6–2 summarizes some of the phase III trials in chemotherapy in recurrent and metastatic SCCHN. Multiple randomized controlled trials have compared cisplatin-based combination chemotherapy to monotherapy. Although some have been associated with higher response rates, there has not been an associated survival benefit for the combination regimens in comparison to the single agent therapy.[47,51]

NOVEL TARGETED THERAPIES

The development of head and neck squamous cell carcinoma occurs as a result of the accumulation of genotypic and phenotypic alterations, including those related to the regulation of cell signaling pathways, angiogenesis, and apoptosis.[52] The epidermal growth factor receptor (EGFR), a member of the ErbB family of receptor tyrosine kinases, is an integral part of cell signaling pathways and regulation of cell growth. The EGFR and its ligand, transforming growth factor alpha (TGF-α), have been shown to be upregulated in the majority of squamous cell cancers of the head and neck, and to be associated with poor clinical outcome in some trials.[53-56] The EGFR is thus a rationale target for therapeutic intervention.

Cetuximab, a monoclonal antibody against EGFR, inhibits receptor activity by blocking the ligand binding site. In phase II trials, patients with recurrent or metastatic SCCHN and platinum-refractory disease, were treated with cetuximab (initial dose of 400 mg/m-2 followed by subsequent weekly doses of 250 mg/m-2) followed by the same dose and schedule of platinum chemotherapy at which progression of disease had occurred.[57,58] Overall response rates ranged from 10 to 12% in the platinum-refractory population. Cetuximab also produced objective responses in a multicenter phase II study designed to investigate the efficacy of cetuximab as monotherapy in patients with platinum-refractory SCCHN.[59] The most common toxicities were anemia, acneiform skin rash, leukopenia, fatigue and malaise, and nausea and vomiting.

The Eastern Cooperative Oncology Group (ECOG) conducted a phase III trial in which patients with recurrent or metastatic SCCHN were randomly assigned to receive cisplatin every 4 weeks, with either weekly cetuximab or placebo.[60] The objective response rate was 26% for the combination arm and 10% for the placebo-controlled arm (p = .03). Despite the improvement in response rate, the two groups did not differ with respect to progression-free survival, the primary endpoint, or overall survival. A correlation was noted between the development of a skin rash and an improvement in survival (p = .03).

The benefit of cetuximab as a radiosensitizer was tested in a multinational phase III trial in which patients with stage III or IV locoregionally advanced head and neck cancer were randomized to receive radiotherapy alone (n = 213) versus radiotherapy plus weekly cetuximab (n = 211).[61] The cetuximab was given at an initial dose of 400 mg/m-2 prior to radiation therapy, followed by weekly doses of 250 mg/m-2 during the course of radiotherapy. With a median follow-up of 54 months, the combination therapy group had a significant improvement in the median duration of locoregional control, the primary study endpoint (24.4 months in the cetuximab arm vs 14.9 months in the radiation alone arm, HR 0.68; p = .005). The progression-free survival and the median overall survival were better in the cetuximab-treated arm (OS 49.0 months vs 29.3 months, HR 0.74; p = .03). Cetuximab did exacerbate some of the adverse effects associated with radiation, including mucositis, xerostomia, dysphagia, pain, and weight loss; however, with the exception of acneiform rash and infusion-related events, the incidence of severe side-effects did not differ among the groups.

The FDA-approved indication for cetuximab is in combination with radiation therapy for patients with locally or regionally advanced SCCHN, or as a single agent in the treatment of metastatic or recurrent SCCHN that is refractory to platinum-based chemotherapy.

Early studies that investigated the small molecule tyrosine kinase inhibitors, gefitinib[62] and erlotinib,[63] showed some activity in pretreated patients with recurrent and/or metastatic SCCHN. Further randomized controlled trials are needed to evaluate whether these agents may augment existing therapies.

FUTURE DIRECTIONS

The role of systemic chemotherapy in squamous cell cancers of the head and neck is growing and many questions remain to be answered. Ongoing research will define better approaches for the optimal delivery of cytotoxic chemotherapy and targeted agents, radiation therapy, and surgical techniques, as part of the multimodality approach to the treatment of this disease.

REFERENCES

1. Kotwall C, Sako K, Razack MS, et al. Metastatic patterns in squamous cell cancer of the head and neck. *Am J Surg.* 1987;154(4):439–442.
2. Vokes EE, Weichselbaum RR, Lippman SM, et al. Head and neck cancer. [see Comment]. *New Engl J Med.* 1993;328(3):184–194.
3. Lefebvre JL. Current clinical outcomes demand new treatment options for SCCHN. *Ann Oncol.* 2005;16(suppl 6):vi–vi.
4. Adelstein DJ. Induction chemotherapy in head and neck cancer. *Hematol-Oncol Clin North Am.* 1999; 13(4):689–698.
5. Vokes EE, Mick R, Lester EP, et al. Cisplatin and flurorouracil chemotherapy does not yield long-term benefit in locally advanced head and neck cancer: results from a single institution. *J Clin Oncol.* 1991;9(8):1376–1384.
6. Anonymous. Induction chemotherapy plus radiation compared with surgery plus radiation in patients with advanced laryngeal cancer. The Department of Veterans Affairs Laryngeal Cancer Study Group. [see Comment]. *New Engl J Med.* 1991;324(24):1685–1690.
7. Cohen EE, Lingen Mw, Vokes EE. The expanding role of systemic therapy in head and neck cancer. *J Clin Oncol.* 2004;22(9):1743–1752.
8. Zorat PL, Paccagnella A, Cavaniglia G, et al. Randomized phase III trial of neoadjuvant chemotherapy in head and neck cancer: 10-year follow-up. [see Comment]. *J Natl Cancer Inst.* 2004;96(22): 1714–1717.
9. Adelstein DJ, Leblanc M. Does induction chemotherapy have a role in the management of locoregionally advanced squamous cell head and neck cancer? *J Clin Oncol.* 2006;24(17):2624–2628.

10. Paccagnella A, Orlando A, Marchiori C, et al. Phase III trial of initial chemotherapy in stage III or IV head and neck cancers: a study by the Gruppo di Studio sui Tumori della Testa e del Collo. [see Comment]. *J Natl Cancer Inst.* 1994; 86(4):265–272.

11. Forastiere AA. Randomized trials of induction chemotherapy. A critical review. *Hematol-Oncol Clin North Am.* 1991;5(4):725–736.

12. Domenge C, Hill C, Lefebvre JL, et al. Randomized trial of neoadjuvant chemotherapy in oropharyngeal carcinoma. French Groupe d'Etude des Tumeurs de la Tete et du Cou (GETTEC). *Br J Cancer.* 2000;83(12):1594–1598.

13. Anonymous. Adjuvant chemotherapy for advanced head and neck squamous carcinoma. Final report of the Head and Neck Contracts Program. *Cancer.* 1987;60(3):301–311.

14. Schuller DE, Metch B, Stein DW, et al. Preoperative chemotherapy in advanced resectable head and neck cancer: final report of the Southwest Oncology Group. *Laryngoscope.* 1988;98(11):1205–1211.

15. El-Sayed S, Nelson N. Adjuvant and adjunctive chemotherapy in the management of squamous cell carcinoma of the head and neck region. A meta-analysis of prospective and randomized trials. *J Clin Oncol.* 1996;14(3):838–847.

16. Pignon JP, Bourhis G, Domenge C, et al. Chemotherapy added to locoregional treatment for head and neck squamous-cell carcinoma: three meta-analyses of updated individual data. MACH-NC Collaborative Group. Meta-Analysis of Chemotherapy on Head and Neck Cancer. [see Comment]. *Lancet.* 2000;355(9208):949–955.

17. Munro AJ. An overview of randomised controlled trials of adjuvant chemotherapy in head and neck cancer. [see Comment]. *Br J Cancer.* 1995;71(1):83–91.

18. Browman GP. Evidence-based recommendations against neoadjuvant chemotherapy for routine management of patients with squamous cell head and neck cancer. *Cancer Investig.* 1994;12(6):662–670.

19. Bourhis JAC, Pignon JP, on behalf of the MACH-NC Collaborative Group; Institut Gustave-Roussy, Villejuif, France. update of MACH-NC (Meta-Analysis of Chemotherapy in Head & Neck Cancer) database focused on concomitant chemoradiotherapy. 2004 ASCO Annual Meeting Proceedings (Post-Meeting Edition). *J Clin Oncol.* 2004;22(14S):5505.

20. Smith RE, Thornton DE, Allen J. A phase II trial of paclitaxel in squamous cell carcinoma of the head and neck with correlative laboratory studies. *Semin Oncol.* 1995; 22(3 suppl 6):41–46.

21. Catimel G, Verweig J, Mattijssen V, et al. Docetaxel (Taxotere): an active drug for the treatment of patients with advanced squamous cell carcinoma of the head and neck. EORTC early clinical trials. *Group Ann Oncol.* 1994;5(6):533–577.

22. Dreyfuss AI, Clark JR, Norris CM, et al. Docetaxel: an active drug for squamous cell carcinoma of the head and neck. *J Clin Oncol.* 1996;14(5):1672–1678.

23. Couteau C, Chouaki N, Leyvraz S, et al. A phase II study of docetaxel in patients with metastatic squamous cell carcinoma of the head and neck. *Br J Cancer.* 1999; 81(3):457–462.

24. Forastiere AA, Shank D, Neuberg D, et al. Final report of a phase II evaluation of paclitaxel in patients with advanced squamous cell carcinoma of the head and neck: an Eastern Cooperative Oncology Group trial (PA390). *Cancer.* 1998;82(11):2270–2274.

25. Remenar E, Van Herpen C, Germa Lluch J, et al. A randomized phase III multicenter trial of neoadjuvant docetaxel plus cisplatin and 5-fluorouracil (TPF) versus neoadjuvant PF in patients with locally advanced unresectable squamous cell carcinoma of the head and neck (SCCHN). Final analysis of EORTC 24971. [abstract 5516]. *Proc Am Soc Clin Oncol.* 2006;24(185).

26. Posner MR, Le HD, Lann L, et al. *TAX 324: a phase III trial of TPF vs. PF induction chemotherapy followed by chemoradiotherapy in locally advanced SCCHN.* Presentation at the 42nd Annual Meeting of the American Society of Clinical Oncology; June 2–6, 2006; Atlanta, Ga.

27. Hitt R, Lopez-Pousa A, Martinez-Truforo J, et al. Phase III study comparing cisplatin plus fluorouracil to paclitaxel, cisplatin, and fluorouracil induction chemotherapy followed by chemoradiotherapy in locally advanced head and neck cancer. [see Comment]. *J Clin Oncol.* 2005;23(34):8636–8645.

28. Lefebvre JL, Chevalier D, Luboinski B, et al. Larynx preservation in pyriform sinus cancer: preliminary results of a European Organization for Research and Treatment of Cancer phase III trial. EORTC Head and Neck Cancer Cooperative Group. [see Comment]. *J Natl Cancer Inst.* 1996;88(13):890–899.

29. Gupta NK, Pointon RC, Wilkinson PM. A randomised clinical trial to contrast radiotherapy with radiotherapy and methotrexate given synchronously in

head and neck cancer. *Clin Radiol.* 1987;38(6): 575-581.

30. Knowlton AH, Percarpio B, Bobrow S, et al. Methotrexate and radiation therapy in the treatment of advanced head and neck tumors. *Radiology.* 1975;116(3):709-712.

31. Smid L, Lesnicar H, Zakotnik B, et al. Radiotherapy, combined with simultaneous chemotherapy with mitomycin C and bleomycin for inoperable head and neck cancer—preliminary report. *Intl J Radiat Oncol Biol Physics.* 1995;32(3):769-775.

32. Haffty BG, Son YH, Papac R, et al. Chemotherapy as an adjunct to radiation in the treatment of squamous cell carcinoma of the head and neck: results of the Yale Mitomycin Randomized Trials. *J Clin Oncol.* 1997;15(1):268-276.

33. Lo TC, Wiley AL, Ansfield FJ, et al. Combined radiation therapy and 5-fluorouracil for advanced squamous cell carcinoma of the oral cavity and oropharynx: a randomized study. *AJR Am J Roentgenol.* 1976;126(2):229-235.

34. Sanchiz F, Milla A, Torner J, et al. Single fraction per day versus two fractions per day versus radiochemotherapy in the treatment of head and neck cancer. [see Comment]. *Intl J Radiat Oncol Biol Physics.* 1990;19(6):1347-1350.

35. Browman GP, Cripps C, Hodson DI, et al. Placebo-controlled randomized trial of infusional fluororacil during standard radiotherapy in locally advanced head and neck cancer. *J Clin Oncol.* 1994;12(12): 2648-2653.

36. Forastiere AA, Maor M, Weber RS, et al. Long-term results of Intergroup RTOG 91-11: A phase III trial to preserve the larynx - Induction cisplatin/5-FU and radiation therapy versus concurrent cisplatin and radiation therapy versus radiation therapy. *J Clin Oncol.* 2006 ASCO Annual Meeting Proceedings. Part I. *J Clin Oncol.* 2006;24(18S [June 20] suppl):5517.

37. Jeremic B, Shibamoto Y, Milicic B, et al. Hyperfractionated radiation therapy with or without concurrent low-dose daily cisplatin in locally advanced squamous cell carcinoma of the head and neck: a prospective randomized trial. [see Comment]. *J Clin Oncol.* 2000;18(7):1458-1464.

38. Al-Sarraf M, LeBlanc M, Giri PG, et al. Chemoradiotherapy versus radiotherapy in patients with advanced nasopharyngeal cancer: phase III randomized intergroup study 0099. *J Clin Oncol.* 1998;16(4):1310-1317.

39. Browman GP, Hodson DI, Mackenzie RJ, et al. Choosing a concomitant chemotherapy and radio-therapy regimen for squamous cell head and neck cancer: a systematic review of the published literature with subgroup analysis. *Head Neck.* 2001; 23(7):579-589.

40. Budach W, Hehr T, Budach V, et al. A meta-analysis of hyperfractionated and accelerated radiotherapy and combined chemotherapy and radiotherapy regimens in unresected locally advanced squamous cell carcinoma of the head and neck. *BMC Cancer.* 2006;6:28.

41. Brockstein B, Haraf DJ, Rademaker AW, et al. Patterns of failure, prognostic factors and survival in locoregionally advanced head and neck cancer treated with concomitant chemoradiotherapy: a 9-year, 337-patient, multi-institutional experience. *Ann Oncol.* 2004;15(8):1179-1186.

42. Laramore GE, Scott CB, Al-Sarraf M, et al. Adjuvant chemotherapy for resectable squamous cell carcinomas of the head and neck: report on Intergroup Study 0034. [see Comment]. *Intl J Radiat Oncol Biol Physics,* 1992;23(4):705-713.

43. Bernier J, Domenge C, Ozsahin M, et al. Postoperative irradiation with or without concomitant chemotherapy for locally advanced head and neck cancer. [see Comment]. *New Engl J Med.* 2004; 350(19):1945-1952.

44. Cooper JS, Pajak TF, Forastiere AA, et al. Postoperative concurrent radiotherapy and chemotherapy for high-risk squamous-cell carcinoma of the head and neck. [see Comment]. *New Engl J Med.* 2004; 350(19):1937-1944.

45. Winquist E, Oliver T, Gilbert R, et al. Postoperative chemoradiotherapy for advanced squamous cell carcinoma of the head and neck: A systematic review with meta-analysis. *Head Neck.* 2007; 29(1):38-46.

46. Colevas AD. Chemotherapy options for patients with metastatic or recurrent squamous cell carcinoma of the head and neck. *J Clin Oncol.* 2006; 24(17):2644-2652.

47. A phase III randomised trial of cisplatinum, methotrexate, cisplatinum + methotrexate and cisplatinum + 5-FU in end stage squamous carcinoma of the head and neck. Liverpool Head and Neck Oncology Group. [erratum appears in *Br J Cancer* 1990 Jul;62(1):171]. *Bri J Cancer.* 1990;61(2): 311-315.

48. Clavel M, Vermorken JB, Cognetti F, et al. Randomized comparison of cisplatin, methotrexate, bleomycin and vincristine (CABO) versus cisplatin and 5-fluorouracil (CF) versus cisplatin (C) in recurrent or metastatic squamous cell carcinoma of the

head and neck. A phase III study of the EORTC Head and Neck Cancer Cooperative Group. *Ann Oncol.* 1994;5(6):521–526.

49. Forastiere AA, Metch B, Schuller DE, et al. Randomized comparison of cisplatin plus fluorouracil and carboplatin plus fluorouracil versus methotrexate in advanced squamous-cell carcinoma of the head and neck: a Southwest Oncology Group study. *J Clin Oncol.* 1992;10(8):1245–1251.
50. Williams SD, Velez-Garcia E, Essessee I, et al. Chemotherapy for head and neck cancer. Comparison of cisplatin + vinblastine + bleomycin versus methotrexate. *Cancer.* 1986;57(1):18–23.
51. Vogl SE, Schoenfeld DA, Kaplan BH, et al. A randomized prospective comparison of methotrexate with a combination of methotrexate, bleomycin, and cisplatin in head and neck cancer. *Cancer.* 1985;56(3):432–442.
52. Cowan JM, Beckett MA, Ahmed-Swan S, et al. Cytogenetic evidence of the multistep origin of head and neck squamous cell carcinomas. *J Natl Cancer Inst.* 1992;84(10):793–797.
53. Santini J, Formento JL, Francoual M, et al. Characterization, quantification, and potential clinical value of the epidermal growth factor receptor in head and neck squamous cell carcinomas. *Head Neck.* 1991;13(2):132–139.
54. Dassonville O, Formento JL, Francoual M, et al. Expression of epidermal growth factor receptor and survival in upper aerodigestive tract cancer. *J Clin Oncol.* 1993;11(10):1873–1878.
55. Rubin Grandis J, Melhem MF, Gooding WE, et al. Levels of TGF-alpha and EGFR protein in head and neck squamous cell carcinoma and patient survival. [see Comment]. *J Natl Cancer Inst.* 1998;90(11):824–832.
56. Ang KK, Berkey BA, Tu X, et al. Impact of epidermal growth factor receptor expression on survival and pattern of relapse in patients with advanced head and neck carcinoma. *Cancer Res.* 2002;62(24):7350–7356.
57. Herbst RS, Arquette M, Shin DM, et al. Phase II multicenter study of the epidermal growth factor receptor antibody cetuximab and cisplatin for recurrent and refractory squamous cell carcinoma of the head and neck [see Comment]. *J Clin Oncol.* 2005;23(24):5578–5587.
58. Baselga J, Trigo JM, Bourhis J, et al. Phase II multicenter study of the antiepidermal growth factor receptor monoclonal antibody cetuximab in combination with platinum-based chemotherapy in patients with platinum-refractory metastatic and/or recurrent squamous cell carcinoma of the head and neck. [see Comment]. *J Clin Oncol.* 2005;23(24):5568–5577.

59. Trigo JM, Hitt R, Koralewski P, et al. Cetuximab monotherapy is active in patients (pts) with platinum-refractory recurrent/metastatic squamous cell carcinoma of the head and neck (SCCHN): Results of a phase II study. ASCO Annual Meeting Proceedings, 2004. *J Clin Oncol.* 2004;14 S (July 15 suppl): p. 5502.
60. Burtness B, Goldwasser MA, Flood W, et al. Phase III randomized trial of cisplatin plus placebo compared with cisplatin plus cetuximab in metastatic/recurrent head and neck cancer: an Eastern Cooperative Oncology Group study [Erratum appears in *J Clin Oncol.* 2006 Feb 1;24(4):724]. *J Clin Oncol.* 2005;23(34):8646–8654.
61. Bonner JA, Harari PM, Giralt J, et al. Radiotherapy plus cetuximab for squamous-cell carcinoma of the head and neck. [see Comment]. *New Engl J Med.* 2006;354(6):567–578.
62. Cohen EE, Rosen F, Stadler WM, et al. Phase II trial of ZD1839 in recurrent or metastatic squamous cell carcinoma of the head and neck. *J Clin Oncol.* 2003;21(10):1980–1987.
63. Soulieres D, Senzer NN, Vokes EE, et al. Multicenter phase II study of erlotinib, an oral epidermal growth factor receptor tyrosine kinase inhibitor, in patients with recurrent or metastatic squamous cell cancer of the head and neck. *J Clin Oncol.* 2004;22(1):77–85.
64. Wendt TG, Grabengauer GG, Rodel CM, et al. Simultaneous radiochemotherapy versus radiotherapy alone in advanced head and neck cancer: a randomized multicenter study. *J Clin Oncol.* 1998;16(4):1318–1324.
65. Brizel DM, Albers ME, Fisher SR, et al. Hyperfractionated irradiation with or without concurrent chemotherapy for locally advanced head and neck cancer. [see Comment]. *New Engl J Med.* 1998;338(25):1798–1804.
66. Adelstein DJ, Lavertu P, Saxton JP, et al. Mature results of a phase III randomized trial comparing concurrent chemoradiotherapy with radiation therapy alone in patients with stage III and IV squamous cell carcinoma of the head and neck. *Cancer.* 2000;88(4):876–883.
67. Calais G, Alfonsi M, Bardet E, et al. Randomized trial of radiation therapy versus concomitant chemotherapy and radiation therapy for advanced-stage oropharynx carcinoma. [see Comment]. *J Natl Cancer Inst.* 1999;91(24):2081–2086.

68. Jacobs C, Lyman G, Velez-Garcia E, et al. A phase III randomized study comparing cisplatin and fluorouracil as single agents and in combination for advanced squamous cell carcinoma of the head and neck. *J Clin Oncol.* 1992;10(2):257–263.

7

Pretreatment and Posttreatment Dental Considerations in Head and Neck Oncology

Zafrulla Khan
Allan G. Farman

INTRODUCTION

Pre- and post-treatment oral mucosal and dental assessments, including monitoring both during and after therapy for head neck cancer, are critical elements of comprehensive oncologic dentistry. The following are learning objectives for the chapter.

■ Understand the role of a Maxillofacial/ Oncologic Dentist in the treatment of head and neck cancers
■ Define related terms referring to head and neck radiotherapy, chemotherapy, and maxillofacial prostheses
■ Describe oral care for preradiation and postradiation therapy patients
■ Describe oral care for prechemotherapy and postchemotherapy patients
■ Understand the care of the oral cavity for the oncology patient
■ Gain a basic knowledge of comprehensive oral and dental care for the head and neck cancer patient using the three different modalities of treatment; namely: surgery, radiation therapy, and chemotherapy.

This chapter emphasizes the pretreatment and post-treatment dental considerations for the head and neck cancer patient and focuses on the prevention and treatment of specific oral and dental complications related to radiation therapy and chemotherapy.

TREATMENTS OF THE ORAL CAVITY AND DENTITION FOR PATIENTS RECEIVING HEAD AND NECK RADIOTHERAPY AND CHEMOTHERAPY

Patients diagnosed with head and neck cancer ideally should be seen in a multidisciplinary clinic made up of head and neck surgeons, radiation oncologists, medical oncologists, maxillofacial/oncologic dentists, dieticians, and speech therapists. Historically, cancers of the head and neck have been treated with surgery and in advanced stages with radiation to decrease local and regional occurrences. Chemotherapy was limited to palliation or recurrence and metastatic disease.

However, during the past 2 decades combined modality treatments including radiation and chemotherapy have been developed[1] in an effort to enhance local and regional disease control, reduced distant metastasis, preserve anatomic structures, and improve overall survival and quality of life. This treatment includes addressing patient's oral needs to avoid or reduce subsequent complications. The oral and dental comprehensive evaluation should be completed as part of initial medical workup so the necessary dental procedures can be incorporated into the overall cancer treatment plan.

The head and neck region contains many vital structures, the protection of which are critical to minimizing and even eliminating the radiation and chemotherapy sequels. The dental treatment aim is to render a healthy and maintainable oral and dental environment prior to the commencement of radiation and chemotherapy, during and after treatment, and to continue throughout the patient's life. This will have a direct impact on the cancer treatment and future quality of life for the head and neck cancer patient.

The oncologic dentist plays an important role in the prevention, stabilization, and treatment of oral problems that can compromise the cancer patient's systemic health and quality of life. Radiation treatment for head and neck cancers can result in several complications. The dental goal is to restore the oral tissues to a reasonable state of health prior to radiation and to maintain oral health during and after radiation.

Short-term effects of head and neck radiation therapy include oral mucositis[2] (Figs 7–1B and 7–1C), infection[2] (secondary infections, candidiasis, bacterial, mycotic and viral), dysgeusia, reduced salivary flow (Fig 7–2), xerostomia, and oral discomfort, which may lead to nutritional deficiency.

Long-term effects of head and neck radiation therapy include xerostomia,[3] radiation caries (Figs 7–3A and 7–3B), osteoradionecrosis and soft tissue necrosis (Figs 7–3C and 7–3D), trismus, tooth sensitivity (rare), and nutritional deficiency due to xerostomia, mucositis, dysgeusia, and periodontal disease.[4] An alteration in maxillofacial development may occur in children.

The oncologic dentist can prevent or decrease in severity several serious side effects of cancer therapy, such as radiation caries, oral mucositis, xerostomia, trismus, and osteoradionecrosis and help

to treat symptomatically several inevitable consequences of cancer therapy. It may be possible to eliminate oral infection prior to radiation therapy or chemotherapy, and subsequently also control post-cancer treatment pain in the oral cavity. The oncologic dentist can implement a program of long-term oral health care and improve the oral status of the cancer patient, decrease the likelihood of deterioration of the natural teeth, and prevent or reduce the incidence of bone and soft tissue necrosis after radiotherapy to the jaws. The dentist's role in cancer therapy is to improve and maintain oral hygiene to reduce the risk of these complications, and thus maintain and improve dentition.

DENTAL AND ORAL HEALTH CARE RECOMMENDATIONS

The oncologic dentist should establish a healthy dentition that the patient will be able to maintain for the rest of his or her life by applying the following criteria: (1) Determine whether any remaining teeth should be restored, reshaped, or removed. (2) All unsustainable teeth within the field of radiation should be removed prior to start of radiation. (3) Oral surgery may also be necessary to remove potential sources of infection or anatomic interferences with future prosthesis placement.

Dental and Oral Management Prior to Radiation

After obtaining referral from the radiation oncologist including a radiation field diagram (Fig 7–1A), a comprehensive oral and dental screening, which includes a panoramic radiograph is essential. Hard and soft tissue examinations should include periodontal and caries examination and charting. These inspections are necessary for planning dental treatment in preparation of the oral cavity prior to radiation and chemotherapy. They are important to reduce subsequent complications of cancer therapy.[5–7] Formulation of a treatment plan is necessary because all teeth (including root fragments) in the field of radiation where long-term maintenance is questionable

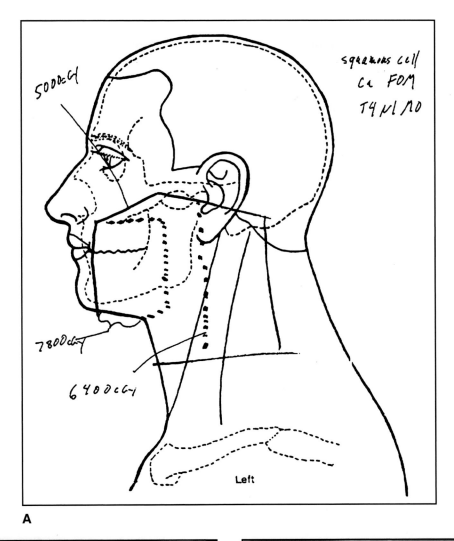

A

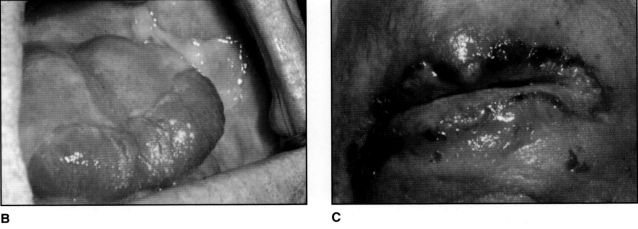

B   **C**

Fig 7–1. A. Radiation field diagram showing involved teeth and jaws, **B.** Mucositis, postradiation showing desquamation of mucosa of dorsal surface of tongue and cheek. **C.** Keratitis of the lips, due to chemotherapy component of the treatment regimen as the lips were outside the radiation field.

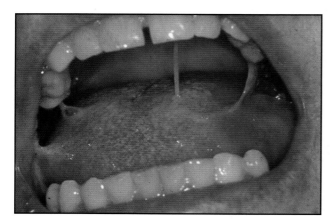

Fig 7–2. Thickened saliva due to radiation-reduced salivary flow.

must be removed. Preprosthetic surgery should be performed, if necessary, allowing adequate healing time prior to radiation. Oral prophylaxis and home care instructions should be provided.

Current prostheses if any need to be evaluated and possible sources of irritation removed. Fabrication of new prostheses must be delayed until at least 3 to 6 months after radiation therapy concludes, depending on mucosal status and the degree of xerostomia present. Nutritional counseling is also necessary.

Radiation intraoral shields, carriers, and positioners should be fabricated if requested by the radiation oncologist (Figs 7-4, 7-5, and 7-6). These appliances help in positioning the radiation beam, shield tissues, carry radioactive material, protect and displace vital structures, and locate tissues in repeatable position.

Patient education instructions concerning possible side effects must stress the need for oral health care and maintenance to avoid periodontal disease (Fig 7-7). Marques and Dib studied periodontal changes in patients undergoing head and neck radiation therapy. Clinical periodontal parameters (probing depth, clinical attachment level, gingival recession, plaque index, and bleeding on probing) were assessed on 27 patients before and 6 to 8 months following radiation therapy. The greatest changes occurred in clinical attachment level: overall, 70% of the patients showed a loss, with 92% of

these having loss in the mandible. Attachment loss was directly related to the field of radiation and was greater when the jaws were actually included in the irradiated area. It was concluded that periodontal status should be evaluated prior to and following radiation therapy in the oral and maxillofacial region to help ensure that periodontal health is maintained in oncology patients. For tooth extraction versus retention, consideration should be given to the radiation fields and dosage, presence of periodontal disease, presence of periapical pathology, caries index, and patient's ability to cooperate in preventive measures.

Dental and Oral Management During and Following Radiation

Following head and neck radiation therapy the following complications are possible:

Mucositis

Mucositis or stomatitis is a painful inflammatory mucosal reaction and is caused by the disruption of cell growth and proliferation of the rapidly dividing basal layer of oral epithelial cells and becomes evident usually in the 2nd or 3rd week of radiation. It is associated with pain which can be severe and occasionally radiation treatments might have to be suspended to allow soft tissues to heal (see Fig 7-1B). Patients with impaired renal and hepatic function are especially at increased risk as a result of reduced metabolism. The combination of radiation with chemotherapy can dramatically increase the degree of mucositis (see Fig 7-1C), usually affecting the soft tissues of the lip, buccal mucosa, tongue, soft palate and pharyngeal mucosa, and to a lesser extent the keratinized tissues of the gingival and palate.

Mucositis is associated with decreased ability to taste, chew, and xerostomia progressing to difficulty in swallowing. This will ultimately impact the patient's nutritional status and lead to difficulty with speech.

If mucositis develops, symptoms may be relieved by treatment including Xylocaine Viscous rinses or Maalox® suspension with equal parts of Benadryl Elixir® and Xylocaine Viscous® used as a rinse. Oratect Gel® or Orabase B® can be used as a topical oral anesthetic.

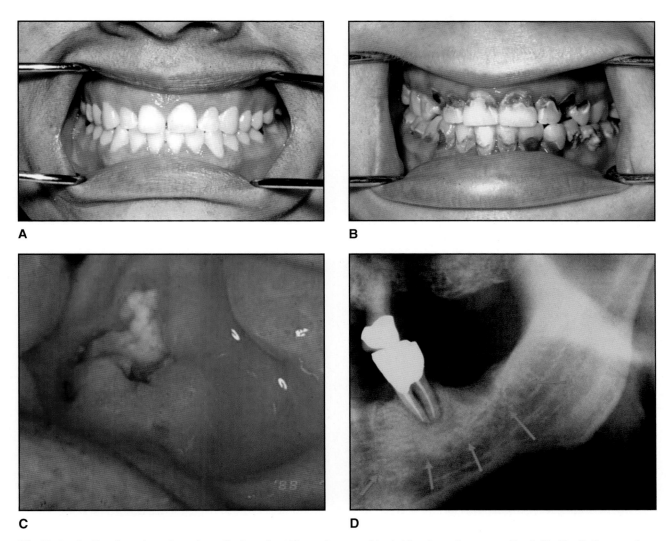

Fig 7–3. A. Pre head and neck radiation dentition of a non-Hodgkins lymphoma patient. **B.** Radiation caries, 24 months postradiation due to dental neglect, same patient. **C.** Clinical features of osteoradionecrosis include ulceration, erythema of soft tissues, and bony sequestration. **D.** Radiographic features of osteoradionecrosis include increased radio-opacity of affected portion of bone.

Infection

Infections of the oral cavity may be odontogenic, periodontal, or mucosal soft tissue in origin. They may be caused by opportunistic or normal oral flora bacteria, fungi, and virus or by combination of these due to reduced immunocompetence in the host. Such infections may be due to bacterial plaque and calculus resulting in periodontal abscess, pericoro-

nitis with bacterial colonies under a flap of tissue (the operculum) covering the occlusal surface of partially erupted teeth, or alternatively an apical dental abscess.

Oral infection is a natural consequence of mucositis as the patient, due to pain on brushing, may ignore oral hygiene. This, in turn, will permit bacterial multiplication, and ulceration consequent to cancer therapy will allow normal oral flora to

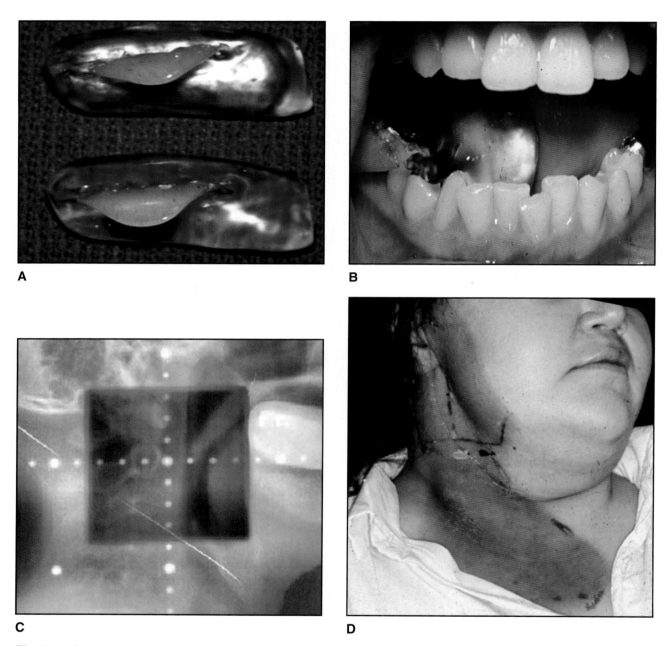

Fig 7–4. A. Intraoral shield for unilateral radiation. **B.** Shield in position in the mouth. **C.** Planning radiograph with shield in place. **D.** Patient on completion of unilateral field radiation.

invade underlying soft tissue and perhaps even bone. Consequences can be severe.

Diagnosis of oral infections is based on clinical findings and medical history, in combination with local and blood cultures to determine the identity of the causative agents, so appropriate treatment can be administered.

For infection control, suspected infections should be cultured and treatment prescribed in cooperation with the radiation oncologist. Peridex®

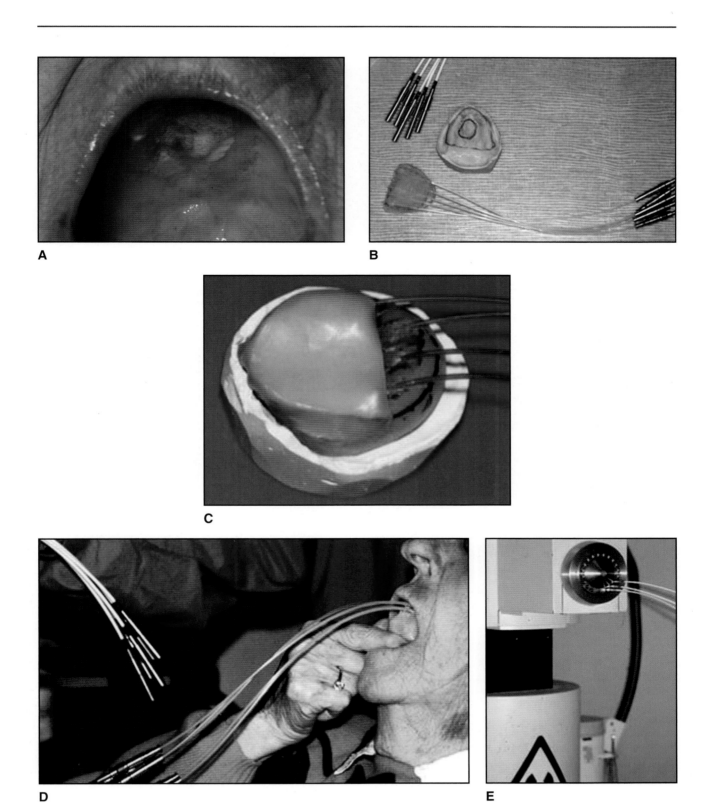

Fig 7–5. A. Squamous cell carcinoma of hard palate to receive brachytherapy. **B.** Radiation carrier to deliver intraoral brachytherapy radiation. **C.** Radiation carrier with wax to protect tongue from radiation. **D.** Radiation carrier in place in the mouth. **E.** HDR machine for delivery of radiation.

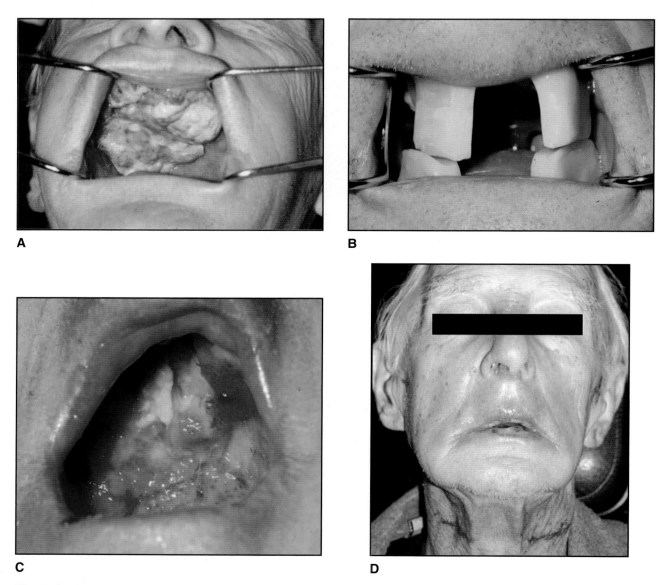

Fig 7–6. A. Advanced squamous cell carcinoma of the maxilla. **B.** Intraoral positioner in the mouth used to protect tongue and mandible from radiation. **C.** Tumor response to radiation and chemotherapy. **D.** Clinical picture shows the positioner sparing the mandible from radiation.

(chlorhexidine 12%) may be used when necessary as a preventive measure. Treatment may include: Mycostatin® (nystatin), 5 mL of 100,000 units/mL 3 to 4 times a day; or Mycelex® (clotrimazole), one troche 5 times daily for 14 days; or Nizoral® (ketoconazole), one tablet daily for 14 days; Diflucan® (fluconazole), 100 mg tablets for 7 days; Zovirax® (acyclovir), 200 mg, 2 capsules 3 times daily for 10 days.

Trismus

Trismus sometimes occurs secondary to surgical procedures such as a maxillectomy due to wound healing and contracture of muscles. Head and neck radiation that involves the temporomandibular joint and the muscles of mastication will also produce trismus secondary to fibrosis.

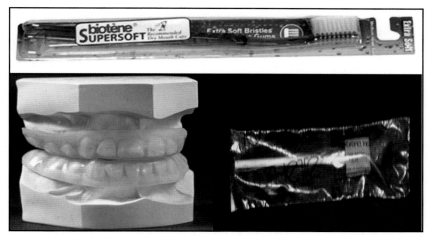

A

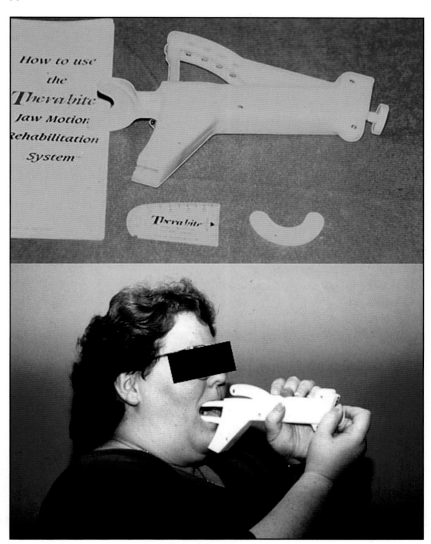

Fig 7–7. **A.** Custom fluoride trays and soft tooth brush and toothette for cleaning teeth during severe mucositis. **B.** Therabite appliance for oral exercise.

B

To avoid trismus, exercise the muscles a few times daily by opening and closing the mouth against pressure as far as possible without pain. Therabite® (a mechanical device) may improve the range of motion during mouth opening (see Fig 7-7B). Oral exercises to be done throughout the radiation treatment and a couple of months posttreatment.

Xerostomia

Radiation may involve the salivary glands, which are responsible for saliva production, which is a complex fluid made up of 94% water and the rest comprising enzymes, proteins, immunoglobulins, and so forth, which moisten the oral cavity thus helping in lubrication and binding, solubilizing dry food, initiating starch digestion, providing alkaline buffering, and also protection and repair by destroying certain mouth bacteria. There are three pairs of salivary glands; the submandibular glands which produce 70% of daily saliva, the parotids 25% and the sublingual glands about 5%. These glands produce 1000 to 1500 mL of saliva per day at the rate of 0.1 mL/min at rest and 4 mL/min during active stimulation. Radiation to salivary glands may result in xerostomia (see Fig 7-2) usually developing after the 4th or 5th fraction of radiation. Xerostomia results from qualitative and quantitative changes in saliva, causing mucosal atrophy and difficulty with mastication, speech, and swallowing, which leads to weight loss and nutritional deficiency. This also predisposes the oral cavity to chronic candidiasis and eventually rampant tooth decay and increased periodontal disease. Xerostomia will also compromise the comfort and retention of any oral prosthesis. Permanent xerostomia is likely to occur if the major salivary glands receive more than 45 Gy.

Relief of symptoms may include artificial saliva substitutes (Xerolube®, Salivart®, Moi-ster®). Frequent sips of water are helpful, and sugarless gum and candy may stimulate salivation. Pilocarpine hydrochloride (Salagen®), 5 mg three times daily, may also produce saliva. These remedies are usually palliative.

Radiation Caries

This rampant form of tooth decay occurs typically on the smooth surfaces of the teeth, such as the cervical margins, and subgingival and incisal edges (see Figs 7-3A and 7-3B). The condition is believed to be the result of radiation-induced xerostomia and the accompanying acidogenic shift of the oral environment. Radiation caries usually occurs 4 to 6 months after radiation is completed with rapid onset and widespread surface involvement, This could lead to pulpal, gingival, and bone infections and ultimately to osteoradionecrosis with severe consequences. Prevention is necessary because this form of tooth decay is difficult to arrest.

Silver amalgam restorations perform better under dry conditions as desiccated composites tend to break down at the margins. Fluoride (Gel-Kam®, Prevident®, TheraFlur®) must be used daily at home using a custom fluoride carrier to prevent caries (see Fig 7-7A).

Use and Care of Dental Prosthesis

Patients should not wear removable prosthesis if any irritation, mucositis, or ulceration develops and limit their use only for eating. Dentures should be cleaned daily and soaked in an antimicrobial denture cleaning solution.

Osteoradionecrosis

Osteoradionecrosis (ORN), although uncommon, is a serious and late complication (see Figs 7-3C and 7-3D) attributed to radiation therapy.[9-11] ORN develops because bone does not heal due to the diminished blood supply caused by radiotherapy-induced endartritis obliterans, reducing tissue vascularity. It usually occurs in the mandible following tooth extraction or bone surgery, but may be associated with denture sores or even occur spontaneously. The incidence of osteoradionecrosis in head and neck cancer patients managed with radiation therapy varies widely in the literature from 0.4% to 56%.[9] Although osteoradionecrosis typically occurs in the first 3 years after radiation therapy, patients probably remain at indefinite risk for life. Factors that may be associated with the risk of osteoradionecrosis include treatment-related variables such as radiation therapy dose, field size, and volume of the mandible irradiated with a high dose; patient-related variables such as periodontitis, preirradiation bone surgery, oral hygiene, alcohol and tobacco abuse, and dental extraction following radiation therapy; and tumor-related factors such as lesion size and lesion proximity to bone.

In a recent study, the incidence of osteoradionecrosis of the jaws after irradiation using modern three-dimensional planning as well as hyperfractionation or moderately accelerated irradiation was evaluated and compared with historical control data.[11]

Studer et al[11] reviewed the records of 268 head and neck cancer patients irradiated with a dose to the mandible of at least 60 Gy. All patients had computerized dose calculation with isodose charts. The long-term cumulative incidence of osteoradionecrosis requiring mandibular resection after conventional fractionation was 6.2% for target dose of 60 to 66.6 Gy target dose compared to 20.1% for target doses of greater than 66.6 to 72 Gy. The incidence of ORN was 6.6% after hyperfractionated irradiation with a target dose 72.0 to 78.8 Gy and no cases of OCN were observed after concomitant boost irradiation according to the MD Anderson regime with a dose of 63.9 to 70.5 Gy. Finally, the incidence of ORN was greater than 17% after 6 × 2 Gy/week or 7 × 1.8 Gy/week and a total target dose of 66 to 72 Gy. Comparison of the incidence of osteoradionecrosis during the period 1980 to 1990 with the following period 1990 to 1998 showed a decrease in risk to approximately 5% using modern three-dimensional techniques as well as hyperfractionation or moderately accelerated fractionation.[11]

Oh et al[12] conducted a retrospective chart review in an attempt to establish whether unerupted third molars should be removed or left in place in patients requiring radiation therapy for cancer.[12] Patients were divided into 2 groups on the basis of preirradiation extraction. Group 1 comprised patients who had impacted third molars extracted before radiation therapy (n = 55). Group 2 comprised patients in whom impacted third molars were left in place (n = 38). Before radiation therapy, 99 impacted third molars were extracted from the 55 patients in Group 1, whereas 55 impacted third molars were left in place in the 38 patients in Group 2. Only 4 patients (2 from Group 1 and 2 from Group 2) subsequently developed ORN; therefore, no significant difference in the incidence of osteoradionectosis

could be attributed to prophylactic removal of unerupted third molars prior to radiation therapy.

Sulaiman et al[13] investigated irradiated head and neck patients to evaluate those patients who developed osteoradionecrosis through dental extraction.[13] One hundred ninety-four patients with a history of radiation to the head and neck treated at Memorial Sloan-Kettering were reviewed. Of these patients, 187 had subsequent dental extractions and only 4 of these developed osteoradionecrosis. It could be concluded that healthy teeth should be retained in patients undergoing radiation therapy.

Osteonecrosis is not only a complication of radiation therapy; it can also occur with certain chemotherapeutic regimens.[14] Ruggiero et al reported that long-term use of bisphosphonates, widely used in the management of metastatic disease to the bone and in the treatment of osteoporosis, can also result in osteonecrosis of the jaws. Histologically, the necrosis observed is otherwise typical of osteoradionecrosis.

Sixty-three patients were identified with refractory osteomyelitis and a history of chronic bisphosphonate therapy (56 had received intravenous bisphosphonates for at least 1 year and 7 patients were on chronic oral bisphosphonate therapy).[14] Typical presentation was either a nonhealing extraction socket or an exposed jaw refractory to conservative debridement and antibiotic therapy. Biopsy showed no evidence of metastatic disease. The majority of the patients required surgical removal of the necrotic bone. In view of the widespread use of chronic bisphosphonate therapy, the observation of an associated risk of osteonecrosis of the jaw should alert practitioners to monitor for this potential complication. Early diagnosis might reduce morbidity resulting from advanced destructive lesions of the jawbone. Periodic panoramic radiography is warranted in such patients.

Local application of high concentrations of fluoride gel as well as good oral hygiene are the most appropriate measures to implement for prevention of dental caries and other complications in patients treated by radiation or chemotherapy.[7,15] Pasquier et al[8] carried out a systematic review on the peer-reviewed literature concerning the use of hyperbaric oxygen therapy in the treatment of radiation-induced lesions. They concluded that, although more controlled randomized trials are needed, the level of evidence supports use of hyperbaric oxygen therapy for treatment of osteoradionecrosis, and in prevention of osteoradionecrosis after dental extractions. A parallel systematic review concluded that there is a lack of reliable clinical evidence for or against the use therapeutic use of hyperbaric oxygen for irradiated dental implant patients.

Teeth in the radiation field should not be extracted for at least 1 year following radiation. Some researchers believe the risk of ORN never abates. If tooth extraction is unavoidable, conservative surgery, antibiotic coverage, and hyperbaric oxygen treatment may be necessary. Dietary counseling is essential, along with excellent home care instructions, frequent oral prophylaxis and dental recall with daily fluoride use (see Fig 7-7A).

The regimen presented offers the head and cancer patients the following: control of cariogenic organisms, reduction in radiation caries, remineralization of teeth, tooth sensitivity relief, palliative relief from dry mouth, and oral irritations, thus providing an opportunity for the cancer patient to maintain oral health and improved quality of life.

Oral and Dental Management Prior to Chemotherapy

Chemotherapy patients can become immunosuppressed and myelosuppressed during treatment leading to mucositis and oral infections similar to head and neck radiation patients. Proper oral and dental care can reduce and eliminate the morbidity and mortality of acute dental disease during cancer treatment caused by oral sources.

Side effects from chemotherapy are generally short-term and similar to radiotherapy, but certain long-term effects may cause difficulty. Short-term effects are mucositis, xerostomia, infections, and hemorrhage.

Long-term effects include neurotoxicity. Certain chemotherapeutic drugs, particularly platinum derivatives can cause severe deep pain mimicking maxillary and mandibular toothache, usually bilateral, with no dental or oral source. Chemotherapy can also cause an alteration in maxillofacial development in children.

It is important that the patient is educated concerning possible side effects and the need for oral

health care and maintenance prior to, during, and after chemotherapy. A complete oral and dental evaluation should be conducted, including dental radiographs and a complete hard and soft tissue examination, including periodontal and caries examination, should be performed, as well as charting. With this information a treatment plan that the patient is able and interested in maintaining may be formulated.

Nonrestorable or periodontally compromised teeth, including root fragments, must be extracted to eliminate risks of infection. This is performed in consultation with a medical oncologist as the patient could be immunosuppressed. The patient's periodontal status should be maintained and improved through scaling and root planning. Indicated restorations may be completed, and orthodontic bands considered for removal if chemotherapy is expected to cause problems in the mouth. The infected periodontium (periodontal disease) can act as a focus for systemic infection in cancer patients suffering neutropenia as a result of high-dose chemotherapy.[16] Raber-Durlacher et al[16] concluded that assessment of a patient's periodontal condition before the onset of profound neutropenia is critical to the diagnosis and the management of potentially life-threatening infections.

If salivary dysfunction is anticipated, fluoride is prescribed for home use which includes Gel-Kam® and Prevident®, to be used with fluoride trays.

Oral hygiene instructions include using a soft tooth brush, such as Biotene Supersoft® tooth brush, and dental floss. Frequent recall is necessary along with dietary counseling.

Oral and Dental Management During and Following Chemotherapy

Irrespective of the site of the cancer, the chemotherapy patient should perform routine dental care as his or her hematologic status permits during chemotherapy. All suspicious lesions should be cultured for bacterial, fungal, and viral infections. Treatment is prescribed in cooperation with the medical oncologist. Refer to the section on radiation therapy for medications that apply.

Postchemotherapy maintenance of quality of life requires excellent home care. Follow-up with the dentist is mandatory to prevent or reduce complications between chemotherapeutic cycles.

At the completion of all planned courses of chemotherapy, closely monitor the patient until all side effects of therapy have resolved, including immunosuppression. The patient may then be placed on a normal dental recall schedule. As these patients may need to undergo additional immunosuppressive therapy if they have a cancer relapse in the future, it is very important to maintain optimal oral health. Consultation and coordination with the medical oncologist is mandatory because of hematologic status and the need for antibiotic prophylaxis due to indwelling central venous catheters. Children should receive close lifetime follow-up, with specific attention to growth and development patterns. Oguz et al[17] investigated the late effects of chemotherapy treatment for childhood non-Hodgkin's lymphomas on oral health and dental development. Thirty-six long-term survivors were included in this study and 36 volunteers with similar age and sex distribution served as controls. Both groups underwent a complete oral and dental examination for decayed, missing, and filled teeth and surfaces, gingival and periodontal health according to standard periodontal and plaque indices, enamel defects and discolorations, root malformations, eruption status, agenesis, premature apexifications, and microdontia. Non-Hodgkin's lymphoma patients had significantly higher plaque index, and more enamel discolorations and root malformations than did the controls, oral and dental disturbances that may be attributed to the chemotherapy regimens. It should be noted that patients with non-Hodgkin's lymphoma sometimes receive limited (mantle field) head and neck radiation.

Dental Outcomes

Allison et al[18] studied the relationship between dental status and health-related quality of life in upper aerodigestive tract cancer patients. The investigation aimed to investigate the hypothesis that dental status is a predictor of quality of life. A cross-sectional study design was used with a sample of 188 subjects. Data were collected on sociodemographic, disease, treatment, and dental status. Linear multiple regression analysis was used to determine those variables with a significant independent association with quality of life. Two multivariate models were developed each containing age, gender, employment status, cancer site, and disease stage, plus either the dental status category "partially dentate with no prosthesis" (F-value = 7.31; p <0.0001; r^2 = 0.20) predicting a significantly worse health related life quality, or the dental status category "edentulous with prostheses" (F-value = 7.56; p <0.0001; r^2 = 0.20) predicting a significantly better quality of life. Furthermore, the "partially dentate with no prosthesis" group reported significantly more "problems with their teeth" (ANOVA, p = 0.0004), significantly more "trouble eating" (ANOVA, p = 0.024), and significantly more "trouble enjoying their meals" (ANOVA, p = 0.01). The results of this study indicate that dental status has an important effect on health related quality of life in post-therapeutic upper aerodigestive tract cancer patients. Many head and neck cancer patients are treated with high-dose radiation therapy to the oral cavity and surrounding structures. Significant side effects occur in both the acute phase and in the long term.

A dedicated multidisciplinary team of medical and radiation oncologist, head and neck surgeon, prosthodontist/oncologic dentist, dietician, physical therapist, social worker, and in some instances plastic surgeon, and psychologist are needed to provide the optimal treatment and supportive care for these patients.[18] Osseointegrated implants used in the rehabilitation of patients who have undergone head and neck surgery have provided a reliable means of retaining intraoral and extraoral prostheses.[1] With close communication between the head and neck surgeon and the prosthodontist/oncologic dentist, and careful patient selection, optimized outcomes are more likely.

DAILY ORAL CARE INSTRUCTIONS FOR CANCER PATIENTS (Table 7–1)

1. Remove any partial or complete dentures from mouth.
   a. Use a denture brush and water to clean dentures.

Table 7–1. Treatment Options and Timing

Product	Pre-XRT	During XRT	Post-XRT
Neutral sodium fluoride gels: 5000 ppm	X	X	X
Sodium fluoride varnish	X	X	X
Chlorhexidine	X	X	?
Antibacterial toothpaste	X	X	X
Saliva substitutes/ lubricants		X	X
Soft toothbrush		X	X

    b. Soak dentures in an antimicrobial denture soaking solution, if necessary.

    c. Removable partial dentures and complete dentures should *not* be worn while sleeping.

2. Brush teeth with a soft-bristled toothbrush using toothpaste or baking soda. May use a "Toothette" or cloth if mouth is too sore to use a toothbrush.

3. Floss natural teeth by gently placing dental floss between teeth and sliding the floss up each side of each tooth.

4. Place fluoride on natural teeth for 5 minutes every night, using a fluoride carrier or a toothbrush. Do not rinse mouth, eat, or drink for 30 minutes.

5. Rinse the mouth with baking soda and salt water solutions. Over-the-counter mouthwashes and full strength peroxide solutions should *not* be used due to their drying and irritating effects. Peridex® (chlorhexidine) may be used if prescribed by your doctor.

6. Choose foods easy to chew and swallow, take small bites, sip liquids with meals. Avoid hard and crunchy foods, foods that are hot, spicy, sugary. and acidic (like colas and citrus fruits and drinks)

7. Avoid all tobacco products and alcoholic drinks

8. Do oral exercises (opening and closing of the mouth) several times a day

9. For dry mouth drink a lot of water, use sugarless gum or candy, use saliva substitutes to help moisten the mouth

10. Have your natural teeth cleaned professionally before cancer treatment and every 4 months after completion of treatment.

REFERENCES

1. Maureen S. The expanding role of dental oncology in head and neck surgery. *Surg Oncol Clin North Am.* 2004;13:37–46.

2. Luglie PF, Mura G, Mura A, Angius A, Soru G, Farris A. Prevention of periodontopathy and oral mucositis during antineoplastic chemotherapy. *Minerva Stomatol.* 2002;51:231–239.

3. Guggenheimer J, Moore PA. Xerostomia: etiology, recognition and treatment. *J Am Dent Assoc.* 2003;134:61–69.

4. Marques MA, Dib LL. Periodontal changes in patients undergoing radiation therapy. *J Periodontol.* 2004;75:1178–1187.

5. Harrison JS, Dale RA, Haveman CW, Redding SW. Oral complications in radiation therapy. *Gen Dent.* 2003;51:552–560.

6. Huber MA, Terezhalmy GT. The head and neck radiation oncology patient. *Quintessence Int.* 2003;34:693–717.

7. Barillot I, Horiot JC. Prevention of caries and osteoradionecrosis in patients irradiated in oncology. Critical review. *Rev Belge Med Dent.* 1999;54:205–207.

8. Pasquier D, Hoelscher T, Schmutz J, et al. Hyperbaric oxygen therapy in the treatment of radio-induced lesions in normal tissues: a literature review. *Radiother Oncol.* 2004;72:1–13.

9. Jereczek-Fossa BA, Orecchia R. Radiation therapy-induced mandibular bone complications. *Cancer Treat Rev.* 2002;28:65–74.

10. Reuther T, Schuster T, Mende U, Kubler A. Osteoradionecrosis of the jaws as a side effect of radiation therapy of head and neck tumour patients—a report of a thirty year retrospective review. *Int J Oral Maxillofac Surg.* 2003;32:289–295.

11. Studer G, Gratz KW, Glanzmann C. Osteoradionecrosis of the mandible in patients treated with different fractionations. *Strahlenther Onkol.* 2004;180:233–240.

12. Oh HK, Chambers MS, Garden AS, Wong PF, Martin JW. Risk of osteoradionecrosis after extraction of

impacted third molars in irradiated head and neck cancer patients. *J Oral Maxillofac Surg.* 2004;62: 139-144.

13. Sulaiman F, Huryn JM, Zlotolow IM. Dental extractions in the irradiated head and neck patient: a retrospective analysis of Memorial Sloan-Kettering Cancer Center protocols, criteria, and end results. *J Oral Maxillofac Surg.* 2003;61:1123-1131.

14. Ruggiero SL, Mehrotra B, Rosenberg TJ, Engroff SL. Osteonecrosis of the jaws associated with the use of bisphosphonates: a review of 63 cases. *J Oral Maxillofac Surg.* 2004;62:527-534.

15. Piret P, Deneufbourg JM. Mandibular osteoradionecrosis: sword of Damocles of radiation therapy for head and neck cancers? *Rev Med Liege.* 2002; 57:393-399.

16. Raber-Durlacher JE, Epstein JB, Raber J, et al. Periodontal infection in cancer patients treated with high-dose chemotherapy. *Support Care Cancer.* 2002;10:466-473.

17. Oguz A, Cetiner S, Karadeniz C, Alpaslan G, Alpaslan C, Pinarli G. Long-term effects of chemotherapy on orodental structures in children with non-Hodgkin's lymphoma *Eur J Oral Sci.* 2004;112:8-11

18. Allison PJ, Locker D, Feine JS. The relationship between dental status and health-related quality of life in upper aerodigestive tract cancer patients. *Oral Oncol.* 1999;35:138-143.

19. Choong N, Vokes E. Expanding role of the medical oncologist in the management of the head and neck cancer. *Cancer J Clinicians.* 2008;58:1:32-53.

8

Anesthesia Consideration in Head and Neck Surgery

Steven B. Edelstein
Timothy J. Hughes

INTRODUCTION

In this chapter we discuss some of the pertinent issues that arise when faced with the perioperative care of the oncology patient undergoing otolaryngologic procedures. Many issues come to the surface when determining the optimal management of these patients including appropriate preoperative assessment, airway management, selection of anesthetic techniques, fluid management, and perioperative antibiotic therapy. This review should allow the nonanesthesiologist to obtain a further understanding of some of the complex issues that arise when faced with the care of these patients.

PREOPERATIVE ASSESSMENT

Many patients who present for the surgical resection of head and neck tumors have significant past medical histories that should be elucidated prior to arrival in the operating room. Assuming that surgical resection of the otolaryngologic tumor is not an emergency, a thorough evaluation for significant comorbidities is essential. The cardiac and respiratory systems are areas of particular focus.

Cardiac Assessment

Many patients have pre-existing cardiac disease or have significant risk factors for coronary artery disease and should therefore undergo risk stratification. Multiple risk stratification methods have been developed over the years; including the Goldman,[1] the Detsky,[2] the Lee Revised Cardiac Risk Assessment Index,[3] and the American College of Cardiology and American Heart Association Guidelines.[4,5]

For brevity we focus on the ACC/AHA guidelines that were developed recognizing that many patients with significant coronary disease present for noncardiac surgery (Fig 8-1[5]). These guidelines serve to help the practitioner stratify coronary risk and allow the physician to have an informed discussion with the patient prior to the procedure.

Whenever faced with a patient who presents for noncardiac surgery, a few significant questions must be answered. First, is the surgical case an emergency or elective in nature? What cardiac risk factors does the patient have? What is the extent and type of surgery? What is the patient's exercise tolerance? The preoperative assessment is meant to identify those patients who are at an unacceptable risk for perioperative cardiac morbidity and mortality.

In a recent version of the ACC/AHA guidelines, specific clinical predictors have been identified

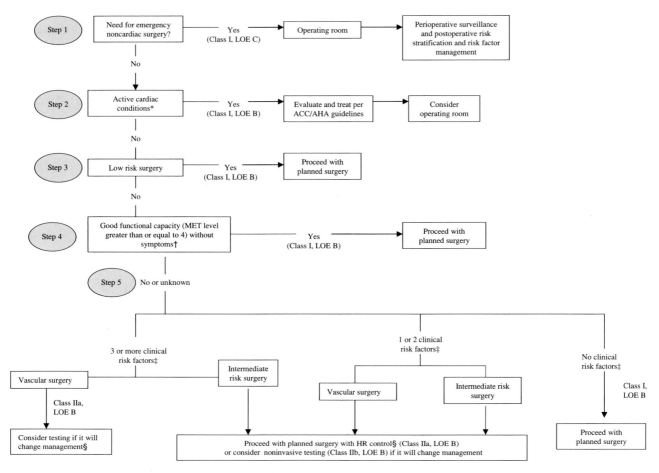

Fig 8–1. Cardiac evaluation and care algorithm for noncardiac surgery, based on active clinical conditions, known cardiovascular disease, or cardiac risk factors for patients 50 years of age or older. ACC/AHA indicates American College of Cardiology/American Heart Association; HR, heart rate; LOE, level of evidence; MET, metabolic equivalent. Reproduced with permission from Fleisher et al.[5] Copyright © 2007 by the American College of Cardiology Foundation and the American Heart Association, Inc.

regarding the likelihood of coronary artery disease. Active cardiac conditions that have been identified as requiring cardiac evaluation prior to noncardiac surgery include the following: unstable coronary syndromes, decompensated heart failure or new onset heart failure, significant arrhythmias (high grade atrioventricular block, Mobitz II atrioventricular block, supraventricular arrhythmias with uncontrolled ventricular rate and symptomatic bradycardia), and severe valvular heart disease (severe aortic stenosis or symptomatic mitral stenosis). Other intermediate

clinical predictors include: history of heart disease, history of compensated or prior heart failure, history of cerebrovascular disease, diabetes mellitus, and renal insufficiency. In addition there are also identified minor clinical predictors: advanced age (greater than 70 years), abnormal ECG, rhythm other than sinus, and uncontrolled hypertension.

Once predictors are determined one must assess the type of surgery, each of which carries a different set of risks. Emergency surgeries, vascular surgeries, and prolonged surgeries with large amounts of volume shifts are noted to have a high cardiac risk. Head and neck surgery has been determined to be an intermediate risk procedure, whereas endoscopic procedures are deemed low risk with a reported incidence of cardiac events of less than 1%. Taking this information into account as well as functional capacity, one can make informed decisions regarding who would benefit from noninvasive testing and those who may proceed to surgery.

As with all forms of noninvasive testing, the question arises as to what to do with the data. If patients have significant risk factors but personally decide against interventions, then risk assessment essentially plays little role other than indicating the need for maximization of medical therapy to reduce perioperative risk. Currently, there are no studies that support coronary revascularization (surgical or percutaneous) prior to high-risk surgical procedures.[6] As such, many in the literature feel that cardiovascular interventions should be performed only in those patients who have symptoms or risk factors that in normal circumstances would indicate the need for risk stratification.[7]

If there is a decision to proceed with coronary revascularization, then timing of the main surgical procedure will be impacted. Patients who undergo percutaneous coronary interventions (PCI) must be placed on antiplatelet therapy for a significant length of time. Complications have been seen when surgery is performed within 2 weeks of a PCI with bare metal stents.[8] As such, recommendations state that at least 4 to 6 weeks of antiplatelet therapy should be performed for bare metal stents (ACC/AHA guidelines) and at least 12 months for drug-eluting stents such as paclitaxel or sirolimus (Cypher®) (Figs 8–2 and 8–3).[5,9,10]

The role of pharmacologic agents to reduce risk is also controversial. The use of β-1 antagonists,[11] statins,[12] and alpha-blocking agents[13] has been examined; however, no definitive trial has determined their long-term usefulness. Currently, a large multicenter trial is focusing on the role of β-blockade and long-term outcomes. The POISE trial,[14] with its approximately 10,000 enrollees promises to shed some light on this controversial topic.

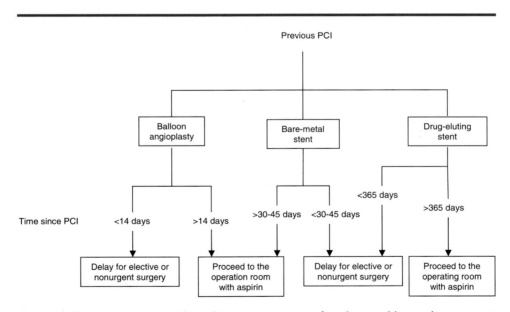

Fig 8–2. Proposed approach to the management of patients with previous percutaneous coronary intervention (PCI), who require noncardiac surgery based on expert opinion. Reproduced with permission from Fleisher et al.[5] Copyright © 2007 by the American College of Cardiology Foundation and the American Heart Association, Inc.

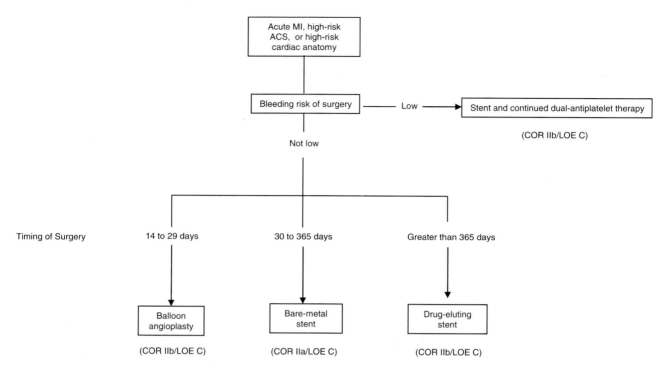

Fig 8–3. Treatment of patients requiring percutaneous cardiac intervention who need subsequent surgery. ACS indicates acute coronary syndrome; COR, class of recommendation; LOE, level of evidence; and MI, myocardial infarction. Reproduced with permission from Fleisher et al.[5] Copyright © 2007 by the American College of Cardiology Foundation and the American Heart Association, Inc.

Pulmonary Assessment

Many patients presenting for head and neck surgery have a significant history of tobacco abuse. As such, this patient population may have a higher overall incidence of pulmonary dysfunction that can affect the perioperative course. It is well known that patients over the age of 70 with pulmonary problems have a higher risk of long-term mortality during 2 years of follow-up.[15]

A complication from smoking is the development of chronic obstructive pulmonary disease (COPD) such as emphysema or bronchial asthma. The presence of COPD puts the patient at risk for postoperative pulmonary complications at rates quoted from 6% to 28% depending on the severity of airflow obstruction. In addition, smokers can see a 1.4- to 4.3-fold greater risk for complications.[16]

Assessment consists usually of obtaining a thorough history and physical along with chest radiography. The value of the chest radiograph is to detect evidence of significant anatomic changes related to emphysema such as flattening of the diaphragm or presence of bullous changes. Occult lung disease such as carcinoma can be frequently detected by simple radiography. The role for pulmonary function tests in head and neck procedures is limited at best. Essentially, the tests have the value of showing whether the patient will respond to bronchodilator therapy. Baseline arterial blood gas measurements should be performed in patients with a significant pulmonary history. These measurements will reveal those patients with significant hypoxia or hypercarbia and allow for appropriate management in the postoperative period. Significant hypoxia will also put the patient at risk for the development of pulmonary hypertension. The existence of pulmonary hypertension (and possibly right ventricular dysfunction) is important to recognize as anesthetic agents, fluid management, positive pressure ventilation, and temperature may have significant impact on this disease state.

AIRWAY

The approach to the airway in head and neck oncologic surgery is best performed as a team approach. Appropriate communication between the anesthesiologist and the otolaryngologist is essential, as various lesions may make securing the airway impossible under conventional techniques. We review the basic anatomy of the airway, as it is important to understand the structures and how they may impact not only the surgical resection, but also the intubation approach.

The upper aerodigestive tract consists of the nasal cavity, nasopharynx, oral cavity, oropharynx, hypopharynx, supraglottis, and glottis. The nasal cavity is designed to both heat and humidify inspired air. The nasal septum is composed of cartilage anteriorly (quadrangular cartilage) and bone posteriorly. The perpendicular plate of the ethmoid bone forms the septum superiorly and the vomer accounts for the inferior portion. The nasal turbinates arise from the lateral walls of the nasal cavity. The inferior, middle, and superior turbinates are bony projections that are covered with mucosa. The turbinates increase nasal surface area to aid in warming and humidifying inspired air. The nasal cavities communicate with the nasopharynx posteriorly.

Access to the nasopharynx during nasal intubation, placement of a nasal trumpet, or placement of a nasogastric tube is achieved by inserting these devices along the floor of the nose inferior to the inferior turbinate (parallel to the horizontal plane). Care must be taken to avoid trauma to the highly vascular nasal septum during these procedures to prevent epistaxis. The nasopharynx is the area posterior to the choana and extends inferiorly to the level of the soft palate. The medial openings of the

eustachian tubes are found on the lateral walls of the nasopharynx and adenoid tissue is found in the midline in the pediatric population.

The oral cavity extends from the lips to the junction of the hard and soft palate and circumvallate papillae. It is the most common site of malignancy of the head and neck. The oral cavity consists of seven subsites: lips, buccal mucosa, alveolar ridge, retromolar trigone (triangle-shaped region with the base at the last mandibular molar and the apex at the maxillary tuberosity), hard palate, floor of mouth, and oral tongue.[17] The oral tongue (anterior 2/3 of the entire tongue) receives its general sensation innervation from the lingual nerve (CN V$_3$), taste sensation from the chorda tympani nerve (CN VII), and the entire tongue receives its motor supply from the hypoglossal nerve (CN XII). The otolaryngologist will refer to these subsites to describe locations of lesions/masses. Primary lesions of the oral cavity may not allow for oral endotracheal intubation because the tube would present an impediment to resection of the lesion. As such, an awake tracheostomy may be necessary and can be performed with sedation and local anesthetic infiltration.

The hard palate and soft palate junction, located above, and the circumvallate papillae, located below, bind the oropharynx anteriorly. The superior boundary is at the level of the hard palate and is continuous with the nasopharynx. Inferiorly it is continuous with the hypopharynx and its boundary is at the level of the pharyngoepiglottic folds. The subsites of the oropharynx are the soft palate (the uvula is its most distal extension), tonsils, lateral pharyngeal walls, posterior pharyngeal wall, and base of tongue/vallecula.

The tonsil is the subsite with the highest incidence of malignancy of the oropharynx. The base of tongue ends caudally at the anatomic region called the vallecula. This area is the space that resides between the base of tongue and epiglottis. The Macintosh laryngoscope blade (curved) is placed in the vallecula during intubation. The base of tongue receives its general sensation and taste sensation innervation from the glossopharyngeal nerve (CN XI). The base of tongue lesions must be approached with care. Difficulty with placement of Macintosh laryngoscope blades or Miller laryngoscope blades (straight) may commonly occur in patients with these lesions. It is important to understand the extent of tumor, the mobility of the tongue, and the friability of tumor. Routine laryngoscopy may cause significant bleeding resulting in obscuring of the airway. As such, other methods of securing the airway such as awake fiberoptic guided intubation or awake tracheostomy may be necessary.

The hypopharynx is inferior to the oropharynx and it surrounds the larynx. Its cephalocaudal extension is from the level of the upper border of the epiglottis to the esophageal inlet. The subsites of the hypopharynx are the piriform sinuses, the posterior pharyngeal wall, and the posterior cricoid region. The piriform sinuses lay posterolaterally to the larynx. They are roughly triangular and conelike in shape with an open base at the cephalad end, which narrows as it extends caudally.[18] The piriform sinus has the highest incidence of malignancy of the hypopharyngeal subsites. Tumors within this region may make anesthetizing of the airway difficult, especially if the anesthesiologist routinely instills local anesthetic into the piriform sinus to anesthetize the internal branch of the superior laryngeal nerve.

The larynx is divided into the supraglottis, glottis, and the subglottis. The role of the larynx is threefold: (1) protect the airway from aspiration, (2) serve as a conduit to the lungs for respiration, and (3) phonation. The supraglottis consists of the epiglottis, aryepiglottic folds, arytenoids, and false vocal folds (cords). The epiglottis has a lingual surface (anterior) and a laryngeal surface (posterior). The supraglottis extends from the superior aspect of the epiglottis to the ventricle. The ventricle is the space that lies between the false vocal folds and the true vocal folds. The internal branch of the superior laryngeal nerve (CN X) is responsible for laryngeal sensation of the false vocal folds and laryngeal mucosa superior to them.

The glottis consists of the true vocal folds. The true vocal folds consist of the thyroarytenoid muscle and the vocalis muscle. These muscles are covered by three layers of lamina propria (superficial, intermediate, and deep). The superficial lamina propria, which is covered by epithelium, is known as Reinke's space. This space provides the vocal folds with fluidity that allows for the mucosal wave that is needed for proper vibration of the vocal folds during phonation.[19]

The vocal folds attach to the arytenoids posteriorly. This area is known as the posterior commissure. The anterior commissure is the area where the true vocal folds oppose each other anteriorly and are attached to the thyroid cartilage. Movement of the true vocal folds is accomplished by muscular action of the lateral cricoarytenoid muscles (adduction), posterior cricoarytenoid muscles (abduction), interarytenoid muscle (adduction), cricothyroid muscles (increases vocal fold tension, adduction), and the thyroarytenoid (increases vocal fold tension, adduction). The motor innervation to the above intrinsic laryngeal muscles is the recurrent laryngeal nerve (CN X), except the cricothyroid muscles, which are innervated by the superior laryngeal nerve. The recurrent laryngeal nerve supplies sensory innervation of the laryngeal mucosa inferior to the false vocal folds. The subglottis is defined as the area below the true vocal folds and extends inferiorly to the inferior border of the cricoid cartilage.

When preoperatively assessing the airway, a decision must be made by the entire surgical team as to the best approach to secure the trachea. There are many accepted techniques such as laryngeal mask facilitated intubation, retrograde intubation, awake direct look laryngoscopy, and lighted stylet, in addition to fiberoptic techniques. Description of these approaches is beyond the scope of this chapter; however, for patient comfort it may be of value to secure the airway prior to tracheostomy. If this is the decision, careful sedation and localization of the airway structures, noted above, are necessary for success. Drying agents, such as anticholingerics, may facilitate topicalization with local anesthetics.

The risk, if inadequate topicalization has occurred, is the development of laryngospasm during the procedure. Laryngospasm is caused by irritation sensed by the recurrent laryngeal nerve that then triggers an exaggerated adduction vocal fold reflex. This may lead to progressive hypoxia unless the reflex is broken and may necessitate emergency cricothyroidotomy to avoid cardiovascular collapse. The laryngospasm reflex can sometimes be broken with positive pressure or small doses of neuromuscular blocking agents.

POSITIONING

Supine

The majority of head and neck procedures are performed in the supine position. For the anesthesiologist, this is the easiest position to maintain and is associated with the most stable hemodynamic profile. The supine position has limited effects on the cardiovascular system; however, there can be significant ventilation to perfusion mismatching in the presence of positive pressure ventilation. When neuromuscular blocking agents are utilized the diaphragm will elevate and abdominal contents may push into the thoracic cavity. This can result in an increase in atelectasis in the lung bases and exaggerate changes in PaO_2.

The patient also tends to be 180° from the anesthesiologist, known in the anesthesia literature as airway avoidance. This makes visual inspection of the airway and endotracheal tube difficult. The remote positioning of the endotracheal tube also causes difficulty in assessing ventilation problems that may occur during the position as well as the ability to suction the endotracheal tube if the need arises.

If the procedure is long, special attention to padding pressure points is necessary. It is especially important to focus on the heels as they are prone to pressure induced ischemia during long periods of immobility.[20] Backache can also be seen during the postoperative period, as neuromuscular blocking agents may relax the tone of paraspinal musculature. To avoid this complication many anesthesiologists will place a pillow beneath the knees to relieve the stretch of the paraspinal musculature.

Lateral

Sometimes the lateral position is chosen, particularly if parascapular, serratus, trapezius or latissimus dorsi flaps are utilized for reconstruction post-tumor resection. The lateral decubitus position is usually well tolerated, but some considerations need to be kept in mind. This position results in a significant change is pulmonary blood flow as the majority of blood will preferentially flow to the dependent portion of the lung.[21] In the meantime, most ventilation will flow to the upright lung, resulting in a significant V/Q mismatch.

Special attention needs to be paid to the dependent arm. The neurovascular bundle of the dependent arm may be compromised by compression and this can be avoided by the proper utilization of a chest roll (also known as an axillary roll). These rolls can be foam, gel, or fabric in nature and need to be placed distal to the axilla, not in the axilla. The upper arm is supported with either pillows or support devices. Attention must be paid to the final position so that stretch on the upper or lower brachial plexus is not present. It is also essential to maintain a neutral position of the cervical spine, as excessive flexion will also result in brachial plexus stretch.

The position of the lower extremities also requires attention. With improper padding, peroneal palsy of the down leg may occur. As such, it is common to flex the lower leg and place a pad between the knees. The top leg is usually positioned straight with the end result of less stretch on the lower extremity nerves.

MONITORING

Standard monitors for head and neck surgery include noninvasive blood pressure monitoring, electrocardiography, end-tidal carbon dioxide ($ETCO_2$), oxygen monitoring (as well as other gases—such as inhalational agents), pulse oximetry (SpO_2), and temperature. Electrocardiography is important as many times surgery occurs near the carotid artery and severe bradycardia may be seen when traction is applied to the artery. As such, we recommend invasive blood pressure monitoring during extensive head and neck procedures. In addition, invasive blood pressure monitoring allows for frequent assessment of hemoglobin and glucose levels as well as beat-to-beat assessment of perfusion.

Because during many head and neck procedures the head is elevated slightly above the heart, there exists a risk for venous air embolism (VAE). If significant entrainment of air occurs, hypotension and cardiac dysrhythmias may follow. Some of the monitors for VAE include precordial Doppler, transesophageal echocardiography, multiorifice central venous catheters, and end-tidal gas monitoring. However, it is obvious that many of these monitors may be difficult or impossible to place given the nature of the surgery. Transesophageal echocardiography, though highly sensitive, is essentially impossible to utilize as surgery will be performed around the probe. Precordial Dopplers may also be in the surgical field, especially if a pectoral flap reconstruction is planned.

Central venous catheters, which can also guide fluid therapy as well as aspirate air from venous air embolisms, have their own set of problems. Placement in the internal jugular system is not possible during neck dissections and subclavian vein placement also may be contraindicated secondary to the planned reconstruction. Brachial venous catheters have been advocated, but, may be difficult to place. However, for the right atrial aspiration catheter to be most effective, it must be in the correct position of the right atria.[22] Position can be confirmed by electrocardiography, fluoroscopy, or echocardiography; but the catheter may be shifted if the patient is moved during the procedure. It is possible to use femoral catheters, but these necessitate radiologic confirmation and may again be difficult to place. As such, unless the patient has a significant medical indication for central venous or pulmonary artery monitoring these devices are not routinely utilized.

At times, neurophysiologic monitoring, especially electromyography (EMG) of the facial nerve may be necessary. This is performed when integrity of the facial nerve is at jeopardy and routine use may affect perioperative outcome.[23] Direct stimulation of the facial nerve by hand-held electrodes or by stimulation needles can be performed by the surgeon and neurophysiologist, respectively. If there is a decision to utilize EMG monitoring, avoidance of long-acting neuromuscular blocking agents is preferred.

ANESTHETIC AGENTS

The selection of anesthetic agents will depend on balancing the risks and benefits of each agent with the medical condition of the patients. Many anesthetic agents adversely affect blood pressure as a result of their vasodilatory and cardiodepressant features. As such, intravenous fluid requirements are increased to maintain adequate perfusion pressure. However, excessive fluid administration will lead to significant peripheral edema that may interfere with the surgical repair.

Induction Agents

Typically, an induction agent is utilized at the start of anesthesia. Induction agents are usually ultrashort acting medications that will induce unconsciousness in the patient and allow for a smooth transition from the awake state to the physiologic state necessary to allow surgery to take place. The ultrashort action of these intravenous drugs is usually related to redistribution and not metabolism. The induction agent will rapidly achieve its effect in the brain, and then rapidly redistribute to tissues of lower blood flow. Once this has taken place, the patient will awaken, unless additional doses of the agent or another agent to sustain unconsciousness have been given.

Propofol (2,6-diisopropylphenol)

Currently, a very popular induction agent, is an isopropyl phenol hypnotic dissolved in a lipid emulsion. Propofol has a very quick onset with a resolution of symptoms in approximately 8 to 10 minutes. As with most induction agents, propofol causes a decrease in the cerebral metabolic requirements for oxygen ($CMRO_2$) by interfering with the gamma aminobutyric acid chloride channel. The GABA-chloride activation results in cell hyperpolarization resulting in the subsequent prevention of depolarization of neurons.[24]

The resulting decrease in $CMRO_2$ will also cause a decrease in cerebral blood flow. This, however, is not the only affect propofol has on blood flow. A major side effect of propofol is hypotension with administration. Propofol is also known to interfere with calcium influx in the heart leading to a decrease in contractility, which may result in a significant decrease in cardiac output with its administration. Propofol administration leads also to a significant vasodilation, which ultimately adversely effects preload and can accentuate hypotension. Compensatory increases in heart rate are not seen with propofol and, in fact, case reports of bradycardia and asystole have been attributed to the drug's administration.[25]

Propofol has a high plasma clearance and undergoes extensive extrahepatic metabolism, which explains the drugs utility as an infusion for prolong sedation. Currently, research has revealed that the kidneys may play a role in the extrahepatic clearance.[26]

Other complications with the administration of propofol include pain on injection (most likely secondary to the emulsion), hyperlipidemia, sepsis (especially if care is not taken when withdrawing the drug as the solution supports bacterial growth), and propofol infusion syndrome. Propofol infusion syndrome is a rare but deadly complication seen in the pediatric and adult population. The syndrome manifests itself by the presence of an unexplained severe metabolic acidosis and may have to do with propofol's effect on mitochondrial structures.[27] Propofol may also be used as an infusion for the maintenance of anesthesia in a total intravenous anesthetic technique. It requires a much higher infusion rate than that required for sedation, and as such, may be costly.

Etomidate

Etomidate is a carboxylated imidiazole hypnotic that acts by potentiating the GABA-mediated chloride currents.[28] The drug, which is dissolved in a glycol-containing solution, is metabolized by ester hydrolysis and is rapidly redistributed from the central nervous system (CNS). The key feature of etomidate is in its unique ability to preserve cardiovascular hemodynamics. At induction doses, there is no significant change in myocardial contractility and heart rate, and minimal effects on systemic vascular resistance. As such, cardiac output is maintained. The patient's $CMRO_2$ and cerebral blood flow are also significantly decreased, as seen with propofol. However, etomidate has no analgesic properties; thus, it does a poor job at blunting the hemodynamic effects seen with laryngoscopy.

Etomidate has a significant number of side effects associated with its use. The drug has been associated with an increase incidence of postoperative nausea, can be painful on injection, and can cause myoclonus. The most significant side effect associated with etomidate administration is transient adrenocortical suppression, which may or may not have clinical significance.[29]

Thiopental

Thiopental is the most popular thiobarbiturate hypnotic utilized in anesthesia. It has a rapid onset and a short duration of action of approximately 5 to 10 minutes. Thiopental has been extensively studied and has many desirable properties. The reduction of $CMRO_2$ and CBF is profound and thiopental has been found to be neuroprotective in times of focal cerebral ischemia.[30] However, on the negative side, thiopental has some significant side effects. Because the elimination half-time is long, approximately 11.9 hours, repeated doses of thiopental may result in delayed emergence. It also causes significant changes in blood pressure secondary to vasodilation, negative inotropy, and reduction in sympathetic outflow. However, there is usually a reflex tachycardia seen with the administration of thiopental, thus the hypotension seen with thiopental tends to be less than that of propofol.

Thiopental is very alkaline in nature, and as such will precipitate acidic medications that may be present in the intravenous line. Also, if accidentally administered via an artery, crystalline precipitation may occur resulting in severe vasospasm and ischemia. In addition, histamine release may occur leading to an accentuation of the hypotension seen with routine administration.

Ketamine

Ketamine is a unique agent that can be utilized for the induction of anesthesia. It is a phencyclidine derivative with significant analgesic properties. The value of the agent is in the fact that it causes an increase in sympathetic outflow, resulting in an increase in blood pressure, heart rate, and cardiac output. As such, it is an ideal agent for patients who have a low cardiac output and hypovolemia. Ketamine can also cause significant bronchial dilation and tends to maintain minute ventilation, so may serve a role as an induction agent in the asthmatic patient.

However, the increase in heart rate and afterload makes ketamine's administration in the presence of cardiovascular disease contraindicated. Other problems associated with ketamine include an increase in cerebral blood flow (CBF), in $CMRO_2$, in salivation, nystagmus, and emergence delirium.

Recently, ketamine has gained popularity as an analgesic. Small subhypnotic doses are effective as an analgesic and have been used successfully to enhance propofol sedation. In addition, ketamine may be useful for in reducing opioid-induced hypergalgesia.[31]

Midazolam

Midazolam is a benzodiazepine sedative-hypnotic that has characteristics that make it a valuable agent during anesthesia. In large doses, it can induce anesthesia while maintaining favorable hemodynamics with only minimal effects on the cardiovascular and respiratory system. The true benefit with midazolam is its anti-anxiolytic and amnestic properties (induces anterograde amnesia). Midazolam is a hydrophilic compound, which at physiologic pH becomes a ring structure, thus lipid soluble. This allows for easy intravenous (IV) administration and intramuscular (IM) administration. As a benzodiazepine, midazolam also has a role as an anticonvulsant agent (Table 8–1).

INHALATIONAL AGENTS

Inhalational agents are typically nonflammable halogenated compounds that are relatively insoluble and poorly metabolized. Inhalational anesthetic agents are the only solitary agents that provide amnesia, analgesia, and muscle relaxation. Thus, technically speaking, they are the only true anesthesic drugs. Currently inhalational agents on the market include: nitrous oxide, halothane, desflurane, enflurane, sevoflurane, and isoflurane.

When discussing inhalational anesthetic agents one must be aware of the term MAC (minimum alveolar concentration). MAC is described as the level of inhalational anesthesia agent necessary to render approximately 50% of the population immobile to surgical stimulation. Many physiologic and pharmacologic features will affect MAC and must be taken into account. Hyperthermia, hypernatremia, and elevated central nervous system catecholamine levels cause some of the increases in MAC. Decreases are seen with the utilization of opioids, increasing age, hypothermia, and alpha-2 agonists. Ultimately the terminology is utilized as a guide of potency, with those agents with a low MAC being the most potent drug. The least potent is nitrous oxide (with a MAC of 104 vol%—obtained in a hyperbaric situation), whereas the most potent agent currently used is halothane (with a MAC of 0.75 vol%).[32]

The mechanism of action of inhalational agents is currently under investigation, but what is known is that it is the partial pressure of the agent in the brain that exerts the effect. As such, the partial pres-

Table 8–1. Agents Utilized for Induction of Anesthesia

Propofol	Induction: 1.5–2.5 mg/kg IV	Sedation: 25–100 mcg/kg/min
Etomidate	Induction: 0.2–0.4 mg/kg IV	Sedation: not recommended
Thiopental	Induction: 3–5 mg/kg IV	Sedation: not recommended
Ketamine	Induction: 1–2 mg/kg IV, 4–8 mg/kg IM	Analgesia: 0.2–0.5 mg/kg IV
Midazolam	Induction: 0.1–0.2 mg/kg	Sedation: 0.5–4 mg IV 1–7 mg/hr infusion

sure of the agent seen in the alveolus equates with that which is seen in the brain. Ultimately, the alveolar concentration (or end-tidal anesthetic concentration) serves as a marker of concentration in the brain. Highly insoluble agents will achieve parity between the alveolus and the brain quicker than more soluble agents; thus, their effects will be faster. This is the situation seen with the newer generation inhalational agents such as sevoflurane and desflurane. Both inhalational agents, due to their highly insoluble nature, have a quick onset of action and allow for easy titration and quick emergence. Sevoflurane has the added benefit of being well tolerated for inhalational induction of anesthesia. This makes the agent the ideal drug for children without intravenous access and for patients in which avoidance of positive pressure ventilation is desired, such as patients with compressive anterior mediastinal masses.

All inhalational agents with the exception of nitrous oxide cause a dose-dependent decrease in blood pressure. This change in blood pressure may be secondary to changes in systemic vascular resistance or inotropy. In addition inhalational agents may affect heart rate by either inducing a reflex tachycardia or bradycardia and appear to sensitize the myocardium to epinephrine.

Inhalational agents blunt the respiratory response to hypoxia that is mediated by the carotid bodies. This may place a patient at risk for hypoxia in the postoperative period as the effect is seen with very small amounts of inhalational anesthetics. Cerebral blood flow is increased even though $CMRO_2$ is slightly decreased; thus autoregulation is uncoupled. This situation can be problematic in the presence of existing intracranial abnormalities.

Choosing which inhalational agent will depend on the duration of the case, the medical condition of the patient, and the side effects of each drug. A unique feature of these agents is that the MAC is additive. In other words, by adding nitrous oxide, an agent which has a low incidence of cardiovascular side effects, to isoflurane, an agent which has significant vasodilatory properties, the anesthesiologist is able to use less of both drugs, and thus have less side effects.

Typically, large doses of inhalational agents will cause profound vasodilation and as such, significant drops in blood pressure. This may result in an increase in fluid administration to maintain adequate perfusion pressures, but lead to increases in third spacing and edema at the surgical site. The utilization of vasoactive substances to allow for deep planes of inhalational anesthesia are controversial and may lead to an increased incidence of perioperative myocardial ischemia in patients at risk.[33] High doses required for surgical immobility may also adversely affect somatosensory evoked potentials and other forms of neurophysiologic monitoring.[34]

Because of these issues, inhalational agents usually serve the purpose as a background anesthetic, namely, to ensure amnesia, whereas other agents such as opioids or neuromuscular blocking agents are used for analgesia and skeletal muscle relaxation.

OPIOIDS

Opioid administration is common during the management of the patient for head and neck surgery. Not only does it provide analgesia for the surgical stimulation, but also provides pain relief for the postoperative period. Opioids have specific characteristics and side effects but elicit their analgesic effect via Mu receptors in the central nervous system. Mu_1 receptors are associated with supraspinal and spinal analgesia, euphoria, and miosis, whereas the Mu_2 receptors are associated with spinal analgesia, depression of ventilation, physical dependence, and constipation.

In general, all opioids have the side effect of dose-dependent, gender-specific ventilatory depression. There is a decreased responsiveness of the ventilation centers to carbon dioxide as demonstrated by a rightward shift in the carbon dioxide response curve. Other complications of opioid administration include nausea and vomiting secondary to stimulation of the chemoreceptor trigger zone in the floor of the fourth ventricle, constipation, urinary retention, cough suppression, biliary colic, and delayed gastric emptying. Antagonists to opioid stimulation of the Mu receptors do exist, notably naloxone. However, care must be taken when administering naloxone, as the unmasking of pain may lead to a surge of sympathetic outflow resulting in pulmonary edema, delirium, and arrhythmias.

Morphine

Morphine is the classic opioid utilized and has value especially as an analgesic in the postoperative period, usually administered via patient-controlled analgesia devices. Intraoperative usage of opioids requires an agent that has a quick onset of action and relatively short duration of effect. As morphine has an onset and peak time of effect that is slow, it is not the ideal drug for intraoperative opioid use. The metabolite of morphine, morphine-6-glucoronide, is excreted via the renal system and has analgesic and respiratory depressant qualities. As such, it should be used with caution in patients with preexisting renal disease. Other complications of morphine administration include histamine release (which can result in hypotension, bronchospasm, or rash) and drug-induced bradycardia.

Fentanyl

One of the more popular opioids utilized in anesthesia is fentanyl. Fentanyl is a phenylpiperidine-derivative opioid that has an analgesic potency that is 75 to 125 times that of morphine. The onset time for fentanyl is quite fast and has a shorter duration of action compared with morphine. Small intravenous doses around 1 to 2 mcg/kg are routinely used for analgesia, whereas doses of 2 to 20 mcg/kg are used to decrease the sympathetic output seen with surgical stimulation or laryngoscopy. Routinely, for prolonged head and neck procedures, fentanyl is administered as an infusion. Because of fentanyl's context-sensitive half-time, prolonged administration may lead to large drug accumulations. It is important to realize that the context-sensitive half-time is the time necessary for the plasma concentration to decrease 50% after discontinuation of the infusion and should be taken into consideration whenever choosing an agent for prolong infusion.[35]

Skeletal muscle rigidity has been seen with the administration of fentanyl and other opioids; however, this rigidity typically is found in the supraglottic musculature. The muscular stimulation may lead to difficult in ventilation and has been given the misnomer of "chest-wall rigidity." Studies, utilizing fiberoptic observation, noted significant movement of supraglottic structures and vocal fold closure with opioid administration and explain the difficulty with mask ventilation.[36,37] Fentanyl has also been associated with bradycardia, but histamine release is not seen. Hypotension seen with the administration of fentanyl is related to its ability to blunt sympathetic outflow.

Remifentanil

Remifentanil is an ultrashort-acting opioid agonist that requires administration via infusion. Typically remifentanil is given by loading with an infusion rate of 0.5 to 1.0 mcg/kg/min, followed by a reduction to a rate of 0.25 to 0.125 mcg/kg/min after stimulation has occurred. Remifentanil has the benefit of being metabolized by esterases, and is well tolerated in patients with a history of liver or kidney disease. The major feature, however, is the rapid onset and short duration of remifentanil. There is no significant accumulation of the drug over long administration due to its context-sensitive half-time.[38] Thus, the drug works well in situations in which respiratory depression is to be avoided.

Remifentanil works exceptionally well for procedures of intense stimulation such as direct laryngoscopy/esophagoscopy and bronchoscopies. Significant bradycardia can be seen with the administration of remifentanil along with hypotension, secondary to a decrease is sympathetic outflow. Other anesthetic agents must therefore be reduced in dose when administered along with remifentanil. Remifentanil has also been utilized as an adjunct to sedation with propofol or midazolam and can be used for postoperative analgesia. However, the utilization of remifentanil for postoperative pain control is limited by its short duration of action.

NEUROMUSCULAR BLOCKING AGENTS

Neuromuscular block agents are routinely utilized during anesthesia to facilitate intubation of the trachea and to provide relaxation of skeletal muscle to enhance surgical exposure. Two general types of blocking agents exist, depolarizing and nondepolarizing neuromuscular agents. Both act on the nicotinic acetylcholine receptors at the neuromuscular junction, leading to an interruption of transmission of nerve impulses to the neuromuscular junction. Depolarizing agents act similar to or mimic the actions of acetylcholine, by opening the junction and causing muscle contraction followed by relaxation. Nondepolarizing agents act by competing with acetylcholine for the receptor site and are easily displaced by large concentrations of acetylcholine. There is an exhaustive list of neuromuscular blocking drugs but we discuss only a couple of those currently utilized.

Succinylcholine

Succinylcholine is a depolarizing neuromuscular blocking agent that has a very short duration of action. The onset time is quick, the relaxation intense, (especially with the musculature around the vocal folds), and the duration around 10 minutes. Succinylcholine is rapidly metabolized into succinic acid and choline by pseudocholinesterase, an esterase found in the plasma. Succinylcholine is characterized by the fasciculation of muscle groups when neuromuscular receptors are stimulated. The drug keeps the channels open for a prolonged period of time, leading to relaxation.

A clinician would think that the features of fast onset, fast offset would make succinylcholine an ideal agent for tracheal intubation; however, it has many major side effects. Succinylcholine, as its structure is similar to acetylcholine, can modestly stimulate the nicotinic receptors in the autonomic ganglia of the sympathetic chain and the cardiac muscarinic receptors.[39] This may lead to significant arrhythmias such as bradycardia and asystole, increases in gastric motility, increases in intraocular pressure, and increases in intracranial pressure. The skeletal muscle fasciculations may lead to myalgias, myoglobinuria, and subsequent renal failure or renal dysfunction. Other complications include significant hyperkalemia (especially in patients with extrajunctional receptors such as burn patients), masseter jaw rigidity, and malignant hyperthermia. Succinylcholine has been used in the past as an infusion to provide relaxation for direct laryngoscopy/esophagoscopy procedures. However, this technique has been all but abandoned secondary to the multiple complications seen with the drug's administration.

Nondepolarizing Neuromuscular Blocking Agents

Vecuronium and rocuronium are examples of nondepolarizing neuromuscular blocking drugs that compete with acetylcholine at the site of the neuromuscular junction. These drugs have limited cardiovascular side effects, and as such, have tremendous value in patients with significant coronary artery disease. Both are classified as intermediate duration drugs with duration of action of approximately 20 minutes. Each can be used for facilitating tracheal intubation; however, rocuronium has a significantly faster onset time as compared to vecuronium. The fast onset time for rocuronium (90–120 seconds) makes it a choice for rapid sequence induction, a technique in which an induction agent followed by a neuromuscular blocking agent and cricoid pressure is administered prior to endotracheal intubation to decrease the possibility of aspiration. However, the longer duration of action is an unattractive feature of rocuronium as compared to succinylcholine.

Atracurium and cisatracurium are also nondepolarizing agents of intermediate duration. These drugs are metabolized by Hoffman elimination and esterases and do not rely on liver metabolism or renal excretion. Therefore, cisatracurium or atracurium has a role in patients with end-stage liver or renal disease. Atracurium has been associated with histamine release when administered in a large and rapid manner, which is not seen with the administration of cisatracurium.

The antagonism of nondepolarizing neuromuscular blocking agents is achieved by administering an agent that will cause a rise in acetylcholine in the neuromuscular junction. These agents are typical acetylcholinesterase inhibitors, which have the function of blocking the breakdown of acetylcholine. Acetylcholinesterase inhibitors are not site specific, so administration of these agents leads to the systemic side effects of excessive acetylcholine, such as bradycardia and nausea. As such, these agents (eg, edrophonium or neostigmine) are administered along with an anticholinergic (eg, atropine or glycopyrrolate, respectively).

The challenge exists to create a nondepolarizing neuromuscular agent that acts similar to succinylcholine, that is, has intense relaxation and a rapid onset and offset. Early agents, such as rapacuronium (removed from the market because of case reports of intense bronchospasm associated with administration) have been unsatisfactory. However, new antagonism agents in development such as sugammadex (Org 25969) may help in this situation. Sugammadex is a novel antagonist to rocuronium that characteristically binds the agent and inhibits rocuronium's effects.[40] Sugammadex has the added benefit of not raising systemic acetylcholine and can be administered shortly after administration of rocuronium. The drug is currently under investigation, but may eventually be of value as part of a succinylcholine replacement therapy.

PERIOPERATIVE ANTIBIOTIC THERAPY

The final steps in the preoperative preparation of the patient for head and neck are the selection and timely administration of the correct antibiotic(s). Antibiotics are prophylactically administered parentally prior to the beginning of surgery to prevent the contaminating of the surgical wound and the development of local wound sepsis. The development of a postoperative wound infection increases the morbidity after head and neck surgery. Patients with head and neck malignancies may have conditions that make them more susceptible to infection including malnutrition due to dysphagia and/or alcoholism, previous radiation to the head and neck, and previous chemotherapy. The use of prophylactic antibiotics depends on the level of wound contamination expected or encountered during the procedure. The majority of oncologic head and neck procedures are either class I surgical wounds (clean) and class II surgical wounds (clean-contaminated). Clean surgical wounds of the head and neck consist of procedures in which the mucosa of the upper aerodigestive tract is not opened or involved in the surgical field (ie, thyroidectomy, parotidectomy, solitary neck dissection). In clean wounds, infection risk without perioperative antibiotic therapy is less than 1%.[41] Previous chemotherapy treatment for

head and neck malignancy has been shown to be a risk factor for wound infection after clean surgical procedures. Penel et al[42] reported a 90% wound infection rate in this specific patient population with the majority of pathogens being gram-positive aerobes. Antibiotic prophylaxis with gram-positive coverage (ie, cefazolin) should be administered in this setting.

The majority of head and neck oncologic procedures involve class II surgical wounds because of their location in the upper aerodigestive tract. Surgical treatment of malignant and benign tumors of the nasal cavity, paranasal sinuses, oral cavity, nasopharynx, oropharynx, hypopharynx, and larynx all involve a breach of the mucosal barrier. This breach allows for contamination of the surgical wound and field with gram-positive aerobes, gram-negative aerobes, and anaerobic pathogens arising from oropharyngeal secretions. The incidence of wound infections without preoperative antibiotics in head and neck clean-contaminated procedures range from 30 to 80%.[43] Comparative studies of perioperative antimicrobial prophylaxis in head and neck cancer surgery have clearly documented the efficacy of antimicrobial prophylaxis and reducing postoperative infections and patient morbidity following head and neck surgery. Johnson et al[44] compared 1.5 g ampicillin/sulbactam and 600 mg clindamycin therapy in the perioperative period. It was shown that 14% in each group developed postoperative wound infection. This study shows ampicillin/sulbactam is as effective as clindamycin in preventing infection. Ampicillin/sulbactam has also been shown to be more cost effective compared to clindamycin.[45] In our institution, ampicillin/sulbactam is the drug of choice and clindamycin is used for those with penicillin allergy. A number of studies have shown that 1-day antibiotic therapy is as effective as prolonged therapy.[46,47]

FLUID MANAGEMENT

Maintaining a state of normovolemia is desirable for any patient undergoing surgery. Head and neck surgery is no exception; however, aggressive fluid resuscitation may lead to peripheral edema and hamper attempts at surgical reaction and repair. During most otolaryngology cancer surgeries, large areas in the neck region are exposed to air. As such, there is significant fluid loss by evaporation. In addition, many of the vascular surfaces are disrupted leading to blood loss and third spacing of crystalloid. The anesthesiologist has to balance the effects of inhalational anesthetics and their side effect of vasodilation. This is especially important as many of the patients presenting for surgery are volume depleted from preoperative fasting or diseases such as hypertension.

There is currently no definitive measure of left ventricular preload, that is, left ventricular end-diastolic volume. Invasive monitors such as central venous pressure and pulmonary artery pressure are only rough estimates and have complications associated with placement. In addition, invasive monitors are affected by afterload, variations in ventricular compliance, positive pressure ventilation, and the presence of positive end-expiratory pressure.[48] Transesophageal echocardiographical (TEE) images of the left ventricle in the short axis, mid-papillary view may give an estimate of preload; however, as mentioned earlier, TEE is technically impossible to perform during these surgeries.

Measuring urine output is a popular way to assess fluid status; however, this too has problems. A history of diuretic use, pre-existing renal or liver disease, hypotension, and low cardiac output states may distort the amount of volume obtained. Commonly, practicing anesthesiologists may feel that urine flow rates of greater than 0.25 to 0.5 mL/kg/hr are signs of adequate fluid status, but this has not been substantiated. Other disease states may also affect urine output such as, the syndrome of inappropriate antidiuretic hormone (SIADH) and diabetes insipidus (DI). Surgical stimulation and intraoperative hypotension are known to elicit release of antidiuretic hormone;[49] thus, urine output may be low, but volume status is adequate.

The goal for fluid therapy is to maintain perfusion to tissue and thus maintain adequate oxygen transport. Early fluid therapy is indicated for hypotension not related to anesthetic dosing. Tracking arterial blood gases and the anion gap may be helpful in detecting the presence of lactic acidosis, a sign of anaerobic metabolism. Fluid administration also is essential to maintain hemodynamic stability which is especially important in this patient population given the high incidence of pre-existing cardiovascular disease.

There is a long-standing debate over the utilization of crystalloid or colloid therapy. There is currently no evidence that a purely crystalloid approach or purely colloid approach to fluid resuscitation make a difference in outcome. Crystalloid therapy is inexpensive and easy to administer. However, complications can occur depending on the crystalloid chosen. Large administrations of normal saline (0.9%) solutions are known to lead to hyperchloremic metabolic acidosis,[50] whereas excess administration of Lactated Ringer's (LR) solution may lead to hyperkalemia because of the presence of potassium and lactic acidosis because of the exogenous lactate buffer. Another problem with LR is that the crystalloid contains calcium. This calcium interacts with the citrate anticoagulant found in blood products; thus, it is contraindicated for slowly administered blood transfusions. Hypertonic saline solutions have been advocated in acute resuscitation as they cause an influx of water from the extracellular space, but can adversely affect cerebral water balance. Other crystalloid solutions such as Plasmalyte® and Normosol-R® have been advocated as they can be administered with blood and contain a lower concentration of chloride, unlike normal saline.

There are many who advocate a combination of colloid and crystalloid due to the fact that excess crystalloid therapy may dilute oncotic pressure and lead to increased peripheral edema. Two colloids are frequently utilized, namely, albumin and heta-starch—a synthetic high molecular weight starch. Colloids have the advantage of staying intravascular for longer periods of time, whereas crystalloids quickly spread throughout the intravascular and extravascular space.[51] Several studies have been performed to assess the safety of colloid therapy such as the Saline versus Albumin Fluid Evaluation study (SAFE) trial. The value of colloid therapy and safety appears to be present.[52] However, these agents are not without problems. Albumin is derived from human donors and, as such, though heat-treated, cares the possible remote risk of viral infection. Hetastarch may lead to coagulopathy when administered in concentrations greater than 20 mL/kg secondary to its interaction with Factor VIII and platelets. Hetastarch has also been associated with anaphylaxis, persistent pruritus, renal failure, and possible hepatic dysfunction.[53]

BLOOD THERAPY

During head and neck surgery significant blood loss can take place. It is prudent at least to have a blood type and screen sent to the blood bank. If a type and screen has been performed, type-specific uncrossmatched blood can be made quickly available if rapid unexpected blood loss occurs. The incidence of significant hemolytic reactions to type-specific uncrossmatched blood is exceedingly low; however, frequent following of the hematocrit during the procedure, as well as observation of the surgical field, can guide the anesthesiologist as to the need for crossmatched blood.

When to transfuse is subject to debate. Obviously, when there are signs of impaired oxygen delivery to the tissues, red blood cell administration is essential. However, one must balance the risks and benefits of transfusion therapy, and there are significant risks. Red blood cell administration has been associated with viral/bacterial infection, immunomodulation, delayed hemolytic reactions, and transfusion-related acute lung injury.[54] Thus, it is important to weigh the risks and benefits of transfusion therapy in each patient. Normovolemic anemia is usually well tolerated; however, the general consensus is that transfusion is indicated for hemoglobin values of less than 7.0 mg/dL in healthy patients and for values of less than 9.0 or 10.0 mg/dL in patients with significant cardiopulmonary disease.[55]

Blood conservation measures also may be taken, such as normovolemic hemodilution or hypotensive anesthesia, assuming there are no medical contraindications to these procedures. The role of cell salvage is limited as the nature of the surgery is that of cancer resection. It remains unclear whether there is a role for antifibrinolytics or preoperative erythropoietin therapy.[56] Namely, the side effects of antifibrinolytics, such as thromboembolism, and the cost and implementation of erythropoietin therapy limit their usefulness.

RECOVERY

Once the surgical procedure is completed, the patient is allowed to emerge from anesthesia. The nature of the procedure, length of procedure, the anesthetic utilized, and possibility of fluid shifts in the postoperative period will affect the decision regarding the need for mechanical ventilation. Physiologically, it is in the patient's best interest to resume spontaneous ventilation as soon as possible. However, care must be taken, especially if excessive manipulation of the airway has occurred without the establishment of a tracheostomy.

Postoperative laryngeal edema, tongue edema, and the presence of blood may make emergency reintubation difficult, if not impossible. Airway maneuvers in the postsurgical patient may disrupt delicate repairs and cause brisk and difficult to control hemorrhage. As such, it is important to ensure that the patient meets specific criteria prior to discontinuation of mechanical ventilation and intubation. The patient must be awake, alert, and appropriate without signs of respiratory distress as evident by the lack of tachypnea, maintenance of oxygen saturation, avoidance of severe hypercarbia, and a low work of breathing. Routine assessment of oxygenation and ventilation by arterial blood gas monitoring may be indicated.

If the patient has a tracheostomy placed during the procedure, care must be taken when manipulating the surgical site. Coughing is commonly seen, as is reflective of the irritating nature of the tracheostomy device. Local anesthetics such as lidocaine or tetracaine can be instilled via the trachea and may temporarily blunt the coughing reflex. At times, bleeding may occur around the tracheostomy site, necessitating surgical revision. It is also important to remember that as the tracheostomy site has not had time to mature, inadvertent removal (without the presence of tracheal identification sutures) may lead to a loss of airway and an inability to reinsert the airway device.

Hemodynamic control is also important in the recovery phase. Excessive changes in afterload and heart rate will affect myocardial oxygen consumption and may lead to myocardial ischemia and infarction. In addition, uncontrolled hypertension may stress suture lines and lead to postoperative hemorrhage. Vasodilators such as the mixed alpha- and beta-blocking agent, labetolol, may serve as an adjunctive to blood pressure control. The clinician must also rule out easily reversible contributors to hypertension, for example, pain, urinary retention, hypercarbia, and hypoxia.

In the immediate postoperative period, attention must also be paid to the maintenance of normothermia and glucose control. Avoidance of hypothermia is essential as hypothermia may lead to coagulopathies, arrhythmias, delayed metabolism of neuromuscular blocking agents, and depression of mental status.[57] Forced air warmers can be effective in maintaining normothermia intraoperatively and postoperatively and will help to avoid shivering, a physiologic response to changes in temperature, which may increase myocardial oxygen consumption. Recent studies involving patients in critical care settings have indicated that tighter glucose control may improve perioperative outcome; therefore, in patients with a history of diabetes mellitus, appropriate glucose management is important.[58]

SUMMARY

There are many issues facing the entire health care team when dealing with patients undergoing head and neck oncologic surgery. Appropriate preoperative assessment of medical diseases, as well as development of a team approach to airway management, is necessary. In addition, balancing the effects of the anesthetic provided along with the comorbidities of the patient is essential to ensure a satisfactory outcome. Providers must have an understanding of the effects of drugs and fluid management utilized during the perioperative period and how these medical interventions interact with the patient's physical status.

REFERENCES

1. Goldman L, Caldera DL, Nussbaum SR, et al. Multifactorial index of cardiac risk in noncardiac surgical procedures. *New Engl J Med.* 1977;297:845-850.

2. Detsky AS, Abrams HB, Forbath N, Scott JG, Hilliard JR. Cardiac assessment for patients undergoing noncardiac surgery: a multifactorial clinical risk index. *Arch Intern Med.* 1986;146:2131-2134.

3. Lee TH, Marcantonio ER, Mangione CM, et al. Derivation and prospective validation of a simple index for prediction of cardiac risk of major noncardiac surgery. *Circulation.* 1999;100:1043-1049.

4. Eagle KA, Berger PB, Calkins H, et al. ACC/AHA guideline update for perioperative cardiovascular evaluation for noncardiac surgery—executive summary: a report of the American College of Cardiology/American Heart Association Task Force on Practice Guidelines (Committee to Update the 1996 Guidelines on Perioperative Cardiovascular Evaluation for Noncardiac Surgery). *Circulation.* 2002;105:1257-1267.

5. Fleisher LA, Beckman JA, Brown KA, et al. ACC/AHA 2007 guidelines on perioperative cardiovascular evaluation and care for noncardiac surgery: executive summary: a report of the American College of Cardiology/American Heart Association Task Force on Practice Guidelines (Writing Committee to Revise the 2002 Guidelines on Perioperative Cardiovascular Evaluation for Noncardiac Surgery). *Circulation.* 2007;116:1971-1996.

6. Kertai, MD, Bogar L, Gal J, Poldermans D. Preoperative coronary revascularization: an optimal therapy for high-risk vascular surgery patients? *Acta Anaesthesiol Scand.* 2006; 50:816-827.

7. Grayburn PA, Hillis LD. Cardiac events in patients undergoing noncardiac surgery: shifting the paradigm from noninvasive risk stratification to therapy. *Ann Intern Med.* 2003;138(6):506-511.

8. Kaluza GL, Joseph J, Lee JR, Raizner ME, Raizner AE. Catastrophic outcomes of noncardiac surgery soon after coronary stenting. *J Am Coll Cardiol.* 2000;35:1288-1294.

9. Dupuis JY, Labinaz M. Noncardiac surgery in patients with coronary artery stent: what should the anesthesiologist know? *Can J Anesth.* 2005; 52(4):356-361.

10. Berger PB, Wilson SH, Fasseas P, Orford J. Reply re: Clinical outcomes of patients undergoing noncardiac surgery in the two months following coronary stenting. *J Amer Coll Card.* 2004;43(4):714-715.

11. Giles JW, Sear JW, Foex P. Effect of chronic β-blockade on perioperative outcome in patients undergoing noncardiac surgery: an analysis of observational and case control studies. *Anaesthesia.* 2004;59:574-583.

12. Poldermans D, Bax JJ, Kertai MD, et al. Statins are associated with a reduced incidence of periopera-

tive mortality in patients undergoing major non-cardiac vascular surgery. *Circulation.* 2003;107: 1848-1851.

13. Wallace AW, Galindez D, Salahieh A, et al. Effect of clonidine on cardiovascular morbidity and mortality after noncardiac surgery. *Anesthesiology.* 2004; 101(2):284-293.

14. Clinical Trial. POISE trial: Perioperative ischemic evaluation study. Retrieved November 27, 2006 from: http://www.clinicaltrials.gov/ct/gui/show/NCT00182039

15. Manku K, Bacchetti P, Leung JM. Prognostic significance of postoperative in- hospital complications in elderly patients. I. Long-term survival. *Anesth Analg.* 2003;96:583-589.

16. Smetana GW. Preoperative pulmonary evaluation. *N Engl J Med.* 1999;340:937-944.

17. Pasha R, Yoo GH, Jacobs JR. Head and neck cancer. In: Pasha R., ed. *Otolaryngology Head and Neck Surgery: Clinical Reference Guide.* San Diego, Calif: Singular; 2001.

18. MacComb WS, Healey JE, McGraw JP, Fletcher GH, Gallager HS, Paulas DD (1967). Hypopharynx and cervical esophagus. In: MacComb WS, Fletcher G H, eds. *Cancer of the Head and Neck.* Baltimore, Md: Williams & Williams; 1967:217-219.

19. Pasha R, Dworkin JP, Meleca RJ. Laryngology. In: Pasha R, ed. *Otolaryngology Head and Neck Surgery: Clinical Reference Guide.* San Diego, Calif.: Singular; 2001:84-87.

20. Warner MA. Supine positions. In: Martin JT, Warner MA, eds. *Positioning in Anesthesia and Surgery,* 3rd ed. Philadelphia, Pa: WB Saunders; 1997:39-46.

21. Lee JW, Cassorla L. In: Stoelting RK, Miller RD, eds. *Basics of Anesthesia,* 5th ed., Philadelphia, Pa: Churchill Livingstone-Elsevier; 2007:294-296.

22. Kerr RHE, Applegate RL. Accurate placement of the right atrial air aspiration catheter: a descriptive study and prospective trial of intravascular electrocardiography. *Anesth Analg.* 2006;103: 435-438.

23. Edwards BM, Kileny PR. Intraoperative neurophysiologic monitoring: indications and techniques for common procedures in otolaryngology-head and neck surgery. *Otolaryngol Clin North Am.* 2005; 38:631-642.

24. Lynch C, Pancrazio JJ. Snails, spiders and stereospecificity—is there a role for calcium channels in anesthetic mechanisms? *Anesthesiology.* 1994;81:1-5.

25. Egan TD, Brock UJG. Asystole after anesthesia induction with fentanyl, propofol and succinylcholine sequence. *Anesth Analg.* 1991;73:818-820.

26. Takizawa D, Hiraoka H, Goto F, Yamamoto K, Horiuchi R. Human kidneys play an important role in the elimination of propofol. *Anesthesiology.* 2005; 102:327-330.

27. Vasile B, Rasulo F, Candiani A, Latronico N. The pathophysiology of propofol infusion syndrome: a simple name for a complex syndrome. *Intensive Care Med.* 2003;29:1417-1425.

28. Stoelting RK, Hillier SC. Nonbarbiturate intravenous anesthetic drugs. *Pharmacology and Physiology in Anesthetic Practice.* 4th ed. Philadelphia, Pa: Lippincott Williams & Wilkins; 2006:155-178.

29. Fragen RT, Shanks CA, Molteni A, et al. Effects of etomidate on hormonal responses to surgical stress. *Anesthesiology.* 1984;61:652-656.

30. Stoelting RK, Hillier SC. Barbiturates. *Pharmacology and Physiology in Anesthetic Practice.* 4th ed. Philadelphia, Pa: Lippincott Williams & Wilkins; 2006:127-139.

31. Himmelseher S, Durieux ME. Ketamine for perioperative pain management. *Anesthesiology.* 2005; 102:211-220.

32. Stoelting RK, Hillier SC. Inhaled anesthetics. *Pharmacology and Physiology in Anesthetic Practice.* 4th ed. Philadelphia, Pa: Lippincott Williams & Wilkins; 2006:42-86.

33. Smith JS, Roizen MF, Cahalan MK, et al. Does anesthetic technique make a difference? Augmentation of systolic blood pressure during carotid endarterectomy: effects of phenylephrine versus light anesthesia and of isoflurane versus halothane on the incidence of myocardial ischemia. *Anesthesiology.* 1988;69(6):846-853.

34. Banoub M, Tetzlaff J E, Schubert A. Pharmacologic and physiologic influences affecting sensory evoked potentials: implications for perioperative monitoring. *Anesthesiology.* 2003;99(3):716-737.

35. Stoelting RK, Hillier SC. Opioid agonists and antagonists. *Pharmacology and Physiology in Anesthetic Practice.* 4th ed. Philadelphia, Pa: Lippincott Williams & Wilkins; 2006:87-126

36. Bennett JA, Abrams JT, Van Riper DF, Horrow JC. Difficult or impossible ventilation after sufentanil-induced anesthesia is caused primarily by vocal cord closure. *Anesthesiology.*1997;87:1070-1074.

37. Vincenzo F, Baldassare M, Francesco M, Spinelli F, Santamaria LB. Tramadol and vocal cord closure. *Anesthesiology.* 2005;102:227-229.

38. Egan TD, Lemmens HJM, Fiset P, et al. The pharmacokinetics of the new short-acting opioid Remifentanil (G187084B) in healthy adult male volunteers. *Pediatr Neurosurg.* 1993;79:881-892.

39. Stoelting RK, Hillier SC. Neuromuscular-blocking drugs. *Pharmacology and Physiology in Anesthetic Practice.* 4th ed. Philadelphia, Pa: Lippincott Williams & Wilkins; 2006:208–250.

40. Kopman AF. Sugammadex: a revolutionary approach to neuromuscular antagonism. *Anesthesiology.* 2006;104:631–633.

41. Johnson JT, Wagner RL. Infection following uncontaminated head and neck surgery. *Arch Otolaryngol Head Neck Surg.* 1987;113:368–369.

42. Penel N, Fournier C, Lefebvre D, et al. Previous chemotherapy as a predictor of wound infections in nonmajor head and neck surgery: results of a prospective study. *Head Neck.* 2004; 26:513–517.

43. Penel N, Lefebvre D, Fournier C, Sarini J, Kara A, Lefevre JL. Risk factors for wound infection in head and neck cancer surgery: a prospective study. *Head Neck.* 2001;23:447–455.

44. Johnson JT, Kachman K, Wagner RL, Myers EN. Comparison of ampicillin/sulbactam versus clindamycin in the prevention of infection in patients undergoing head and neck surgery. *Head Neck.* 1997;19:367–371.

45. Weber RS, Raad I, Frankenthaler R, et al. Ampicillin/sulbactam vs. clindamycin in head and neck oncologic surgery: the need for gram-negative coverage. *Arch Otolaryngol Head Neck Surg.* 1992;118: 1159–1163.

46. Coskun H, Erisen L, Basut O. Factors affecting wound infection rates in head and neck surgery. *Otolaryngol Head Neck Surg.* 2000;123:328–333.

47. Righi M, Manfredi R, Farneti G, Pasquini E, Cenacchi V. Short-term versus long-term antimicrobial prophylaxis in oncologic head and neck surgery. *Head Neck.* 1996;18:399–404.

48. Magder, S. Central venous pressure: a useful but not so simple measurement. *Crit Care Med.* 2006; 34:2224–2228.

49. Treschan T, Peters J. The vasopressin system. *Anesthesiology.* 2006;105:599–612.

50. Scheingraber S, Markus R, Sehmisch C, Finsterer U. Rapid saline infusion produces hyperchloremic acidosis in patients undergoing gynecologic surgery. *Anesthesiology.* 1999;90:1265–1270.

51 Grocott MPW, Mythen MG, Gan TJ. Perioperative fluid management and clinical outcomes in adults. *Anesth Analg.* 2005;100:1093–1106.

52. Finfer S, Bellomo R, Boyce N, French J. A comparison of albumin and saline for fluid resuscitation in the intensive care unit. *N Engl J Med.* 2004;350: 2247–2256.

53. Barron ME, Mahlon MW, Navickis RJ. A systemic review of the comparative safety of colloids. *Arch Surg.* 2004;139:552–563.

54. Goodnough LT. Risks of blood transfusion. *Anesthesiol Clin North Am.* 2005;23:241–252.

55. Kuriyan M, Carson JL. Anemia and clinical outcomes. *Anesthesiol Clin North Am.* 2005;23: 315–325.

56. Goodnough LT, Monk TG, Andriole GL. Erythropoietin therapy. *N Engl J Med.* 1997;336: 933–938.

57. Sessler D. Complications and treatment of mild hypothermia. *Anesthesiology.* 2001;95: 531–543.

58. Ouattara A, Lecomte P, Le Manach Y, et al. Poor intraoperative blood glucose control is associated with a worsened hospital outcomes after cardiac surgery in diabetic patients. *Anesthesiology.* 2005; 103:687–694.

9

Medical Malpractice and Head and Neck Cancer

Daniel D. Lydiatt
Ryan K. Sewell
William M. Lydiatt

INTRODUCTION

Medical malpractice has reached crisis proportions in the United States. The literature is rife with references to the increased economic medical costs resulting from malpractice insurance and defensive medicine. Unfortunately, costs are not incurred by the health care system as a whole, as medical malpractice has a significant impact on the psychological and professional status of the individual practitioner(s). This chapter examines the history of medical malpractice and offers a tool, litigation analysis, to identify common themes in medical malpractice as it relates to head and neck surgery. We conclude by analyzing tort reform efforts in the United States and considering alternative schemes used in other countries.

HISTORY

The historical basis for medical malpractice has several sources. The Code of Hammurabi is regarded as the first codification of law to cite clinical malpractice. The Romans further developed medical malpractice and were the first to regard law as a science.[1] The origin of medical malpractice in the United States can be traced to English common law.[2] Common law, as opposed to statutory law, develops legal principles and rules based on judicial judgments and decrees. In Anglo-Saxon England, judges were appointed by the king. To promote efficiency and reproducibility, decisions were written down and principles decided previously were applied when similar circumstances arose. This doctrine, called "stare decisis" or let the decision stand, remains a guiding principle in American jurisprudence. During the development of the legal system in the United States, this process of accepting a law based on previous use was a simple extension of natural selection and resulted in a state of "natural law,"[3] thus leading to the belief that this state of "natural law" was both innate and unalienable. This concept of "natural law" was not new, however, and was most fully developed in Roman civil law. Although Roman and English law certainly differed, each contributed to the development of tort law in the United States.

The actual litigation of medical malpractice in the United States was rare until the middle of the Nineteenth century.[4] From 1840 to 1860, malpractice cases experienced a 950% increase. The change in malpractice during this time period is likely multifactorial, with contributions from the decline in religious fatalism, increased efforts to improve the general welfare, and increased advertising by those on the periphery of medicine.[4] Physicians often supported these cases in an attempt to discourage untrained individuals.

The "modern" malpractice crisis initially surfaced during the 1970s. The original crisis was one of coverage as many carriers opted to drop out of the malpractice insurance market. The second phase began during the 1980s which saw the cost of coverage increase. This left few affordable options available to practitioners. The present situation, some have argued, is really a combination of the previous crises with problems with both availability and affordability. For example, in 2001, St. Paul Companies, the largest malpractice insurer at the time covering 9% of all physicians, dropped out of the malpractice insurance market.[5] This time period has also seen malpractice premiums far outpace the rate of inflation, with annual increases in the 10% to 20% range and some regions experiencing nearly 100% increases. The net result is a lack of affordable malpractice insurance.[5]

THE CURRENT STATE OF MEDICAL MALPRACTICE

To better understand medical malpractice law, a general understanding of tort law is required. Medical malpractice is a subset of tort law. In general, torts can be defined as "a civil wrong, wherein one person's conduct causes compensable injury to the person, property, or recognized interest of another, in violation of a duty imposed by law."[6] The purpose of torts is to compensate the injured party by the party responsible for the injury. The goal is to make the person as near to whole as possible, considering both current and future damages.

Within this larger scheme of tort law, medical malpractice seeks to compensate patients who are injured by physicians who act negligently. To satisfy a negligence claim, the plaintiff must satisfy a four-part test. The plaintiff must prove a duty existed between the parties, the defendant breached his or her duty, the plaintiff suffered an injury, and the breach of the duty was the cause of the injury. Once

this test is satisfied, the focus turns to compensation. The goal in tort law is to return the plaintiff to a "state of wholeness," generally achieved by assessing financial damages. Damages are then divided into economic and noneconomic damages. Economic damages include lost wages and increased cost of medical care. Noneconomic damages are more nebulous and include pain and suffering as well as loss of consortium. These damages are then assessed against the party or parties found to be negligent.

Medical malpractice, in theory, provides both a deterrent and punishment to the negligent practice of medicine. Punishment comes in the form of a public accounting (ie, trial) of the error and financial compensation for any negligence found. The deterrent effect works by providing an incentive to avoid the public forum and costs associated with medical malpractice. Deterrence also occurs by allowing other physicians to learn of the negligence and take steps to prevent similar occurrences in their practice. In this way medical malpractice can result in improved medical care.

Although these theoretical attributes may exist in some form, current malpractice system appears to be losing its effectiveness and becoming increasingly expensive. The expense of the system has resulted in a 2002 U.S. Department of Health and Human Services report describing the system as "broken" and a "threat to health care quality for all Americans."[7] A closer examination of the crisis reveals a threat on several fronts.

The most obvious threat to the health care system is the legal system itself. Americans spend more per person on litigation costs than any other country in the world.[7] One estimate has placed the average cost of defending a medical malpractice claim, meritorious or not, at $28,801 per case.[8] Successful plaintiffs have seen huge increases in award amounts from 1995 to 2001, with the median jury award doubling from $500,000 to $1,000,000.[8] Although plaintiffs do see some of these increased awards, they are far from the primary beneficiaries. A recent study found that plaintiffs receive only 38% of the total amount of money in the malpractice litigation system, whereas the remaining 62% goes to plaintiff's lawyers, expert witnesses, insurers' claims adjustment, and the cost of defending claims.[8] This small percentage indicates not only an inefficient economic system of compensating those injured in the medical system, but also the financial stake attorneys and insurers have in maintaining the present system.

Insurance premiums comprise a significant portion of the malpractice costs. A 1995 study by the General Accounting Office found that insurance premiums cost medical providers between $4.86 and $9.2 billion annually.[9] In 2003, the General Accounting Office examined changes in medical malpractice insurance rates in a sampling of seven states beginning in 1999. The study found "dramatic" increases for some physicians with considerable variation based on both specialty and location. The cause of the increase, not surprisingly, was deemed to be multifactorial. The study identified falling investment income and rising reinsurance rates as contributing to the increases. The single most significant factor identified, however, were losses attributed to malpractice claims. From 1998 to 2001 inflation adjusted losses increased by an annual average rate of 18.7% with nearly $7 billion dollars in incurred losses in 2001.[10] The large losses have resulted in several large commercial insurers leaving the market.[8] This has resulted in difficulty finding malpractice coverage in some locations.

As a result of this crisis and the threat of litigation, physician behavior has changed. The resulting defensive medicine has also resulted in increased costs. Definitions for defensive medicine vary, with one source defining it as "services and procedures that are provided largely or entirely to avoid potential liability."[11] With the varying definitions, there are large disparities in the estimated prevalence and cost. One poll found 79% of practicing physicians have ordered unnecessary tests and 74% made referrals despite not believing the referral was medically necessary due to fear of possible litigation.[12] Cost estimates, like the definitions, vary widely but appear to range from $4.2 to $12.7 billion a year.[9]

The threat is not limited to the financial aspects of medical care. The high cost of malpractice insurance and risk of malpractice have resulted in physicians choosing lower risk specialties and geographic regions. An American Medical Association survey of medical students indicated medical malpractice situation was a factor in specialty choice for 50% and residency location for 39%.[13] A U.S. Health and Human Services study found states with caps on noneconomic damages experienced about 12% more physicians per capita than states without a cap. When examined closely, states with lower caps experienced a higher increase than those states with higher caps.[14] The resulting changes in physician specialties and locations have left some parts of the country without adequate specialized medical care.[7,12]

Another noneconomic concern actually implicates the purported strengths of the medical malpractice system. Some experts fear the threat of litigation actually makes it more difficult to identify and report medical mistakes.[15,16] The ability to prevent future errors is also diminished by the length of time it takes to resolve cases, which is currently just under 4 years.[8] Due to the pace of medical advancement, this long time frame may make any conclusions from a particular case obsolete.

It must be noted that the overwhelming majority of patients do not bring medical malpractice claims. One study found less than 0.2% of all hospital discharges actually result in a negligence claim.[15] An even more striking number occurs when just adverse events are identified, with only 2% of patients with adverse events bringing a medical malpractice claim.[15] Another study examined the link between potential adverse events and risk management claim files and found no rational link between the tort system and the reduction of adverse events.[17] These studies indicate the medical malpractice system does little to deter or prevent medical errors. The low rate of claims prevents the identification of any statistically significant number of events to aid in prevention. In addition, the lack of any connection between the adverse events and claim files further questions the accuracy of the process.

The current malpractice crisis has left physicians seeking malpractice reform. The lack of any national reform, however, has left physicians working on multiple fronts to combat the crisis. Previous efforts have focused on education and risk management strategies. A new tool, litigation analysis, attempts to more objectively study medical malpractice claims in order to identify trends in those who initiate lawsuits and which suits are successful.[18-26]

LITIGATION ANALYSIS

Internet-based legal databases, such as Westlaw and Lexis-Nexis, can obtain and analyze past summaries of suits. Attorneys use these databases to examine cases that have been litigated for precedents, summary content, verdict outcomes and size of judgments. Precedents set by previous cases are considered strongly persuasive in predicting the outcome of future cases. Cases that are settled or dropped prior to going to court, however, are unavailable for examination under the Internet-based research sites.

Litigation analysis can review individual disease states such as certain cancers or specific anatomic sites.[18-27] We analyzed several specific cancers at specific head and neck sites, and several common factors emerged that predicted likely litigation. The four most important predictive factors included a delay in diagnosis, a younger patient age than is typical for the disease, a poor oncologic outcome, and informed consent issues.[19-23,26]

Delay in Diagnosis

Patients with cancer at various sites in the head and neck were studied, and delay in diagnosis was a frequent factor alleged in the initiation of litigation.[19-22] For the head and neck, we found a delay alleged in 19 of 23 (83%) cases involving the larynx, 43 of 50 (86%) cases involving the oral cavity, 6 of 7 (75%) cases involving the thyroid, and 54 of 99 (54%) cases involving the skin.[19-22] In cases alleging delays, verdicts for the defendant occurred in 50% of laryngeal, 47% of oral cavity, 57% of thyroid, and 56% of skin cases.[19-22] Analysis of these studies revealed the following. Fifty-three percent of suits involving cancer of the larynx alleged physicians failed to evaluate hoarseness or in 16% a neck mass.[20] Although we could not always tell from the analysis the defendant's specialty, when it was known, 9/18 (50%) were otolaryngologists.[20] Errors of omission were alleged because plaintiffs thought biopsies were indicated, but not taken. This occurred in 11/19 (58%) with cancer of the larynx, 21/43 (49%) with cancer of the oral cavity, 4/7 (57%) with cancer of the thyroid, and 26/54 (48%) with cancer of the skin.[19-22]

We asked the question, "Why did these defendants fail to investigate rather straightforward symptoms of cancer?"[26] Our analysis points to the fact that the mean age of the patients in these studies was many years younger than the peak incidence of cancer for that anatomic site. We must all be vigilant in investigating signs of cancer irrespective of how likely the patient before us would seem to have the disease.

Young Patient Age

The mean and median ages for plaintiffs with cancers at head and neck sites was 49/46 for laryngeal, 45/47 oral cavity, 45/41 thyroid, and 48/50 cutaneous malignancies.[19-22] These ages are younger than expected, being approximately 15 years younger than the average age for presentations of cancer at that site in the general population. Only the age of thyroid cancer patients was similar to the age of presentation in the general population. For cancer of the larynx, the median age for plaintiff was 46 years old, with a peak incidence in the general population of between 70 to 74 years of age. This emphasizes that patients with persistent symptoms of cancer should be evaluated irrespective of their age. Sixty-three percent of patients with laryngeal carcinoma who alleged a delay in diagnosis thought they required the more radical treatment of a laryngectomy as a result or complication of the delay.[20] Nearly one-half of these suits resulted in significant monetary verdicts or settlements, indicating the difficulty in defending such claims. Delays occur for a variety of reasons; however, several studies show a decline in defense verdicts with increasing length of delay.[21,26,28] In Kern's study,[26] defense verdicts were handed down in 64% with delays less than 3 months, in 42% delayed from 4 to 6 months, and then stabilized at 26% for those delayed for greater than 7 months. Delays in the diagnosis and treatment of head and neck cancers also can be the result of health care system delays; Canada and the United Kingdom have recorded health care system delays that may have implications on prognosis.[29-31] Clinical guidelines should ideally strive to secure a definitive diagnosis as timely as possible.

Although intuitive, a prolonged delay may not always correlate with outcome as plaintiff attorneys would have us believe. Studies with breast cancer patients alleging a delay in diagnosis revealed that the patients also had a biologically aggressive disease.[32] These studies showed a high incidence of young patients (similar to head and neck studies), negative mammograms, painful breast masses, rapidly progressive diseases, and a short time to death.[32] This suggests a more aggressive biology might be playing a role in addition to the delays. Dennis et al[33] found no significant relationship between delay and survival in breast cancer patients presenting with a painful mass. Kern[18] found breast cancer patients bringing malpractice suits had no significant correlation between tumor size at final diagnosis and diagnostic delay. Head and neck cancer may also present in a young patient with a biologically aggressive disease. Although the results are mixed, several studies indicate that younger patients with head and neck cancer have an overall worse prognosis than older patients.[34-36] Timely diagnosis should certainly be the goal, but patients with biologically aggressive cancer may simply do poorly. Delayed diagnosis for cancer of the larynx resulted in a mortality rate of 35% and alive with disease of 12%, indicating that 47% had a bad outcome.[20] How important the delay was to the overall survival is unknown. What is known, however, is that delays in diagnosis for cancer account for a significant percentage of claims, 19% in a 1990 report of the Physician Insurers Association of America and 31% in Kern's study.[26] The importance of biology to outcome must be accounted for in future studies.

Clinical guidelines should reflect the fact that cancer can occur in all patients and persistent hoarseness must be followed to resolution or stabilization, irrespective of patient age. All patients with neck masses must be followed to a definitive diagnosis, and repeated examinations may be necessary to diagnose head and neck cancers.

Informed Consent Issues

Suits brought for lack of informed consent related to nerve injuries were analyzed and found to be alleged in facial nerve paralysis in 16/53 (30%) cases, recurrent laryngeal nerve injury in 7/9 (78%) cases, and lingual nerve injury in 17/33 (52%) cases.[19,24,25]

Regarding facial nerve injuries, the debilitating nature of a facial nerve paralysis makes it unlikely that surgeons would not inform the patients of this potential complication, yet 30% of patients did not feel they were adequately informed. Studies measuring patients recall of information given to them preoperatively report patient retain 35 to 57% of the information provided.[37-39] Hekkenberg et al[40] studied informed consent for patients undergoing either a thyroidectomy, parathyroidectomy, or a parotidectomy. The risks discussed for parotidectomy included facial scar, greater auricular nerve paresthesia, Frey's syndrome, and facial nerve weakness/paralysis. Patients were interviewed 1 to 8 weeks after the informed consent was obtained. Recall was 27% for scar and Frey's syndrome, 60% for greater auricular nerve injury, and 93% for facial nerve paralysis.[40] How much information is remembered later is really not germane as to whether the patient was truly "informed" at the time the consent was obtained, only that the patient understands the risks at the time the decision was made to undergo surgery.

It seems likely that a high percentage of patients do understand the gravity and likelihood of facial nerve paralysis. Adequate documentation should always be the goal, and written forms listing the major complications and signed and received by both parties provides documentation to educate patients, to protect against the decline of information remembered over time, and the extended litigation times.[37] It also may be perceived by patients as a good idea.[39]

Poor Outcome

In the United States, a medical malpractice claim must establish a physician acted in a negligent manner. In order to prove negligence, a plaintiff must satisfy a four-part test: a duty existed between the parties, a breach of the duty occurred, the patient was injured, and the breach was the cause of the injury.[41] Three components are usually straightforward; the surgeon has a duty to the patient he or she operated on, damages are assessable, and postoperative injuries would reasonably be assumed to be the result of the operation. The breach of duty or the standard of care is more difficult to prove. A lay jury cannot be expected to have adequate knowledge to understand a medical malpractice suit, and the courts and juries must depend on expert advice.

Despite the plaintiff's burden to show a breach of duty, a decline in defense verdicts often correlates more with a poor outcome. In our head and neck studies, plaintiffs were considered to have a poor oncologic result if they were either dead of disease or alive with disease. Plaintiffs had a poor outcome by this standard in cancer of the larynx 8/17 (47%), oral cavity 23/49 (47%), thyroid 7/7 (100%), and skin 17/56 (30%).[19-22] Defendant verdicts were rendered in 6/8 (75%), 11/24 (46%), 3/7 (43%), and 6/17 (35%), respectively.[19-22]

Our study evaluating facial nerve paralysis after surgical procedures found 53 patients.[24] All patients with any other allegation such as informed consent issues, failure to diagnose, failure of nerve monitor to function, operation beyond the scope of the surgeon, excessive blood loss, and so forth, were excluded. Nineteen suits alleged a surgical misadventure alone negligently caused the facial nerve paralysis. Twelve of the 19 plaintiffs received a verdict award or settlement. A total of 31 plaintiffs alleged malpractice, admitting that they had received informed consent that they may suffer a facial nerve paralysis, with plaintiffs winning awards in 20 (65%) of the suits. Facial nerve paralysis rates vary, but the incidence for parotidectomy, rhytidectomy, and most elective otologic procedures is around 5%.[42-46] All of these procedures have evolved to avoid or otherwise protect and preserve the facial nerve. Proper training and careful surgical technique are indispensable, but facial nerve injuries happen to all surgeons operating in this area. Dawes et al state that patients are more inclined to sue for an unsatisfactory outcome.[47] Our study agrees with this finding, with many suits seeming to hinge on the poor outcome alone.

Perhaps the surgeon had inadequate scope of training, or that errors in judgment were made intraoperatively, but many[19] of the suits seem to hinge on the poor outcome alone. A facial nerve paralysis is a devastating injury and doubtless makes a compelling site in court. Awards and settlements can be large, and occur frequently, with one study showing a combined plaintiff award and settlement rate of 64%.[24] Morris[17] found that patients with a disability of greater than 6 months or with death accounted for 98% of their institutional liability. The size of the settlement was more associated with the degree of disability than the presence of negligence. We believe these findings require further study and should be a part of much needed tort reform.

MALPRACTICE REFORM

The malpractice crisis within the United States is well documented. Multiple efforts to reform the system have been in place for over 30 years. As tort law is based on state law, and not federal law, reform efforts have focused on the state level. California has a long history of malpractice reform with the passing of Medical Injury Compensation Reform Act (MICRA) in 1975. MICRA was passed in response to a medical malpractice crisis in the state of California. Among the provisions is a cap on noneconomic damages of $250,000 and limits on contingency fees charged by attorneys. Other states have followed suit with a variety of reform efforts with 37 states having some form of medical malpractice reform. It has remained a fertile area of legislation, with 32 states enacting over 60 bills in 2005.[48]

Current reform efforts have focused on modifying existing elements of the medical malpractice system. States have employed multiple malpractice reform schemes. The most commonly reported reform effort is caps on damage awards. As of 2005, approximately 32 states have enacted some form of limitation on damage awards. The most frequently used cap places limits on noneconomic damages. The amount of the cap depends on the particular state, with ranges from $250,000 to $650,000. Other states have imposed limits on the total amount of damages awarded, typically close to $1 million.

Despite the publicity of caps on noneconomic damages, the most popular reform effort is to modify or eliminate joint-and-several liability. As of 2005, 37 states had employed reform efforts focused on altering joint and several liability. Joint and several liability is a principle when multiple parties are found to be negligent, recovery for the whole amount can be imposed on one of the negligent parties regardless of his or her assigned fault. In general, if multiple defendants have been identified and are found to be negligent, each party is assigned a percentage of the fault. Under a system that has not been reformed, a party found to be 10% at fault can be forced to pay all of the damages and then attempt to recover any excess damages from the other negligent parties. Reform efforts generally limit damages to the percentage of fault assigned to the party or by limiting joint and several liability to cases where a party is found to be at least 50% at fault.

Another reform effort has attempted to limit attorney fees. Typically, malpractice attorneys work on a contingency basis. Under this scheme, attorneys do not receive payment unless the plaintiff is successful receiving a settlement or jury award. There are no defined limits on the percentage an attorney can charge as a contingency fee; however, one-third is a generally accepted amount. States have begun to examine this practice and several states have imposed limits attorneys can charge. There are currently 19 states which have imposed some form of limit. Some states have placed the traditional one-third contingency fee as the maximum allowed. Other states have initiated a sliding scale, with larger percentages for smaller awards and smaller percentages for larger awards.

Statutes of limitations laws also have been an area of reform in the states. Statutes of limitations place a time limit on when a suit can be initiated for a claimed injury. Once a statute of limitation has run (ie, expired) that case can no longer be claimed. States have modified statute of limitation laws by decreasing the time plaintiffs have to bring a cause of action.

The federal government has recently become involved in the reform discussion. Congress has debated several pieces of legislation over the last several years. Proponents of this effort contend national malpractice reform will result in a more uniform system and will aid states unable to pass meaningful reform. Opponents argue, alternatively, the national measure may not be as strong as laws already passed in some states. The recently proposed measures include limiting noneconomic damages to $250,000, limiting contingency fees, and decreasing the statute of limitations to 2 years or 1 year from discovery. These efforts, however, have not been successful to date.[49]

Other proposed measures make more dramatic changes. These proposals do not attempt to alter the current medical malpractice system, but rather look to fundamentally change it. One option is to develop alternative dispute resolution systems. These proposals focus on the use of arbitration or administrative bodies as an initial measure for a medical malpractice claim.[50] Other countries utilize such measures. Austria employs voluntary administrative bodies, called *Schiedsstellen*, which function as the initial forum for malpractice litigation if both the plaintiff and defendant agree to use the panel. The recommendation from the panel is nonbinding with the plaintiff retaining the right to later file suit.[51] Germany uses a mediation-based system to resolve medical malpractice claims. Regional physician councils, called *Arztekammer*, hear cases of alleged malpractice and determine if malpractice has occurred. If malpractice is found, damages are later determined during negotiation.[51]

A more fundamental change removes fault from the system. A "no-fault" system tries only to determine whether a patient is injured by the health care system. Sweden and New Zealand have used no-fault compensation systems since the mid-1970s. This type of system has several advantages. One, the amount paid for a specific injury is often predetermined. This makes for a more uniform system with much less disparity in award amounts. Second, it lessens a possible adversarial relationship between the patient and physician. In theory, physicians would be more willing to admit to iatrogenic injuries. Patients truly injured by the medical system would therefore be compensated and the system would be able to document those injuries, providing a better opportunity to study and prevent repeat injuries to other patients. This most significant disadvantage of this system is the cost. Both Sweden and New Zealand have been forced to reform the system in order to reduce the costs.[52-54]

The multiple reform efforts employed by the states all indicate no single solution has been found for the medical malpractice crisis. Further reform efforts continue both on a state and national level. Examining conflict resolution strategies from other countries provides alternative approaches for consideration, but none has been shown to control the costs associated with medical malpractice.

CONCLUSION

The problems with the current medical malpractice system are well documented. Solutions to the current situation will require efforts on multiple fronts. One front works to reform the medical malpractice system through political action. Many states have passed various medical malpractice reform legislation and new national efforts are underway. To date, these measures have worked to alter the current negligence-based system through caps on damages, modifying joint and several liability, placing limits on attorney's fees, and amending statutes of limitation.

A second effort attempts to better study the malpractice system. Litigation analysis is a tool which studies medical malpractice cases to better identify those patients who are likely to bring negligence claim. Our examination of head and neck patients indicated that delay in diagnosis, young patient age, and poor outcomes were important factors. Further research is needed not only in head and neck surgery, but also in broader patient populations. This information can lead to the development of clinical guidelines and risk management strategies to reduce the number of malpractice claims.

These efforts will ultimately support one another. Any solution will require innovative thinking backed with good research. Physicians play a central role in this effort to reform the medical malpractice system, working as provider, researcher, and advocate. As the ultimate patient advocate, physicians must continue their work to ensure that safe and affordable health care is delivered to patients.

REFERENCES

1. Justinian. *The Digest of Roman Law: Theft, Rapine, Damage and Insult.* London, England: Penguin Books; 1979:7.
2. Nora PF. *Professional Liability/Risk Management: A Manual for Surgeons.* Chicago, Ill: American College of Surgeons; 1991.
3. Richard CJ. *The Founders and the Classics: Greece, Rome, and the American Enlightenment.* Cambridge, Mass: Harvard University Press; 1994: 173–182.
4. Mohr JC. American medical malpractice litigation in historical perspective. *JAMA.* 2000; 283:1731–1737.
5. Mello MM, Studdert DM, Brennan TA. The new medical malpractice crisis. *New Engl J Med.* 2003; 348(23):2281–2284.
6. Kionka EJ. *Torts.* 2nd ed. St. Paul, Minn: West Publishing; 1992:1–5.
7. United States Department of Health and Human Services. *Confronting the new health care crisis: improving health care quality and lowering costs by fixing our medical liability system.* Retrieved May 22, 2007 from http://aspe.hhs.gov/daltcp/reports/litrefm.pdf
8. Employment Policy Foundation. *Medical malpractice litigation raises health care cost, reduces access and lowers quality of care.* Retrieved May 15, 2007 from http://www.epf.org/research/newsletters/2003/ib20030619.pdf
9. United States General Accounting Office. *Medical liability: impact on hospital and physician costs extends beyond insurance.* Retrieved May 27, 2007 from http://www.gao.gov/archive/1995/ai95169.pdf
10. United States General Accounting Office. *Medical malpractice insurance: multiple factors have contributed to increased premium rates.* Retrieved May 27, 2007 from http://www.gao.gov/new.items/d03702.pdf
11. Congressional Budget Office. *Medical malpractice tort limits and health care spending.* Retrieved May 22, 2007 from http://www.cbo.gov/ftpdocs/71xx/doc7174/04-28-MedicalMalpractice.pdf
12. Taylor H. *Most doctors report fear of malpractice liability has harmed their ability to provide quality care: caused them to order unnecessary tests, provide unnecessary treatment and make unnecessary referrals.* Harris Interactive Web site. Retrieved May 15, 2007 from http://www.harrisinteractive.com/harris_poll/index.asp?PID=300
13. AMA Survey: *Medical students' opinions of the current medical liability environment.* Retrieved May 18, 2007 from http://www.ama-assn.org/ama1/pub/upload/mm/15/mss-mlr-survey.pdf
14. Hellinger FJ, Encinosa WE. U.S. Department of Health and Human Services. *The impact of state laws limiting malpractice awards on the geographic distribution of physicians.* July 3, 2003. Retrieved May 20, 2007 from http://www.ahrq.gov/RESEARCH/tortcaps/tortcaps.htm.
15. Localio AR, Lawthers AG, Brennan TA, et al. Relation between malpractice claims and adverse events due to negligence: results of the Harvard Medical Practice Study III. *New Engl J Med.* 1991;325:245–251.

16. Joshi M, Anderson JF, Marwaha S. A systems approach to improving error reporting. *J Health Inf Manag.* 2002; 16(1):40-45.

17. Morris JA, Carrillo Y, Jenkins JM, et al. Surgical adverse events, risk management and malpractice outcome: morbidity and mortality review is not enough. *Ann Surg.* 2003;237(6):844-852.

18. Kern KA. Causes of breast cancer malpractice litigation: a 20-year civil court review. *Arch Surg.* 1992;127:542-547.

19. Lydiatt DD. Medical malpractice and the thyroid gland. *Head Neck.* 2003;25:429-431.

20. Lydiatt DD. Medical malpractice and cancer of the larynx. *Laryngoscope.* 2002;112:445-448.

21. Lydiatt DD. Cancer of the oral cavity and medical malpractice. *Laryngoscope.* 2002;112:816-819.

22. Lydiatt DD. Medical malpractice and cancer of the skin. *Am J Surg.* 2004;187(6):688-694.

23. Kern KA. Preventing the delayed diagnosis of breast cancer through medical litigation analysis. *Surg Oncol Clin North Am.* 1994;3:101-123.

24. Lydiatt DD. Medical malpractice and facial nerve paralysis. *Arch Otolaryngol Head Neck Surg.* 2003;129:50-53.

25. Lydiatt DD. Litigation and the lingual nerve. *J Oral Maxillofac Surg.* 2003;61:197-200.

26. Kern KA. Medicolegal analysis of the delayed diagnosis of cancer in 338 cases in the United States. *Arch Surg.* 1994;129:397-404.

27. Hollows P, McAndrew PG, Perini MG. Delays in the referral and treatment of oral squamous cell carcinoma. *Br Dent J.* 2000;188(7):262-265.

28. Allison P, Locker D, Feine JS. The role of diagnostic delays in the prognosis of oral cancer: a review of the literature. *Oral Oncol.* 1998;34(3):161-170.

29. Jones TM, Hargrove O, Lancaster J, et al. Waiting times during the management of head and neck tumors. *J Laryngol Otol.* 2002;116:275-279.

30. Fortin A, Bairati I, Albert M, et al. Effect of treatment delay on outcome of patients with early-stage head-and-neck carcinoma receiving radical radiotherapy. *Int J Radia Oncol Biol Phys.* 2002; 52(4):929-936.

31. Mackillop WJ, Zhou Y, Quirt CF. A comparison of delays in the treatment of cancer with radiation in Canada and the United States. *Int J Radia Oncol Biol Phys.* 1995;32(2):531-539.

32. Diercks DB, Cady B. Failure to diagnose breast cancer suits: tumor biology in causation and risk management strategies. *Surg Oncol Clin North Am.* 1994;3:125-140.

33. Dennis CR, Gardner B, Lim B. Analysis of survival and recurrence vs. patient and doctor delay in treatment of breast cancer. *Cancer.* 1975;35:714-720.

34. Vargas H, Pitman KT, Johnson JT, Galati LT. More aggressive behavior of squamous cell carcinoma of the anterior tongue in young women. *Laryngoscope.* 2000;110:1623-1626.

35. Sarkaria JN, Harari PM. Oral tongue cancer in young adults less than 40 years of age: rationale for aggressive therapy. *Head Neck.* 1994;16:107-111.

36. Friedlander Pl, Schantz SP, Shaha AR, Yu G, Shah JP. Squamous cell carcinoma of the tongue in young patients: a matched-pair analysis. *Head Neck.* 1998; 20:363-368.

37. Hutson MM, Blaha JD. Patient's recall of preoperative instruction for informed consent for an operation. *Bone Joint Surg (Br).* 1991;73:160-162.

38. Leeb D, Bowers DG, Lynch JB. Observations on the myth of "informed consent." *Plast Reconstr Surg.* 1976;58:280-282.

39. Priluck IA, Robertson DM, Buettner H. What patients recall of the pre-operative discussion after retinal detachment surgery. *Am J Ophthalmol.* 1976;87:620-623.

40. Hekkenberg RJ, Irish JC, Rotstein LE, Brown DH, Gullane PJ. Informed consent in head and neck surgery: how much do patients actually remember? *J Otolaryngol.* 1997;26:155-159.

41. Sanbar SS, Gibofsky A, Firestone MH, LeBlang TR. *Legal Medicine.* St. Louis, Mo: Mosby; 1998: 123-131.

42. Sullivan CA, Masin J, Maniglia AJ, Stepnick DW, Complication of rhytidectomy in an otolaryngology training program. *Laryngoscope.* 1999;109(2 pt 1): 198-203.

43. Witt RL. Facial nerve monitoring in parotid surgery: the standard of care? *Otolaryngol Head Neck Surg.* 1999;119(5):468-470.

44. Green JD, Shelton C, Brackman DE. Iatrogenic facial nerve injury during otologic surgery. *Laryngoscope.* 1994;109(8 pt 1):922-926.

45. Dulguerov P, Marchal F, Lehmann W. Post parotidectomy facial nerve paralysis: possible etiologic factor and results with routine facial nerve monitoring. *Laryngoscope.*1999;109(5):754-762.

46. Beahrs OH. The surgical anatomy and technique of parotidectomy. *Surg Clin North Am.* 1977;57(3): 477-493.

47. Dawes PJD, O'Keefe L, Adcock S. Informed consent: using a structured interview changes patients' attitudes towards informed consent. *J Laryngol Otol.* 1993;107:775-779.

48. National Conference of State Legislatures. Medical Malpractice Tort Reform. Retrieved May 17, 2007 from http://www.ncsl.org/standcomm/sclaw/med maloverview.htm

49. American Medical Association Web site. Medical Liability Reform—NOW! Available at http://www .ama-assn.org/ama1/pub/upload/mm/450/mlrn owdec032004.pdf

50. HR 534. Available at http://thomas.loc.gov/cgi-bin/ bdquery/z?d109:h.r.00534

51. Koch BA. Austrian cases on medical liability. *Eur J Health Law.* 2003;1:91–114.

52. Magnus U, Micklitz H. Comparative analysis of national liability systems for remedying damage caused by defective consumer services: a study commissioned by the European Union. Available at http://europa.eu.int/comm/consumers/cons_ safe/serv_safe/liability/reportabc_en.pdf

53. Adelman SH, Westerlund L. The Swedish Patient Compensation System: A viable alternative to the U.S tort system? *Bull Am Coll Surgeons.* Jan. 2004. Available at http://www.facs.org/fellows_info/bul letin/2004/adelman0104.pdf

54. Cunningham W, Crump R, Tomlin A. The characteristics of doctors receiving medical complaints: a cross-sectional survey of doctors in New Zealand. *NZ Med J.* 2003: 116(1183). Available at http:// www.nzma.org.nz/journal/116-1183/625/

10

Skin Cancer of the Head and Neck*

Brian A. Moore
Randal S. Weber

INTRODUCTION

Skin cancer is the most common cancer in the United States, and it is rapidly becoming an epidemic, with significant morbidity and mortality. Cutaneous melanoma and aggressive nonmelanoma skin cancers (NMSC) of the head and neck often require a multidisciplinary approach that includes surgery, radiation, and systemic therapy. Health care providers who care for patients with disorders of the head and neck will be increasingly faced with patients with these cancers. This chapter focuses on the evaluation and management of the patient with aggressive cutaneous malignancy of the head and neck, including the principles of surgical resection, reconstruction, management of the regional lymphatics, applications for radiation therapy, and indications for systemic therapy. Prevention and screening are also noted, because the answer to this public health dilemma is prevention and early detection.

DEFINITIONS OF UNIQUE TERMS

Nonmelanoma skin cancer (NMSC) refers to squamous cell carcinoma (SCC), basal cell carcinoma (BCC), Merkel cell carcinoma, and adnexal carcinoma of the skin. Squamous cell carcinoma arises from keratinocytes in the spinous layer of the epidermis, whereas BCC has its cell of origin in the basal layer. Merkel cell carcinoma is thought to arise from neuroendocrine cells in the basal layer of the epidermis. Other rare NMSC include dermatofibrosarcoma protuberans (DFSP) that evolves from dermal fibroblasts, in addition to carcinomas arising from sebaceous glands, eccrine sweat glands, or apocrine glands. Melanoma arises from melanocytes that are scattered throughout the epidermis.

A common feature of aggressive cutaneous SCC, as well as certain types of melanoma, is perineural invasion (PNI). Perineural invasion represents invasion of tumor cells into the nerve sheath, a potential space, with subsequent antegrade or retrograde spread along the nerve. Because lymph node metastases are common in skin cancer of the head and neck, patients may undergo lymphoscintigraphy or sentinel node biopsy as a diagnostic and prognostic measure. Lymphoscintigraphy refers to the localization of lymph nodes following cutaneous injection of dye or radionuclides in which the particles travel through the lymphatic system to one or more lymph nodes—the sentinel node(s)—that are identified visually or with a gamma counter. The sentinel nodes are then removed for histopathologic analysis.

---

*The views expressed in this article are those of the author(s) and do not reflect the official policy or position of the United States Air Force, Department of Defense, or U.S. Government.

EPIDEMIOLOGY

Nonmelanoma skin cancer affects over 1.3 million people in the United States each year, and this incidence has risen significantly over the last 30 years.[1,2] Because NMSC is often triggered by ultraviolet light exposure, these lesions occur on sun-exposed areas of the body, with 75% on the head and neck.[3] Men over the age of 50 are at greatest risk of developing NMSC, but these cancers are on the rise in women and younger patients.[4]

Basal cell carcinoma accounts for 80% of NMSC, and squamous cell carcinoma comprises nearly 20%. Although over 95% of NMSC may be cured by a variety of surgical and nonsurgical therapies, aggressive variants exist that are marked by recurrence, metastases, increased morbidity, and at least 2500 deaths per year.[5] Aggressive NMSC must be identified early to optimize patient outcomes.

The incidence of cutaneous melanoma has increased over 600% since 1950, with an attendant increase of 165% in annual mortality.[6] Cutaneous melanoma affected more than 55,000 Americans in 2004 and led to over 7900 deaths.[7] It afflicts a younger population than NMSC and constitutes the second leading cause of lost productive years and the most common cancer in women ages 20 to 29.[6] Cutaneous melanoma arises in the head and neck in up to 30% of cases.[8] Because of the frequency and severity of distant metastases, multidisciplinary care is paramount for cutaneous melanoma of the head and neck.

ANATOMY

Skin Anatomy

The skin is the largest organ, serving to protect the body against infection, exposure, and injury. Although its thickness varies throughout the body, with extremes of thickness occurring in the head and neck, it maintains a laminar structure with epidermis, dermis, and fat. The epidermis consists of an outer stratum corneum, a keratinocyte layer (divided into granular and spinous cell layers), and a basal cell layer, with melanocytes interspersed throughout. The dermis contains blood vessels, lymphatics, nerve endings, hair follicles, and sweat glands, and it primarily composed of collagen. The subcutaneous layer is chiefly composed of collagen and fat.

Lymphatic Drainage Pathways

Lymphatic drainage from cutaneous sites in the head and neck is highly complex, as depicted in Figure 10-1.[9] Deviations from this general framework are demonstrated by studies that reveal a discordance of up to 34% between the clinical prediction and lymphoscintigraphy.[10] In general, lesions anterior to a vertical line extending toward the vertex from the auricle will drain to the ipsilateral parotid gland and upper cervical lymph nodes, including lymph nodes along the external jugular chain. Lesions posterior to this line will drain to the postauricular, occipital and posterior cervical

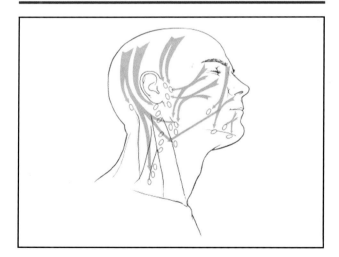

Fig 10–1. Patterns of lymphatic drainage for cutaneous sites in the head and neck. The periparotid lymph nodes, external jugular nodes, and upper jugular nodes constitute the typical first echelon of drainage for most subsites. Bilateral drainage is common in midface and lower lip lesions. Image adapted from Moore BA, Kies M, Rosenthal D, Weber RS. Skin Cancer of the Head and Neck. In: Genden E, ed. *Head and Neck Cancer.* New York: Thieme, In Press.

nodes.[8] Midface and lower lip tumors drain to bilateral anterior cervical nodes, including the perifacial nodes, submental nodes, and submandibular nodes. Lesions on the neck will likely drain to the closest underlying lymph nodes and the external jugular vein nodes.

CRITICAL ELEMENTS IN THE HISTORY AND PHYSICAL EXAMINATION

Patients with fair skin, a history of early or severe sunburns, recreational or occupational exposure to ultraviolet light, a family history of skin cancer, previous skin cancers, prior radiation treatment, and immunosuppression should undergo comprehensive cutaneous exams on a regular basis. Exposure to ultraviolet (uv) light, particularly the combination of uvA and uvB light, is the main factor leading to melanoma and nonmelanoma skin cancer. Early, intermittent, or excessive sun exposure, in a society that values a tanned appearance, and a history of blistering sunburns correlate with development of skin cancer.[4] Cellular and molecular events that promote skin cancer include uv light-induced mutations in keratinocyte or melanocyte DNA, inadequate or failed DNA repair mechanisms, pyrimidine dimer formation in the p53 tumor suppressor gene, local immunosuppression, loss of the Fas-Fas ligand interaction, activation of proto-oncogenes (*ras*), activation of the mitogen-activated protein kinase signal transduction pathway (MAPK) via *BRAF* or other mechanisms, inactivation of tumor suppressor genes including *PTCH* and *INK4a/ARF*, and abnormalities in the nuclear factor kappa B (NFκB) signaling pathway.[11,12] Risk factors for the development of skin cancer of the head and neck are listed in Table 10–1.[2,6]

Growth or change in appearance of an existing lesion is the most common complaint in skin cancer. Other symptoms such as itching, formication, bleeding, ulceration, and pain indicate advanced disease. Actinic keratoses (AK) are common precursor lesions for cutaneous squamous cell carcinoma, with an annual risk of progression to invasive cancer of 0.025 to 20%.[2] Other precursor lesions for cutaneous SCC include Bowen's disease, bowenoid papulosis, and epidermodysplasia verruciformis. At least 81% of patients with cutaneous melanoma also describe a change in a pre-existing lesion.

The presence of numerous freckles or pigmented lesions carries a higher theoretical risk of malignant melanoma. Large congenital nevi, sporadic dysplastic nevi, and lentigo maligna transform to malignant melanoma in 5 to 33% of cases.[8] In Familial Melanoma/Dysplastic Nevus Syndrome (FM/DNS, mapped to chromosome 9p21 at the p16 gene), the lifetime risk of melanoma for family members with dysplastic nevi approaches 100%.[8] Lentigo maligna is an atypical proliferation of melanocytes within the basal layer of the epidermis, and it is commonly regarded as a precursor lesion for melanoma—it frequently arises on the cheek, or other sun-exposed areas, of older patients.[13]

A simple "ABCD" evaluation may identify suspicious lesions. **A**symmetry, **B**order irregularities, **C**olor variegation, and **D**iameter greater than 6mm have been shown to correlate with malignancy, particularly melanoma.[14] A Wood's lamp may delineate subclinical extension of melanoma.[13] Close inspection of surrounding areas may identify satellite lesions. Photodocumentation is a useful adjunct to memory and written documentation, and images may be readily stored in secure databases for later comparison, with patient informed consent.

In a patient with presumed skin cancer of the head and neck, a comprehensive cutaneous exam should be performed, including close inspection of the scalp. Patients may also be referred to dermatologists for full-body exams, due to the risk of second primary tumors. Motor and sensory cranial nerve function should be assessed to detect perineural invasion (PNI), although most cases of PNI are asymptomatic. Palpation of the parotid glands and cervical lymphatics should also be performed to detect regional metastases.

APPROPRIATE DIAGNOSTIC OFFICE-BASED PROCEDURES

Unlike many other subsites in the head and neck, skin lesions are particularly amenable to biopsy, and this is the definitive step in the patient evaluation. All suspicious lesions should be biopsied with a

Table 10–1. Risk Factors for Developing Skin Cancer of the Head and Neck

Melanoma and NMSC	Melanoma	NMSC
Childhood sun exposure	Family history of melanoma	Ionizing radiation exposure
Intermittent sun exposure	Pre-existing pigmented lesions	Genodermatoses
Severe sunburns	Large congenital nevi	Albinism
Fair complexion	Sporadic dysplastic nevi	Xeroderma pigmentosus
Blond or red hair	Lentigo maligna	Basal cell nevus syndrome
Blue or green eyes		Bazex syndrome
Fitzpatrick class 1–2		Actinic keratoses
Previous skin cancer		Immunosuppression*
		Organ transplantation
		Chronic lymphocytic leukemia
		Lymphoma
		Chemical exposures
		Polycyclic hydrocarbons
		Arsenic
		Coal tar
		Psoralens
		Human papillomavirus infection
		Chronic irritation
		Burn scars
		Prior skin cancer (incl. melanoma)
		Bowen's disease
		Bowenoid papulosis
		Epidermodysplasia verruciformis

*Veness MJ, Quinn DI, Ong CS, et al. Aggressive cutaneous malignancies following cardiothoracic transplantation: the Australian experience. *Cancer.* 1999;85:1758–1764.

technique that allows for an assessment of the depth of the lesion. Either excisional biopsy with 1 to 2-mm margins or incisional techniques such as punch biopsy (2, 4, or 6-mm punch) are acceptable methods. For an incisional biopsy, the sample should be taken from the thickest and most pigmented area.[13] The biopsy site may heal by secondary intention or be sutured in either a linear or purse-string fashion. Shave or partial-thickness biopsies are inadequate and should not be performed—they provide no information on the depth of invasion.[8] Whether an incisional or excisional biopsy is performed, the surgeon must maintain close communication with colleagues in pathology to ensure that important information is included in the pathology report. The contents of an ideal pathology report are summarized in Table 10-2.[5]

RECOMMENDED IMAGING STUDIES

Although most patients with skin cancer of the head and neck present with limited, local disease and do not require diagnostic studies other than tissue biopsy, advanced imaging studies are often indicated in aggressive NMSC and melanoma. Computed tomography (CT) and magnetic resonance imaging

Table 10–2. The Complete Pathology Report for Skin Cancer

Nonmelanoma Skin Cancer	Melanoma
Histologic type	Histologic type
Differentiation	Depth of invasion
Depth of invasion	Clark level
Clark level	Breslow thickness (mm)
Breslow thickness (mm)	Patterns of growth
	Vertical phase present/absent
Perineural invasion	Radial phase present/absent
Lymphovascular invasion	Ulceration
	Perineural invasion
Inflammation	Regression
Margins	Margins
Lesion Size	Satellitosis
	Special stains
	S-100
	MART-1
	HMB-45

(MRI) complement one another and facilitate tumor staging and treatment planning, and CT scans comprise an excellent first-line modality. A contrasted CT scan of the head and neck may help determine the extent of a clinically advanced lesion, detect bone involvement, identify nodal metastases, and suggest advanced perineural invasion. MRI can detect perineural invasion, deep extension into subcutaneous tissues, and evidence of involvement of important sensory and neural structures, such as the orbital contents.[15] Ultrasound and positron emission tomography (PET) scanning, as well as emerging metabolic techniques, demonstrate great potential due to their noninvasive character, but their routine use remains unproven. Detection of systemic metastases may be accomplished with simple laboratory tests including a liver panel and a chest radiograph, although PET-CT is becoming more widespread in this application.

The workup of patients with melanoma follows guidelines that may be obtained from the National Comprehensive Cancer Network (NCCN, http://

www.nccn.gov) and the National Cancer Institute (NCI, http://www.nci.nih.gov). Patients with lentigo maligna melanoma and those with thin lesions with favorable signs (no ulceration, no extension to the reticular dermis) classified as stage 0 and stage IA, do not require additional testing. In early stage melanoma, the recommended workup includes a lactate dehydrogenase level (LDH) and a chest radiograph (CXR). As in NMSC, routine use of PET scans in melanoma remains investigational.[16]

STAGING OF SKIN CANCER OF THE HEAD AND NECK

Accurate clinical staging provides useful prognostic information for the patient and providers, often guides treatment, allows communication between treatment team members, and promotes comparison of outcomes. The staging systems proposed by the American Joint Committee on Cancer (AJCC) are designed for use in primary lesions arising on all cutaneous surfaces, potentially limiting their application in the head and neck. Melanoma staging incorporates contemporary techniques and has undergone extensive validation. Recent endeavors have attempted to overcome weaknesses and expand NMSC staging in the head and neck.

Staging of Nonmelanoma Skin Cancer

The 2002 AJCC staging system for NMSC is depicted in Table 10-3.[17] The system focuses on lesion size, extracutaneous extension, and metastases. The combination of clinical staging and the histopathologic features of the primary lesion essentially guide planning and prognosis. Although uncommon, regional metastases are a hallmark of aggressive NMSC, with significant implications for disease control and survival.[18] Perceived weaknesses in the staging of regional metastases have recently been addressed, and a revised system for staging lymphatic metastases to the parotid and cervical nodes has been proposed. The revised system for cervical lymphatic metastases has demonstrated useful prognostic information, and it appears in Table 10-4.[19,20]

Table 10–3. 2002 American Joint Commission on Cancer (AJCC) System for Nonmelanoma Skin Cancer

Primary Tumor (T)

Tx	Primary tumor cannot be assessed
T0	No evidence of primary tumor
Tis	Carcinoma in situ
T1	Tumor 2 cm or less in greatest dimension
T2	Tumor more than 2 cm but not more than 5 cm in greatest dimension
T3	Tumor more than 5 cm in greatest dimension
T4	Tumor invades deep extradermal structures (ie, cartilage, skeletal muscle, or bone)

Regional Lymph Nodes (N)

Nx	Regional lymph nodes cannot be assessed
N0	No regional lymph node metastases
N1	Regional lymph node metastases

Distant Metastases (M)

Mx	Distant metastases cannot be assessed
M0	No distant metastases
M1	Distant metastases

Stage Grouping

Stage 0	Tis	N0	M0
Stage 1	T1	N0	M0
Stage 2	T2	N0	M0
	T3	N0	M0
Stage 3	T4	N0	M0
	Any T	N1	M0
Stage 4	Any T	Any N	M1

Source: Adapted from the *AJCC Cancer Staging Manual, Sixth Edition (2002)*. New York: Springer-Verlag; 2002.

Staging of Melanoma

Clinical staging in melanoma has emerged as a reliable therapeutic and prognostic tool, but rudimentary risk stratification based on location and depth of invasion remains valid. Head and neck melanomas have higher rates of recurrence and lower survival rates than lesions elsewhere.[21] Likewise, scalp and temporal lesions appear to be more aggressive than other head and neck subsites.[22] Over time, the Clark

Table 10–4. Modified Staging for Regional Metastases of Cutaneous Squamous Cell Carcinoma

Stage	Features
P1	Single metastatic node in parotid <3 cm in diameter
P2	Single 3 to 6 cm in diameter parotid metastasis
P3	Parotid mass >6 cm Skull base involvement Facial nerve involvement
N0	No clinical neck metastases
N1	Single metastatic cervical node <3 cm in diameter
N2	Single metastatic cervical node >3 cm in diameter Multiple ipsilateral cervical metastases Contralateral cervical metastases

Source: Adapted from O'Brien CJ, McNeil EB, McMahon JD, et al. Significance of clinical stage, extent of surgery, and pathologic findings in metastatic cutaneous squamous cell carcinoma of the parotid gland. *Head Neck.* 2002;24:417–422.

depth of invasion and Breslow thickness of cutaneous melanoma have been validated to correlate with biologic behavior (Table 10–5).[23,24]

The 2002 AJCC staging system for cutaneous melanoma (Table 10–6) relies on contemporary techniques and important clinicopathologic features.[17,25] The new system utilizes both clinical staging and pathologic staging, fusing histopathologic detail from both the primary lesion and regional nodes, as determined by sentinel lymph node biopsy (SLNB) or regional lymphadenectomy.[26]

Tumor thickness and ulceration determine T stage. Clark levels are used in T1 lesions because of the high predictive value for level of invasion on survival for melanomas thinner than 1.0 mm. For all thicker lesions, the Breslow depth in millimeters correlates more strongly with prognosis.[25] Within each stage, tumors are assigned an a- or a b-designation, indicating the presence or absence of ulceration, because ulceration indicates more aggressive disease and diminished survival. Patients with localized melanoma are classified as stage I or stage II.

Table 10–5. Clark and Breslow Levels of Invasion for Cutaneous Melanoma

Clark Levels	
I	In situ melanoma, lesion confined to the epidermis
II	Invasion of papillary dermis. No extension to papillary-reticular junction
III	Invasion throughout papillary dermis. No penetration of reticular dermis
IV	Invasion into reticular dermis but not subcutaneous tissue
V	Invasion into subcutaneous tissue

Breslow Thickness	
Stage I	≤ 0.75 mm
Stage II	≥ 0.76 mm, ≤1.50 mm
Stage III	≥ 1.51 mm, <4.0 mm
Stage IV	≥ 4.0 mm

Patients with clinical evidence of nodal metastases are classified as stage III disease. The clinical or pathologic status of the regional lymph nodes is the most important index of recurrence and survival. Further, the extent of regional metastases has a tremendous impact on outcomes of patients with stage III melanoma.[25,27,28] Ulceration remains the only feature of the primary that retains prognostic import in stage III melanoma.

Patients with distant metastases have stage IV disease, and differences in the survival rates of patients with cutaneous, subcutaneous, distant lymph node, lung, and other visceral metastases vary, with 1-year survival rates ranging from 40 to 60%. Elevated serum lactate dehydrogenase carries the poorest prognosis, signifying hepatic or osseous metastases.[17,25]

Intense research continues to focus on other serum biomarkers for melanoma diagnosis and follow-up: S100B protein, C-reactive protein, tyrosinase, loss of heterozygosity at tumor suppressor gene loci, and elevated levels of or antibodies to a 90-kd (kilodalton) glycoprotein antigen called TA90.[12,29,30] However, continued investigation is required before routine biomarker assessment becomes clinically applicable.

Table 10–6. Staging of Cutaneous Melanoma

Primary Tumor (T)	
Tx	Primary tumor cannot be assessed
T0	No evidence of primary tumor
Tis	Melanoma in situ
T1	Tumor = 1.0 mm thick
a	Without ulceration and Clark level II/III
b	With ulceration or Clark level IV/V
T2	Tumor 1.01–2.0 mm thick
a	Without ulceration
b	With ulceration
T3	Tumor 2.01–4.0 mm thick
a	Without ulceration
b	With ulceration
T4	Tumor >4.0 mm thick
a	Without ulceration
b	With ulceration

Regional Lymph Nodes (N)	
Nx	Regional lymph nodes cannot be assessed
N0	No regional lymph node metastases
N1	One positive lymph node
a	Micrometastasis
b	Macrometastasis
N2	Two or three positive lymph nodes
a	Micrometastases
b	Macrometastases
c	In transit metastases/satellites without metastatic nodes
N3	Four or more positive nodes, matted nodes, or in-transit/satellite nodes with metastatic node(s)

Distant Metastases (M)	
Mx	Distant metastases cannot be assessed
M0	No distant metastases
M1	Distant metastases
a	Distant skin, subcutaneous, or lymph node metastasis
b	Lung metastasis
c	All other visceral metastases
	Or any distant metastasis with an elevated serum LDH*

*serum lactate dehydrogenase

Source: Adapted from the 2002 American Joint Committee on Cancer (AJCC) melanoma staging system (Greene F, Page DL, Fleming ID, et al. *AJCC Cancer Staging Manual, Sixth Edition.* New York: Springer-Verlag, 2002.

EXAMPLES OF
REPRESENTATIVE HISTOLOGY

Nonmelanoma Skin Cancer

Basal Cell Carcinoma

Basal cell carcinoma exists in several histologic subtypes: superficial, nodular, infiltrative, and micronodular. Superficial BCC (25% of cases) tend to occur as plaquelike lesions on the trunk with sharp borders. Nodular BCC (60%) constitute the characteristic "rodent ulcer," with raised edges around central ulceration—nodular BCC are common on the head and neck. Peripheral palisading is the histopathologic hallmark of these subtypes. Infiltrative, formerly known as morpheaform, and micronodular BCC comprise only 2% to 5%, and 15% of BCC, respectively, and they have a tendency for local recurrence. Infiltrative lesions are characterized by subclinical spread, tumor islands, and ill-defined projections. Micronodular lesions are small nodules with peripheral palisading.[31]

Some lesions demonstrate more than one histologic pattern, and treatment is directed at the more aggressive pathology. Aggressive BCC have been defined as lesions with a diameter greater than 1 cm; multiply recurrent lesions, and deep lesions.[32] Although basal cell carcinoma rarely metastases, neglected lesions may be locally aggressive and can result in significant morbidity (Fig 10–2).

Squamous Cell Carcinoma

Cutaneous SCC appear as firm, pale-pink textured lesions, often in the setting of a pre-existing actinic keratosis. Variants of SCC include verrucous carcinoma, a slow-growing, exophytic, locally aggressive lesion; spindle cell SCC; desmoplastic SCC; and basosquamous carcinoma.[2] Spindle cell carcinoma often demonstrates perineural invasion, local recurrence, and regional metastases. Hallmark spindle cells are poorly differentiated and surrounded by collagen; electron microscopy and immunohistochemical may facilitate a difficult diagnosis.[33]

In desmoplastic SCC, fine peripheral branches of tumor cells are surrounded by a desmoplastic

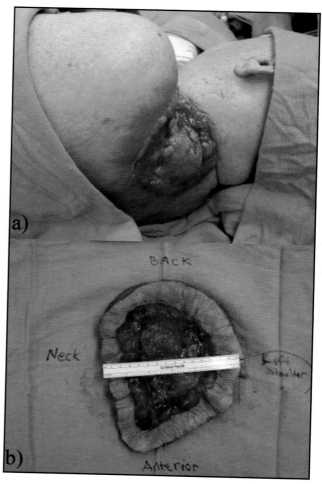

Fig 10–2 (A and B). Neglected basal cell carcinoma of the neck and shoulder. Radical surgery and complex reconstruction were required for local control. The patient received postoperative radiation therapy due to the extent of her disease.

stroma. Desmoplastic SCC exhibits 6 times the rate of metastasis and 10 times the rate of local recurrence as nondesmoplastic cutaneous SCC.[34] Basosquamous carcinoma, also known as basaloid squamous (cell) carcinoma, exhibits features of both SCC and BCC. Malignant basal cells with peripheral palisading nuclei are intermixed with malignant squamous cells without a transition zone. Although these lesions account for only 1 to 2% of skin cancers, they are marked by local recurrence, lymphatic metastasis, and perineural invasion.[33]

Aggressive Nonmelanoma Skin Cancer

Both basal cell carcinoma and squamous cell carcinoma of the skin can demonstrate clinically aggressive behavior in which lesions are prone to recurrence and metastasis, with attendant morbidity and mortality, and these lesions share certain features (Table 10-7).[35,36] Lesions larger than 4 cm, perineural invasion, and invasion beyond the subcutaneous tissues have been associated with significant decreases in disease-specific survival (Fig 10-3).[37] Early identification and aggressive treatment, including consideration for treating the regional lymphatics, are integral for patient survival with minimized morbidity in aggressive NMSC.

Melanoma

As in NMSC, there are several subtypes of cutaneous melanoma, including lentigo maligna (discussed as a precursor lesion), lentigo maligna melanoma, superficial spreading melanoma, desmoplastic melanoma, nodular, and acral lentiginous melanoma.

Lentigo maligna melanoma is the least common type of melanoma (5-10%), but it comprises 50% of cutaneous melanomas of the head and neck, often on the cheek of older patients.[13] Lentigo maligna melanoma exhibits a prolonged radial growth phase, with invasion into the papillary dermis. Superficial

spreading melanoma is the most common subtype, and it exhibits a radial growth phase that is followed by a vertical growth phase, heralding more aggressive disease (Fig 10-4).[8]

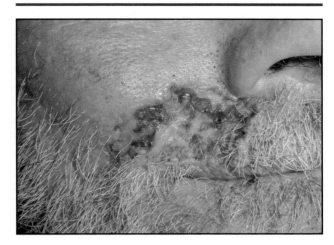

Fig 10–3. Aggressive cutaneous squamous cell carcinoma of the cheek.

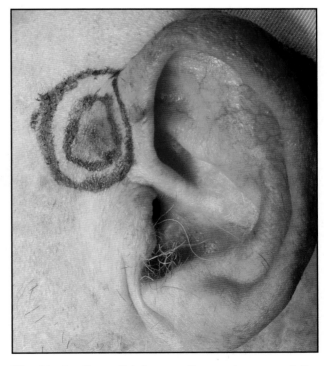

Fig 10–4. Superficial spreading melanoma of the preauricular skin.

Table 10–7. Hallmarks of Aggressive Nonmelanoma Skin Cancer

Clinical Signs	Histopathologic Features
Recurrent lesions	Poor differentiation
Regional metastases	Histology
Size >2 cm	Desmoplastic SCC
Rapid growth	Spindle cell SCC
	Basosquamous carcinoma
Location	Infiltrative BCC
Central H-zone of the face	Lymphovascular invasion
	Inflammation
	Invasion to/beyond the subcutaneous layer

Desmoplastic melanoma is uncommon—in incidence, appearance, and behavior. The lesions may be nonpigmented and frequently occur on the head and neck. The lesions demonstrate infiltrates of spindle cells in a fibrous or myxoid stroma, and special staining for S-100 protein may be required for accurate diagnosis.[8,38] Desmoplastic melanoma is characterized by local recurrence, perineural invasion, and distant metastases, but an unexpectedly low risk of regional metastases.[38] Nodular melanoma comprises less than 15% of lesions, and it is characterized by an early vertical growth phase. Acral lentiginous melanoma merits mention only for completeness; it is encountered on the palms and soles and demonstrates large malignant cells in the basal layer.[8]

IDENTIFICATION OF CRITICAL DECISION POINT

When evaluating a patient with a history of significant sun exposure or other risk factors for skin cancer, a high index of suspicion must be maintained. Following a comprehensive cutaneous exam and thorough head and neck exam searching for evidence of parotid or regional metastases, incisional or excisional biopsy is imperative. The tissue diagnosis will determine what, if any, additional diagnostic tests are indicated, as well as the appropriate treatment options. Identification of the features of aggressive NMSC or melanoma should prompt a multidisciplinary evaluation and aggressive treatment. Because regional metastases often present in a delayed fashion, a history of locoregional skin cancer must be elicited from patients presenting with neck or parotid masses. Problems arise in the management of patients with skin cancer of the head and neck because aggressive features are not identified, or because the high index of suspicion is not maintained.

TREATMENT OPTIONS AND COMPLICATIONS

A multidisciplinary approach is required to treat aggressive nonmelanoma skin cancer and cutaneous melanoma of the head and neck. The primary lesion may receive definitive treatment (wide excision) whereas the "workup" continues with the sentinel node biopsy. Although there are more options for treating early NMSC, the foundations of local control are the same for NMSC and melanoma: excise the lesion using sound oncologic principles while attempting to minimize morbidity and preserve options for reconstruction.

Treatment of Nonmelanoma Skin Cancer

Over 90% of patients with cutaneous basal cell and squamous cell carcinoma have an excellent prognosis, regardless of treatment type. As such, these lesions are treated by a variety of providers, including family physicians, dermatologists, general surgeons, plastic surgeons, head and neck surgeons, and radiation oncologists. These various doctors have an equally diverse armamentarium to treat the majority of BCC and SCC: electrodissection and curettage, cryosurgery, wide local excision, Mohs' micrographic surgery, photodynamic therapy, laser ablation or resection, radiation therapy, and certain topical agents. Eradicating the lesion is not the challenge in nonmelanoma skin cancer—the difficulty is identifying in advance which lesions merit more aggressive or multidisciplinary treatment.

Cryotherapy

Cryotherapy, cooling the lesion with liquid nitrogen, is effective for actinic keratoses and low-risk NMSC, and it is readily performed in the clinic setting on patients with low-risk lesions who are poor operative candidates.[2] Because cryotherapy does not provide tissue for pathologic analysis, it must be used with extreme caution in NMSC, and it is not indicated for melanoma.

Electrodissection and Curettage

In this technique, tumor is scraped from the bed with a curette and the bed is cauterized, with several cycles to maximize tumor removal. Because margin assessment is not performed, this technique should be used with caution in NMSC and is not indicated for melanoma.[2,33]

Wide Excision

Wide local excision, in a circumferential or elliptical fashion without compromising margins to facilitate reconstruction, has been the traditional standard for managing skin cancer of the head and neck. Because of important neurosensory and functional structures such as the eye, ear, nose, and mouth, plus cosmetic concerns, wide excision is performed with the narrowest margin that does not compromise cure (Table 10–8). The pathology and histopathologic features of the tumor determine the margin size. Margins of 2 to 10 mm and 4 to 15 mm are common for basal cell carcinoma and squamous cell carcinoma, respectively, leading to local control rates of 96 to 97%.[39] Larger margins of at least 6 mm are mandatory for SCC larger than 20 mm.[40]

Surgical excision remains the primary method for treating primary cutaneous melanoma. Historically, surgical margins were wide for melanoma; recent clinical trials support narrower, 1- to 2-cm margins, without a decrement in survival or local control.[8,41,42] Lentigo maligna requires a 5- to 10-mm margin, and lesions less than 1 mm in diameter need a 1-cm margin.[13] Intermediate thickness lesions (1–4 mm) merit 2-cm margins, but the poor prognosis associated with failure at other sites in thick (>4 mm) melanoma does not justify margins exceeding 2 cm (Fig 10–5).

The primary limitation of wide excision is the traditional bread-loaf or four-quadrant sectioning techniques that do not allow complete assessment of the peripheral margin. Tumor cells may be missed in the setting of irregular shapes or significant subclinical spread.[43] Comprehensive 360-degree margin assessment may be accomplished, however, by working closely with pathology and assessing margins en face. Although frozen section diagnosis may be readily accomplished in NMSC, this technique remains controversial in melanoma.

Mohs' Micrographic Surgery

This extirpative technique was developed in the 1930s by a medical student named Frederic Mohs. Lesions are excised in a sequential fashion in the outpatient setting, with resection, orientation of the specimen, assessment of horizontal margins, mapping of residual tumor, and re-excision repeated until the margins are clear.[43] The process is labor intensive, but effective in select NMSC, with cure rates in primary BCC approaching 99%.[44] Similar results have been noted in recurrent BCC, as well as

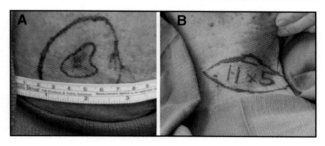

Fig 10–5 (A and B). Margins of resection for Clark level V melanoma of the scalp with regression. A previous biopsy had been performed, and the surrounding skin showed actinic damage. Margins are 2 cm from the actual biopsy site and at least 1.5 cm from the surrounding focal actinic damage. The defect was reconstructed with a full-thickness skin graft obtained from the neck.

Table 10–8. Minimum Margins for Resection of Skin Cancer of the Head and Neck

Basal Cell Carcinoma	Squamous Cell Carcinoma (and Other Aggressive Variants)	Melanoma
Routine = 4 mm	<2 cm diameter = 5 mm	Lentigo maligna = 5–10 mm
Basosquamous/Infiltrative = 10 mm	>2 cm = 10 mm	<1 cm diameter = 10 mm
>2 cm diameter = 10 mm		1–4 mm thick = 20 mm
		>4 mm thick = 20 mm

in primary and recurrent SCC. Mohs' micrographic surgery has demonstrated long-term control rates of 90% in selected, recurrent SCC.[45]

Although MMS effectively controls many NMSC, it is not indicated in patients with aggressive NMSC and deep invasion to or beyond the subcutaneous tissues. Patients with aggressive NMSC are best treated with en bloc surgical resection as opposed to the Mohs' technique that emphasizes maximum tissue conservation. The proximity of major neurovascular structures and the inadequacy of MMS for clearing tumor from bone and muscle complicate margin assessment. Aggressive lesions require aggressive treatment by a head and neck oncologic surgeon because radical surgery is often required to maximize outcomes.

This philosophy pervades discussions on local treatment for melanoma as well because there is increasing interest within the dermatology community about the potential for MMS in melanoma. Despite the objections of some dermatopathologists to frozen section assessment in cutaneous melanoma because of discordance between en face frozen section and permanent section margin assessment, experienced MMS practitioners have achieved 100% sensitivity and 90% specificity with frozen section evaluation of margins in melanoma.[46,47]

From a practical standpoint, experience with MMS in melanoma remains limited to lentigo maligna melanoma, and its efficacy in malignant melanoma remains investigational.[46] Because multidisciplinary treatment is often required in aggressive NMSC and melanoma, practitioners of MMS *must* collaborate regularly with head and neck surgical oncologists, radiation oncologists, and medical oncologists to optimize patient outcomes.

Combination Techniques

The potential to achieve microscopic margin control, eliminate subclinical disease, and minimize destruction of normal tissue makes MMS a potentially attractive adjunct for aggressive NMSC and melanoma, provided that the subtle histopathologic findings of each may be reliably and reproducibly detected on frozen section analysis. Additional investigation into mapped serial excision, immunohistochemical

staining of frozen section specimens, and rapid permanent section analysis may ultimately maximize local control in NMSC and melanoma with minimal morbidity, but wide excision remains the standard for aggressive NMSC and melanoma.

Special Considerations

Temporal Bone and Skull Base Involvement. Auricular and peri-auricular NMSC often invade the temporal bone, requiring sleeve, lateral, subtotal, or total temporal bone resection to achieve gross tumor clearance. Temporal bone invasion carries a poor prognosis, with overall survival of 63% at a mean follow-up of 26.7 months.[48] Involvement of the anterior skull base and calvarium may develop from direct extension, invasion along embryonic fusion planes, or via perineural spread. The true incidence is difficult to determine—this often occurs in patients with recurrent tumors who have undergone multiple prior treatment modalities. These patients may be amenable to craniofacial resection with adjuvant radiation, if possible. Poorer outcomes are associated with intracranial extension, perineural invasion, and previous radiation therapy.[49]

Radiation Therapy

Primary Radiation Therapy. Radiation therapy (XRT) remains a popular means of treating cutaneous malignancies, particularly for elderly patients, those deemed to be poor surgical candidates, and in cosmetically important areas such as the eyelids or nose. Radiation therapy for NMSC includes external beam radiation with orthovoltage x-rays, megavoltage x-rays, electron beam, and interstitial therapy with cesium afterloading catheters.[50] With the evolution of delivery techniques and fractionation schedules, radiation doses are increasingly focused on the tumor and high-risk areas, with decreasing collateral damage. Results from treating NMSC with radiation therapy are comparable to the methods previously discussed, particularly in advanced tumors, but local control and cosmetic outcomes may be inferior to surgical excision.[51-55]

Despite the perception that melanoma is radioresistant, primary radiotherapy achieved local control of 93% in patients with lentigo maligna and lentigo maligna melanoma.[13] By increasing the dose per fraction and decreasing the number of fractions (hypofractionated therapy, typically 30 Gray in 5 fractions), radiation therapy has resulted in durable locoregional responses, albeit in unresectable patients or poor surgical candidates.[56] Nonetheless, the hypofractionated techniques should be avoided in proximity to neural or sensory tissues, due to the potential for neurotoxicity.[8]

Adjuvant Radiation Therapy. Despite the limitations and challenges of treating NMSC and melanoma with primary XRT, adjuvant radiation therapy plays a significant role in the comprehensive management of these lesions. Common indications for radiation therapy to the primary lesion following surgical extirpation include positive margins, advanced lesions, temporal bone or skull base involvement, recurrent lesions at presentation, nodal metastases, and perineural invasion.[57,58] Thick primary melanomas, ulcerated lesions, satellitosis, desmoplastic histology, and patients at high risk for regional metastases but are poor candidates for elective neck dissection or sentinel node biopsy constitute additional indications for adjuvant radiotherapy in cutaneous melanoma.[59-61] Selected application of postoperative hypofractionated radiation in melanoma has improved locoregional control in stage I and II disease, compared to historical controls.[61-62]

Regardless of the histology or the treatment setting, complications following radiation therapy for skin cancer of the head and neck include cutaneous depigmentation, telangiectasias, scar contracture, lipodystrophy, tissue necrosis or atrophy, and damage to neurosensory structures.[55] Furthermore, the potential to trigger a radiation-induced second primary tumor or other tumor constitutes more than a theoretical risk, particularly in young patients.[63]

Other Techniques

Photodynamic therapy (PDT), which involves the administration of photosensitive drugs that are activated by light exposure, selectively destroys malignant cells. Common photosensitizing agents include benzoporphyrin, 5-aminolevulinic acid, meta-tetrahydroxyphenylchlorin (Foscan), and porfirmer sodium (Photofrin).[64] Complete clinical responses have been achieved in 92% of BCC and 100% of SCC in a highly selected population using PDT alone or in conjunction with surgery—there is no reported experience with PDT in melanoma.[65] Delayed wound healing, discomfort, and photosensitivity constitute recognized complications of PDT.[64,65] Carbon dioxide laser ablation has been used to successfully treat superficial BCC and for palliation of cutaneous melanoma metastases, but the lack of a surgical margin prohibits its routine use in primary disease.[66] Systemic therapy has traditionally played little role in the treatment of skin cancer of the head and neck, but innovations in targeted molecular therapy demonstrate great promise in phase II trials.[67]

Topical Therapy

The use of topical agents to treat superficial NMSC and even lentigo maligna is increasing in popularity. Topical therapy with 5-fluorouracil or the immune response modifier imiquimod (Aldara™) appears to be useful in treating precursor or superficial NMSC.[68-70] Imiquimod has also successfully eradicated Bowen's disease (SCC in situ), extramammary Paget's disease, cutaneous T-cell lymphoma, and, anecdotally, lentigo maligna.[13,68] Other medical interventions for skin cancer of the head and neck include intralesional injection of interferon-alpha and retinoids.[68]

RECONSTRUCTION OF CUTANEOUS DEFECTS OF THE HEAD AND NECK

Regardless of the histopathology and the extirpative technique, surgical treatment of head and neck skin cancer creates a cosmetic and often functional defect. As such, reconstructive surgeons are key members of the multidisciplinary team. Thorough surgical planning will incorporate potential reconstructive options without compromising oncologic cure. Reconstruction of head and neck cutaneous defects comprises a wide array of techniques that vary according to the involved subsites, and no summary can be exhaustive.

An overview of potential reconstructive modalities, by anatomic site, appears in Table 10–9. The chosen technique for a given defect must address the following challenges: restoration of form and function; color, texture, and thickness match; coverage of key structures such as the great vessels, calvarium, and dura; preservation of oral competence; and minimized ocular distortion. Often the best reconstructive technique employs adjacent, like tissue, although the entire reconstructive ladder from primary closure to free tissue transfer may be required.

DETECTION AND MANAGEMENT OF REGIONAL DISEASE

Regional metastases to parotid and cervical lymph nodes are a feature of advanced disease, contributing to diminished disease control and survival in both nonmelanoma skin cancer and melanoma. Despite the risk and implications of nodal spread, the general philosophies toward nodal metastases differ in that assessment and control of regional metastases

Table 10–9. Options for Reconstruction of Head and Neck Cutaneous Defects

Location	Challenges and Special Considerations	Reconstructive Choices

Lip	Focal point of appearance
	Oral competence
	Projection of emotion
	Access to oral cavity for food and dental appliances
	Meticulous approximation of vermilion border
		Wedge excision with primary closure
		Local advancement flaps
		  V-Y advancement
		  Stairstep advancement
		  A-T closure
		Lip/Cheek advancement
		  Webster-Bernard flap
		  Karapandzic flap
		  Gilles fan flap
		  Melolabial flap
		Lip switch procedures
		  Abbe flap
		  Estlander flap
		Free tissue transfer

Nose	Three layers: cover, support, mucosa
	Remember nasal subunits
	Multiple procedures are common
		Mucosal coverage
		  Skin grafts on flap undersurface
		  Turnover cutaneous flaps
		  Hinge flaps from septum/turbinate
		  Free flaps
		Support
		  Cartilage grafts from septum, auricle, rib
		  Full-thickness auricle grafts
		Cover
		  Secondary intention
		  Primary closure
		  Small defects (<1.5 cm)
		    Banner (note) flap
		    Dorsal nasal flap
		    Bilobed flap
		    Full-thickness grafts from auricle
		  Larger defects
		    Paramedian forehead flap
		    Melolabial flap
		    Free tissue transfer
		    Prosthetics

Table 10–9. *continued*

Location	Challenges and Special Considerations	Reconstructive Choices

Orbital/Periorbital	Thin skin
	Risk of ectropion, exposure keratopathy
	Remember concepts of anterior and posterior lamella
	Ensure meticulous alignment of the tarsus
		Small wounds
		  Secondary intention
		  Primary closure (<50% marginal defect)
		  Full-thickness grafts from upper lid
		Larger wounds
		  Single or bipedicled transposition flaps
		  Cross lid techniques
		    Hughes tarsoconjunctival flap
		    Cutler-Beard composite flap
		  Cervicofacial flaps
		Lateral defects
		  Primary closure
		  V-Y advancement flap
		  Rhomboid flap
		Posterior lamella
		    Free cartilage grafts
		    Free mucosal grafts

Auricle	Anatomic detail requires planning
	Multiple procedures are common
	Size of reconstructed ear may be sacrificed for normal appearance
	Prosthetics are an option
		Small rim defects
		  Primary closure
		  Star excision
		Large rim defects
		  Antia-Buch advancement flaps
		Conchal bowl defects
		  Secondary intention
		  Full/split thickness skin grafts
		  Postauricular flaps
		Extensive defects of temporal bone
		  Temporalis flap
		  Pedicled trapezius or latissimus flap
		  Free tissue transfer

Cheek	Primary goal is optimal color and texture match
	Orient in concert with relaxed skin tension lines
	Complex wounds must address mucosal lining and external cover
		Small wounds
		  Secondary intention
		  Primary closure
		  Local flaps
		    Banner (note) flaps
		    Rhomboid flaps
		    Bilobed flaps
		Larger wounds
		  Cervicofacial flap
		  Free tissue transfer

Scalp	Tissue has limited flexibility
	Tissue expansion may be an option
	Must preserve perichondrium for skin graft survival
	Beware of skin grafts in a radiated field
		Small wounds
		  Secondary intention
		  Primary closure
		  Full/split thickness skin grafts
		Larger wounds
		  Scalp flaps
		  Local transposition flaps
		Extensive defects
		  Free tissue transfer

in melanoma is a proactive concept. Because lymphatic drainage pathways are not specific to histology, sentinel lymph node biopsy and molecular analysis of specimens are increasingly applied to aggressive NMSC, rendering neck management more proactive in this condition as well.

Risk Factors for Regional Metastases

Nonmelanoma Skin Cancer

The reported incidence of metastatic squamous cell carcinoma of the skin ranges from <1% to over 20%, although the most frequently quoted rate is 5%.[18,45,71] Given the low risk of regional metastases, nodal NMSC metastases typically are treated after they develop. Because patients with nodal metastases have diminished overall survival, disease-free survival, and disease-specific survival at 5 years compared to patients without nodal metastases, there is an increased emphasis on identifying high risk lesions early in order to minimize future morbidity and mortality.[18] Risk factors for nodal metastases in NMSC include recurrent lesions, lesions larger than 2 cm or deeper than 4 mm, invasion into Clark level IV and V or the subcutaneous tissues, poorly differentiated histology, perineural invasion, lymphovascular invasion, inflammation, infiltrative tumor strands or single cells, acantholysis, and lesions that arise in existing scars or on the ear or lip.[18,35,45,72]

Melanoma

Nodal metastases in cutaneous melanoma portend a worse prognosis, with sentinel node-positive patients having a 3-year DFS of 56% compared to sentinel node-negative patients with similar primary lesions (3-year DFS 88%). The status of the regional nodes is a more reliable prognostic feature than Clark level, Breslow thickness, and ulceration status in melanoma.[27]

Depth of the primary melanoma constitutes the strongest predictor for regional metastases—less than 5% of lesions <1 mm thick metastasize, in contrast to 30% to 50% of lesions >4 mm thick.[28,73] Additional risk factors for regional metastasis in head and neck melanoma include Breslow thickness, Clark level >III, ulceration, and patient age <60, histology other than superficial spreading, lymphovascular invasion, and a present vertical growth phase.[74,75]

Management of the Clinically N0 Neck

Options for managing the clinically N0 neck in skin cancer of the head and neck include watchful waiting, elective neck dissection, sentinel lymph node biopsy, and elective radiation. Because of the perceived low risk for regional metastases in NMSC, the nodal basins are typically observed for signs of recurrence, which is then dealt with aggressively. On the other hand, expectant management of the neck in melanoma is reserved solely for stage Ia lesions.[28]

Elective Neck Dissection

Elective neck dissection may be considered in skin cancer of the head and neck based on the features of the primary lesion: recurrent NMSC in previously radiated patients, NMSC exhibiting multiple features of aggressive disease listed in Table 10–7, direct invasion of the neck or parotid capsule, intermediate thickness melanoma in patients younger than 60, and, potentially, patients with intermediate or thick melanoma, based on the poor prognosis for patients who manifest regional failure.[8,76,77] Although elective neck dissection in melanoma identifies about 20% of patients with occult disease, there is no clear survival benefit for elective dissection.[78,79]

Clinical assumptions about the pattern(s) of lymphatic metastases often guide the extent of elective neck dissection, with a 93% correlation between predicted basins and proven metastases.[80] Clinicopathologic studies of regional disease have demonstrated common drainage patterns. However, recent efforts have identified significant variability from predictions; therefore, preoperative lymphoscintigraphy may facilitate more accurate elective dissections.[81]

In general, a superficial parotidectomy and lateral neck dissection encompassing levels II to IV should be performed for lesions located on the face and scalp anterior to a vertical line from the external auditory canal.[8] Because the parotid contains paraglandular lymph nodes on the capsule and intraglandular nodes that are predominately located lateral to the facial nerve and retromandibular vein, a superficial parotidectomy is sufficient in the clinically negative gland. Total parotidectomy is reserved for extensive intraglandular metastases, and the facial nerve should be preserved unless it is clinically involved or there is gross evidence of perineural invasion.[82,83] A posterolateral neck dissection including the postauricular and occipital nodes, in addition to levels II to V, is indicated for lesions located posterior to the vertical line of the external auditory canal.[8,84] Bilateral supraomohyoid dissection should be considered for lesions of the medial orbit, central midface, and lips.

Sentinel Lymph Node Biopsy

Sentinel lymph node mapping and biopsy (SLNB) is based on the premise that metastasizing tumor cells will spread first to the draining lymphatic basin, with the sentinel node reflecting the status of the entire basin.[85] Identification of a positive sentinel lymph node (SLN) has emerged as the most important prognostic factor for recurrence and survival in cutaneous melanoma, and it has been validated with SLN identification rates exceeding 92%.[27,86,87] The feasibility of SLB in NMSC has been suggested by several case series.[81,88,89] Success rates for SLNB may be increased by adhering to the "10% Rule" proposed by McMasters and colleagues: remove all blue lymph nodes, all clinically suspicious nodes, and all nodes that are = 10% of the ex vivo radioactive count of the most radioactive sentinel node.[75]

Sentinel lymph node biopsy is indicated for intermediate thickness melanoma from 0.8 mm to 4 mm thick, as well as for ulcerated lesions of any thickness less than 4 mm.[27,90] There is no benefit to sentinel node biopsy in lesions thicker than 4 mm because of the high presumed rate of regional metastases. It should be considered in aggressive NMSC, high-risk SCC, and Merkel cell carcinoma.[81,91]

Preoperative lymphoscintigraphy with technetium-99m sulfur colloid or technetium-99m antimony trisulfide colloid injected intradermally in the periphery of the lesion, followed by intraoperative lymphatic mapping, is the cornerstone of SLNB.[86,92] Immediate and delayed images are then performed to identify the draining lymphatic basins. Radiolabeled tracer may be augmented by intraoperative,

intradermal injection of isosulfan blue dye for visual guidance.[27]

A gamma counter is used to obtain baseline radioactivity levels and levels after excision of the primary (or biopsy scar); increased radioactivity is then used to guide incision and blunt dissection of the sentinel lymph nodes (SLNs), as depicted in Figure 10-6. Facial nerve monitoring, or a nerve

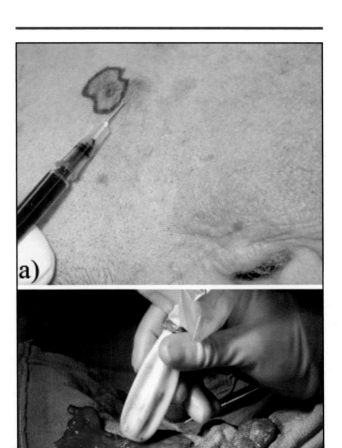

Fig 10–6 (A and B). Sentinel lymph node biopsy. The patient has already undergone radionuclide injection and lymphatic mapping. Isosulfan blue dye is injected in the periphery of the lesion prior to excision. Dissection is guided by increased radioactivity (and blue color) in sentinel lymph nodes—this patient manifested a confluence of nodes with increased uptake.

stimulator, may be used for lesions in the area of the parotid or spinal accessory nerve.[81,86] Excised SLNs are subjected to routine hematoxylin and eosin (H&E) staining, as well as immunohistochemical staining for proteins such as S-100, MART1, Melan-A, and HMB-45, or cytokeratins in SCC. Advanced molecular techniques such as polymerase chain reaction for tyrosinase, MART1, Mage3, and gp100 demonstrate improved sensitivity compared to standard assessments, and their use is becoming more widespread to identify patients at increased risk of failure.[12,29] Patients with microscopic disease after SLNB require a comprehensive neck dissection.

The benefits of SLNB include detection of occult regional metastases while sparing the majority of patients the morbidity of comprehensive neck dissection, improved accuracy of staging in melanoma, and identification of those patients who may benefit the most from systemic therapy.[27,86,87,92,93] Complications include injury to the facial nerve or spinal accessory nerve, seroma, sialocele formation, reactions to blue dye, and failure to identify sentinel nodes, but adverse events are rare in experienced hands.[81]

Management of the Positive Neck

Comprehensive neck dissection with preservation of vital neurovascular structures, when possible, is indicated for clinical nodal metastases or those detected by sentinel lymph node biopsy. The dissection must address the location of the primary and the metastatic focus with all intervening lymphatics.[8] Selective neck dissections may be performed if adjuvant radiotherapy is planned to cover undissected areas, but modified radical neck dissections or comprehensive neck dissections are required when postoperative radiation is not an option.[18]

Multimodality Therapy of Neck Metastases

Identification of regional metastases demands aggressive treatment in order to maximize locoregional control (LRC) and survival. Adjuvant radiation has been shown to improve LRC in metastatic SCC (80% vs 57%) and 5-year disease-free survival (74% vs 54%) versus neck dissection alone.[94] Postoperative

radiation therapy is recommended for patients with parotid or cervical metastases from NMSC with undissected levels included in the radiation portals.[18] Concurrent chemotherapy and radiation therapy may emerge as a viable treatment option in patients with multiple positive nodes, extracapsular spread or positive margins, based on the success of a similar approach to lymphatic metastases from the upper aerodigestive tract.[95,96]

Adjuvant radiation therapy for metastatic cutaneous melanoma after comprehensive neck dissection has been achieved 94% regional control at 10 years, with 10-year disease-specific survival and distant metastasis-free survival of 48% and 43%, respectively, in patients with clinical stage III disease. Common indications for adjuvant radiation therapy in melanoma include extracapsular spread, lymph nodes larger than 3.0 cm, multiple involved lymph nodes, recurrent disease, and less than radical or modified radical neck dissection.[97]

Radiation Therapy as the Sole Means of Regional Treatment

Elective radiation of the neck in patients with cutaneous melanoma has been performed on a hypofractionated schedule, achieving 5-year rates of local control, regional control, locoregional control, disease-specific survival, and disease-free survival of 94%, 89%, 86%, 68%, and 58%, respectively. As a result, elective neck radiation may be an alternative strategy for patients with intermediate or deep melanoma, or even positive sentinel nodes, who are poor candidates for neck dissection or systemic therapy.[98,99]

Management of the Unknown Primary with Neck Metastases

In both NMSC and melanoma, regional metastases without a clear primary lesion constitute a clinical challenge. A careful history must focus on a prior history of skin cancer or even skin lesions that were previously removed. Although an index lesion is often identified, other patients require a thorough physical examination, including an assessment for ocular or mucosal sites, to detect a source lesion, and one may not be found. Neck dissection followed by XRT is indicated for regional metastases from an unknown (but presumed cutaneous) primary of NMSC. Similarly, patients with nodal melanoma of unknown primary have stage III disease and require neck dissection followed by an evaluation for systemic therapy and potential XRT.[100,101]

THE MANAGEMENT OF ADVANCED AND SYSTEMIC DISEASE

Nonmelanoma Skin Cancer

Experience is limited with the management of advanced or metastatic NMSC, due to the relative rarity of this condition. Systemic chemotherapy has been shown to decrease tumor burden in patients with unresectable disease, but there are no randomized studies to support neoadjuvant chemotherapy in NMSC or to provide clear guidelines for systemic therapy.[102,103] Phase II studies of combinations of interferon-alpha (IFN-α), retinoic acid, and cisplatin have demonstrated overall responses and complete responses of 34% and 17%, respectively, in patients with locally advanced or metastatic NMSC.[104,105] Recent innovations in chemotherapy, such as the taxanes, may exhibit some promise in NMSC, and targeted molecular therapy against the epidermal growth factor pathway has successfully been applied to aggressive lesions, with a noteworthy response.[67] However, further investigation is required in this promising arena.

Melanoma

Distant metastases (DM) develop in roughly 30% of patients with localized melanoma, and patients with stage IIB, IIC, and III melanoma are at highest risk of systemic metastases and death.[106] Patients at increased risk of DM are identified by the 2002 AJCC staging system for potential systemic therapy, with intent to prevent metastases and subsequent death. The immunogenic properties of melanoma have been extensively exploited as potential targets for systemic therapy in the form of biologic response modifiers, vaccines, and immune stimulants.[8]

High-dose interferon alpha-2b (IFNα-2b) is the only adjuvant treatment approved by the Food and Drug Administration (FDA) to minimize the risk of recurrence and metastasis in Stage IIB-III melanoma, although the benefit of IFNα-2b for overall survival remains controversial. With a documented improvement in relapse-free survival of 20 to 30% in several trials, recent efforts have suggested that high-dose interferon (HDI) therapy is actually cost effective in patients younger than 60 with stage IIIC disease.[107-110] High-dose interferon treatment involves a 4-week induction period of 20 million units/m^2/day subcutaneously (SC) 5 days per week followed by 10 million units/m^2/day SC three times per week for 48 weeks. Toxicities from HDI include constitutional symptoms, fatigue, headache, nausea, weight loss, depression, hepatic injury, and myelosuppression.[6,111]

Other strategies, including intermediate- and low-dose regimens, have been investigated, along with combinations of interferon with melanoma vaccines, interleukin-2 (IL-2), gene therapy, and chemotherapeutics such as dacarbazine, cisplatin, temazolamide, and vinblastine. Adjuvant therapy of high-risk cutaneous melanoma remains an area of intense research, and patients with stage IIB to III disease should be encouraged to participate in clinical trials.[6,8]

Patients with stage IV melanoma have a poor prognosis, with about 5% to 20% 5-year survival.[106] Common sites for metastases include the lung, skin and subcutaneous tissues, brain, gastrointestinal tract, adrenal glands, bone, and liver.[112] Patients with distant skin, subcutaneous, and nodal metastases have a better prognosis than patients with lung or visceral metastases, accounting for the subdivision of stage IV in the 2002 AJCC staging system. Aggressive chemotherapy regimens have evolved for stage IV melanoma, with minimal success these include high dose IL-2, surgical resection of isolated metastases, and cytotoxic therapy with dacarbazine or temazolamide.[6,106] Biochemotherapy with IL-2 or IFNα-2b and cytotoxic agents have been attempted, but severe toxicities have limited its widespread acceptance, underscoring the need for novel approaches.[113]

PREVENTION

Avoidance, protective clothing, and sunscreen are the most common strategies to minimize sun and ultraviolet radiation exposure and subsequent risk of developing skin cancer of the head and neck.[114] The limitations of early sunscreen formulations against UVA or the sense of false confidence imparted by sunscreens has led to the contention that sunscreen does not prevent skin cancer.[115] Educational programs designed to alter sun behaviors and increase awareness of skin cancer among lay people and medical professionals alike may lead to earlier detection of suspicious lesions, and, ultimately, a decrease in the incidence of skin cancer.[116]

Preventive strategies for individuals with genetic, occupational, or recreational risk factors for developing skin cancer continue to evolve. Retinoids, nonsteroidal anti-inflammatory medications (NSAIDS), and inhibitors of cyclooxygenase (COX) have been studied as preventative measures, as have homeopathic interventions such as a low-fat diet, beta-carotene, vitamins C and E supplementation, extracts from green tea and grape seeds, and analogs of 1,25-dihydroxyvitamin D3.[68] A recent randomized trial of adjuvant 13-*cis*-retinoic acid and interferon alfa in patients with aggressive skin squamous cell carcinoma did not demonstrate any benefit towards preventing recurrent disease or second primary tumors, but it did generate renewed interest in systemic strategies for treating and preventing advanced skin cancer.[117,118]

SUMMARY

Skin cancer, both nonmelanoma and melanoma, is a rising global health problem that leads to significant morbidity and mortality, and these lesions commonly appear on the head and neck, due to the strong association between ultraviolet light exposure and skin cancer. Given its high prevalence, patients and providers must remain a high index of suspicion for skin cancer, focusing not only on the primary lesion but also the risk of metastatic disease in the cervical lymph nodes and parotid. Although the vast majority of NMSC may be cured by a variety of methods, aggressive lesions demand precise excision—traditional wide local excision and Mohs' micrographic surgery constitute the most common techniques—as well as meticulous assessment to identify the features of aggressive disease such as perineural invasion, deep invasion, and lymphovascular invasion. Wide excision remains the standard of care for cutaneous melanoma, but continued innovations in histopathologic techniques and less ablative therapies like topical therapy may ultimately lead to equivalent or improved local control with less tissue destruction in both NMSC and melanoma. Resulting tissue defects are best reconstructed with local tissue to optimize function and cosmesis, and a variety of flaps and techniques are available, encompassing all levels of the reconstructive ladder.

The potential for lymphatic metastases to the cervical and parotid nodes in both NMSC and melanoma should not be underestimated. Sentinel lymph node biopsy with traditional, immunohistochemical, and even molecular analysis of nodal specimens constitutes the best available means to detect regional metastases, promoting the identification of high-risk patients for potential adjuvant radiation therapy or systemic therapy. Although traditional cytotoxic therapies are most commonly used in advanced or metastatic NMSC, future work will highlight targeted molecular therapy. Similarly, IFNα-2b is the primary systemic option for advanced melanoma, but this remains an area of intense research. Nonetheless, the key to limiting the impact of the skin cancer epidemic is prevention, with an increased focus on novel strategies for prevention and early detection.

REFERENCES

1. Santmyire BR, Feldman SR, Fleischer AB Jr. Lifestyle high-risk behaviors and demographics may predict the level of participation in sun-protection behaviors and skin cancer primary prevention in the United States: Results of the 1998 national health interview survey. *Cancer.* 2001; 92:1315–1324.

2. Alam M, Ratner D. Primary care: cutaneous squamous cell carcinoma. *N Engl J Med.* 2001;344: 975-983.

3. Johnson TM, Rowe DE, Nelson BR, Swanson NA. Squamous cell carcinoma of the skin (excluding lip and oral mucosa). *J Am Acad Dermatol.* 1992; 26:467-484.

4. Christenson LJ, Borrowman TA, Vachon CM, et al. Incidence of basal cell and squamous cell carcinomas in a population younger than 40 years. *JAMA.* 2005;294:681-690.

5. Khanna M, Fortier-Riberdy G, Dinehart SM, Smoller B. Histopathologic evaluation of cutaneous squamous cell carcinoma: results of a survey among dermatopathologists. *J Am Acad Dermatol.* 2003;48:721-726.

6. Tsao H, Atkins MB, Sober AJ. Medical progress: management of cutaneous melanoma. *N Engl J Med.* 2004;351:998-1012.

7. Jemal A, Tiwari RC, Murray T, et al. Cancer statistics, 2004. *CA Cancer J Clin.* 2004;54:8-29.

8. Lentsch EJ, Myers JN. Melanoma of the head and neck: current concepts in diagnosis and management. *Laryngoscope.* 2001;111:1209-1222.

9. Moore BA, Kies M, Rosental D, Weber RS. In: Genden E, ed. *Head and Neck Cancer.* New York, NY: Thieme; in press.

10. O'Brien CJ, Uren RF, Thompson JF, et al. Prediction of potential metastatic sites in cutaneous head and neck melanoma using lymphoscintigraphy. *Am J Surg.* 1995;170:461-466.

11. Melnikova VO, Ananthaswamy HN. Cellular and molecular events leading to the development of skin cancer. *Mutation Res.* 2005;571:91-106.

12. Fecher LA, Cummings SD, Keefe MJ, Alani RM. Toward a molecular classification of melanoma. *J Clin Oncol.* 2007;25:1606-1620.

13. Arlette JP, Trotter MJ, Trotter T, Temple CLF. Management of lentigo maligna and lentigo maligna melanoma: seminars in surgical oncology. *J Surg Oncol.* 2004;86:179-186.

14. Friedman RJ, Rigel DS, Kopf AW. Early detection of malignant melanoma: the role of physician examination and self-examination of the skin. *CA Cancer J Clin.* 1985;35:130-151.

15. Ginsberg LE. MR imaging of perineural tumor spread. *Neuroimaging Clin North Am.* 2004;14: 663-677.

16. Wagner JD, Schauwecker D, Davidson D, et al. Inefficacy of F-18 fluorodeoxy-D-glucose-positron emission tomography scans for initial evaluation in early-stage cutaneous melanoma. *Cancer.* 2005;104:570-579.

17. Greene F, Page DL, Fleming ID, et al. *AJCC Cancer Staging Manual.* 6th ed. New York, NY: Springer-Verlag; 2002.

18. Moore BA, Weber RS, Prieto V, et al. Lymph node metastases from cutaneous squamous cell carcinoma of the head and neck. *Laryngoscope.* 2005; 115:1561-1567.

19. O'Brien CJ, McNeil EB, McMahon JD, et al. Significance of clinical stage, extent of surgery, and pathologic findings in metastatic cutaneous squamous carcinoma of the parotid gland. *Head Neck.* 2002;24:417-422.

20. Palme CE, O'Brien CJ, Veness MJ, et al. Extent of parotid disease influences outcome in patients with metastatic cutaneous squamous cell carcinoma. *Arch Otolaryngol Head Neck Surg.* 2003; 129:750-753.

21. Morton DL, Wen DR, Wong JH, et al. Technical details of intraoperative lymphatic mapping for early stage melanoma. *Arch Surg.* 1992;127: 392-399.

22. Ballantyne AJ. Malignant melanoma of the skin of the head and neck: an analysis of 405 cases. *Am J Surg.* 1970;120:425-431.

23. Clark WH Jr., From L, Bernardino EA, Mihm MC. The histogenesis and biologic behavior of primary human malignant melanomas of the skin. *Cancer Res.* 1969;29:705-727.

24. Breslow A. Thickness, cross-sectional areas and depth of invasion in the prognosis of cutaneous melanoma. *Ann Surg.* 1970;172:902-908.

25. Balch CM, Buzaid AC, Soong S-J et al. New TNM melanoma staging system: linking biology and natural history to clinical outcomes. *Semin Surg Oncol.* 2003;21:43-52.

26. Petro A, Schwartz J, Johnson T. Current melanoma staging. *Clin Dermatol.* 2004;22:223-227.

27. Gershenwald JE, Thompson W, Mansfield PF, et al. Multi-institutional melanoma lymphatic mapping experience: the prognostic value of sentinel lymph node status in 612 stage I or II melanoma patients. *J Clin Oncol.* 1999;17:976-983.

28. Balch C, Soong S-J, Gershenwald JE, et al. Prognostic factors analysis of 17,600 melanoma patients: validation of the American Joint Committee on Cancer melanoma staging system. *J Clin Oncol.* 2001;19:3622-3634.

29. Torabian S, Kashani-Sabet M. Biomarkers for melanoma. *Curr Opin Oncol.* 2005;17:167-171.

30. Litvak DA, Gupta RK, Yee R, et al. Endogenous immune response to early- and intermediate-stage melanoma is correlated with outcomes and is independent of locoregional relapse and standard prognostic factors. *J Am Coll Surg.* 2004; 198:27–35.

31. Wong CSM, Strange RC, Lear JT. Basal cell carcinoma. *BMJ.* 2003;327:794–798.

32. Vico P, Fourez T, Nemec E, et al. Aggressive basal cell carcinoma of head and neck areas. *Eur J Surg Oncol.* 1995;21:490–497.

33. Rudolph R, Zelac DE. Squamous cell carcinoma of the skin. *Plast Reconstr Surg.* 2004;114: 82e–94e.

34. Breuninger H, Schaumberg-Lever G, Holzschuh J, Horny H-P. Desmoplastic squamous cell carcinoma of the skin and vermilion surface. *Cancer.* 1997;79:915–919.

35. Lai SY, Weinstein GS, Chalian AA, et al. Parotidectomy in the treatment of aggressive cutaneous malignancies. *Arch Otolaryngol Head Neck Surg.* 2002;128:521–526.

36. Panje WR, Ceilley RI. The influence of the midface on the spread of epithelial malignancies. *Laryngoscope.* 1979;89:1914–1920.

37. Clayman GL, Lee JJ, Holsinger FC, et al. Mortality risk from squamous cell skin cancer. *J Clin Oncol.* 2005;23:759–765.

38. Lens MB, Newton-Bishop JA, Boon AP. Desmoplastic malignant melanoma: a systematic review. *Br J Dermatol.* 2005;152:673–678.

39. Thomas DJ, King AR, Peat BG. Excision margins for nonmelanoma skin cancer. *Plast Reconstr Surg.* 2003;112:57–63.

40. Brodland DG, Zitelli JA. Surgical margins for excision of primary cutaneous squamous cell carcinoma. *J Am Acad Dermatol.* 1992;27:241–248.

41. Balch CM, Soong SJ, Smith T, et al. Long-term results of a prospective trial comparing 2 cm vs. 4 cm excision margins for 740 patients with 1–4 mm melanomas. *Ann Surg Oncol.* 2001;8: 101–108.

42. Khayat D, Rixe O, Martin G, et al. Surgical margins in cutaneous melanoma (2 cm versus 5 cm for lesions measuring less than 2.1 mm-thick. *Cancer.* 2003;97:1941–1946.

43. Nelson BR, Railan D, Cohen S. Mohs' micrographic surgery for nonmelanoma skin cancer. *Clin Plast Surg.* 1997;24:705–718.

44. Rowe DE, Carroll RJ, Day CL Jr. Long-term recurrence rates in previously untreated (primary) basal cell carcinoma: implications for patient follow-up. *J Dermatol Surg Oncol.* 1989;15: 315–328.

45. Rowe DE, Carroll RJ, Day CL Jr. Prognostic factors for local recurrence, metastasis, and survival rates in squamous cell carcinoma of the skin, ear, and lip. *J Am Acad Dermatol.* 1992;26:976–990.

46. Zitelli JA, Brown CD, Hanusa BH. Surgical margins for excision of primary cutaneous melanoma. *J Am Acad Dermatol.* 1997;37:422–429.

47. Prieto VG, Argenyi ZB, Barnhill RL, et al. Are en face frozen sections accurate for diagnosing margin status in melanocytic lesions? *Am J Clin Pathol,* 2003;120:203–208.

48. Gal TJ, Futran ND, Bartels LJ, Klotch DW. Auricular carcinoma with temporal bone invasion: outcomes analysis. *Otolaryngol Head Neck Surg.* 1999;121: 62–65.

49. Backous DD, DeMonte F, El-Naggar A, et al. Craniofacial resection for nonmelanoma skin cancer of the head and neck. *Laryngoscope.* 2005;115: 931–937.

50. Mendenhall WM, Parsons JT, Mendenhall NP, Million RP. T2–T4 carcinoma of the skin of the head and neck treated with radical irradiation. *Int J Radiation Oncol Biol Phys.* 1987;13: 975–981.

51. Wilder RB, Kittelson JM, Shimm DS. Basal cell carcinoma treated with radiation therapy. *Cancer.* 1991;68:2134–2137.

52. Shimm DS, Wilder RB. Radiation therapy for squamous cell carcinoma of the skin. *Am J Clin Oncol.* 1991;14:383–386.

53. Al-Othman MOF, Mendenhall WM, Amdur RJ. Radiotherapy alone for clinical T4 skin carcinoma of the head and neck with surgery reserved for salvage. *Am J Otolaryngol.* 2001;22:387–390.

54. Avril M-F, Auperin A, Margulis A, et al. Basal cell carcinoma of the face: surgery or radiotherapy? Results of a randomized study. *Br J Cancer.* 1997; 76:100–106.

55. Petit JY, Avril MF, Margulis A, et al. Evaluation of cosmetic results of a randomized trial comparing surgery and radiotherapy in the treatment of basal cell carcinoma of the face. *Plast Reconstr Surg.* 2000;105:2544–2551.

56. Ang KK, Byers RM, Peters LJ, et al. Regional radiotherapy as adjuvant therapy for head and neck melanoma: preliminary results. *Arch Otolaryngol Head Neck Surg.* 1990;116:169–172.

57. Morrisson WH, Garden AS, Ang KK. Radiation therapy for nonmelanoma skin cancers. *Clin Plast Surg.* 1997;24:719–729.

58. Fowler BZ, Crocker IR, Johnstone PAS. Perineural spread of cutaneous malignancy to the brain: a review of the literature and five patients treated with stereotactic radiotherapy. *Cancer.* 2005; 103:2143–2153.

59. Ballo MT, Ang KK. Radiotherapy for cutaneous malignant melanoma: rationale and indications. *Oncology (Williston Park).* 2004; 18:99–107.

60. Vongtama R, Safa A, Gallardo D, et al. Efficacy of radiation therapy in the local control of desmoplastic malignant melanoma. *Head Neck.* 2003; 25:423–428.

61. Ang KK, Peters LJ, Weber RS, et al. Postoperative radiotherapy for cutaneous melanoma of the head and neck region. *Int J Radiation Oncol Biol Phys.* 1994;30:795–798.

62. Stevens G, Thompson JF, Firth I, et al. Locally advanced melanoma: results of postoperative hypofractionated radiation therapy. *Cancer.* 2000;88:88–94.

63. Perkins JL, Liu Y, Mitby PA, et al. Nonmelanoma skin cancer in survivors of childhood and adolescent cancer: a report from the childhood cancer survivor study. *J Clin Oncol.* 2005;23:3733–3741.

64. Schweitzer VG. Photofrin-mediated photodynamic therapy for treatment of aggressive head and neck nonmelanomatous skin tumors in elderly patients. *Laryngoscope.* 2001;111:1091–1098.

65. Kubler AC, Haase T, Staff C, et al. Photodynamic therapy of primary nonmelanomatous skin tumours of the head and neck. *Laser Surg Med.* 1999;25:60–68.

66. Gibson SC, Byrne DS, McKay AJ. Ten-year experience of carbon dioxide laser ablation as treatment for cutaneous recurrence of malignant melanoma. *Br J Surg.* 2004;91:893–895.

67. Weber RS, Lustig R, Glisson B, et al. A phase II trial of ZD 1869 for advanced cutaneous squamous cell carcinoma of the head and neck. *J Clin Oncol.* 2007; ASCO Annual Meeting Proceedings Part I (25: Abstract No. 6038).

68. Chakrabarty A, Geisse JK. Medical therapies for non-melanoma skin cancer. *Clin Dermatol.* 2004;22:183–188.

69. Sterry W, Herrera E, Takwale A, et al. Imiquimod 5% cream for the treatment of superficial and nodular basal cell carcinoma: randomized studies comparing low-frequency dosing with and without occlusion. *Br J Dermatol.* 2002;147:1227–1236.

70. Urosevic M, Dummer R. Role of Imiquimod in skin cancer treatment. *Am J Clin Dermatol.* 2004;5:453–458.

71. Lund HZ. How often does squamous cell carcinoma of the skin metastasize? *Arch Dermatol.* 1965;92:635–637.

72. Cherpelis BS, Marcusen C, Lang PG. Prognostic factors for metastasis in squamous cell carcinoma of the skin. *Dermatol Surg.* 2002;28:268–273.

73. Singluff CL Jr., Stidham KR, Ricci WM, Stanley WE, Seigler HF. Surgical management of regional lymph nodes in patients with melanoma: experience with 4682 patients. *Ann Surg.* 1994;219: 120–130.

74. McMasters KM, Wong SL, Edwards MJ, et al. Factors that predict the presence of sentinel lymph node metastasis in patients with melanoma. *Surgery.* 2001;130:151–156.

75. McMasters KM, Noyes RD, Reintgen DS, et al. Lessons learned from the Sunbelt Melanoma Trial. *J Surg Oncol.* 2004;86:212–223.

76. Balch CM, Soong S-J, Bartolucci AA, et al. Efficacy of elective regional lymph node dissection of 1 to 4 mm thick melanomas for patients 60 years of age and younger. *Ann Surg.* 1996;224:255–266.

77. Cascinelli N, Morabito A, Santinami M, et al. Immediate or delayed dissection of regional nodes in patients with melanoma of the trunk: a randomized trial. *Lancet.* 1998;351:798–796.

78. Veronesi U, Adamus J, Bandiera DC, et al. Inefficacy of immediate node dissection in stage I melanoma of the limbs. *N Engl J Med.* 1977; 297:627–630.

79. Sim FH, Taylor WF, Pritchard DJ, Soule EH. Lymphadenectomy in the management of stage I malignant melanoma: a prospective randomized study. *Mayo Clin Proc.* 1986;61:697–705.

80. Pathak I, O'Brien CJ, Petersen-Schaeffer K, et al. Do nodal metastases from cutaneous melanoma of the head and neck follow a clinically predictable pattern? *Head Neck.* 2001;23:785–790.

81. Civantos FJ, Moffat FL, Goodwin WJ. Lymphatic mapping and sentinel lymphadenectomy for 106 head and neck lesions: contrasts between oral cavity and cutaneous malignancy. *Laryngoscope.* 2006;116(suppl 109):1–15.

82. Conley J, Arena S. Parotid gland as a focus of metastasis. *Arch Surg.* 1963;87:757–764.

83. McKean ME, Lee K, McGregor IA. The distribution of lymph nodes in and around the parotid gland: an anatomical study. *Br J Plast Surg.* 1985; 38:1–5.

84. Goepfert H, Jesse RH, Ballantyne AJ. Posterolateral neck dissection. *Arch Otolaryngol.* 1980;106: 618–620.

85. Morton DL, Wen Dr, Wong JH, et al. Technical details of intraoperative lymphatic mapping for early stage melanoma. *Arch Surg.* 1992;127:392-399.

86. Schmalbach CE, Nussenbaum B, Rees RS, et al. Reliability of sentinel lymph node mapping with biopsy for head and neck cutaneous melanoma. *Arch Otolaryngol Head Neck Surg.* 2003;129:61-65.

87. Shpitzer T, Segal K, Schachter J, et al. Sentinel node guided surgery for melanoma in the head and neck region. *Melanoma Res.* 2004;14:283-287.

88. Weisberg NK, Bertagnolli MM, Becker DS. Combined sentinel lymphadenectomy and Mohs micrographic surgery for high-risk cutaneous squamous cell carcinoma. *J Am Acad Dermatol.* 2000;43:483-488.

89. Michl C, Starz H, Bachter D, Balda B-R. Sentinel lymphonodectomy in nonmelanoma skin malignancies. *Br J Dermatol.* 2003;149:763-769.

90. Zapas JL, Coley HC, Beam SL, et al. The risk of regional lymph node metastases in patients with melanoma less than 1.0mm thick: recommendations for sentinel lymph node biopsy. *J Am Coll Surg.* 2003;197:403-407.

91. Schmalbach CE, Lowe L, Teknos TN et al. Reliability of sentinel lymph node biopsy for regional staging of head and neck Merkel cell carcinoma. *Arch Otolaryngol Head Neck Surg.* 2005;131:610-614.

92. de Wilt JHW, Thompson JF, Uren RF, et al. Correlation between preoperative lymphoscintigraphy and metastatic nodal disease sites in 362 patients with cutaneous melanomas of the head and neck. *Ann Surg.* 2004;239:544-552.

93. Doubrovsky A, de Wilt JHW, Scolyer RA, et al. Sentinel node biopsy provides more accurate staging than elective lymph node dissection in patients with cutaneous melanoma. *Ann Surg Oncol.* 2004;11:829-836.

94. Veness MJ, Morgan GJ, Palme CE, Gebski V. Surgery and adjuvant radiotherapy in patients with cutaneous head and neck squamous cell carcinoma metastatic to lymph nodes: combined treatment should be considered best practice. *Laryngoscope.* 2005;115:870-875.

95. Cooper JS, Pajak TF, Forastiere AA, et al. Postoperative concurrent radiotherapy and chemotherapy for high-risk squamous cell carcinoma of the head and neck. *N Engl J Med.* 2004;350:1937-1944.

96. Bernier J, Domenge C, Ozsahin M, et al. Postoperative irradiation with or without concomitant chemotherapy for locally advanced head and neck cancer. *N Engl J Med.* 2004;350:1945-1952.

97. Ballo MT, Bonnen MD, Garden AS, et al. Adjuvant irradiation for cervical lymph node metastases from melanoma. *Cancer.* 2003;97:1789-1796.

98. Bonnen MD, Ballo MT, Myers JN, et al. Elective radiotherapy provides regional control for patients with cutaneous melanoma of the head and neck. *Cancer.* 2004;100:383-389.

99. Ballo MT, Garden AS, Myers JN, et al. Melanoma metastatic to cervical lymph nodes: can radiotherapy replace formal dissection after local excision of nodal disease? *Head Neck.* 2005;27:718-721.

100. Nasri S, Namazie A, Dulguerov P, Mickel R. Malignant melanoma of cervical and parotid lymph nodes with an unknown primary site. *Laryngoscope.* 1994;104:1194-1198.

101. Katz K, Jonasch E, Hodi FS, et al. Melanoma of unknown primary: experience at Massachusetts General Hospital and Dana-Farber Cancer Institute. *Melanoma Res.* 2005;15:77-82.

102. Denic S. Preoperative treatment of advanced skin carcinoma with cisplatin and bleomycin. *Am J Clin Oncol.* 1999;22:32-34.

103. Sadek H, Azli N, Wendling JL, et al. Treatment of advanced squamous cell carcinoma of the skin with cisplatin, 5-fluoruracil, and bleomycin. *Cancer.* 1990;66:1692-1696.

104. Lippman SM, Parkinson DR, Itri LM, et al. 13-cis-retinoic acid and interferon-alpha-2a: effective combination therapy for advanced squamous cell carcinoma of the skin. *J Natl Cancer Inst.* 1992;84:235-241.

105. Shin DM, Glisson BS, Khuri F, et al. Phase II and biologic study of interferon alfa, retinoic acid, and cisplatin in advanced squamous skin cancer. *J Clin Oncol.* 2002;20:364-370.

106. Essner R, Lee JH, Wamek LA, Itakura H, Morton DL. Contemporary surgical treatment of advanced-stage melanoma. *Arch Surg.* 2004;139:961-967.

107. Kirkwood JM, Strawderman MH, Ernstoff MC, et al. Interferon alfa-2b adjuvant therapy of high-risk resected cutaneous melanoma: the Eastern Cooperative Oncology Group trial EST 1684. *J Clin Oncol.* 1996;14:7-17.

108. Kirkwood JM, Ibrahim JG, Sondak VK, et al. High and low-dose interferon alfa-2b in high risk melanoma: first analysis of Intergroup trial E1690/S9111/C9190. *J Clin Oncol.* 2000;18:2444-2458.

109. Kirkwood JM, Ibrahim JG, Sosman JA, et al. High-dose interferon alfa-2b significantly prolongs

relapse-free and overall survival compared with the GM2–KLH/QS-21 vaccine in patients with resected stage IIB-III melanoma: results of Intergroup trial E1694/S9512/C509801. *J Clin Oncol.* 2001;19:2370–2380.

110. Cormier JN, Xing Y, Ding M, et al. Cost effectiveness of adjuvant interferon in node-positive melanoma. *J Clin Oncol.* 2007;25:2442–2448.

111. Muggiano A, Mulas C, Fiori B, et al. Feasibility of high-dose interferon alpha-2b adjuvant therapy for high-risk resected cutaneous melanoma. *Melanoma Res.* 2004;14(suppl 1):S1–S7.

112. Daryanani D, Plukker JT, de Jong MA, et al. Increased incidence of brain metastases in cutaneous head and neck melanoma. *Melanoma Res.* 2005;15:119–124.

113. Chapman PB, Panageas KS, Williams L, et al. Clinical results using biochemotherapy as a standard of care in advanced melanoma. *Melanoma Res.* 2002;12:381–387.

114. Rodenas JM, Delgado-Rodriguez M, Herrantz MT, et al. Sun exposure, pigmentary traits, and risk of cutaneous malignant melanoma: a case-control study in a Mediterranean population. *Cancer Causes Control.* 1996;7:275–283.

115. Autier P, Dore JF, Schifflers E, et al. Melanoma and use of sunscreens: an EORTC case-control study in Germany, Belgium, and France. *Int J Cancer.* 1995;61:749–755.

116. Marks R. Two decades of the public health approach to skin cancer control in Australia: why, how and where we are now? *Austral J Dermatol.* 1999;40:1–5.

117. Brewster AM, Lee JJ, Clayman GL, et al. Randomized trial of adjuvant 13–cis-retinoic acid and interferon alfa for patients with aggressive skin squamous cell carcinoma. *J Clin Oncol.* 2007;25:1974–1978.

118. Pfister DG, Halpern AC. Skin squamous cell cancer: the time is right for greater involvement of the medical oncologist. *J Clin Oncol.* 2007;25:1953–1954.

11

Nasopharyngeal Carcinoma

Sheng-Po Hao
Ngan-Ming Tsang

DEFINITIONS OF UNIQUE TERMS

Nasopharyngeal carcinoma (NPC) is a squamous cell carcinoma arising from the nasopharynx. The tumor originates from the epithelial cells lining the nasopharyngeal space.[1] The definition of NPC strictly excludes all other nasopharyngeal malignancies arising from lymphoid tissue or connective tissue, such as lymphoma and sarcoma, or glandular type carcinoma from minor salivary glands. NPC is a unique malignancy with an endemic distribution among certain well-defined ethnic geographic groups.[2] NPC is a frequent cancer among Chinese. Its close relationship with Epstein-Barr virus (EBV) makes NPC a model for viral carcinogenesis of humans.[1] NPC shows various degrees of differentiation and is frequently seen at the pharyngeal recess (Rosenmüller's fossa) posteromedial to the medial crura of the eustachian tube opening in the nasopharynx.

EPIDEMIOLOGY AND PREVALENCE

NPC is one of the most common head and neck cancers among the Chinese population, particularly the residents in the southeastern provinces of China, such as Guang Dong, Guang Xi, and Fu Kien. These regions also have the highest incidence of NPC around the world. NPC is also known as "Cantonese cancer" with reported cases of 10 to 20 per 100,000 men and 5 to 10 per 100,000 women, respectively, is highest.

NPC is seen in all parts of the world but varies in incidence and dominant histologic type among different ethnic groups. Chinese are the most frequently affected population. NPC are classified to have 3 subtypes: type I: differentiated, type II: poorly differentiated, and type III: undifferentiated carcinoma.[3] Moderate risk of NPC are seen in Taiwan, Singapore, North Africa, and in the Eskimo population. People in Taiwan, as part of Southeast Asia region, are affected at a rate of 5 to 10 per 100,000 per year. In such endemic areas, almost all of the tumors were classified histologically as poorly differentiated or undifferentiated carcinoma NPC, the latter being more common. NPC also tends to show extensive lymphocytic infiltration and has been described as lymphoepitheliomas. The type II poorly differentiated and type III undifferentiated subtypes of NPC are closely related to EBV and are frequently considered as a single pathogenetic entity.[1] In the other parts of the world, NPC is a rare disease where tumors are more frequently classified histologically as type I differentiated NPC.

NPC is a tumor of multifactorial etiologies involving virologic, environmental, and genetic components.[2] Although NPC becomes a rare cancer among whites in North America, a high incidence of NPC is still noted in American-born Chinese.[4] The reported incidence is lower than in Chinese immigrants or who people reside in the southeastern part of China.[4] These findings impose an interaction among geographic, ethnic, and environmental etiologic factors.

Epstein-Barr virus (EBV), a double-stranded DNA virus, is closely related to NPC.[1] Almost every NPC tumor cell carries clonal EBV genomes and expresses EBV proteins.[1] EBV is a ubiquitous infectious agent that infects greater than 90% of the world's population.[5] The infected individuals carry the virus in a persistent, lifelong infection, but are completely asymptomatic in the vast majority of cases.[5] Most NPC tumors arise in long-term virus carriers many years after primary EBV infection reflecting the multistep nature of the oncogenic process.[6] EBV infection can be characterized in three phases: acute, latent, and reactivated.[1,7] The peripheral blood and lymphoid organs are ordinarily the sites of dormancy for latently EBV-Infected lymphocytes.[5,6,8] In vivo, most human EBV infection initiates in the oropharyngeal epithelium.[5] Early in the course of primary infection, EBV infects B lymphocytes. Among the circulating B lymphocytes, the EBV somehow escapes from the immune surveillance system and becomes a latent infection.[1] These infected cells are permissive for virus replication. A persistent lytic infection ensues that continues at some level for many years or even for life.[6]

B lymphocytes are the major site of latent infections and are important in the dissemination of infection to distal epithelial surfaces, including the nasopharynx, and in continuously reseeding the oropharyngeal epithelium.[1,5] The presence of EBV in NPC is well documented. Initial studies using hybridization kinetic analyses revealed that NPC contained EBV DNA[9] and that the viral DNA and EBV nuclear antigen complex (EBNAs) were detected in the malignant epithelioma cells rather than in the abundant infiltrating lymphoid cells.[10]

The etiologic link between NPC and EBV was first suggested based on serologic evidence. Several serologic studies demonstrated that patients bearing NPC had elevated levels of antibodies to EBV antigens, usually IgA antibodies to viral capsid antigen (VCA) and IgA antibodies to early antigens (EA).[11,12] Several large population-based screening studies have validated the use of EBV serology for NPC detection in high-risk groups in southern China.[13] Although it has been claimed that elevated titers of anti-VCA IgA and anti-EA IgA can predict the presence of NPC,[13] the use of serologic titers as a screening method for NPC has been quite disappointing in some reports.[14,15] The sensitivity and specificity of using EBV antibody titers in screening patients for early detection of NPC were unsatisfactory at different cutoff points.[15] In one report, only 7(5.4%) out of 130 asymptomatic individuals who had elevated anti-VCA IgA (above 10) had early NPC after randomized biopsy of 6 different sites in the nasopharyngeal space.[16]

In addition to anti-VCA IgA antibody, the neutralizing antibody against EBV DNase has been reported to be a useful serologic marker for the diagnosis of NPC. Recently, a population-based prospective cohort study using a combination of detection of IgA antibodies against EBV VCA and anti-EBV DNase antibodies revealed that these two serologic markers are strong predictors of the risk of NPC, even when the tumor developed more than 5 years after recruitment.[17]

MOLECULAR DIAGNOSIS WITH NASOPHARYNGEAL SWAB

It has been reported that 3 latent membrane proteins are expressed in NPC and nearly all NPC tumor cells contain the EBV-derived latent membrane protein 1 (LMP-1) gene.[18,19] LMP-1 gene is a classic oncogene with transformation properties[20] and is an ideal target for screening purposes.[8] It has been reported that detecting EBV-derived LMP-1 gene by nasopharyngeal swab verifies NPC with a sensitivity of 87.3% and specificity of 98.4%.[8] The nasopharyngeal swab coupled with PCR-based EBV LMP-1 gene detection is a useful screening tool in high-risk populations.[8] Only 7 (2%) of 256 patients with a diagnosis other than NPC had LMP-1 gene detected in the nasopharyngeal space.[8] The LMP-1 gene is also a potential marker to differentiate between recurrent NPC and osteoradionecrosis (ORN).[21] The presence of the LMP-1 gene in patients with ORN may indicate local recurrence.[22] In one study of detecting LMP-1 gene in middle ear aspirates, the results reveal no detection of LMP-1 in patients diagnosed with middle ear effusion but without NPC.[23] The detection of LMP-1 in middle ear aspirates may indicate petrous apex invasion.[23] In the study to detect LMP-1 in various head and neck cancers, the results show the presence of LMP-1 gene detected by PCR in the tumor cells is significantly associated only with tumors located in nasopharynx, implying that EBV plays a trifling role in the tumorigenesis of carcinomas arising from other head and neck locations.[24,25] Another study on population screening of NPC, based on a study of 437 adults, detecting EBV genomic LMP-1 genes and EBNA genes by nasopharyngeal swab verifies NPC with a sensitivity of 91.4% and specificity of 98.3%.[26]

Nasopharyngeal swab with LMP-1 and EBNA-1 gene detection is a useful and reliable method to monitor local recurrence in NPC patients. It helps to detect recurrence early and may improve local control and survival rate.[22] Based on a follow-up study of 84 NPC patients after radiation therapy, detection of LMP-1 gene followed by verification with the EBNA-1 gene from nasopharyngeal swabs predicted local recurrence with a sensitivity of 91.7% and specificity of 98.6%.[22] The time frame of the EBV LMP-1 gene to disappear in nasopharyngeal swabs after initiation of primary radiotherapy is proved to be an independently significant prognostic factor predicting local control for patients with nasopharyngeal carcinoma.[27] The patients with late regression had a significantly worse local control than those with intermediate or early regression.[27] Another study on the LMP-1 gene was also applied to the follow-up of NPC after radiation therapy; it showed that the median LMP-1 remission time after the beginning of irradiation was 4.3 weeks.[28] Patients with early LMP-1 disease remission (= 4 weeks after beginning irradiation) and delayed LMP-1 disease remission (>4 weeks) had 3-year local control rates of 93.5% and 76.9%, respectively, in one study.[28] By detecting re-LMP-1 using nasopharyngeal swabs, mucosal recurrence was diagnosed with a sensitivity of 100% and a specificity of 98.4%.[22]

Recently, quantitative analysis of plasma cell-free DNA with RT PCR technique have been applied for early diagnosis, predict treatment outcome and monitoring recurrence of NPC.[29,30,31]

The incidence of NPC increases with a high level of consumption of preserved salted fish.[32] The carcinogenic nitrosamine components in salted fish may be the real etiology.[32] A gradual decline in the incidence of NPC is noted in Taiwan; changes in lifestyle and environment are likely to be the contributory factors.

ANATOMIC BOUNDARIES AND SUBDIVISIONS OF THE REGION

The nasopharynx lies deep and central in the skull. The nasopharynx is the most cephadad portion of the upper aerodigestive tract. It is located beneath the sphenoid sinus and upper clivus, anterior to the lower clivus and the body of the first cervical vertebra, and medial to the medial pterygoid plate. The posterior wall is separated from the basiocciput and clivus by the pharyngobasilar fasciae. The nasopharynx measures approximately 4 cm in transverse diameter and height and 2 cm in its anterior-posterior dimension. It communicates freely with the posterior nasal choanae anteriorly, and with the oropharynx inferiorly. The nasopharynx is surrounded by pharyngobasilar fasciae in its posterior and lateral wall.

The lateral wall of the nasopharynx is formed by the torus tubarius—the bulging cartilage of the medial end of eustachian tube. The opening of the eustachian tube is formed by an incomplete cartilaginous ring that is deficient inferolaterally.

The eustachian tube and accompanying levator palatine muscle travel through a congenital pharyngobasilar fasciae defect over the lateral pharyngeal wall named sinus of Morgagni.

The superior recess above the torus tubarius, just between the roof and the lateral wall, is the fossa of Rosenmüller where NPC is commonly located.

NPC commonly originates from the Rosenmüller fossa and may extend laterally through the sinus of Morgagni to invade the parapharyngeal space. Skull base extension by destruction of the pterygoid base is common, and the tumor may extend superiorly to involve the cavernous sinus or invade laterally to involve the foramen ovale. The pharyngobasilar fasciae surrounding nasopharynx are tough fasciae and can be a strong barrier against tumor. In rare instances, NPC may invade these fasciae to involve the clivus. NPC is notorious for submucosal extension and it is not surprising to see the aggressiveness of tumor spread several centimeters away from the visible tumor.

The mucosa of nasopharynx is composed of ciliated stratified columnar epithelium. Mucous-secreting glands are scattering around the submucosal lamina propria. These glandular structures may give rise to salivary gland type nasopharyngeal carcinomas, such as adenoid cystic carcinoma, or mucoepidermoid carcinoma which are infrequently encountered. The lamina propia of nasopharyngeal mucosa contains abundant lymphoid tissue. The adenoids are residual lymphoid tissue located in the central portion of nasopharyngeal roof, which may be mistaken for superficial NPC.

Deep to the mucosa layer is the pharyngobasilar fascia. The fascia is a tough membrane surrounding the superior, posterior, and lateral wall. It is inserted to the basisphenoid superiorly and medial pterygoid plate laterally. It continues inferiorly as the buccopharyngeal fascia. The eustachian tube pierces through a natural defect of the pharyngobasilar fascia and superior constrictor muscle known as the sinus of Morgagni on the lateral wall of nasopharynx to reach the middle ear space.

Two groups of muscle, the tensor and levator palatini muscles control soft palate and eustachian tube functions. The tensor veli palatini muscle arises from the lateral side of the eustachian tube and the floor of the scaphoid fossa. It does not travel through the sinus of Morgagni, rather its fibers converge to a tendon and curve around the pterygoid hamulus with attachment to the palatine aponeurosis of the soft palate. When the tensor veli palatini contracts, the lateral wall of auditory tube is pulled laterally and the lumen opens. The levator palatini muscle arises from the inferior surface of the petrous temporal bone. It passes through the sinus of Morgagni along with the eustachian tube and inserts into the palatine aponeurosis.

CRITICAL ELEMENTS OF THE HISTORY AND PHYSICAL EXAMINATION

Nasopharyngeal carcinoma affects relatively younger patients, with a median age of 46 years in Taiwanese.[33,34] NPC is a male-predominant disease with a male-to-female ratio of 3:1.[34] NPC is a great masquerader., patients typically exhibit with vague symptoms such as enlarged upper neck nodes, bloody nasal discharges, stuffy ear, diplopia, and headaches. Most patients are already at stage III or IV of the disease at the time of diagnosis.[35] The clinical symptomatology of patients with NPC can be categorized into four main aspects.[36]

1. *Nasal symptoms:* As NPC is located posteriorly in the nasopharyngeal space, and may approach the posterior nasal choanae, unilateral nasal obstruction with occasional blood-tinged nasal discharges is common. There is rarely a severe epistaxis, whereas the patients are more frequently presented with early morning blood stained postnasal discharge.

2. *Aural symptoms:* NPC arises from the fossa of Rosenmüller, and may infiltrate laterally along the eustachian tube to involve the tensor veli palatini muscle and/or levator palatini muscle, or the nerves which innervate these muscles. Thus, it is not surprising to see the auditory tube dysfunction in NPC patients, which may lead to middle ear effusion with possible subsequences of conductive hearing loss and occasionally tinnitus. In endemic area of NPC, such as Taiwan, adults presented with middle ear effusion without obvious upper respiratory tract infection symptoms should alert physicians to the possibility of NPC.

3. *Neck masses:* The most common mode of presentation of NPC is one or more painless unilateral, sometimes bilateral, upper cervical masses, accounting for 60% of the chief complaints of the NPC population. Although the first echelon node of NPC is actually the retropharyngeal node, which is not palpable clinically, the subdigastric and jugulodigastric nodes are commonly presented as the first palpable nodes. The lymphatic metastasis then can be spread along the spinal accessory nerve to the posterior cervical

triangle and supraclavicular fossa or less commonly along the jugular chain to the lower neck. In endemic area of NPC, such as Taiwan, adults presented with painless upper neck mass should undergo a thorough head and neck examination, including nasopharyngoscopy to exclude the possibility of NPC.

4. *Skull base and cranial nerves involved symptoms:* Patients may exhibit intractable headaches when the skull base or dura are involved. Abducent palsy from cranial nerve VI involvement are not uncommon, as NPC may damage the skull base bone and directly involve the cavernous sinus within which cranial nerve VI has a long and tortuous course. Patients may also present with unilateral facial numbness when the foramen ovale and/or foramen rotundum are involved.

Other unusual symptoms may include trismus which is related to pterygoid muscle involvement, velopharyngeal insufficiency due to levator palatini muscle involvement, tinnitus, or sensorineural deafness due to inner ear or cochlear involvement.

Although NPC tends to have a high distant metastatic rate, mainly to bone, liver, and lung, rarely patients initially present with severe bone pain, or other distant metastatic symptoms.

APPROPRIATE DIAGNOSTIC OFFICE-BASED PROCEDURES

Because NPC typically arise from the fossa of Rosenmüller, a relatively obscure space, they are not easily seen directly. Inspection of the nasopharynx requires the use of a mirror or a fiberoptic nasopharyngoscope. There is no doubt that fiberoptic nasopharyngoscopy, either flexible or rigid, are important tools in office examination. Rigid nasopharyngoscopy is invaluable to guide a biopsy in patients suspicious for NPC.[16] These scopes can also be adapted for office photography, documentation, and follow-ups.

Middle ear effusion is frequently encountered in patients with NPC.[23] Middle ear effusions can be easily detected under otoscopy. Subsequent pure tone audiometry and tympanogram are mandatory to confirm the diagnosis.

In cases with enlarged painless upper cervical nodes without visible evidence of mucosal tumor, serologic test of EBV titers, especially anti-EBV VCA IgA, and DNase may help to detect NPC. Fine-needle aspiration cytology or cutting biopsy of neck masses under ultrasound guide also is crucial to delineate the nature of some unknown primaries.

RECOMMENDED IMAGING STUDIES

Head and neck, including skull base, imaging with high-resolution computed tomography (CT) and magnetic resonance imaging (MRI) has become more accurate and useful tools for patients with NPC. CT and MRI are widely used in diagnosis, clinical staging, treatment planning, and follow-up of NPC. These imaging modalities can provide details which cannot be afforded by mirror inspection and/or fiberoptic nasopharyngoscopy. The skull base erosion can be greatly appreciated with CT, whereas MRI appears to be better to delineate soft tissue or perineural invasion. CT and MRI should be complementary rather than competitive (Figs 11-1, 11-2, 11-3, and 11-4). When comparing MRI with CT, 20% to 30% of T2 and T3 NPC lesions are upstaged.[37] MRI of head and neck including skull base should be the imaging modality of choice for NPC.

Positron emission tomography (PET) is overwhelmingly used nowadays to detect distant metastasis in NPC patients. However, it is not justified to use PET in routine staging purposes especially in low-risk groups of distant metastasis group. In high-risk groups of distant metastasis such as T4 or N3, however; pretreatment workup may include chest x-ray, liver ultrasound, bone scan, or PET to detect possible distant metastasis.

As for monitor of post-treatment recurrence, MRI is better than CT.[38] However, locally recurrent NPC can exhibit a variety of signal intensities and can mimic skull base osteoradionecrosis, for which even PET has a low sensitivity and specificity.[39,40] Regularly repeated MRI examinations are perhaps the best option to follow postirradiated patients. The role of PET in the follow-up of past treatment patients need to be further studied.

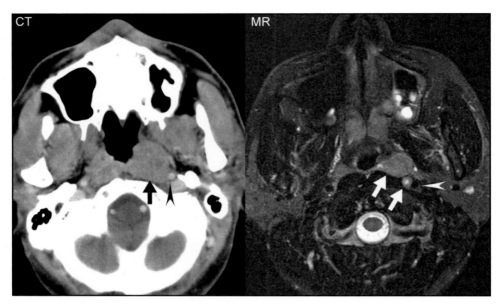

Fig 11–1. The 45-year-old male was a victim of nasopharyngeal carcinoma. CT shows a tumor invading left lateral pharyngeal recess but poor distinction between the tumor, left longus colii muscle (*black arrow*), and internal carotid artery (*black arrowhead*). However, axial T2-weighted MR image clearly depicts the relationships of tumor mass (*medial white arrow*), longus colii muscle, ipsilateral retropharyngeal node (*lateral white arrow*), and internal carotid artery (*white arrowhead*). Eventually, the patient was staged as T1 rather than T3.

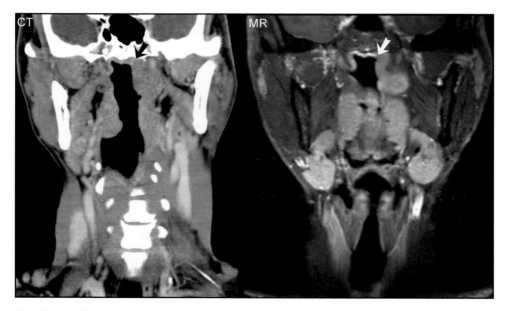

Fig 11–2. The 45-year-old male is a victim of nasopharyngeal carcinoma with T1 stage. CT cannot demonstrate the extent of tumor (*black arrow*) but coronal MR with contrast enhancement well differentiates normal mucosa from the tumor (*white arrow*).

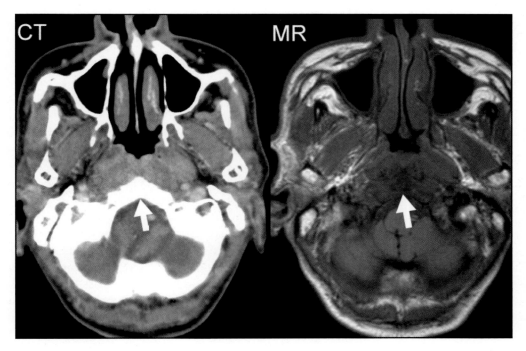

Fig 11–3. This 59-year-old male was a patient of advanced nasopharyngeal carcinoma with skull base invasion. Although CT shows intact outline of clivus (*white arrow*), axial T1-weighted MR image more clearly demonstrates tumor infiltration with loss of normal high-signal marrow, so-called marrow replacement.

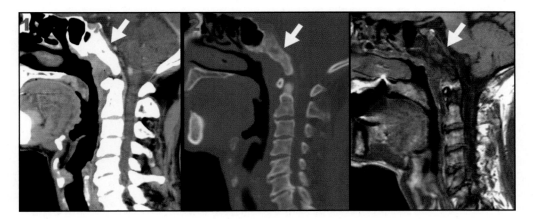

Fig 11–4. The 59-year-old male suffered from advanced nasopharyngeal carcinoma with skull base invasion and intracranial extension (staging as T4). Enhanced reconstructed CT (1) fails to demonstrate the extent of clivus (*white arrow*) invasion. CT with bone window (2) shows more central osteolytic change of clivus but remaining uncertain extent. Sagittal T1-weighted MR image (3) displays extensive tumor infiltration, total marrow replacement of clivus and retroclival tumor growth. The information is crucial for planning of radiotherapy.

AJCC STAGING OF NPC

The 2002 AJCC staging of NPC is presented in Tables 11-1 and 11-2.[41]

Table 11–1. American Joint Committee on Cancer TNM Classification of Neopharygeal Cancer*

Primary tumor, T	
TX	Primary tumor cannot be classified.
T0	No evidence of primary tumor
Tis	Carcinoma in situ
T1	Tumor confined to nasopharynx
T2	Tumor extends to soft tissues of oropharynx or sinuses
T2a	without a parapharyngeal extension
T2b	with a pharyngeal extension
T3	Tumor invades bony structure and/or paranasal sinuses
T4	Tumor with intracranial extension and/or involvement of cranial nerves, infratemporal fossa, hypopharynx, orbit, or masticator space
Regional lymph nodes, N	
NX	Regional lymph nodes cannot be assessed
N0	No regional lymph node metastasis
N1	Unilateral metastasis in lymph node(s), 6 cm or less in greatest dimension, above the supraclavicular fossa
N2	Bilateral metastasis in lymph node(s), 6 cm or less in greatest dimension above the supraclavicular fossa
N3	Metastasis in a lymph node(s)
N3a	Greater than 6 cm in dimension
N3b	Extension to the supraclavicular fossa
Distant metastasis, M	
MX	Distant metastasis cannot be assessed
M0	No distant metastasis
M1	Distant metastasis

*Reprinted with permission from *AJCC Cancer Staging Manual.* 6th ed. Published by Springer-Verlag, Inc., New York, NY.

EXAMPLES OF REPRESENTATIVE HISTOPATHOLOGY

The classification of nasopharyngeal carcinoma that enjoys widespread usage is the World Health Organization (WHO) terminology. The first edition of the classification of nasopharyngeal carcinoma was published in 1978.[3] Three subtypes of nasopharyngeal carcinoma were acknowledged as squamous cell carcinoma (WHO type 1; Fig 11-5), nonkeratinizing carcinoma (WHO type 2; Fig 11-6), and undifferentiated carcinoma (WHO type 3; Fig 11-7). The second edition followed in 1991.[42] The nomenclature was simplified to squamous cell carcinoma and nonkeratinizing carcinoma. Nonkeratinizing carcinoma was further classified into differentiated and undifferentiated types. Lymphoepithelioma-like carcinoma was a variant of undifferentiated carcinoma. The numerical indication of WHO types 1, 2, and 3 is no longer used. The histopathologic features of nonkeratinizing carcinoma comprise sheets of tumor cells intermingled with lymphocytes and

Table 11–2. American Joint Committee on Cancer Stage Groupings for Nasopharyngeal Cancer*

Stage 0	Stage III
Tis (in situ), N0, M0	T1, N2, M0
	T2a, N2, M0
Stage I	T2b, N2, M0
T1, N0, M0	T3, N0, M0
	T3, N1, M0
Stage IIB	T3, N2, M0
T2a, N0, M0	
	Stage IVA
Stage IIB	T4, N0, M0
T1, N1, M0	T4, N1, M0
T2, N1, M0	T4, N2, M0
T2a, N1, M0	
T2b, N0, M0	**Stage IVB**
T2b, N1, M0	Any T, N3, M0
	Stage IVC
	Any T, any N, M1

*Reprinted with permission from *AJCC Cancer Staging Manual.* 6th ed. Published by Springer-Verlag, Inc., New York, NY.

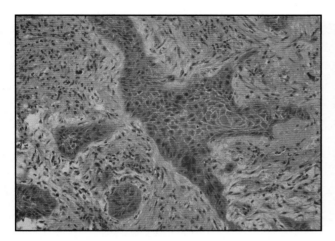

Fig 11–5. Keratinizing squamous cell carcinoma. Irregular invasive nests of tumor cells with squamous differentiation.

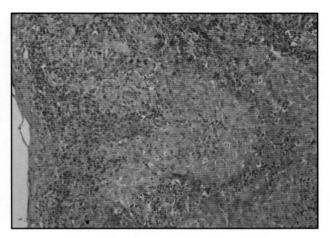

Fig 11–7. Nonkeratinizing carcinoma, differentiated subtype.

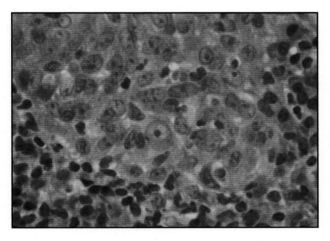

Fig 11–6. Nonkeratinizing carcinoma, undifferentiated subtype. Sheets of large tumor cells with prominent nucleoi with adjacent lymphocytes.

plasma cells. The undifferentiated subtype shows syncytial patterns of large tumor cells with vesicular nuclei and prominent nucleoli. The current WHO classification was published in 2005. [43] Three subtypes were recognized as nonkeratinizing carcinoma, keratinizing squamous cell carcinoma, and basaloid squamous cell carcinoma. The terminology was the same as the 1991 edition, with the addition of basaloid squamous cell carcinoma.

IDENTIFICATION OF CRITICAL DECISION POINTS

Preliminary results suggested that chemotherapy concurrent with radiotherapy using an accelerated fractionation scheme could significantly improve locoregional tumor control when compared with conventional RT alone in NPC patients with 1997 AJCC stage T3-4N0-1M0 diseases.[44] Another similar randomized controlled trial demonstrated that concurrent chemotherapy for regionally advanced NPC improved tumor control compared with the radiotherapy alone arm in the patients with advanced nodal disease which was classified as AJCC stage T1-4N2-3M0.[45] Both trials employed the same chemotherapy regimens as that used in the Intergroup Study 0099, in which cisplatin (CDDP) and 5-fluorouracil (5-FU) were administered concurrently with radiotherapy.

ANALYSIS OF VARIOUS TREATMENT OPTIONS

Efficacy

Potential complications

Cost-benefit analysis (if possible)

Current available therapies for primary NPC are radiotherapy and chemotherapy, or a combination of both. The mainstay treatment for NPC is radiotherapy, as most NPCs are undifferentiated or nonkeratinizing carcinomas, both radiosensitive. NPC is highly radiosensitive and patients presenting with early disease have a high cure rate after radiotherapy. Concurrent cisplatin-radiotherapy with or without adjuvant chemotherapy has been demonstrated to significantly improve survival and is currently the standard treatment strategy for patients with locoregionally advanced disease.[44] The 5-year actuarial survival rate is greater than 76%, whereas the local control rate is over 81%. [46] The specific radiation dose required for controlling NPC can be as high as 66 Gy for certain patients.[47] Even for patients who exhibit no palpable neck disease, full-dose irradiation is still recommended for the effective management of NPC.[48] Imaging is required for the correct staging and treatment planning of NPC.

In conventional radiotherapy, NPC patients received a dosage of 46 Gy in 23 separate fractions by means of ^{60}Co or 6-MV photon therapy to the nasopharynx, the base of the skull, and the upper neck lymphatic through two parallel opposing ports.[49] Meanwhile, the whole lower whole neck was irradiated by an anterior portal. The nasopharynx was then boosted with 6- to 10-MV photon irradiation to a level of additional 24 Gy in a series of 12 fractions. For the patients with initial node-positive necks, the radiation regimens included a neck boost with electron beams to a total of 24 Gy in 12 fractions. Finally, the nasopharynx was treated with intracavitary brachytherapy, which could confer treatment benefits for the patients with T1 to T2 lesions confined to the nasopharynx.[50] At the time of completion of radiotherapy, the nasopharynx per se should have received a total dose of 76 Gy. Instead of intracavitary brachytherapy, the application of stereotactic radiosurgery in NPC patients was used as an alternative booster treatment as part of the initial therapy for persistent or recurrent diseases.[51] The characteristics of stereotactic radiosurgery substantially are to deliver a high and homogeneous dose distribution to the tumor mass, while limiting the unnecessary dose delivered to the surrounding normal tissues.[52] The main effects brought about by the radiosurgery boost not only increase the external RT dose, but also possibly decrease the complication rate.

In recent years, based on the advances in medical imaging and the use of modern computerized treatment planning systems, RT technique has improved greatly. Three-dimensional conformal RT (3DCRT) technique spares normal tissues from a heavy radiation dose, thereby decreasing complications.[53] The most recent advanced radiation treatment technique is IMRT.[54] By using dynamic control of the collimator in a linear accelerator, IMRT delivers a more conformal radiation dose to the target area. The pituitary gland, mandible, spinal cord, brainstem, and parotid gland are spared by IMRT technique.[54] The ability to spare the parotid gland is a promising improvement for treatment of patients with early stage disease. IMRT can offer excellent tumor control and fewer complications. During the past several years, the conventional radiotherapy has been largely replaced by the IMRT in the treatment of NPC.[54] One of the main goals of IMRT is to optimally spare the critical organs, thus reducing the adverse effects caused by radiation. By taking advantage of IMRT which can discriminate normal tissue from the tumor, dose escalation focusing on the tumor might be achieved while decreasing the risk of normal tissue toxicity. Previous studies on the management in NPC patients have shown that better local control is yielded by a higher radiation dose.[55]

Chemotherapy

Concurrent chemotherapy is aimed at enhancing the radiation effect by administrating chemotherapy with radiation-sensitizing drugs such as 5-fluorouracil and cisplatin. The actual benefits associated with the administration of adjuvant chemotherapy remained quite controversial until several years ago when concomitant chemotherapy proved to be effective in systemic control of NPC and prolonging patient survival.[56-58] Computed tomography (CT) and/or magnetic resonance imaging (MRI) are recommended for the diagnostic process and evaluation of tumor extent. MRI appears to be better than CT imaging for visualizing soft tissue invasion outside the nasopharynx, demonstrating involved retropharyngeal nodes, and identifying skull base involvement. Because asymptomatic distant metastases are not uncommon, a pretherapeutic workup including chest x-ray, liver ultrasound, and bone scans are recommended for all patients with nodal disease.

Recurrent NPC

Nasopharyngeal carcinoma, compared with other epithelial cancers of the upper aerodigestive tract, has a high incidence of distant metastasis. However, locoregional failure is still the main cause of death. Although overall survival in NPC patients ranges from 50 to 80% after radiation, local failure unfortunately occurs in 10% to 30% of patients.[59] The majority of local recurrence occurs within the first 5 years after treatment. Patients with NPC local recurrence without salvage treatment have dismal survival. On average, the local salvage rate might range from 18 to 66% if aggressive treatment is given.[59] A variety of therapeutic options, including surgical resection,[60] intracavitary brachytherapy,[61] IMRT, interstitial implantation,[62] and radiosurgery,[63] have been used to manage local recurrence in the nasopharyngeal region.

Although the incidence of local persistent or recurrent disease has decreased following the introduction of concurrent chemoradiotherapy,[64] it still results in a dismal prognosis. Reirradiation of the primary recurrence of NPC has been reported,[65-67] but it was accompanied by significant morbidity caused by complications such as severe xerostomia, trismus, deafness, and neurologic sequelae.[68,69] Other pitfalls include the complications of ORN following reirradiation.[70] The patient may experience foul odor, severe pain, and massive bleeding. Furthermore, it cannot be assumed that NPC cells surviving the first course of radiotherapy will respond to further radiotherapy. Salvage nasopharyngectomy has been the mainstay of treatment after radiation failure.[60,71] Various surgical approaches to the nasopharynx have been developed, such as transpalatal,[72,73] transmaxillary,[74] midline mandibulotomy,[73] facial translocation,[60,71] and infratemporal fossa approaches.[75] Using the maxillary swing approach for the surgical resection of local recurrence, Wei et al reported

actuarial rates of tumor control and overall survival at 3.5 years of 42 and 36%, respectively.[76] Recently, King et al reported their 12-year experience in the surgical treatment of recurrent NPC in 31 patients. They concluded that surgical resection with postoperative RT was a better salvage treatment than reirradiation alone for selected cases of recurrent NPC.[77] Hao reported 18 consecutive patients with primary recurrence of NPC after radiation underwent nasopharyngectomy via a facial translocation approach.[60] The tumor stages included rT1 (8 patients), rT2b (1 patient), rT3 (5 patients), and rT4 (4 patients). Five patients with skull base invasion required a combined neurosurgical approach to treatment. The actuarial 3-year survival was 57%, whereas the local control was 78%.[60] Four of 5 patients who had skull base invasion achieved local control. No surgical mortality occurred and the morbidity rate was 22%. The advances in skull base surgery make possible the effective control of primary recurrence of NPC possible, with acceptable mortality and morbidity.[60] A subsequent report based on 38 patients of recurrent NPC who underwent nasopharyngectomy, showed the actuarial 3-year survival and local control rate was 60% and 72.8%, respectively.[71] Ten (83.3%) of twelve patients with intracranial and skull base invasion achieved local control in the report. There was no surgical mortality, and the morbidity rate was only 13.2%. The results of that study concluded a better outcome after salvage surgery as compared to most published literatures of reirradiation for recurrent NPC.[71] With the adequate exposure provided by the transfacial approach, an integrated concept of skull base surgery, and the collaboration of different specialties such as head and neck surgeons, plastic reconstructive surgeons, and neurosurgeons, surgeons now can extend surgical indications of salvage surgery and resect many advanced lesions with acceptable mortality and morbidity.[60,71]

In the facial translocation approach, the facial osteotomy can be localized based on the location of the tumor. If the tumor is confined to the nasopharynx or has paranasal extension, a naso-orbitomaxillary osteotomy will suffice, and the infraorbital neurovascular bundle can be preserved.[78] However, when the tumor has invaded the parapharyngeal space, a larger facial osteotomy, optionally including part of the zygoma, is created to remove the tumor.[78] If the tumor has invaded the pterygoid plate base, a combined preauricular infratemporal subtemporal approach is used.[79] This approach offers superior and lateral approaches to the nasopharyngeal and parapharyngeal space. After temporal craniotomy, the temporal lobe is retracted to expose the temporal base. The foramen ovale can be decompressed, and the transverse portion of the petrous internal carotid artery lying behind the foramen ovale is located and protected. The tumor can then be removed from the superior, lateral, and anterior directions.[78]

Anterior craniofacial resection is carried out if recurrent NPC involves the cribriform plate or the planum sphenoidale.[60,71]

COMPLICATIONS OF THERAPY

Irradiation alone or in combination with chemotherapy is the major treatment strategy for NPC. It is inevitable that tumor control is often compromised by the tolerance of normal tissue to irradiation, because dose delivery is usually restrained by critical organs such as eyeballs, brain, brainstem, or spinal cord. RT-related complications includes xerostomia,[79] hearing impairment,[80] endocrine dysfunction,[81] temporal lobe radionecrosis,[82] cranial nerve palsy,[83] radiation myelopathy[84] and osteoradionecrosis.[85,86]

The incidence of all potential complications after conventional irradiation has ranged from 6% in temporal lobe necrosis to 91% in xerostomia.[87] IMRT has been recommended to reduce late adverse effects such as xerostomia.[54]

SUMMARY

NPC is one of the most common cancers among Chinese. It is an epithelial tumor with endemic distribution among well-defined ethnic groups and geographic regions. Its close relationship with EBV makes the effective screening, molecular diagnosis, and monitoring possible. The advent of modern technology, including CT, MRI, and PET and improvement in therapeutic approach, including 3D conformal radiation therapy, IMRT, and chemotherapy have improved the local-regional control as well as survival rate, but at the same time, decreased the complication rate. Early detection of relapse disease and prompt management by salvage skull base surgery have rendered recurrent NPC a curable disease. Future studies can be focused on large-scale population screening with EBV-derived genes or proteins and anti-viral gene therapy for target populations.

REFERENCES

1. Cohen JI. Epstein-Barr virus infection. *New Engl J Med.* 2000;343:481–492.
2. William Wei. Nasopharyngeal carcinoma. *Lancet.* 2005;365:2041–2054.
3. Shanmugatatnam K. Sobin LH. *Histological Typing of Upper Respiratory Tract Tumours.* Geneva, Switzerland: World Health Organization; 1978.
4. Buell P. The effect of migration on the risk of nasopharyngeal cancer among *Chinese. Cancer Res.* 1974;34:1189–1191.
5. Rickinson A, Kieff E. Epstein-Barr virus. In: Field B, Knipe B, Howley P, eds. *Field Virology.* 3rd ed. Philadelphia, Pa: Lippincott Raven Publishers; 1996: 2397–2446.
6. Lin HJ, Lin JC. Pathogenesis and therapy of Epstein-Barr virus-associated nasopharyngeal carcinoma. *J Chinese Oncol Soc.* 2004;20(1):1–17.
7. Lin SY, Tsang NM, Kao SC, et al. Presence of Epstein-Barr virus latent membrane protein 1 gene in the nasopharyngeal swabs from patients with nasopharyngeal carcinoma. *Head Neck.* 2001;23:194–200.
8. Hao SP, Tsang NM, Chang KP. Screening nasopharyngeal carcinoma by detection of LMP-1 gene from nasopharyngeal swab. *Cancer.* 2003;97: 1909–1913.
9. Nonoyama M, Huang EH, Pagano JS, Klein, Singh S. DNA of Epstein-Barr virus detected in tissue of Burkitt's lymphoma and nasopharyngeal carcinoma. *Proc Natl Acad Sci USA.* 1973;70:3265–3268.
10. Klein G, Giovanella BC, Lindahl T, Fialkow PJ, Singh S, Stehlin JS. Direct evidence for the presence of Epstein-Barr virus DNA and nuclear antigen in the malignant epithelial cells from patients with poorly differentiated carcinoma of the nasopharynx. *Proc Natl Acad Sci USA.* 1974;71:4797–4741.
11. Zong YS, Sham JST, Ng MHI. Immunoglobulin a against viral capsid antigen of Esstein-Barr virus and indirect mirror examination of the nasophar-

ynx in the detection of asymptomatic nasopharyngeal carcinoma. *Cancer.* 1992;69:3–7.

12. Liu MT, Lin LS, Yu Y. Use of recombinant Epsteini Barr virus early antigen for detection of antibody in patients with nasopharyngeal carcinoma. *Chin Med J Taipei.* 1996;57:7–15.

13. Deng H, Zeng Y, Lei Y, et al. Serological survey of nasopharyngeal carcinoma in 21 cities of south China. *Chin Med J.* 1995;108:300–303.

14. Liu MY, Chang YL, Ma J. Evaluation of multiple antibodies to Epstein-Barr virus as markers for detecting patints with nasopharyngeal carcinoma. *J Med Virol.* 1997;52:262–269.

15. Sheen TS, Ko JY, Chang YS, Huang YT, Chang Y. Nasopharyngeal swab and PCR for the screening of nasopharyngeal carcinoma in the endemic area: a good supplement to the serologic screening. *Head Neck.* 1998;20:732–738.

16. Wei WI, Sham JS, Zong YS, Choy D, Ng MH. The efficacy of fiberoptic endoscopic examination and biopsy in the detection of early nasopharyngeal carcinoma. *Cancer.* 1991;(12):3127–3130.

17. Chien YC, Chen JY, Liu MY, et al. Serologic markers of Epstein-Barr virus infection and nasopharyngeal carcinoma in Taiwanese men. *N Engl J Med.* 2001; 345:1877–1882.

18. Jeng KC, Hsu CY, Liu MT, et al. Prevalence of Taiwan variant of Epstein-Barr virus in throat washings from patients with head and neck tumors in Taiwan. *J Clin Microbiol.* 1994;32:28–31.

19. Li Sn, Chang YS, Liu ST. Effect of a 10-amino acid deletion on the oncogenic activity of latent membrane protein 1 of Epstein-Barr virus. *Oncogene.* 1996;12:2129–2135.

20. Baichwal VR, Sugden B. The multiple membrane-spanning segments of the BNLF-1 oncogene from Epstein-Barr virus are required for transformation. *Oncogene.*1989;4:67–74.

21. Hao SP, Tsang NM, Chang KP. Differentiation of recurrent nasopharyngeal carcinoma and skull base osteoradionecrosis by Epstein-Barr virus-derived latent membrane protein-1 gene. *Laryngoscope.* 2001;111:650–652.

22. Hao SP, Tsang NM, Chang KP. Monitoring tumor recurrence with nasopharyngeal swab and LMP-1 and EBNA-1 gene detection in treated patients of NPC. *Laryngoscope.* 2004;114(11):2027–2030.

23. Hao SP, Tsang NM, Chen YL, Chang KP, Su JL. Detection of LMP-1 gene in middle ear effusion of NPC. *Oral Oncol.* 2003;39(3):296–300.

24. Pai PC, Tsang CK, Tsang NM, et al. Prevalence of LMP-1 gene in tonsils and non-neoplastic naso-

pharynxes by nest-polymerase chain reaction in Taiwan. *Head Neck.* 2004;26:619–624.

25. Tsang NM, Chang KP, Lin SY, et al. Detection of Epstein-Barr virus-derived latent membrane protein-1 gene in various head and neck cancers: is it specific for nasopharyngeal carcinoma? *Laryngoscope.* 2003;113:1050–1054.

26. Hao SP, Tsang NM, Chang KP, Ueng SH. Molecular diagnosis of nasopharyngeal carcinoma-detecting LMP-1 and EBNA by nasopharyngeal swab. *Otolaryngol Head Neck Surg.* 2004;131(5):651–654.

27. Tsang NM, Chuang CC, Tseng CK, et al. Presence of the latent membrane protein 1 gene in nasopharyngeal swabs from patients with mucosal recurrent nasopharyngeal carcinoma. *Cancer.* 2003; 198:2385–2392.

28. Lin SY, Chang KP, Hsieh MS, et al. The time frame of Epstein-Barr virus latent membrane protein-1 gene to disappear in nasopharyngeal swabs after initiation of primary radiotherapy is an independently significant prognostic factor predicting local control for patients with nasopharyngeal carcinoma. *Int J Radiat Oncol Biol Phys.* 2005;63(5):1339–1346.

29. Shao JY, Li YH, Gao HY, et al. Comparison of plasma Epstein-Barr virus (EBV) DNA levels and serum EBV immunoglobulin A/virus capsid antigen antibody titers in patients with nasopharyngeal carcinoma. *Cancer.* 2004;100(6):1162–1170.

30. Lin JC, Wang WY, Chen KY, et al. Quantification of plasma Epstein-Barr virus DNA in patients with advanced nasopharyngeal carcinoma. *N Engl J Med.* 2004;350(24):2461–2470.

31. Wei WI, Yuen AP, Ng RW, et al. Quantitative analysis of plasma cell-free Epstein-Barr virus DNA in nasopharyngeal carcinoma after salvage nasopharyngectomy: a prospective study. *Head Neck.* 2004;26(10):878–883.

32. Yu MC, Ho JHC, Lai SH, et al. Cantonese-style salted fish as a cause of nasopharyngeal carcinoma: Report of a case-control study in Hong Kong. *Cancer Res* .1986;46:956–961.

33. Department of Health. Leading causes of death from cancer in Taiwan area from 1991 to 1996. Health and vital statistics of Republic of China. Taipei: *Executive Yuan, ROC.* 1997;72–77.

34. Chen YP, Tsang NM, Tsang CK, et al. Nasopharyngeal Cancer Registry in sixteen years. *Therapeut Radiol Oncol.* 1996;3:233–237.

35. Huang SC, Lui LT, Lynn TC. Nasopharyngeal carcinoma, III. a review of 1206 patients treated with combined modalities. *Int J Radiat Oncol Biol Phys.* 1985;11:1789–1793.

36. Lee AW, Poon YF, Foo W, et al. Retrospective analysis of 5037 patients with nasopharyngeal carcinoma treated during 1976–1985: overall survival and patterns of failure. *Int J Radiat Oncol Biol Phys.* 1992;23:261–270.

37. Chong VF, Mukherji SK, Ng SH, et al. Nasopharyngeal carcinoma: review of how imaging affects staging. *J Comput Assist Tomogr.* 1999;23:984–993.

38. Ng SH, Chang JT, Ko SF, et al. MRI in recurrent nasopharyngeal carcinoma. *Neuroradiology.* 1999; 41:855–862.

39. Kao CH, Shiau YC, Shen YY, et al. Detection of recurrent or persistent nasopharyngeal carcinomas after radiotherapy with technetium-99m methoxy-isobutylisonitrile single photon emission computed tomography and computed tomography:comparison with 18-fluoro-2-deoxyglucose positron emission tomography. *Cancer.* 2002;94:1981–1986.

40. Yen RF, Hung RL, Pan MH, et al. 18-fluoro-2-deoxyglucose positron emission tomography in detecting residual/recurrent nasonance imaging. *Cancer.* 2003;98:283–287.

41. AJCC *Cancer Staging Manual.* 6th ed. New York, NY: Springer-Verlag, Inc; 2002.

42. Shanmugatatnam K. *Histological Typing of Tumours of the Upper Respiratory Tract and Ear.* 2nd ed. Berlin, Germany: Springer-Verlag; 1991.

43. Barnes L, Everson JW, Reichart P. Sidransky D, eds. *World Health Organization Classification of tumours: Pathology and Genetics of Head and Neck Tumours.* Lyon, France: IARC Press; 2005

44. Lee AW, Tung SY, Chan AT, et al. Preliminary results of a randomized study (NPC-9902 Trial) on therapeutic gain by concurrent chemotherapy and/or accelerated fractionation for locally advanced nasopharyngeal carcinoma. *Int J Radiat Oncol Biol Phys.* 2006;66(1):142–151.

45. Lee AW, Lau WH, Tung SY, et al. Preliminary results of a randomized study on therapeutic gain by concurrent chemotherapy for regionally-advanced nasopharyngeal carcinoma: NPC-9901 Trial by the Hong Kong Nasopharyngeal Cancer Study Group. *J Clin Oncol.* 2005;23(28):6966–6975.

46. Al-Sarraf M, LeBlanc M, Giri PG, et al. Chemoradiotherapy versus radiotherapy in patients with advanced nasopharyngeal cancer: phase III randomized intergroup study 0099. *J Clin Oncol.* 1998;16(4):1310–1317.

47. Yi JL, Gao L, Huang XD, et al. Nasopharyngeal carcinoma treated by radical radiotherapy alone: ten-year experience of a single institution. *Int J Radiat Oncol Biol Phys.* 2006;65(1):161–168.

48. Teo PM, Leung SF, Tung SY, et al. Dose-response relationship of nasopharyngeal carcinoma above conventional tumoricidal level: a study by the Hong Kong nasopharyngeal carcinoma study group (HKNPCSG). *Radiother Oncol.* 2006;79(1):27–33.

49. Chua DT, Ma J, Sham JS, et al. Improvement of survival after addition of induction chemotherapy to radiotherapy in patients with early-stage nasopharyngeal carcinoma: subgroup analysis of two phase III trials. *Int J Radiat Oncol Biol Phys.* 2006;65(5):1300–1306.

50. Leung WM, Tsang NM, Chang FT, Lo CJ. Lhermitte's sign among nasopharyngeal cancer patients after radiotherapy. *Head Neck.* 2005;27(3):187–194.

51. Lu JJ, Shakespeare TP, Tan LK, Goh BC, Cooper JS. Adjuvant fractionated high-dose-rate intracavitary brachytherapy after external beam radiotherapy in T1 and T2 nasopharyngeal carcinoma. *Head Neck.* 2004;26(5):389–395.

52. Low JS, Chua ET, Gao F, Wee JT. Stereotactic radiosurgery plus intracavitary irradiation in the salvage of nasopharyngeal carcinoma. *Head Neck.* 2006; 28(4):321–329.

53. Teo PM, Ma BB, Chan AT. Radiotherapy for nasopharyngeal carcinoma—transition from two-dimensional to three-dimensional methods. *Radiother Oncol.* 2004;73(2):163–172.

54. Kam MK, Teo PM, Chau RM, et al. Treatment of nasopharyngeal carcinoma with intensity-modulated radiotherapy: the Hong Kong experience. *Int J Radiat Oncol Biol Phys.* 2004;60(5):1440–1450.

55. Kwong DL, Sham JS, Leung LH, et al. Preliminary results of radiation dose escalation for locally advanced nasopharyngeal carcinoma. *Int J Radiat Oncol Biol Phys.* 2006;64(2):374–381.

56. Chan AT, Teo PM, Ngan RK, et al. Concurrent chemotherapy-radiotherapy compared with radiotherapy alone in locoregionally advanced nasopharyngeal carcinoma: progression-free survival analysis of a phase III randomized trial. *J Clin Oncol.* 2002;20(8):2038–2044.

57. Chua DT, Sham JS, Au GK, Choy D. Concomitant chemoirradiation for stage III–IV nasopharyngeal carcinoma in Chinese patients: results of a matched cohort analysis. *Int J Radiat Oncol Biol Phys.* 2002;53(2):334–343.

58. Lin JC, Jan JS, Hsu CY, et al. Phase III study of concurrent chemoradiotherapy versus radiotherapy alone for advanced nasopharyngeal carcinoma: positive effect on overall and progression-free survival. *J Clin Oncol.* 2003;21(4):631–637.

59. Yu KH, Leung SF, Tung SY, et al. Survival outcome of patients with nasopharyngeal carcinoma with first local failure: a study by the Hong Kong Nasopharyngeal Carcinoma Study Group. *Head Neck.* 2005;27(5):397–405.

60. Hao SP, Tsang NM, Chang CN: Salvage surgery for recurrent nasopharyngeal carcinoma. *Arch Otolaryngol Head Neck Surg.* 2002;128:63–67.

61. Leung TW, Tung SY, Sze WK, et al. Salvage radiation therapy for locally recurrent nasopharyngeal carcinoma. *Int J Radiat Oncol Biol Phys.* 2000;48(5): 1331–1338.

62. Law SC, Lam WK, Ng MF, et al. Re-irradiation of nasopharyngeal carcinoma with intracavitary mold brachytherapy: an effective means of local salvage. *Int J Radiat Oncol Biol Phys.* 2002;54(4): 1095–1113.

63. Pai PC, Chuang CC, Wei KC, et al. Stereotactic radiosurgery for locally recurrent nasopharyngeal carcinoma. *Head Neck.* 2002;24(8):748–753.

64. Cheng SH, Liu TW, Jian JJ, et al. Concomitant chemotherapy and radiotherapy for locally advanced nasopharyngeal carcinoma. *Cancer J Sci Am.* 1997;3:100–106.

65. Wang CC. Re-irradiation of recurrent nasopharyngeal carcinoma: treatment techniques and results. *Int J Radiat Oncol Biol Phys.* 1987;13:953–956.

66. Lee AW, Foo W, Law SC, et al. Reirradiation for recurrent nasopharyngeal carcinoma: factors affecting the therapeutic ration and ways for improvement. *Int J Radiat Oncol Biol Phys.* 1997;28:43–52.

67. Teo PM, Kwan WH, Chan AT, et al. How successful is high-dose (= 60 Gy) reirradiation using mainly external beams in salvaging local failures of nasopharyngeal carcinoma? *Int J Radiat Oncol Biol Phys.* 1998;40:897–913.

68. Chua DT, Sham JS, Kwong DL, et al. Locally recurrent nasopharyngeal carcinoma: treatment results for patients with computed tomography assessment. *Int J Radiat Oncol Biol Phys.* 1998;41: 379–386.

69. Lam KSL, Ho JHC, Lee AWM, et al. Symptomatic hypothalamic pituitary dysfunction in nasopharyngeal carcinoma patients following radiation therapy: a retrospective study. *Int J Radiat Oncol Biol Phys.* 1987;13:1343–1350.

70. Lee AWM, Ng SH, Ho JHC, et al. Clinical diagnosis of late temporal lobe necrosis following radiation therapy for nasopharyngeal carcinoma. *Cancer.* 1988;61:1535–1542.

71. Chang KP, Hao SP, Tsang NM, Wong SH. Salvage surgery for locally recurrent nasopharyngeal carcinoma—a 10-year experience. *Otolaryngol Head Neck Surg.* 2004;131(4):497–502.

72. Fee WE, Gilmer PA, Goffinet DR. Surgical management of recurrent nasopharyngeal carcinoma after radiation failure at the primary site. *Laryngoscope.* 1998;98:1220–1226.

73. Hsu MM, Ko JY, Sheen TS, et al. Salvage surgery for recurrent nasopharyngeal carcinoma. *Arch Otolaryngol Head Neck Surg.* 1997;123:305–309.

74. Wei WI, Lam KH, Sham JST. New approach to the nasopharynx:the maxillary swing approach. *Head Neck.* 1991;13:200–207.

75. Fisch U. The infratemporal fossa approach for nasopharyngeal tumors. *Laryngoscope.* 1983;93:36–44.

76. Wei WI, Ho CM, Yuen PW, et al. Maxillary swing approach for resection of tumors in and around the nasopharynx. *Arch Otolaryngol Head Neck Surg.* 1995;121:638–642.

77. King WW, Ku PK, Mok Co, Teo PM. Nasopharyngectomy in the treatment of recurrent nasopharyngeal carcinoma: a twelve-year experience. *Head Neck.* 2000;22(3):215–222.

78. Hao SP, Pan WL, Chang CN, Hsu YH. The use of the facial translocation technique in the management of tumors of the paranasal sinuses and skull base. *Otolaryngol Head Neck Surg.* 2003;128(4): 571–575.

79. Jen YM, Shih R, Lin YS, et al. Parotid gland-sparing 3-dimensional conformal radiotherapy results in less severe dry mouth in nasopharyngeal cancer patients: a dosimetric and clinical comparison with conventional radiotherapy. *Radiother Oncol.* 2005;75(2):204–209.

80. Low WK, Toh ST, Wee J, Fook-Chong SM, Wang DY. Sensorineural hearing loss after radiotherapy and chemoradiotherapy: a single, blinded, randomized study. *J Clin Oncol.* 2006;24(12):1904–1909.

81. Lam KS, Ho JH, Lee AW, et al. Symptomatic hypothalamic-pituitary dysfunction in nasopharyngeal carcinoma patients following radiation therapy: a retrospective study. *Int J Radiat Oncol Biol Phys.* 1987;13(9):1343–1350.

82. Tsui EY, Chan JH, Ramsey RG, et al. Late temporal lobe necrosis in patients with nasopharyngeal carcinoma: evaluation with combined multi-section diffusion weighted and perfusion weighted MR imaging. *Eur J Radiol.* 2001;39(3):133–138.

83. Lin YS, Jen YM, Lin JC. Radiation-related cranial nerve palsy in patients with nasopharyngeal carcinoma. *Cancer.* 2002 ;95(2):404–409.

84. Lau SK, Wei WI, Choy D, Sham JS, Engzell UC. Brainstem auditory evoked potentials after irradiation

of nasopharyngeal carcinoma—report on two cases with myelopathy of the brainstem. *J Laryngol Otol.* 1988;102(12):1142-1146.

85. Cheng SJ, Lee JJ, Ting LL, et al. A clinical staging system and treatment guidelines for maxillary osteoradionecrosis in irradiated nasopharyngeal carcinoma patients. *Int J Radiat Oncol Biol Phys.* 2006;64(1):90-97.

86. Chang KP, Tsang NM, Chen CY, Su JL, Hao SP. Endoscopic management of skull base osteoradionecrosis. *Laryngoscope.* 2000; 110: 1162-1165.

87. Yeh SA, Tang Y, Lui CC, Huang YJ, Huang EY. Treatment outcomes and late complications of 849 patients with nasopharyngeal carcinoma treated with radiotherapy alone. *Int J Radiat Oncol Biol Phys.* 2005;62(3):672-679.

12

Malignancies of the Nasal Cavity, Paranasal Sinuses, and Orbit

Michael E. Kupferman
Ehab Hanna

INTRODUCTION

Malignancies of the nasal cavity, paranasal sinuses, and orbit are rare, and comprise a wide range of histologic types. With the exception of tumors arising in the orbit, these lesions tend to be clinically silent and are often diagnosed at an advanced stage. High resolution imaging is critical to determine the extent of disease and, in particular, involvement of the orbit and cranial base. Although several staging systems do exist, the lack of a clinically validated system that accurately predicts patient outcomes limits their utility. Surgical resection and, in most cases, postoperative adjuvant radiation has been the primary treatment modality for these cancers. However, a role of neoadjuvant chemotherapy is emerging and may limit the morbidity associated with extensive craniofacial resection often necessary for tumor removal. This chapter reviews the diagnostic and therapeutic management of malignant tumors of the nose, paranasal sinus, and orbit.

EPIDEMIOLOGY

Cancers of the paranasal sinus and nasal cavity account for approximately 3% of all head and neck malignancies, and less than 0.5% of all human malignancies. With an incidence of only 0.5 to 1 per 100,000, these tumors have been difficult to study in large clinical trials, and thus treatments and outcomes are often based on limited retrospective data.[1] In addition to tobacco, epidemiologic evidence suggests an increased risk of sinonasal squamous cell carcinomas and adenocarcinomas among those who have occupational exposures to nickel, wood dust, chromium, and formaldehyde, and to substances that are used in the furniture, textile, leather, and petroleum industries.

ANATOMY

The nasal cavity comprises the nasal vestibules anteriorly, the bony-cartilaginous nasal septum (quadrangular cartilage, maxilla, vomer, ethmoid, and palatine bones) in the midline, the turbinates laterally, the cribriform plate superiorly, and the sphenoid rostrum posteriorly. Excluding cutaneous lesions in the nasal sill, malignancies of the nasal cavity most commonly arise from the nasal septum. Paranasal sinus cancers are most frequently located in the maxillary sinuses, and can invade the orbit superiorly, the oral cavity inferiorly and the nasal cavity medially. Tumors may gain access to the skull base when posterior and posterolateral extension is present, via the pterygopalatine and infratemporal fossae, respectively (Fig 12-1).

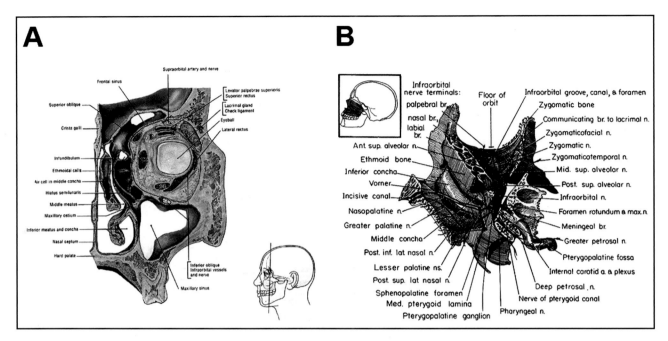

Fig 12–1. A. Anatomic diagram of the nasal cavity, paranasal sinuses and their relationship to the orbit. (Used with permission from Moore K. *Clinically Oriented Anatomy*, 3rd ed. Copyright 1992 Lippincott, Williams and Wilkins.). **B.** The pterygopalatine fossa is an anatomically complex space that contains the internal maxillary artery, branches of V_2 and V_3, and lymphatics. It is a route of tumor spread into the orbit, brain, and infratemporal fossa when invaded by cancers of the paranasal sinuses. (Used with permission from Woodburne R. *Essentials of Human Anatomy*, 6th ed. Copyright 1981 Oxford University Press).

The ethmoid sinuses are a two-tiered labyrinth of air cells medial to the medial orbital walls, and extend in a horizontal plane from the frontal sinuses anteriorly to the sphenoid sinuses posteriorly. The roof of the ethmoid sinuses is defined by the floor of the anterior fossa. Counterintuitively, the bone of the cranial base does not provide a significant barrier to tumor invasion, whereas the dura is rarely penetrated by an advancing tumor front. The sphenoid sinuses are paired cells in the central skull base, surrounded laterally by the carotid artery, the optic nerve, V_2 and the vidian nerve. The planum sphenoidale is the roof of the sphenoid sinus and supports the pituitary gland.

The orbit is a pyramidal-shaped bony cavity, bounded superiorly by the orbital plate of the frontal bone and inferiorly by the roof of the maxillary sinus. The greater wing of the sphenoid defines the lateral wall, and the medial wall is composed of the lamina papyracea of the ethmoid bane, the lacrimal bone, and the frontal process of the maxilla. The posteriorly oriented apex is composed of 3 anatomic foramina: (1) the optic foramen, transmitting the optic nerve and ophthalmic artery (2) the superior orbital fissure, transmitting cranial nerve III, IV, V_1, VI, and (3) the inferior fissure, transmitting V_2.

HISTORY AND PHYSICAL EXAMINATION

All components of a thorough history and physical examination are necessary in the complete evaluation of a patient suspected of harboring a sinonasal or orbital tumor. Complaints of blurred vision, diplopia, parasthesias, or hypesthesias along the branches of the trigeminal nerve should prompt further investigation into possible perineural or ophthalmic involvement. When an orbital tumor is present, or when there is suspicion of orbital extension, a formal ophthalmic evaluation, including slit-lamp examination, is necessary.

No examination of the nasal cavity or sinuses is complete without rigid or flexible nasal endoscopy (Fig 12–2). Rigid endoscopy is advantageous as it may allow for in-office biopsy when the histologic diagnosis is in doubt. The practitioner should be cautioned to avoid a biopsy without formal axial and coronal imaging, or when the superior margin of the tumor cannot be visualized. A cerebrospinal leak or uncontrolled epistaxis is an unwanted complication, particularly in the clinic setting.

RADIOGRAPHIC IMAGING

High-resolution axial and coronal imaging is necessary to adequately stage all sinonasal and orbital malignancies. For these lesions, both computerized tomography (CT) and magnetic resonance imaging (MRI) are complementary and are often both obtained for pretreatment planning. CT offers the advantage of defining the extent of bony invasion, the presence of neural foramina widening, and is a better modality for the identification of metastatic lymphadenopathy (Fig 12–3). MRI, on the other hand, can identify any soft tissue, dural, and perineural invasion (Fig 12–4). Furthermore, MRI can allow the radiologist to distinguish between tumor and retained secretions, a distinction that is difficult to make with CT modality. FDG-PET is valuable when recurrence is suspected, especially in the presence of prior reconstruction or post-treatment anatomic distortion. Angiography is reserved for the evaluation of lesions that abut the carotid artery at the skull base and helps to define the respectability of the tumor. Preoperative embolization is sometimes necessary for hypervascular lesions.

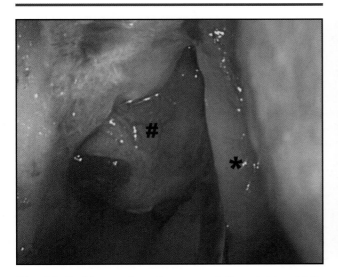

Fig 12–2. Mucosal melanoma of the right middle meatus (#), with distraction of middle turbinate (*) toward the nasal septum.

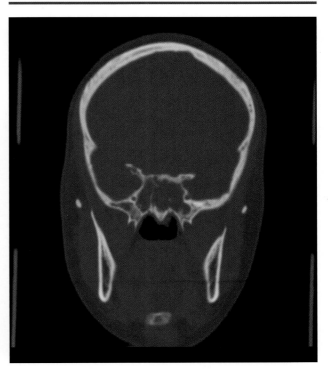

Fig 12–3. Coronal CT of a patient with an osteosarcoma of the sphenoid sinus. An endoscopic-assisted transcranial approach was used for surgical resection.

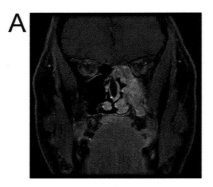 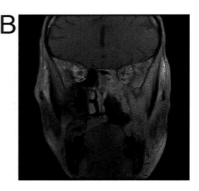

Fig 12–4. A. Coronal MRI of an adenocarcinoma of the left ethmoid sinuses. **B.** Coronal MRI of squamous cell carcinoma of the maxillary sinus.

STAGING

Table 12-1 presents the staging system for paranasal sinus and nasal cavity cancers. Distinct staging systems for olfactory neuroblastomas have been described, and will be elaborated later in this chapter. No staging system for orbital tumors is currently in use; rather, most clinicians utilize the staging system for particular pathologic subtypes (Table 12-2).

HISTOPATHOLOGY

Histologically, squamous cell carcinoma is the most common malignancy of the nasal cavity and paranasal sinuses. It accounts for over 50% of all tumors at these sites. Nonsquamous cancers are typically of salivary gland origin, with adenocarcinoma (Fig 12-5) and adenoid cystic carcinoma predominating.[2] Other less common malignancies include olfactory neuroblastoma, neuroendocrine carcinoma, sinonasal undifferentiated carcinoma (SNUC), mucosal melanoma, lymphoma, sarcoma, and metastases. The rarity of these tumors requires the evaluation by an experienced head and neck pathologist for accurate diagnosis. Further discussion of the management of specific histopathologic subtypes are briefly addressed at the end of this chapter.

Due to the pleotropic tissue types present, lesions of the orbit comprise a spectrum of pathologies. Tumors of the lacrimal gland are typically salivary gland malignancies or lymphoma, whereas rhabdomyosarcomas usually arise from the extraocular musculature. Malignant nerve sheath tumors may arise from the optic nerve.

CRITICAL DECISION POINTS

One of the most critical aspects in the treatment decision process for sinonasal malignancies is determining the extent of orbital, cavernous sinus, and skull base involvement. Surgical planning for an orbital exenteration or a craniofacial resection should be determined early and must be discussed preoperatively with the patient. In addition, nonsurgical modalities may be recommended in elderly or medically unfit patients, in those who are reluctant to undergo extensive resection, or when the disease is deemed unresectable. Clinical signs of orbital or cavernous sinus involvement are suggested by limited globe motion, chemosis, and ophthalmoplegia. However, these findings are usually indicative of extensive disease progression. Coronal and axial imaging are effective in establishing tumor involvement of the medial orbital wall that may not require an extensive resection. Similarly, subclinical skull base and intracranial invasion are difficult to assess on physical examination, and brain parenchymal invasion is often considered unresectable disease. These

Table 12–1. Staging Systems for Paranasal Sinus and Nasal Cavity Cancers

MAXILLARY SINUS	
T1	Tumor limited to maxillary sinus mucosa with no erosion or destruction of bone
T2	Tumor causing bone erosion or destruction including extension into the hard palate and/or middle nasal meatus, except extension to posterior wall of maxillary sinus and pterygoid plates
T3	Tumor invades any of the following: bone of the posterior wall of maxillary sinus, subcutaneous tissues, floor or medial wall of orbit, pterygoid fossa, ethmoid sinuses
T4a	Tumor invades anterior orbital contents, skin of cheek, pterygoid plates, infratemporal fossa, cribriform plate, sphenoid or frontal sinuses
T4b	Tumor invades any of the following: orbital apex, dura, brain, middle cranial fossa, cranial nerves other than maxillary division of trigeminal nerve (V_2), nasopharynx, clivus
NASAL CAVITY AND ETHMOID SINUS	
T1	Tumor restricted to any one subsite, with or without bony Invasion
T2	Tumor invading two subsites in a single region or extending to involve an adjacent region within the nasoethmoidal complex, with or without bony invasion
T3	Tumor extends to invade the medial wall or floor of the orbit, maxillary sinus, palate, or cribriform plate
T4a	Tumor invades any of the following: anterior orbital contents, skin of nose or cheek, minimal extension to anterior cranial fossa, pterygoid plates, sphenoid or frontal sinuses
T4b	Tumor invades any of the following: orbital apex, dura, brain, middle cranial fossa, cranial nerves other than (V_2), nasopharynx, or clivus
REGIONAL LYMPH NODES (N)	
N0	No regional lymph node metastasis
N1	Metastasis in a single ipsilateral lymph node, 3 cm or less in greatest dimension
N2a	Metastasis in a single ipsilateral lymph node, more than 3 cm but not more than 6 cm in greatest dimension
N2b	Metastasis in multiple ipsilateral lymph nodes, none more than 6 cm in greatest dimension
N2c	Metastasis in bilateral or contralateral lymph nodes, none more than 6 cm in greatest dimension
N3	Metastasis in a lymph node, more than 6 cm in greatest dimension
DISTANT METASTASIS (M)	
M0	No distant metastasis
M1	Distant metastasis

issues highlight the importance of thorough clinical and radiographic studies prior to treatment planning.

Most therapeutic options have been extrapolated from the management of squamous cell carcinomas of the sinuses, which comprises the largest percentage of malignancies. However, the treatment must be tailored to the histology, as low-grade salivary gland tumors do not necessarily warrant multimodality therapy. Furthermore, some lesions may be best treated with nonsurgical therapy alone. Thus, a thorough understanding of the unique biology of each tumor type is necessary for effective patient counseling.

Table 12–2. Staging System for Pathologic Subtypes

ESTHESIONEUROBLASTOMA STAGING SYSTEM
Primary Tumor
T1 Tumor isolated to nasal cavity and ethmoid sinuses
T2 Tumor extends to sphenoid sinus or cribriform plate
T3 Tumor extends to anterior cranial fossa or orbit, no dural invasion
T4 Tumor invades dura or brain parenchyma
Regional Lymph Nodes
N0 Lymph node metastases absent
N1 Lymph node metastases present
Metastasis
M0 Distant metastases absent
M1 Distant metastases present

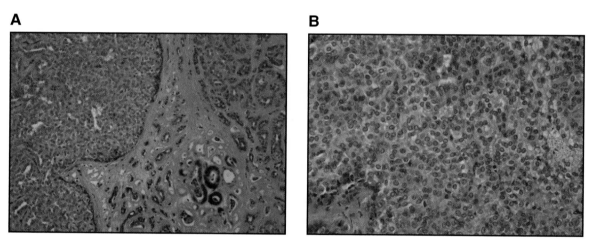

A **B**

Fig 12–5. Histopathology of adenocarcinoma of nasal cavity. **A.** Low-power image. **B.** High-power view.

TREATMENT OPTIONS

Surgery

Surgical resection remains the mainstay therapeutic option for squamous cell carcinomas and salivary gland malignancies of the nasal cavity and paranasal sinuses. It must be stated that operative management is predicated on the ability to obtain negative margins, and the absence of distant metastasis. This section describes the various surgical approaches and resections that can be undertaken to manage these malignancies.

Surgical Approach

A number of surgical approaches have been developed to provide access to the nasal cavity and paranasal sinuses for surgical resection. Both endoscopic and open approaches can provide the needed exposure, but the decision regarding the appropriate one must take into account the extent of the lesion, the need for vascular and intracranial access, and the experience of the surgeon. Most centrally located lesions can be accessed with the lateral rhinotomy incision and provide adequate exposure to the septum, the lateral nasal wall, the medial aspect of the maxillary sinus, ethmoid sinuses, and the sphenoid sinus. This incision can be extended onto the infraorbital rim (Weber-Ferguson) or the supraorbital rim (Lynch incision) for extended access to the maxillary sinus, frontal sinus, orbit, and central skull base. Although facial incisions are necessary, scarring is minimal when incisions are placed along the lines of relaxed skin tension and in natural skin creases (Fig 12–6). Combined approaches, including the subfrontal approach and the craniofacial approach, provide adequate access to the cribriform plate and provide the necessary exposure for an intracranial resection.

The midface degloving approach offers the advantage of requiring no external incisions, but is limited by its superior exposure at the skull base. Endoscopic and endoscopic-assisted resections are gaining popularity among a number of surgeons, but should be utilized judiciously, based on the extent of disease and the feasibility of obtaining negative margins. These approaches offer the advantage of magnified visualization of sinonasal anatomy and offer the ability to perform safe dissection in critical areas, such as the lateral wall of the sphenoid sinus and along the cribriform plate. Endoscopic approaches also may be used in conjunction with open intracranial approaches in selected cases where significant dural resection and reconstruction is needed. The oncologic efficacy and safety of purely endonasal endoscopic resections are currently being evaluated by various groups.

Surgical Resection

For lesions limited to the nasal septum, a near-total or total septectomy can be achieved endoscopically or via a lateral rhinotomy approach. The medial maxillectomy is the ideal procedure for lesions of the lateral nasal wall and turbinates, and selected lesions of the ethmoid sinuses as well. Control of the anterior and posterior ethmoid arteries is critical for hemostatic control, which can be ligated as they penetrate the ethmoid bone along the medial orbital wall. Lesions of the maxillary sinus below Ohngren's line, a plane defined by a line drawn from the angle of the mandible to the medial canthus, are

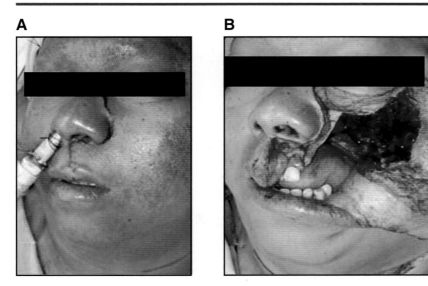

Fig 12–6. A. Lateral rhinotomy incision with subciliary extension for total maxillectomy. **B.** Surgical defect after total maxillectomy via lateral rhinotomy approach.

best managed with an infrastructure maxillectomy. This resection can be extended to a total maxillectomy, with resection of the orbital floor when the lesion is above Ohngren's line. An orbital exenteration is included when there is frank invasion of the orbital periosteum and fat, extraocular musculature or the globe itself. Craniofacial resection is necessary for tumors that involve the cribriform plate.[3] A bicoronal incision with a frontal craniotomy, in conjunction with a transfacial approach, provides wide access to the anterior skull base for resection and reconstruction.[4] The subfrontal approach provides similar exposure but minimizes the need for frontal lobe retraction.

Management of the Neck

Regional metastasis from sinonasal malignancies are generally detected in 10% to 15% of patients at the time of presentation. For lesions arising in the orbit, the parotid bed and levels I and II are most common sites of lymphatic spread. Tumors of the maxillary and ethmoid sinuses metastasize erratically, and it is not uncommon to see metastases in the retropharyngeal nodes, or in levels I or II. Due to the low risk of lymphatic metastasis at presentation for early-staged lesions, elective neck dissection is generally not advocated, unless it is necessary for surgical exposure of the neck vessels for microvascular reconstruction. Elective neck irradiation, even for early stage tumors, should be considered. However, patients with T3 or T4 lesions have a greater risk for the development of cervical metastasis during the course of disease, and thus elective neck management is mandated.

Results

Due to the rarity of these tumors and the heterogeneity of histologic types, the various treatment approaches and the lack of treatment uniformity, an accurate assessment of outcomes based on the published literature is limited. Few centers have had extensive experience with these lesions, and most published reports are retrospective reviews that include patients treated over periods of evolving radiographic, surgical, and reconstructive techniques.

Nonetheless, some general treatment principles have evolved. Surgical resection or radiation therapy is sufficient for early-staged lesions of the nasal cavity. More extensive lesions require a multimodality approach, generally entailing surgical resection followed by radiation therapy.[5] Tumors of the paranasal sinuses, with proximity to the orbit and cranial base, are best managed with a multimodality treatment plan. Although surgical resection and postoperative radiation therapy traditionally have been the approach of choice, the utilization of chemoradiotherapy combinations can offer similar locoregional control rates. Surgical salvage may be necessary for residual or recurrent disease. The ideal treatment paradigm remains to be determined.

Radiation Therapy

The role of external beam in sinonasal malignancies has not been clearly defined. Although some centers advocate postoperative radiotherapy, a number of centers have utilized radiotherapy in the neoadjuvant setting, or as definitive therapy. Additionally, concomitant chemoradiation regimens have been established by some groups for definitive therapy, with surgery reserved for the salvage setting. Radiation as a single modality offers local control rates of 30% to 40%.[6] Nonetheless, for resectable lesions, combined surgery with external beam radiation results in superior local control over other modalities.[7] However, a multi-institutional study has yet to be undertaken to confirm this.

The challenges of radiotherapy for these diseases include: the proximity of the orbits and optic nerve, brain, carotid arteries, and the pituitary gland. Although conformal dosing with intensity modulated radiation therapy (IMRT) and proton beam therapy can limit scatter effect, external beam radiation to these critical structures poses significant treatment-related morbidity.[8] The dosages required postoperatively and for curative intent are in the 60 to 70-Gy range. Proton beam therapy is a modality that is gaining popularity for tumors encroaching on the critical structures of the skull base. The advantages of this modality are (1) the ability to limit radiation to uninvolved structures while

(2) achieving homogeneous therapeutic doses to the tumor bed.

Complications of radiotherapy to the paranasal sinuses and orbit include: optic neuritis, cataracts, blindness, skull base osteoradionecrosis, temporal and frontal lobe necrosis, panhypopituitarism, carotid artery stenosis, and spinal cord necrosis. Morbidity generally increases with doses above 50 Gy.

Systemic Therapy

The role of chemotherapy in sinonasal malignancies is evolving. For undifferentiated carcinomas, small-cell neuroendocrine tumors, rhabodmyosarcoma, and T-cell lymphomas, systemic chemotherapy in combination with external beam radiation is an efficacious treatment modality. Its role in SCC and salivary gland cancers is not as clearly defined. Intra-arterial chemotherapy has been proposed as a novel approach in the management of aggressive, unresectable lesions, but requires further study.[9] Most regimens are platinum-based in combination with 5-fluorouracil or a taxane. Some patients have enjoyed significant reduction in tumor burden when treated with concomitant chemotherapy and radiation therapy, although this approach awaits further validation in larger studies. In the recurrent setting, salvage chemotherapy can be offered for palliation.

SPECIFIC HISTOLOGIC SUBTYPES

Adenocarcinoma

After squamous cell carcinoma, adenocarcinoma is the second most common malignancy of the paranasal sinuses and has been associated with occupational exposure to tin, mercury, wood, and textiles. Adenocarcinomas arise from the minor salivary gland acini and the ethmoid sinuses are most common site of disease. Although three histopathologic subtypes have been described, the prognostic implication of this classification remains unclear. As these tumors may resemble malignancies of gastrointestinal and gynecologic histologic origin, a potential abdominal source should be excluded prior to initiating therapy. Similar to other salivary gland cancers, surgical resection with wide margins is the treatment of choice, which often entails a craniofacial resection. Data from some limited retrospective series demonstrate that postoperative radiation offers improved local control of disease. A role for chemotherapy has not been established to date. Overall survival ranges from 70% to 85%, depending on the stage of disease.

Olfactory Neuroblastoma

Tumors arising from the olfactory neuroepithelium are small-cell carcinomas that have unique biological and clinical behavior. These lesions are locally aggressive with a propensity for skull base invasion. Three staging systems have been proposed, but the TNM system, outlined in Table 12–2, is used most commonly. The evaluation includes confirmation of the pathologic diagnosis, as these may mimic lymphoma, sarcoma, or mucosal melanoma. Furthermore, these must be distinguished from a true small cell neuroendocrine tumor, which may be best managed with chemotherapy alone. Lymphatic metastasis may develop in up to 20% of patients during the course of their disease. Surgical resection to negative margins usually requires an anterior craniofacial approach, and is the preferred treatment modality for oncologic control in most patients.[10] A role for endoscopic tumor resection is emerging at some centers, but this approach should be utilized with caution due to the difficulty in achieving negative margins without complete removal of the cribriform plate. Radiotherapy is added postoperatively for lesions invading the orbit and anterior cranial fossa, but should be considered for all patients to maximize local control. The risk of distant metastasis increases with increasing tumor stage, and thus chemotherapy, is commonly added to the therapeutic plan. The limited data in the literature suggest that, although recurrences are common in higher stage disease, many of them can be successfully salvaged. The overall 5-year survival from this disease ranges from 75% to 95%.[11]

Sinonasal Undifferentiated Carcinoma

One of the most aggressive neoplasms of the paranasal sinuses is sinonasal undifferentiated carcinoma (SNUC), a rare malignancy with a historically fatal outcome. Extension beyond the confines of the paranasal sinuses is common, with intracranial, cranial nerve, and orbital involvement frequently evident on presentation. It is imperative that these tumors be distinguished histologically from other small round blue-cell tumors of the sinuses, as they may be confused with small cell neuroendocrine carcinoma, rhabdomyosarcoma, T-cell lymphoma, and malignant melanoma. Surgical resection alone is ineffective in treating SNUC; rather, induction chemotherapy, followed by definitive radiation or surgical resection may offer acceptable local control. A craniofacial resection is the operative approach of choice for the oncologic control of disease. Preoperative chemoradiotherapy therapy has also been advocated to maximize local control. Despite this multimodality approach, local failure and distant metastasis occurs in approximately 23% and 25% of patients, respectively, and overall survival at 5 years is 65%.[12]

Mucosal Melanoma

Mucosal melanoma (MM) accounts for 6% of head and neck melanomas and occurs primarily in the oral cavity and nasal cavity. Intranasally, the lesions appear pigmented and polypoid and are friable. The biological behavior of mucosal melanoma is characterized by locoregional recurrence and distant metastasis. Evaluation of the patient with MM entails whole-body axial imaging to exclude distant metastasis. The mainstay of treatment entails surgical resection to negative margins. Determinants for an open versus an endoscopic approach include the experience of the surgeon, the location of the tumor, and the ability to achieve a gross total resection. An anterior craniofacial resection is necessary for lesions of the ethmoid and frontal sinuses due to the need for obtaining a negative margin at the skull base. Postoperative radiation has been demonstrated to improve local control, but most patients succumb to distant metastasis. Surgical resection with postoperative radiation can achieve a local control rate of 85%, with the majority of patients succumbing to distant failure.[13] Long-term survivorship beyond 5 years is uncommon.[14] Due to the high risk for distant metastasis among these patients, consideration should be given to immunotherapy or an experimental vaccine trial.

Adenoid Cystic Carcinoma

Although mucoepidermoid carcinoma is the most common malignancy of the salivary glands, adenoid cystic carcinoma (ACC) is the most common cancer of the minor salivary glands, and accounts for 15% of sinonasal cancers. The three histologic subtypes described, ranging from least to most aggressive, are: (1) tubular, (2) cribriform, and (3) solid, although many tumors are composed of a combination of each of these. These tumors are notorious for exhibiting perineural invasion along both named and unnamed nerves, and intracranial spread via branches of V_2 and V_3 is not uncommon. Although ACC has a slow-growth pattern and are often amenable to surgical resection when perineural invasion is absent, distant metastasis may develop in as many as 40% of patients, and recurrences 10 years after initial therapy are not uncommon. Lymphatic spread, however, occurs in 10% to 25% of patients.[15] Primary surgical resection to negative margins remains the treatment of choice for these lesions. Postoperative radiation improves local control but does not improve overall survival. The role of neutron-beam radiation is evolving and may be an important adjunct to the management of persistent or recurrent disease. If surgical resection of perineural microscopic disease at the skull base would lead to significant morbidity, postoperative stereotactic radiation should be considered. Chemotherapy may be beneficial for those with distant metastasis, although patients may have a prolonged symptom-free interval once the metastases are identified. Although 5-year survival from this disease may be as high as 40% to 60%, long-term studies have demonstrated continually declining survivorship, even at the 20-year interval, and thus life-long surveillance for these patients is required.

SUMMARY

Tumors of the paranasal sinuses, nasal cavity and orbit are rare tumors comprising a wide range of histologic types. Most patients will present with advanced disease due to the relatively nonspecific symptoms that ensue. High-resolution imaging with both CT and MR are critical for staging and treatment planning. Surgical resection is the mainstay of therapy for these diseases, whereas radiation is reserved for the postoperative and palliative settings. Novel neoadjuvant chemotherapeutic approaches may be efficacious in decreasing disease burden and in limiting the extent of resection. Nonetheless disease-free and overall survival remains poor, due to the locoregional recurrences. Multi-institutional trials, with standardization of evaluation and management, are necessary to delineate the ideal treatment approaches for these diseases.

REFERENCES

1. Myers EN. *Cancer of the Head and Neck*. 4th ed. Philadelphia, Pa.: Saunders; 2003.
2. Dulguerov P, Jacobsen MS, Allal AS, Lehmann W, Calcaterra T. Nasal and paranasal sinus carcinoma: are we making progress? A series of 220 patients and a systematic review. *Cancer*. 2001;92(12):3012–3029.
3. Lund VJ, Howard DJ, Wei WI, Cheesman AD. Craniofacial resection for tumors of the nasal cavity and paranasal sinuses—a 17-year experience. *Head Neck*. 1998;20(2):97–105.
4. McCutcheon IE, Blacklock JB, Weber RS, et al. Anterior transcranial (craniofacial) resection of tumors of the paranasal sinuses: surgical technique and results. *Neurosurgery*. 1996;38(3):471–479; discussion 479–480.
5. Ketcham AS, Van Buren JM. Tumors of the paranasal sinuses: a therapeutic challenge. *Am J Surg*. 1985;150(4):406–413.
6. Waldron JN, O'Sullivan B, Warde P, et al. Ethmoid sinus cancer: twenty-nine cases managed with primary radiation therapy. *Int J Radiat Oncol Biol Phys*. 1998;41(2):361–369.
7. Jiang GL, Ang KK, Peters LJ, Wendt CD, Oswald MJ, Goepfert H. Maxillary sinus carcinomas: natural history and results of postoperative radiotherapy. *Radiother Oncol*. 1991;21(3):193–200.
8. Duthoy W, Boterberg T, Claus F, et al. Postoperative intensity-modulated radiotherapy in sinonasal carcinoma: clinical results in 39 patients. *Cancer*. 2005;104(1):71–82.
9. Samant S, Robbins KT, Vang M, Wan J, Robertson J. Intra-arterial cisplatin and concomitant radiation therapy followed by surgery for advanced paranasal sinus cancer. *Arch Otolaryngol Head Neck Surg*. 2004;130(8):948–955.
10. Levine PA, Gallagher R, Cantrell RW. Esthesioneuroblastoma: reflections of a 21-year experience. *Laryngoscope*. 1999;109(10):1539–1543.
11. Diaz EM, Jr., Johnigan RH, 3rd, Pero C, et al. Olfactory neuroblastoma: the 22-year experience at one comprehensive cancer center. *Head Neck*. 2005; 27(2):138–149.
12. Rosenthal DI, Barker JL, Jr., El-Naggar AK, et al. Sinonasal malignancies with neuroendocrine differentiation: patterns of failure according to histologic phenotype. *Cancer*. 2004;101(11):2567–2573.
13. Patel SG, Prasad ML, Escrig M, et al. Primary mucosal malignant melanoma of the head and neck. *Head Neck*. 2002;24(3):247–257.
14. Manolidis S, Donald PJ. Malignant mucosal melanoma of the head and neck: review of the literature and report of 14 patients. *Cancer*. 1997;80(8): 1373–1386.
15. Fordice J, Kershaw C, El-Naggar A, Goepfert H. Adenoid Cystic Carcinoma of the head and neck: predictors of morbidity and mortality. *Arch Otolaryngol Head Neck Surg*. 1999;125(2):149–152.

13

Cranial Base Malignancy

William J. Benedict, Jr.
Thomas C. Origitano
Douglas E. Anderson
John P. Leonetti
Guy J. Petruzzelli

The diagnosis and management of patients with malignant tumors of the cranial base represents one of the most challenging aspects of head and neck surgical oncology. The anatomic location, histologic heterogeneity, and overall infrequency of these tumors contribute to the difficulties encountered in their management. Although the first report of combined craniofacial resection by Ketchum in 1963[1] warned of significant operative morbidity and mortality recent data from our own and other institutions indicate an operative mortality of 1% with an overall rate of complications under 20%. Fortunately, these increases in technical safety also translate into improvements in overall and disease-free survival for patients with tumors in these regions.

Improvements in safety and enhanced survival are largely due to technologic advances in the areas of medical imaging including intraoperative navigation, stereotactic delivery of high doses of ionization radiation without serious injury to surrounding uninvolved tissues, more frequent use of radiosensitizing chemotherapy regimens, neuroanesthesia techniques which maximize cerebral protection and neuromonitoring, and a better understanding of the biology and patterns of spread of these tumors. As we discuss, the use of sinonasal endoscopy for both preoperative assessment (including pretreatment biopsy) and transnasal endoscopic definitive resection of these tumors represents the next step in the evolution in management these complex patients (Fig 13-1).

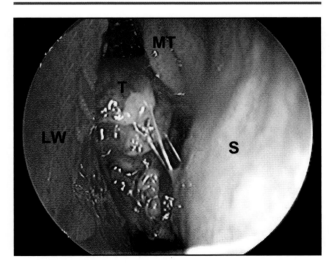

Fig 13–1. Intranasal examination with 0-degree, 4-mm endoscope. Biopsy of this mass revealed olfactory neuroblastoma (LW, lateral nasal wall; MT, middle turbinate, S, nasal septum; T, tumor).

There is no widely accepted definition for what constitutes a "cranial base malignancy." Primary malignancies occurring at the junction of the cranial vault and facial skeleton such as the olfactory neuroblastoma or clival chondrosarcoma are extremely rare neoplasms. More commonly, the skull will be involved secondarily by a primary orbital, paranasal sinus, or jugular foramen malignancies extending superiorly. The common element is that these tumors involve complex anatomic regions that have both an extradural and intradural component, and may involve multiple cranial nerves or the carotid arteries.

The rarity of these tumors makes it extremely difficult for any one surgeon or center to develop large series or experiences with these patients. The lack of uniformly collected and reported data for patents with cranial base malignancies makes the treatment of these patients difficult. Variations in clinical experience and available recourses make the implementation of large clinical trials extremely challenging. The numbers of patients needed to adequately power such trials make them even more daunting to consider. This chapter discusses cranial base malignancies and their surgical and medical treatment. Included is a detailed discussion of skull base anatomy, particularly as it applies to the resection of these neoplasms. The preoperative workup and examination of the patient with cranial base malignancies is discussed including suggested diagnostic tests. Surgical planning and skull base reconstruction are addressed based on the general location of a particular disease, as is the role for either adjuvant or neoadjuvant radiation and chemotherapy.

ANATOMY OF THE CRANIAL BASE

Osteology and Boundaries of the Cranial Base

The skull base is divided into three regions (fossae): anterior, middle, and posterior. The skull base is oriented around the sphenoid bone, which forms the central portion of the middle cranial fossa, connecting the anterior and posterior fossae. The anterior

cranial fossa is bounded rostrally by the frontal lobes and olfactory tracts and caudally by the orbits and ethmoid sinus. The middle cranial fossa contains the sella and pituitary complex, medially, and the squamous and petrous temporal bones laterally. In this region, the temporal lobe is the rostral boundary, and the infratemporal fossa is the caudal boundary. The posterior fossa extends from the posterior aspect of the petrous temporal bone to the inner table of the occipital bone. It includes the anterior aspect of the foramen magnum and the posterior clivus. Rostrally, the posterior fossa is adjacent to the cerebellum, pons, and tentorium cerebelli. Caudal to the posterior fossa, the suboccipital region includes the craniovertebral junction, and posterior-most aspect of the infratemporal fossa, which includes the jugular foramen and its neurovascular complex.

The Anterior Cranial Fossa

The anterior cranial fossa is formed by the frontal, ethmoid, and anterior superior aspects of the body and lesser wing of the sphenoid bone. The medial most portion of the anterior cranial fossa is deeper than lateral regions due to the bilateral fovea ethmoidali of the ethmoid bone. The posterior table of the frontal sinus forms the most anterior portion of this region. Moving posterior, toward the frontal crest, the foramen cecum contains the most distal portion of the superior sagittal sinus. In children, nasal veins will communicate with the superior sagittal sinus through this opening.[2] Posterior to the foramen cecum, centrally, is the superior most aspect of the ethmoid bone.

Approximately 88 cribroethmoid foraminae pierce the cribriform plate, allowing for the olfactory fila to pass from the olfactory bulb to the nasal cavity. Centrally the crista gali connects the falx cerebri to the cranial base. The cribriform plate also allows passage of branches of the anterior and posterior ethmoidal vessels. Meningo-orbital foraminae may persist within the orbital roof, allowing passage of branches from the ophthalmic and middle meningeal arteries.[2] Posterior to the cribriform, the planum sphenoidale serves as the posterior-most aspect of the anterior cranial fossa.

The Middle Cranial Fossa

Greater Wing of the Sphenoid and Lateral Middle Fossa

The middle cranial fossa consists of the sella, the parasellar region, and the floor of the middle skull base, formed by the greater wing of the sphenoid and the temporal bone (petrous and squamous parts). The zygomatic root marks the most lateral and caudal extension of the middle cranial fossa. Separating the anterior and middle fossa, the crista alaris sylvi extends from the posterior border of the lesser wing of the sphenoid laterally.

The classical pterional craniotomy allows access to both the anterior and middle cranial fossae. It is centered on the convergence of the frontal, parietal, squamous temporal, and sphenoid (greater wing) bones.

The middle cranial fossa, contains several anatomic portals through which nerves, vessels, and tumors pass both rostrally and caudally into the infratemporal fossa. The sphenoid bone houses these foraminae, as it forms the central bone of the skull base. Anteriorly, the superior orbital fissure (SOF) is formed by the inferior surface of the lesser wing of the sphenoid, and superior surface of the greater wing. The SOF contains cranial nerves (CNs) III, IV, V_1, and VI and the superior ophthalmic vein.[3]

Nerves of the Superior Orbital Fissure

Cranial nerves entering the SOF are responsible for ocular movement and pupillary function. CN III controls the levator palpebrae, and all extraocular muscles of the eye except the lateral rectus, which is innervated by CN VI (abducens nerve) and the superior oblique, innervated by CN IV. Preganglionic parasympathetic fibers course through CN III from the Edinger-Westphal nucleus to the ciliary ganglion of the orbit via the inferior division of the intraorbital oculomotor nerve. Postganglionic fibers travel in short ciliary nerves to the ciliary muscle and sphincter pupillae muscles of the iris where their constriction causes miosis. Postganglionic sympathetic fibers travel along the internal carotid artery (ICA), passing through the ciliary ganglion via the sympathetic root, coursing via the short ciliary nerves to the dilator pupillae muscle. Sympathetic innervation of the iris results in pupillary dilation. Additional sympathetic innervation derives from the carotid plexus via the nasociliary and long ciliary nerves of V_1. This division along with CN III fibers innervate the superior tarsal muscle of the eyelid.[3] The first division of the trigeminal nerve (ophthalmic nerve), transmits mainly general sensation from the eye, conjunctiva, lacrimal gland, eyelids, forehead, scalp, and parts of the nose.[3] It has two main divisions, the frontal and nasociliary nerves. The frontal nerve further divides into the supraorbital and supratrochlear nerves, which exit the orbit to supply sensation to the forehead and eyelid. The nasociliary nerve branches into anterior ethmoidal, infratrochlear, and posterior ethmoidal branches. These provide sensation to the skin and conjunctiva of the lower eye, lacrimal sac, external lateral nose, and nasal mucosa of the posterior ethmoidal and sphenoid sinuses.[3] Sensory fibers from the ophthalmic nerve synapse in the trigeminal (gasserian) ganglion before entering the pons, where they terminate in several nuclei, including the spinal trigeminal nucleus.

Foramenae Rotundum, Ovale, and Spinosum

Inferomedially to the SOF lies the foramen rotundum, containing the maxillary nerve (V_2). This nerve traverses its foramen to enter the ptergoplatine fossa (within the infratemporal fossa), where it unites with the pterygopalatine ganglion. This ganglia provides postsynaptic parasympathetic input to the lacrimal gland of the orbit, via the zygomatic nerve. Sensation to the face and superior mouth derives from two branches: the infraorbital and zygomatic nerves. The infraorbital nerve passes through the inferior orbital fissure, emerging on the face to supply sensation to the inferior eyelid, nasal alae, and upper lip. The zygomatic nerve divides and enters the maxillary sinus to supply the upper teeth and gums.[3]

The mandibular nerve contains both sensory and motor modalities. Both leave the skull through the foramen ovale, located posterolaterally from foramen rotundum. Sensory and motor components unite within the pterygopalatine fossa, into a short, thick nerve located between the lateral pterygoid muscle and the tensor veli palatine muscle (anterior to the middle meningeal artery).[3] In close association with the mandibular nerve, the otic ganglion provides postganglionic parasympathetic input to the parotid gland.

The mandibular nerve has several sensory and motor branches. The meningeal branch (sensory) courses back into the skull through the foramen spinosum to supply the meninges of the middle cranial fossa. The nerve to the medial pterygoid muscle then passes through the otic ganglion to supply the tensor veli palatine and tensor tympani muscles.[3] Terminal sensory branches of the mandibular nerve may be divided into anterior and posterior portions. Anterior divisions include sensory (buccal nerve) and motor (nerves to the lateral pterygoid, masseter, and temporalis). The posterior division contains fibers that provide motor control to the mylohyoid and anterior belly of the diagastric muscles (mylohyoid nerve). Sensory divisions of the posterior division include the auriculotemporal, lingual, and inferior alveolar nerves.[3]

The foramen spinosum lies posterior and lateral to the foramen ovale. It serves as an anatomic landmark for locating the third division of the trigeminal nerve. Moving posteriorly and medially, at the anterior aspect of the petrous temporal bone, the trigeminal impression extends forward to the foramen lacerum, over which the internal carotid artery (ICA) passes. Below (deep) to the trigeminal impression, the ICA canal moves toward the cavernous sinus. This region was dehiscent in 96% of cases in one series.[2] Other anatomic landmarks in this region include the greater and lesser superficial petrosal nerves (GSPN and LSPN, respectively), which run anteriorly and medially. These nerves are embedded in dura close to the cranial base. The GSPN pierces this dura (inferior petrosphenoid ligament) to join the deep petrosal nerve, forming the nerve of the pterygoid canal which then passes to the ptergopalatine ganglion. Postganglionic parasympathetic fibers from the GSPN exit the ganglion and innervate the lacrimal gland. Deep petrosal nerve fibers (postganglionic from the cervical sympathetic plexi) travel through the pterygopalatine ganglion, providing afferent and efferent autonomic innervation to the pituitary, lacrimal, salivary, and thyroid glands. The lesser petrosal nerve derives from CN IX (glossopharyngeal), where preganglionic parasym-

pathetics ascend through the tympanic canaliculus via the tympanic nerve to the tympanic plexus. The lesser petrosal nerve exits the skull base through its hiatus inferior and rostral to the GSPN to enter the otic ganglion in the pterygopalatine fossa. Postganglionics innervate the parotid gland through auriculotemporal branches[3] (Fig 13-2).

Sellar and Parasellar Regions

Centrally within the skull base, the sella is rostral to the sphenoid sinus. The pituitary gland is within the hypophyseal fossa, the floor of which is the bone of the sphenoid sinus. The posterior boarder of this region is the dorsum sellae, bilaterally terminating in the posterior clinoid processes. Anterior to the hypophyseal fossa just inferior to the chiasmatic sulcus is the tuberculum sellae. The optic chiasm lies within the prechiasmatic sulcus, the anterior boarder of which is the limbus sphenoidalis. Just anterior to this region is the body of the sphenoid (the jugum). The optic canals extend laterally from the prechiasmatic sulci, extending into the lesser wing of the sphenoid. The anterior clinoid processes form the medial most aspects of the lesser wing of the sphenoid, covering the lateral aspects of the optic nerves.[2,3] The optic strut separates the optic canal and SOF. Its rostral extension is the anterior clinoid process.

The transverse dural layer covering the pituitary gland (diaphragma sellae) is pierced by the pituitary stalk. Moving laterally, the tentorial edge is formed by both the anterior petroclinoid fold which attaches to the anterior clinoid, and the posterior petroclinoid fold, which affixes to the posterior clinoids. Thick dural fibers in continuity with the anterior petroclinoid fold extend over the optic nerve, forming the falciform ligament. These are in continuity with dura covering the planum sphenoidale, just anterior to the jugum. There is a small depression between the lateral edge of the sella and the tentorial edge. This region contains traversing cranial nerves entering the SOF, and the intracranial internal carotid artery as it exits the cavernous sinus.

Cavernous Sinus

The lateral wall of the cavernous sinus is formed by dura from the middle cranial fossa. It has an external

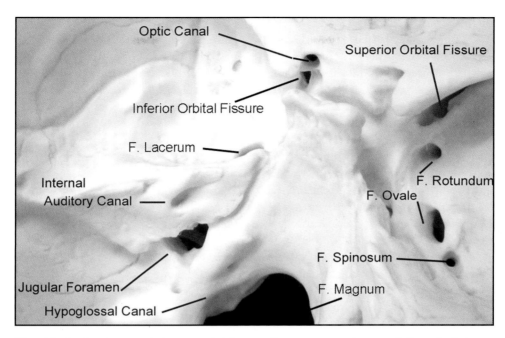

Fig 13–2. Anatomy of the cranial base. Osseous anatomy of the skull base viewed from the intracranial aspect with major foramen labeled. Structures associated with the major foramen include: **optic canal**, optic n, ophthalmic a; **superior orbital fissure**, oculomotor n, trochlear n, ophthmalmic division of trigeminal n., abducens n., ophthalmic v.; **foramen rotundum**, maxillary division of trigeminal n.; **foramen ovale**, mandibular division of trigeminal n, accessory meningeal a, lesser superficial petrosal n; **inferior orbital fissure**, maxillary division of trigeminal n, infraorbital a; **foramen spinosum**, middle meningeal a and v, recurrent branch of mandibular branch. of trigeminal n.; **internal auditory canal**, facial n, cochleovestibular n, internal auditory (labyrinthine) a and v; **jugular foramen**, glossopharyngeal n, vagus n, spinal accessory n, inferior petrosal sinus, sigmoid sinus (forming internal jugular v.); **hypoglossal canal**, hypoglossal n, meningeal branch. of ascending pharyngeal a; **foramen magnum**, medulla, vertebral a, spinal root of accessory n; **foramen lacerum**, internal carotid a, carotid sympathetic plexus, greater superficial petrosal n.

(lamina propria) and internal layer. Between these, CNs III, V_1, V_2, and IV pass as they move toward the superior orbital fissure. CN VI exits the pons, traverses the prepontine cistern, and enters the cavernous sinus from the lateral clivus, inferior to the posterior clinoid. The abducens nerve and inferior petrosal sinus pass beneath a ligamentous attachment (sphenopetrosal ligament) between the lateral dorsum sellae and sphenoidal process of the petrous temporal bone. The space beneath this ligament is known as Dorello's canal.[2] The abducens nerve courses through the cavernous sinus, lateral to the

ICA as it enters the SOF. The internal carotid artery ascends from the foramen lacerum deep to the mandibular nerve to nearly the level of the posterior clinoid. It then bends anteriorly into a horizontal segment, then again into a vertical segment as it pierces the dura to enter the subarachnoid space.

The Inferior Skull Base, Infratemporal Fossa, and Pterygopalatine Fossa

The infratemporal region (fossa) extends from the inferior orbital fissure (IOF) anteriorly to the jugular foramen posteriorly.[4] The IOF is limited anteriorly and inferiorly by the maxillary tuberosity, and superiorly by the greater wing of the sphenoid bone. Thus, the posterolateral maxilla marks the anterior border of the infratemporal fossa. Medially, this region is limited by the anterior aspect of the lateral pterygoid plate. Laterally, the infratemporal fossa is limited by the zygomatic bone, ramus of the mandible, and styloid process.[4,5] The squamous temporal bone provides the posterosuperior boundary of the infratemporal fossa. Anterosuperiorly, the infratemporal fossa is bound by the infratemporal surface of the greater sphenoid wing with its associated foraminae.[6]

The infratemporal fossa can be subdivided into three lateral to medial layers.[4] The outermost layer includes superficial tissues and bone. Structures include the zygomatic arch, temporomandibular joint (TMJ), the mandibular ramus, and the masseter and temporalis muscles.

The intermediate layer is composed of mainly the medial and lateral pterygoid muscles. The lateral pterygoid has two heads, and travels posteriorly. The origin of the infratemporal head is the inferior surface of the greater wing of the sphenoid; the origin of the pterygoid head is the lateral pterygoid plate. Insertions include the temporomandibular joint and the neck of the mandible. The lateral pterygoid functions to displace the mandible and TMJ articular disk forward thus depressing the mandible and opening the mouth. The medial pterygoid arises in the pterygoid fossa, between the medial and lateral plates. It obliquely inserts at the angle of the mandible, assisting in rotational closure of the mandible. The pterygoid hiatus is a triangle formed by the medial and lateral pterygoid muscles and the ramus of the mandible. Through this space, the maxillary artery and lingual, inferior dental, and mylohyoid nerves run. The chorda tympani exits the lingual nerve in this region, moving posteriorly to the petrotympanic fissure. The buccal nerve passes between the two heads of the lateral pterygoid muscle.

The deepest layer of the infratemporal region includes those structures that course within a line drawn from the stylomastoid foramen to the hook of the hamulus of the sphenoid bone.[4] From posterior to anterior, these structures include: the stylomastoid foramen (CN VII), the styloid process, the jugular foramen, the carotid canal, the petrotym-panic fissure of the chorda tympani, the sphenoid spine, the foramen spinosum, the eustacian tube, the foramen ovale and the levator and tensor velum palatine muscles.[4] The sphenoid spine and styloid process are key anatomic landmarks in avoiding the vital structures that pass through many of these foraminae.

Within the infratemporal fossa, the pterygopalatine fossa is formed anteriorly by the maxillary tuberosity, medially by the vertical lamina of the palatine bone, and posteriorly by the pterygoid process. The pterygoid process anteriorly, along with the maxillary tuberosity, form a fissure (pterygomaxillary fissure), forming the lateral opening of the pterygopalatine fossa.[2,7] This region opens into the orbital apex via the IOF. The pterygopalatine fossa contains the pterygopalatine ganglion, the maxillary artery and nerves, and fat. The internal maxillary artery passes from the infratemporal fossa into this region, where it terminates in several branches. Medially, the sphenopalatine foramen opens into the nasal cavity, just above the root of the middle turbinate, allowing passage if the sphenopalatine nerve and vessels into this region. Inferiorly, the pterygopalatine fossa extends into the palatine canals and oral cavity. The vidian nerve enters this region from its canal medial and inferior to the foramen rotundum, traversing the maxillary nerve.[6]

The Posterior Fossa

The posterior fossa extends from the tentorial incisura to the foramen magnum. It is surrounded by the occipital, parietal, temporal, and posterior, inferior sphenoid bones. Its primary foraminae include the jugular foramen, the hypoglossal canal, and the internal acoustic meatus (IOM). The cerebellum, medulla, pons, and midbrain exist within the posterior fossa.

The clivus forms the anterior medial portion of the posterior fossa. It is composed of the posterior sphenoid body and anterior occipital bone. Just lateral, the hypoglossal canal enters the deep infratemporal fossa rostral to the occipital condyle, between the foramen lacerum and carotid canal at the occipitopetrosal suture.[8] Moving posteriorly, within the midline along the rostral skull base, the occipital bone is indented bilaterally, where the transverse sinuses extend to either side. These originate from the confluence of sinuses (bilateral transverse sinuses, and straight sinus). The straight sinus originates from the great cerebral vein of Galen, which receives both internal cerebral veins from the roof of the third ventricle. It passes inferior to the splenium of the corpus callosum, at the level of the entry of the inferior sagittal sinus, where the two merge to form the straight sinus. The straight sinus is a valveless vein formed by the split of dural layers in the midline there the two halves of the tentorium and the falx cerebri merge. The transverse sinus has a similar histologic appearance, formed by dural division where the tentorium meets the lateral skull base dura.

Safe surgical access to the posterior fossa involves primarily passage around large venous structures. The right transverse sinus is generally larger than the left, and the course of this vessel follows the insertion of the paraspinal muscles at the ligamentum nuchae. The transverse sinus turns inferiorly and laterally into the sigmoid sinus at the asterion, the convergence of the occipital, parietal, and temporal bones (mastoid and squamous parts). The inferior petrosal sinus drains from the clival basilar venous plexus along the medial posterior and middle fossae to the jugular bulb. It enters the jugular foramen between CNs IX and X.[8] It is encountered during the middle fossa approach to the midbrain. The superior petrosal sinus drains from the cavernous sinus within the tentorium along the posterior aspect of the petrous ridge, following it to the junction of the transverse and sigmoid junctions.[3,8] The vein of Labbe drains the temporal lobe, arising from the superior sylvian vein. It courses posteriorly to drain into the anterior portion of the transverse sinus.[9] Its insertion determines whether a transpetrosal approach to the cerebellopontine angle is feasible.

The Jugular Foramen

The jugular foramen is formed anterolaterally by the temporal bone, and posteromedially by the occipital bone. This complex region contains CNs IX, X, XI, the sigmoid and inferior petrosal sinuses, meningial branches of the ascending pharyngeal and occipital arteries, Jacobson's nerve, Arnold's nerve, and the cochlear aqueduct.[10] It is a difficult region to access because of surrounding anatomy: anteriorly, the carotid artery; laterally, the facial nerve; medially, the hypoglossal nerve; and inferiorly, the vertebral artery. The jugular foramen has three compartments: the posterolateral sigmoid portion containing the sigmoid sinus; an anteromedial petrosal portion, receiving drainage from the inferior petrosal sinus; and a neural portion for CNs IX, X, and XI. The foramen is divided into anterior and posterior parts by intrajugular processes of the temporal and occipital bones. These are connected by a fibrous bridge, or continuous bone in some cases.[10] The fibrous septum divides the jugular foramen into an anterior petrosal portion (for the inferior petrosal sinus), and a posterior sigmoid portion for the sigmoid sinus. Two sutures lie in line with the jugular foramen. Posterolaterally, the occipitomastoid suture underlies the sigmoid sinus as it approaches the foramen. Medially, the petroclival fissure lies adjacent to the inferior petrosal portion of the foramen.

The dura mater separates both venous compartments from the neural compartment. Anteromedially, the petrosal compartment is separated from the lateral posterior sigmoid area by the intrajugular process of the temporal bone. This protruberance gives rise to the intrajugular ridge, along which the cranial nerves traverse. The intrajugular dura has two perforations, one for the glossopharyngeal nerve, and another for the vagus and accessory spinal nerves.

The glossopharyngeal nerve exits the brainstem, penetrating the dura medial to the cochlear aqueduct, along the medial aspect of the intrajugular process of the temporal bone. As it exits the jugular foramen, the nerve expands as it forms the superior and inferior ganglia (petrossal ganglion) of the ninth nerve. The tympanic branch (Jacobson's nerve) exits just distal to the foramen at the inferior skull base. This branch then enters the tympanic canniculus and tympanic cavity to form the tympanic plexus. From this plexus, fibers forming the lesser petrosal nerve of the infratemporal fossa provide parasympathetic innervation to the parotid gland via postganglionics from the otic ganglion.[10]

The superior and inferior ganglia of the glossopharyngeal nerve receive special visceral afferents (taste) from the posterior third of the tongue and soft palate. General visceral afferents (pain, temp, touch) from the same regions, along with general somatic afferents from postauricular skin and posterior fossa meninges also synapse here on their way to brainstem nuclei. Other visceral afferents from the carotid body via the carotid sinus nerve enter the ganglia as they course ultimately to the brainstem. Motor branches of this nerve include that to the stylopharyngeus muscle of the pharyngeal area.[3]

The vagus and accessory nerves exit the posterior fossa via the vagal meatus, inferior to the ninth nerve. The vagus expands at the level of its superior ganglion within the foramen. A portion of the accessory nerve (CN XI) blends with the 10th nerve just before the auricular branch (Arnold's nerve), exits and is joined by a branch from the inferior ganglion of the glossopharyngeal nerve. This auricular branch enters the mastoid canaliculus, sending an ascending branch to the facial canal, then exiting the temporal bone through the tympanomastoid fissure.[10] This nerve carries afferent sensory modalities from the tympanic membrane and external acoustic meatus to the superior vagal ganglion, then to the brainstem.[3] A recurrent nerve from the superior ganglion carries sensory fibers from posterior fossa dura. The inferior vagal (nodose) ganglion carries visceral afferents from the pharynx, larynx, and carotid sinus and body. This ganglion is in close association with the superior cervical ganglion and hypoglossal nerve. Distal vagal branches descend in the bilateral carotid sheaths to innervate multiple viscera throughout the chest and abdomen. The majority of fibers within the vagal nerves are visceral sensory in modality. Efferents include those to the heart, lungs, GI tract, and genitalia, providing visceral (involuntary) motor function. Additional efferent branches include those to intrinsic laryngeal muscles (branchiomeric muscles) via the right and left recurrent laryngeal nerves.

NEUROLOGIC EXAMINATION, HEAD AND NECK EXAMINATION, AND OUTPATIENT EVALUATION OF PATIENTS WITH SKULL BASE MALIGNANCIES

Depending on the location of the malignancy and associated symptoms, patients may initially seek care with ophthalmology (because of diplopia or visual loss) or with primary care or neurology because of an endocrine disturbance, neurologic deficit, or facial pain syndrome. Hoarseness, dysphagia, and/or nasal symptoms may lead to an examination by an otolaryngologist.

The initial evaluation of the patient with cranial base malignancy includes the history and physical examination. Attention to complaints of endocrine dysfunction may suggest the presence of a parasellar lesion; particularly, polyuria, polydipsia, and fatigue. Change in facial features such as prominence of the nose and jaw with hypertrophy of the hands may suggest gigantism resulting from a growth hormone secreting tumor. Purple stria along the trunk and legs, rounded face, bronzing of the skin, osteoporosis, and thinning of the skin with a propensity to bruise may suggest Cushing's disease secondary to an ACTH-secreting pituitary tumor.

The patient's mental status and speech should be evaluated during the encounter. Subtle deficits can be further evaluated with detailed neuropsychological testing. Attention to ocular motility, visual acuity, visual fields, and pupillary response to direct and indirect light localizes the effects of a malignancy on the optic nerve/chiasm and occulomotor, abducens, and trochlear nerves. Evaluation of facial sensation and symmetry determines if the lesion is within the middle or posterior cranial fossa. The palate, pharynx, and voice should be evaluated for involvement of the lower cranial nerves. Flexible endoscopy allows for detailed study of the vocal folds. Motor and sensory function of the upper and lower extremities suggests involvement or mass effect on cortical structures. When possible, a transnasal biopsy is performed to determine pathology and initial oncologic staging.[11] Examination of the neck is detailed in other chapters of this text, but attention the cervical and adjoining lymphatic chains may suggest extent of disease.

The radiologic workup of patients with skull base malignancies includes CT and MRI imaging with and without contrast media. MRI studies detail neural and adjacent structures, and may allow for determination of extent of disease or spread of tumor along the perineurium of nerves. CT imaging has its greatest benefit in the evaluation of the cranial base. Prior to surgical resection, MRI data is utilized in a frameless stereotaxic computer system to aid resection. These data can be merged with CT data, allowing for toggling between both images during the surgical procedure. To complete the staging process, CT imaging of the chest, abdomen, and pelvis with either bone scanning or who body PET will determine extent of disease and feasibility of primary resection. Angiography allows for evaluation of tumor blood supply and vascularity. In certain lesions such as paraganglioma and angiofibroma, endovascular embolization can minimize operative blood loss. The use of balloon occlusion testing is indicated when large vessel sacrifice may be required. FDG PET imaging has its greatest utility in discerning tumor recurrence from scar tissue following surgery and radiation therapy.

COMMON CRANIAL BASE MALIGNANCIES AND THEIR TREATMENT

Sinonasal Malignancies That May Extend into the Skull Base

Other chapters of this text discuss in greater detail the management of sinonasal malignancies. These tumors, when large enough, may extend into the skull base, necessitating a combined approach for their resection. These neoplasms are briefly discussed, with more detail given to tumors that arise de novo from the cranial base.

Adenoid Cystic Carcinoma

Adenoid cystic carcinoma (ACC) comprises 12% of all salivary tumors, with 40% occurring in the major, and 60% arising in the minor salivary glands. They generally present as slowly growing, painful masses. The most common site of growth is the palate, followed by the sinonasal tract, then the parotid gland.[12,13] The median age of presentation is 52 years, and ACC presents equally in men and women. There are three histologic patterns: tubular, cribriform, and solid. Contrary to its name, adenoid cystic carcinoma rarely forms cysts. Prognosis is based primarily on histologic grade. Table 13-1 details overall survival in patients with ACC, relative to histologic

grade. Survival for tumors of the sinonasal tract is slightly worse with 5-, 10-, and 15-year survival rates of only 50%, 20%, and 8%, respectively.[14]

Local recurrences occur in up to 52% of patients. Lung and bone metastasis may occur in up to 37% of cases. Many of these are solitary, and can be resected. Metastatic disease to the lymph nodes is relatively rare, found in 5 to 15% of patients.[14]

Poor prognosis is related to certain histologic grades (cribriform and solid architectures), advanced clinical stage, large tumors (larger than 4 cm), positive resection margins, bone invasion, local recurrence, and distant metastasis. Cranial nerve invasion predicts poor outcome. The propensity of this insidious disease for perineural spread makes the likelihood of distant recurrence significant. Table 13-2 details the AJCC staging system for ACC.

The imaging characteristics of ACC relate significantly to the cellularity of the tumor. Greater cellularity is associated with adverse outcome. ACC is isointense to muscle on T1-weighted MRI. Cellular tumors have greater water content, and higher signal on T2-weighted MRI imaging. T1-enhanced imaging

Table 13–1. Grading and Prognosis if Adenoid Cystic Carcinoma

Grade	Differentiation	Prognosis
Tubular (Grade I)	Well differentiated	9–12 years
Cribriform (Grade II)	Moderately differentiated	6–9 years
Sold (Grade III)	Poorly differentiated	2–5 years

Table 13–2. AJCC Staging for Adenoid Cystic Carcinoma

T1	Disease confined to nasopharynx
T2a	Extension to oropharynx/nasal cavity soft tissues
T2b	T2a disease with extension to the parapharyngeal space
T3	Paranasal sinus or bony invasion
T4	Intracranial extension or cranial nerve involvement

is best facilitated with fat suppression; particularly when evaluating for intracranial spread of disease.[14] Perineural involvement is suggested by diffuse enlargement of nerves. Sclerosis of the neural foramen with expansion or destruction, also suggests perineural spread from involvement of the connective tissue surrounding the nerve itself.[15] Marrow invasion is also appreciated by CT imaging, manifest by bone destruction and sclerosis. Replacement of fat density or signal in the pterygopalatine fossa can also suggest intracranial extension. Abnormal signal intensity within the cavernous sinus and Meckel's cave may be appreciated with MRI[14,15] (Fig 13–3).

Primary surgery and postoperative radiation is the standard of care for ACC and other minor salivary gland malignancies. Utilizing these combined modalities, 5- and 10-year survival rates range from 60% to 75% and 50% to 65%, respectively.[16,17]

Adenoid cystic carcinomas of the maxillary antrum or palate can extend along the second division of the trigeminal nerve to involve structures within the pterygomaxillary space or cavernous sinus. The standard surgical approach to resection of these lesions is the lateral infratemporal middle fossa approach. This often involves a modified pterional craniotomy with an orbitozygomatic osteotomy. The cranial incision is taken anterior to the ear, into the neck to allow for a modified neck dissection, and control of the great vessels in the carotid sheath.[18]

Chemotherapy has a role in stabilizing disease, rather than promoting its regression. Mitoxantrone, vinorelbine, and epirubicin have some single agent activity in the treatment of ACC. Cisplatin-anthracycline combinations also have some activity in disease management.[19] The tyrosine kinase inhibitor, imantinib, has been used, as a high proportion of these tumors express the gene, c-kit. Again, disease stabilization was noted, but no regression could be proven.

Nasopharyngeal Carcinoma

Nasopharyngeal carcinoma (NPC) is a squamous cell carcinoma that derives from the nasopharyngeal mucosa.[20] The World Health Organization classifies these tumors into two subtypes: Keratinizing squamous cell carcinoma and nonkeratinizing carcinoma, of which there are two subvariants. Of the nonkera-

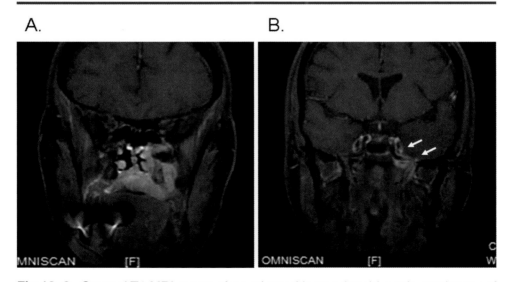

A.

B.

Fig 13–3. Coronal T1 MRI scans of a patient with an adenoid cystic carcinoma of the hard palate. **A.** Contrast-enhanced image identifying tumor of the palate extending across the midline and extending superiorly along the pterygoid plates. **B.** Perineural extension of tumor superiorly along V_2 with enhancement at foramen rotundum and along middle fossa dura (*arrows*).

tinizing variant, there are differentiated and undifferentiated subtypes.[14] Nonkeratinizing NPC is the more common of the two subtypes, and is radiation sensitive. An epidemiologic relationship with the Epstein-Barr virus exists between these two subvariants.

Risk factors for NPC include race, genetic susceptibility, environmental carcinogens, and exposure to the Epstein-Barr virus. There is a higher incidence of NPC in China. Of all cancers in the United States, 0.2% are NPC compared to 18% in patients of Chinese origin. This may be related to ingestion of nitrosamine-rich salted fish, or exposure to smoke or dust inhalants in southern China.[14]

NPC generally presents in the lateral wall of Rosenmüller's fossa (82% of cases). The remaining lesions may be found in the midline (12%) and in normal appearing mucosa (6%).[20] Squamous cell NPC has typical histologic squamous differentiation (poor or moderately differentiated). Nonkeratinizing NPC has cells with well-defined borders, a syncytial growth pattern, and large round or oval nuclei with prominent nucleoli.[14] There are characteristics histologically that resemble lymphoma; however, positive immunohistochemical staining for cytokeratin confirms NPC.[14]

Stage I and II disease may be cured with radiation alone. For patients with locally advanced nasopharyngeal carcinoma, combined radiation with cisplatin and 5-FU yielded a 76% 3-year survival. Surgical resection of NPC follows failure of primary therapies (radiation and chemotherapy). See Chapter 11 for a more detailed discussion of nasophayryngeal carcinoma.

Epithelial Malignancies

Epithelial malignancies of the sinonasal region are relatively uncommon. They constitute 3% of all tumors of the upper aerodigestive tract. The majority arise in the maxillary sinuses (59%), followed by the nasal cavities (24%), then the ethmoid (15%) and sphenoid sinuses (1%).[14] Squamous cell carcinoma (SCC) generally presents in an advanced stage when diagnosed, because of its insidious progression. The mean age of presentation is 60 years, and men are slightly more commonly affected than women. Symptomatology relates to location of tumor and direction of growth. Stage predicts outcome more

significantly than histologic grade. Five-year survival ranges from 20 to 50% according to most studies.[14] Ten percent present with positive cervical nodes. Up to 20% will develop nodal metastasis at some point during their disease course.[14] Local recurrence is the most common manifestation of treatment failure.

Rhabdomyosarcoma

Rhabdomyosarcomas comprise one-fifth of all soft tissue sarcomas, and three-quarters of all soft tissue neoplasms in children. Over one-third of all cases of rhabdomyosarcoma occur in the head and neck. Patients present in the first and second decades of life. The orbit is the most common site of presentation, followed by the nasopharynx, middle ear/mastoid, and sinonasal tract[14] (Fig 13-4).

Histologic classification includes embryonal, alveolar, and pleomorphic types.[21] Embryonal subtypes are most common (85%), followed by alveolar (15%) and pleomorphic (<5%) variants. Table 13-3 demonstrates the clinical staging system for rhabdomyosarcoma, with 5-year survivals depending on extent of disease.

Immunohistologic staining in rhabdomyosarcoma will be positive for desmin and myoglobin. Electron microscopy reveals Z-bands.[22] Intracranially, rhabdomyosarcoma can arise from within the brain parenchyma, or from the meninges.

In general, outcome is determined by the location of primary disease and the presence of intracranial extension (meningeal involvement). Five-year survival in one study in patients with meningeal disease was 57%.[23] Treatment for rhabdomyosarcoma involves confirmatory biopsy followed by surgical resection if possible. Adjuvant treatment involves chemotherapy and radiation. Chemotherapeutic regimens include a combination of dactinomycin, vincristine, and cyclophosphamide. Radiation is given after induction of chemotherapy (6 to 9 weeks later) to a total dose of 59.4 Gy in 1.5 to 1.8-Gy fractions. A meningeal margin of 2 cm may be added if enhancement is noted intracranially. Frank brain involvement may necessitate whole brain radiation (30 Gy in 10 fractions or slightly less in younger patients).[23] In large, unresectable tumors, neoadjuvant treatment may be utilized followed by surgical resection.

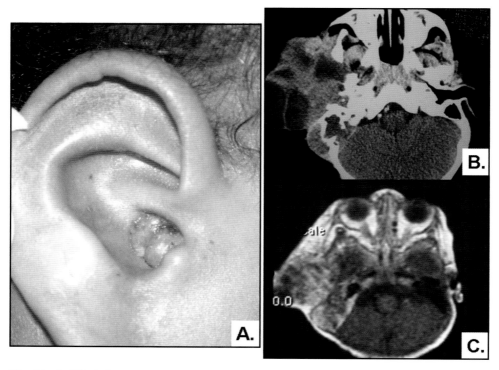

Fig 13–4. Rhabdomyosarcoma of the lateral temporal bone, middle ear and mastoid in a 6-month-old child. **A.** Firm granular mass filling external auditory canal. **B.** CT scan demonstrating large infiltrating tumor mass with destruction of bony external auditory canal and mastoid and eroding into middle and posterior cranial fossae. **C.** Contrast-enhanced T1 MRI demonstrating involvement of posterior cranial fossa.

Table 13–3. Staging and Prognosis of Rhabdomyosarcoma

Stage	Description	Five-Year Survival
Group I	Localized, completely resected disease without nodal involvement	83%
	Localized disease with microscopic residual or regional disease with positive nodes that are completely resected without microscopic residual or regional disease that is resected	
Group II	(with nodes and microscopic residual disease)	70%
Group III	Incomplete resection or biopsy with gross residual disease	52%
Group IV	Metastatic disease at presentation	20%

Chondrosarcoma

Chondrosarcomas comprise 0.15% of all intracranial tumors and 6% of skull base neoplasms.[24] Mean age of presentation is 30 to 50 years, and men and women are equally affected.[24-26] The jaws, larynx, and skull base are the most common sites of presentation in the head and neck. Sites of endochondral ossification in the skull base are thought to be the areas of neoplastic origin. The petro-occipital, sphenooccipital, and spheno-petrosal synchondrosis and the petrous temporal bone all undergo this type of ossification. Another theory suggests that residual mesenchymal cells from skull base development may give rise to chondrosarcomas[27] (Fig 13–5).

There are five histologic variants: conventional, mesenchymal, myxoid, clear cell (malignant chondroblastoma), and dedifferentiated. Each has a different prognosis. Histologically, there are hyaline and/or myxoid areas. The myxoid regions demonstrate chondrocytes within a mucinous matrix. In order to differentiate these tumors from chordomas, immunohistochemical staining is often necessary. Chondrosarcomas stain positive for vimentin and S-100; they remain negative for cytokeratin and epithelial membrane antigen.[28-30] The three histologic grades of chondrosarcoma are discussed in Table 13–4 with associated 5-year survival data. Survival is based in large part on histologic grade.[31]

Hearing loss, visual and gate disturbance, headaches, tinnitus, nausea, and vomiting are all presentations of these lesions. Multiple cranial nerve palsies are often noted on physical examination. On CT scan, chondrosarcoma erodes the skull base, and may form curvilinear calcifications (ringlets).[15] On T1-enhanced MRI, chondrosarcoma has a diffusely

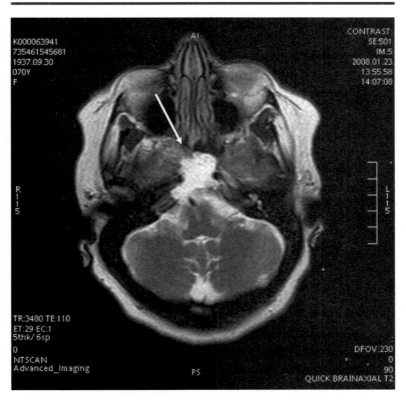

Fig 13–5. T2-weighted MRI demonstrating midline clival chondrasarcoma (*arrow*).

Table 13–4. Histologic Grading for Chondrosarcoma

Grade	Differentiation	Description	Five-Year Survival
I	Well	Small dark nuclei with multiple nuclei per lacuna. Chondroid to myxoid matrix. Calcification and bone formation common. Absent mitoses.	90%
II	Moderately	Moderate vesicular nuclei. Increased cellularity and matrix that is more myxoid. Less than 2 mitoses per 10 high-power field.	81%
III	Poorly	Moderate size vesicular nuclei with pleomorphism and prominent nucleoli. Spindle cell matrix with 2 or more mitoses per 10 high-power fields.	43%

enhancing heterogeneous appearance. Plain T1 images are generally isointense, whereas T2 studies demonstrate high signal.[15]

The majority of these skull base lesions are slow growing, but locally aggressive (grade I or II, histologically). Metastatic disease occurs in about 10% of cases. Survival in most patients is 8 to 10 years. Most patients will recur within 1 to 3 years of initial treatment.[14] The treatment of choice is surgical en bloc resection if possible. Complete resection is often difficult because of the vital neural and vascular structures that often surround these tumors. There are several small series describing complete resection and surgical cure of chondrosarcoma utilizing a combination of skull base approaches and resections.[24,32,33]

Conventional radiotherapy has had mixed results in the treatment of chondrosarcoma. One larger study utilizing proton beam radiation with doses ranging from 64 to 80 Gy in 38 fractions yielded 10-year local control rates of 98% in 200 patients.[29] Stereotactic radiosurgery has been reported to be efficacious in small series of patients. Muthukumar[34] and Debus[35] have reported success utilizing both single dose radiotherapy (24 to 40 Gy to the tumor bed) and fractionated doses of 64.9 Gy over 36 fractions. In a limited study, fractionated therapy seemed to have a greater efficacy, with a reported 5 year survival (and local control) of 100%.[35] Chemotherapy has not been shown to prolong survival, but may have a role in treatment of unresectable lesions or those with more aggressive grade II or III histology.[27]

Chordoma

Chordomas arise from embryologic notochord remnants. They occur in the sacrococcygeal region (50%), the vertebral column (15%), and the skull base, particularly the clivus (35%).[36] Chordomas account for about 4% of all bone tumors, and come in three histologic variants: conventional, chondroid, and dedifferentiated. Men and women are effected equally, and the mean age of presentation is 40 to 50 years.[37,38] Chordomas have been diagnosed in all age groups.[39] Because chordomas arise in the clivus, presentation includes a potential variety of cranial nerve palsies. CN III, IV, V, and VI can all be affected, resulting in diplopia, ptosis, and pupillary abnormalities (cavernous sinus syndrome). The cavernous sinus is involved in 54% to 75% of cases.[35,40] Headaches and diplopia are the most common reasons that patients seek medical attention. Significantly large lesions may cause pontine compression and obstructive hydrocephalus requiring cerebrospinal fluid shunting prior to resection. Table 13–5 describes the anatomic classification of skull base chordoma based on location and extent of disease.

Table 13–5. Classification of Chordoma

Type	Description
I	Chordomas confined to one compartment (bone) of the skull base
II	Chordomas extending to two or more areas of the skull base, but may be reached through one skull base procedure
III	Extensive tumor spread requiring more than one skull base approach for resection

MRI imaging of chordoma demonstrates replacement of the clival marrow with soft tissue. Chordomas demonstrate high signal on T2-weighted imaging, and are isointense to the bone and nasopharynx in T1 plain-imaging sequences. This is in contrast to the high signal of the marrow in the normal clivus. On CT imaging, the clivus is expanded and replaced by this lytic lesion, without evidence of boney sclerosis.[39] Most chordomas enhance to some degree with gadolinium on T1 sequences (Fig 13-6).

The classic histopathologic finding in chordomas, is the physaliferous cell; a vacuolated ("bubble-containing") epithelioid cell within a mucoid matrix. Cells exist in rows or cords and may appear lobular. The cells are polygonal and have an eosinophilic cytoplasm with eccentric nuclei. Chordomas histologically resemble the embryologic notochord.[41] Differentiation of these lesions from chondrosarcomas

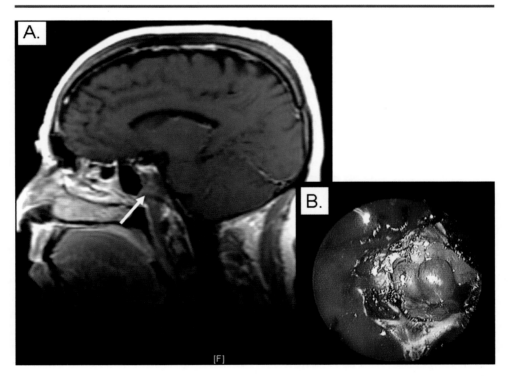

Fig 13–6. A. T1-weighted sagittal MRI of clival chordoma (*arrow*). Note change in signal characteristics of the central portion of the clivus and loss of marrow fat (see text). **B.** Transnasal endoscopic resection of tumor—note "bubblelike" appearance of tumor encountered after removal of posterior wall of sphenoid sinus.

is facilitated by immunohistochemistry. Chordomas stain for cytokeratin and epithelial membrane antigen.[42,43] Normal rests of bone may be noted within pathologic specimens, emphasizing the invasive nature of these tumors. They are not encapsulated, and complete surgical resection is impossible.[39] Chordomas are locally invasive and slow growing. As they progress, the dura is infiltrated and surrounding neural and vascular structures are encased in tumor. Mass effect on vital brainstem and pontine structures complicates resection of these lesions. Ten to 20% of patients will demonstrate systemic metastasis.[44] Dedifferentiated chordoma constitutes 1 to 8% of all chordomas. These contain malignant mesenchymal components such as fibrous histiocytoma, fibrosarcoma, and osteosarcoma.[45] This variant of chordoma may arise de novo, or as the result of irradiation. Survival in most patients is 6 to 12 months following diagnosis because of the aggressive nature of these neoplasms.[14]

Surgical resection combined with irradiation is the treatment of choice for chordoma. Subtotal resection with preservation of neurologic function is paramount. Decompression of the pons and brainstem allow for delivery of high-dose radiotherapy to residual tumor. No studies to date have demonstrated an improvement in survival with aggressive surgical resection compared to subtotal removal with subsequent radiotherapy.[46] The average survival for most patients is 4 to 8 years; however, two groups of patients appear to exist within the chordoma population. Those with an aggressive disease course seem to develop recurrence even within weeks of initial tumor resection, and those with a more indolent course of disease that can result in survival for many years. This emphasizes the unique biology of each tumor, and the variable nature of progression.[37,46-49] Chordomas metastasize in up to 10% of patients, with postmortem evidence of distant disease in as many of 40%.[39] The most common sites of metastasis include the lungs, skeletal bones, lymph nodes, the liver and skin.[14]

There is a clear dose-response relationship with regard to radiotherapy for chordomas. Conventional dosing of 45 to 60 Gy does not improve survival, with recurrence rates ranging from 50% to 100% depending on the series reviewed.[48,50] A survival benefit has been noted in patients receiving 60 Gy

or greater.[51] Proton beam radiation has the advantage of delivering high-dose therapy to a focal region of the skull base with a rapid drop-off that preserves vital surrounding neurologic structures (the Bragg peak effect).[52] A recent study by Hug et al[48] containing 33 patients revealed a 5-year survival of 79% in patients with chordoma, with little radiation-related morbidity. Smaller volumes were associated with better local control, advocating the role for cytoreductive surgery followed by radiation. This observation has been confirmed in other studies utilizing surgery and proton beam radiation.[53] Combination treatment of photon and proton beam radiotherapy (fractionated) has been shown in one study to provide local control with minimal toxicity.[54] Experience with stereotaxic radiosurgery has been limited to studies with few patients.[52]

Angiofibroma

Angiofibromas present in young males, ages 10 to 17 years. They are rare, accounting for 0.05% of head and neck neoplasms. They arise from the posterolateral nasal wall in the region of the sphenoplatine foramen. Histologically benign but locally invasive,[55-57] angiofibromas have histologic characteristics of vascular malformations.[58] The most common presentation of angiofibroma is nasal obstruction and epistaxis. Twenty to 36% of patients will present with intracranial involvement[26,59] (Fig 13-7).

MRI imaging demonstrates a heterogeneous lesion with flow voids. T1-enhanced images demonstrate brisk enhancement in the region of the infratemporal fossa and ptergopalatine region. On CT imaging, there is evidence of bone remodeling and erosion. A Holman Miller sign may be noted on CT or plain film imaging, characterized as anterior bowing of the posterior wall of the maxillary sinus.[20] The blood supply to these lesions comes primarily from the internal maxillary artery nasal branches, the accessory meningeal artery, and the pharyngeal and ascending palatine arteries[15] (Figs 13-8 and 13-9).

Histologically, these tumors demonstrate vascular and stroma elements. Intermixed within the fibrous stroma are gaping vascular channels that are "staghorn" in appearance. They are not encapsulated,[14] and are locally invasive. The majority of

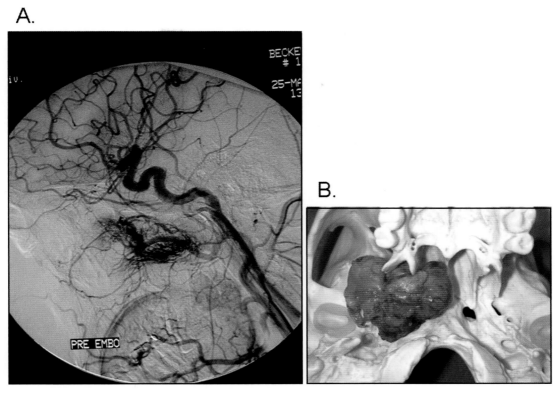

Fig 13–7. Juvenile nasopharyngeal angiofibroma. **A.** Preoperative embolization demonstrating tumor blush with major blood supply arising from sphenopalatine branches of internal maxillary artery. **B.** Intact resected specimen mounted on ventral skull base illustrating origin of tumor from within pterygomaxillary space with infratemporal fossa, pterygomaxillary, nasopharyngeal, and posterior nasal cavity components.

angiofibromas are positive for androgen receptors, thus predominantly presenting in young (pubescent) males.

Treatment is surgical resection with or without radiation therapy. The goal of treatment is removal of as much tumor as possible. Residual disease is generally monitored, as angiofibromas generally arrest or involute as the patient progresses through and completes puberty. Recurrence is defined by disease that progresses or becomes symptomatic after surgical resection. The likelihood of recurrence ranges from 0 to 50% depending on extent of initial disease. Higher recurrence rates are noted in patients with disease that extends beyond the bony confines of the nose. Preoperative endovascular embolization has been advocated to minimize intraoperative blood loss. When there is intracranial invasion, a common approach to this tumor includes a standard pterional craniotomy with zygomatic osteotomy for exposure of the pterygopalatine fossa. Endoscopic transnasal or transfacial exposure may necessary. Radiation therapy has been utilized as both primary and adjuvant treatment.[60-63] When surgical resection is subtotal in extensive disease, the standard dosage protocol is 30 Gy in 22 fractions. This has been shown to control disease locally.

Flutamide (testosterone receptor blocker) has been shown to reduce tumor size an average of 44% according to one study.[64] Other chemotherapeutic agents that have been used to treat angiofibroma include doxorubicin, decarbazine, doxorubicin, vincristine, dactinomycin, and cyclophosphamide.[65,66]

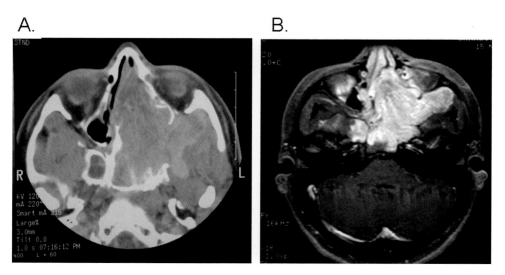

Fig 13–8. Juvenile nasopharyngeal angiofibroma. **A.** Contrast-enhanced axial CT scan demonstrating bony erosion of the lateral wall of the antrum with extension into the infratemporal fossa. **B.** Contrast-enhanced T1-weighted MRI at comparable level to CT scan.

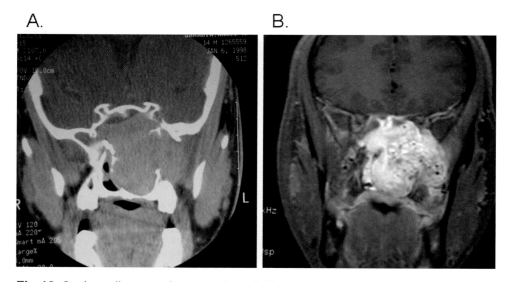

Fig 13–9. Juvenile nasopharyngeal angiofibroma. **A.** Contrast-enhanced coronal CT scan demonstrating bony erosion of the pterygoid plates with extension into the infratemporal fossa. **B.** Contrast-enhanced T1-weighted MRI at comparable level to CT scan with tumor filling pterygomaxillary space. Note presence of significant number and caliber of flow voids within the tumor.

Olfactory Neuroblastoma

Olfactory neuroblastomas originate from neuroectodermal tissue, particularly, the mitotically active basal layer of the olfactory epithelium, located along the superior one-third of the nasal septum, cribriform plate, and superior turbinate.[7] Pathologically, these tumors have either a diffuse or combined diffuse and lobular cellular pattern. Prominent eosinophilic neurofibrillary stroma, hyperchromatic nuclei, and small inconspicuous nucleoli characterize their histology. Mitoses are rare, as are Flexner true rosettes; however, Homer-Wright pseudorosettes are seen in up to 50% of cases.[7] Histologic grading systems such as that proposed by Hyams [67] predicts prognosis to some degree (Table 13-6).

Clinical staging as proposed by Kadish defines disease in relation to the confines of the nasal cavity[68] (Table 13-7). Biller et al[69] describe an alternative classification system that includes lesions that are radiographically unresectabe. Esthesioneuroblastoma is a member of the Ewing sarcoma and PNET (primitive neuroectodermal tumor) families[70] (Fig 13-10).

Treatment of esthesioneuroblastoma includes surgical resection followed by radiation and chemotherapy.[68,71,72] Survival is best predicted by initial Kadish stage, with A, B, and C disease having 5-year survivals of 75, 60, and 41%, respectively.[73] When there is intracranial extension, surgical resection generally involves a bicoronal craniotomy and removal of the supraorbital ridge. The intracranial portion of the tumor is removed along with any involved dura.

Both free and vascularized pericranium are used to close the dural defect. The sinonasal component of the tumor may be removed through the transcranial route, or with endoscopic assistance transnasally. If endoscopic resection in not possible, an open transnasal route may be utilized (Fig 13-11).

Radiation therapy is reserved for patients with high pathologic grade lesions and advanced Kadish stage disease. In a series published from the Mayo Clinic based on 49 patients, overall 5-year survival was found to be 69%.[72] In those with low-grade lesions, survival was 80% over 5 years. For those with high-grade disease, it was 40%. Recommendations from this study suggested that radiation should be administered in patients with low-grade disease in which margins are close, and in all cases of high-grade and recurrent disease. In patients with negative margins and no intracranial extent of disease,

Table 13–7. Kadish Staging of Olfactory Neuroblastoma

Stage	Description	Five-Year Survival
Stage A	Disease confined to nasal cavity	75%
Stage B	Disease confined to nasal cavity and one or more paranasal sinuses	60%
Stage C	Disease extending beyond the nasal cavity (into brain)	41%

Table 13–6. Hyams' Grading of Olfactory Neuroblastoma

Feature	Grade 1	Grade II	Grade III	Grade IV
Architecture	Lobular	Lobular	+/– Lobular	+/– Lobular
Mitotic activity	Absent	Present	Prominent	Marked
Nuclear pleomorphism	Absent	Moderate	Prominent	Marked
Fibrillary matrix	Prominent	Present	Minimal	Absent
Rosettes	+/– Homer Wright	+/– Homer Wright	Flexner	Absent
Necrosis	Absent	Absent	+/– present	Common

A. B.

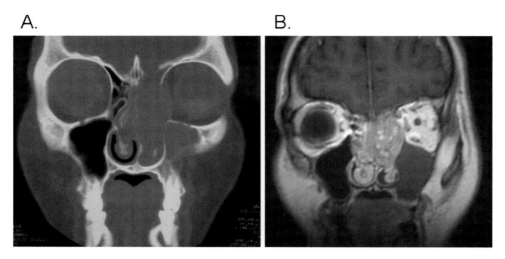

Fig 13–10. Olfactory neuroblastoma of the anterior cranial base. **A.** Bone algorithm coronal CT scan demonstrating erosion of the bone of the cribriform plate, fovea ethmoidalis, and lamina papyracea. **B.** Companion T1 MRI scan demonstrating involvement of the anterior fossa dura with extension into the medial orbit, sparing the orbital fat. Note differential signal characteristics between the tumor in the ethmoid and anterior skull base and the obstructive polyp and secretions in the ipsilateral maxillary antrum.

radiation is deferred and frequent radiographic monitoring proceeds. Other studies have suggested that radiation decreases the likelihood of local recurrence. Local tumor control rates with surgery alone ranged from 44 to 86% compared to combined treatment which decreased local failures to zero in some studies and 40% in others.[68,73-75] Five-year survival is increased from 10 to 15% to as high as 44% with combined surgery and radiation therapy.[76]

Chemotherapy has been reserved for patients with either inoperable disease or recurrence. Various agents such as thiotepa, doxorubicin, cyclophosphamide, vincristine, decarbazine, and nitrogen mustard have been used alone.[71] Cyclophosphamide and vincristine are often used in combination with varied responses.[71] In one series, Goldsweig et al demonstrated improvement in 19 of 20 patients with recurrent esthesioneuroblastoma.[77] For initially unresectable lesions, neoadjuvant therapies such as cyclophosphamide/doxorubicin/vincristine[78] cisplatin/VP-1621, and cisplatin/5-FU have been used as continuous infusions for 6 days (21-day cycles for four cycles) prior to resection.[79] Alternatively, a six-cycle regimen of cyclophophamide and vincristine

prior to surgical resection, has been utilized with some success.[70]

Paraganglioma

Paragangliomas are a diffuse group of tumors that arise from specialized autonomic neural crest cells that normally exist within the adrenal gland and paraganglia. In the adrenal medulla, they are pheochromocytomas. Extra-adrenal paraganglia that may harbor these tumors include the jugulotympanic carotid body; the laryngeal, subclavian, and aorticopulmonary paraganglia; the intravagal (nodose or jugular) ganglion; the aorticosympathetic paraganglia, and the visceral autonomic ganglia.[55,80,81] Carotid body tumors are the most common of the paragangliomas, constituting 60% of all lesions.[80,82] Ten percent are familiar, demonstrating autosomal dominant inheritance. Paragangliomas may present as part of the multiple endocrine neoplasia syndrome. The remainder of this discussion reviews skull base paragangliomas (glomus jugulare tumors) of the tympanic cavity and jugular bulb.

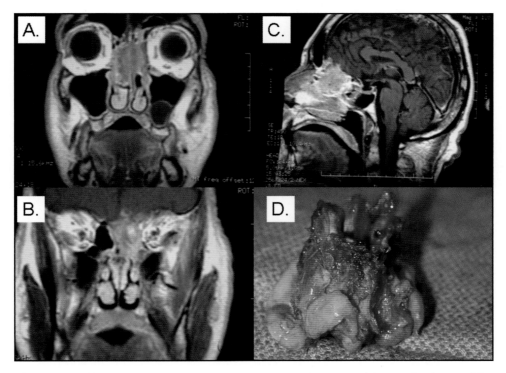

Fig 13–11. Olfactory neuroblastoma on the anterior cranial base. **A.** Coronal T1 MRI at the level of the midportion of the globe. Medial orbital wall is intact and tumor appears to be localized to the ethmoid labyrinth. **B.** Coronal T1 MRI at the level of the orbital apex and posterior ethmoid air cells indicating erosion of the fovea and anterior planum and enhancement of the anterior fossa dura. **C.** Sagittal MRI confirming transcranial extension of the tumor. **D.** En bloc anterior craniofacial resection specimen.

Only 2% to 10% of paragangliomas of the head and neck demonstrate malignant behavior. They tend to be locally aggressive, and recurrence following resection when intracranial involvement is present, occurs in up to 50% of cases.[83] Glomus tympanicum tumors arise from Jacobson's nerve, or from the promontory of the middle ear. Glomus jugulare tumors arise from the jugular bulb region, inferior to Jacobson's nerve. The range of presentation extends from the second to ninth decades of life. There is a female predominance. The most common presentation is unilateral hearing loss with pulsatile tinnitus. Large tumors may cause lower cranial nerve dysfunction, with intracranial hypertension related to occlusion of the sigmoid sinus.[84] Hypertension may be a presenting finding, as 1% to 4% of these tumors secrete catecholamines. Preoperative 24-hour

urine vanillylmandelic acid, metanephrines, and catecholamines should be evaluated so that perioperative blood pressure medications can be titrated.[84]

Imaging of these lesions includes CT and MRI. Paragangliomas briskly enhance in either modality. Angiography reveals a highly vascular lesion fed from the external carotid artery. These are generally selected individually for preoperative embolization (Fig 13-12).

Histologic characteristics of these lesions include two cell types: chief cells arranged in compact nests (Zellballen) and peripheral sustenacular cells which are modified Schwann cells. Chief cells are full of neurosecretory granules. Immunohistologic stains confirm the neuroendocrine origin of these lesions. Chief cells stain for NSE, synaptophysin, and chromogranin.[7]

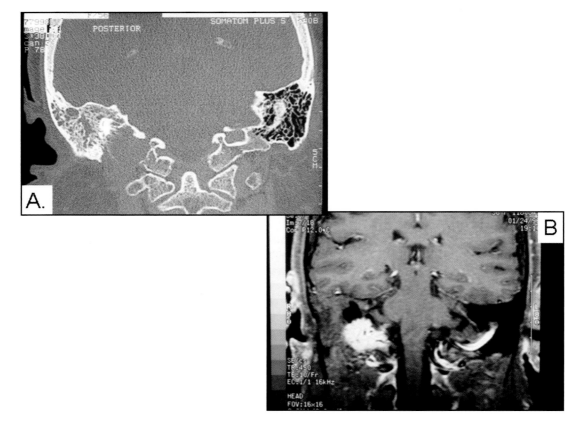

Fig 13–12. Paraganglioma of the temporal bone. **A.** Erosion of the temporal bone and expansion of the jugular foramen caused by large infiltrative glomus jugulare tumor. **B.** Companion coronal T1 MRI with hyperintense tumor localized within jugular foramen.

Glomus jugulare tumors are treated surgically through a lateral skull base approach utilizing a retrosigmoid craniectomy with far lateral extension. A mastoidectomy is performed, as is a lateral neck dissection to isolate the jugular vein in the neck, and the sigmoid sinus cranially. The sigmoid is ligated, and the tumor is dissected from the medial wall of the jugular bulb. This allows for protection of the lower cranial nerves which are medial to the jugular bulb. Gross total resection is possible in 40% to 80% of cases according to one study.[85-87]

Standard external beam radiation has been used in elderly patients or symptomatic tumors considered unresectable. Control has been acheived in 85% to 100% of cases with complication rates around to 10%. These complications include temporal bone necrosis, chronic mastoiditis, and brain necrosis.

Stereotaxic radiosurgery has been used in tumor doses up to 14.9 Gy. According to one study[88] including 41 patients, 37 patients had either stable disease, or evidence of regression at 10 years follow-up. There were no major complications.

RESECTION OF SKULL BASE MALIGNANCIES

Removal of skull base malignancies may be performed through a variety of approaches. The skull base is divided into the anterior, middle, and posterior cranial fossae, and approaches are designed to maximize exposure of each region while maintaining control of important neurovascular structures.

Subfrontal Approaches with Modifications

This approach is ideal for lesions such as chordomas and chondrosarcomas involving the midline cranial base inferiorly to the clivus. Olfactory neuroblastomas are also accessible through variations of this approach. When extended to the level of the clivus, the carotid, trigeminal roots, and hypoglossal nerves are the lateral extents of the dissection. A bicoronal incision is made from zygomatic root to zygomatic root. The pericranium is preserved under both skin flaps. This is elevated and displaced anteriorly, preserving the supraorbital neurovascular complex. A craniotomy is performed with bilateral orbitofrontoethmoidal osteotomies.[89] The frontal lobe is minimally elevated extradurally, or for olfactory neuroblastomas, the dura is incised to expose the intracranial extension of tumor.[89] This is resected, with a dural margin, and the dura is closed with a free pericranial graft from the mobilized vascularized pericranium. If more posterior extension is required for other lesions, the planum sphenoidale can be removed, and the sphenoid sinus opened. The optic nerves and carotids are exposed, and tumors of the clivus may be removed. This approach may be assisted with by an endoscope passed transnasally. The remaining defect is reconstructed with the vascularized aspect of the pericranium which is sutured to the remnants of the planum sphenoidale. The nasal cavity is customarily packed, and drains are left in the epidural and subgaleal spaces (Fig 13-13).

Lateral Approaches

Lateral portions of the anterior cranial fossa, the middle cranial fossa, and the infratemporal fossa and pterygopalatine regions can be approached through modifications of the pterional craniotomy.[90] An incision is made from the level of the root of the zygoma posterior to the hairline to the contralateral superior temporal line. The periosteum is preserved for duraplasty if necessary. The temporalis is mobilized with sharp subperiosteal dissection to preserve blood supply. Bur holes are made posterior to

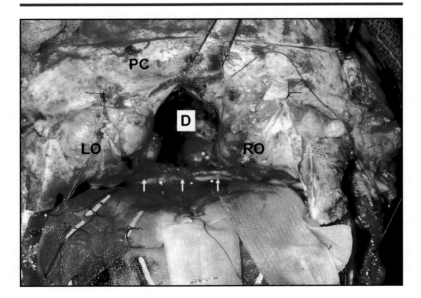

Fig 13–13. Cranial view of traditional open anterior skull base resection (ie, craniofacial resection) (LO, Left orbit; RO, Right orbit: PC, pericranial flap prior to transposition and inset; D, surgical defect; arrows indicate posterior limit of resection at the planum sphenoidale).

the fronto-zygomatic suture at the "keyhole." Additional holes are made just superior to the root of the zygoma, and at the posterior quarter of the superior temporal line. A bone flap is elevated, and the zygoma is separated at its root and anteriorly at the zygomaticofacial foramen. The dural is elevated from the sphenoid ridge and superior and lateral orbit. The orbital rim is then cut either medial or lateral to the supraorbital neurovascular bundle. This cut is extended posteriorly about 2 cm, and then turned laterally to include the superior and lateral orbit. This cut is taken to the inferior orbital fissure, separating the zygoma and superior orbital rim. The masseter is detached from the zygoma prior to removal. The temporalis may now be mobilized inferiorly to expose the infratemporal fossa and pterygopalatine fossa.[90] Subfrontal exposure is facilitated by removal of the orbital rim as needed. Extension of the preauricular incision into the neck allows for control of the carotid artery and jugular vein. For more posterior exposure, the petrous apex can be removed either intra- or extradurally, through retraction of the temporal lobe (subtemporal exposure). Important landmarks in this approach are the greater superficial petrosal nerve arising from the geniculate ganglion. It traverses the middle fossa from posterior to anterior toward the vidian canal. It overlies the petrous carotid which passes toward the cavernous sinus under the third division of the trigeminal nerve.

Reconstruction involves microplating of the zygoma and bone flap. For large skull base defects, free tissue grafts are utilized. The facial artery and vein serves as the blood supply for these tissue transfers.

Lateral and Posterior Fossa Approaches

Lesions of the petroclival region that cannot be reached through modifications of anterolateral approaches may be accessed through a petrosal approach.[91] A mastoidectomy is generally performed, and the sinodural angle is exposed along with the superior petrosal sinus. The lateral, superior, and posterior canals are exposed, but not entered. The petrous temporal bone is drilled medially, with the semicircular canals the limits of anterior and infe-

rior exposure. The petrosal sinus is ligated, and the dura is incised along the axis of the temporal lobe. The tentorium is incised, exposing the petroclival region, the midbrain/pons, the posterior cerebral artery, and CNs III, IV, V, and VI.

This exposure may be taken posteroinferiorly with removal of the semicircular canals. With translabyrinthine craniotomies alone, the petrosal sinus is not ligated. The presigmoid dura is exposed from the level of the jugular bulb to the sinodural angle. The facial nerve is identified and preserved in a shell of bone. This exposure allows for more anterior pontine exposure than that facilitated by a retrosigmoid craniectomy.

Posterior fossa exposure is facilitated by a retrosigmoid craniotomy, which involves removal of bone from posterior to the transverse-sigmoid junction to the midline. The cerebellopontine angle including CNs XII through V can be exposed with this craniotomy. It is one of three customary craniotomies used for removal of vestibular schwannomas. Most of these approaches are closed with an abdominal fat graft.

Inferior exposure of the lower cranial nerves with control of the jugular vein and carotid artery may be achieved with a modified far lateral approach as in the exposure for removal of a glomus jugulare tumor, as described by Fisch.[90] A posterior auricular incision is made, preserving the greater auricular nerve for grafting (if necessary). The ear canal is oversewn and the skin flap is mobilized anteriorly. In the neck, the carotid artery and jugular vein are identified and isolated. The facial nerve exiting the stylomastoid foramen is identified. A mastoidectomy and pre and post sigmoid bone dissection isolates this sinus. Translabyrinthine and transcochelar extension of this exposure may be added for tumors extending further into the tympanic region of the temporal bone.

RECONSTRUCTION OF THE CRANIAL BASE

In addition to the techniques described above, reconstruction of the cranial base involves a wide range of techniques, from the simple pericranial flap to a free tissue vascularized flap. Large dural defects can be closed with local pericranium, which is preserved in most craniotomies. If the defect is too large, porcine pericardial grafts may be utilized. In the anterior cranial fossa, small defects in the lateral skull base can be filled with split temporalis grafts.[92] The temporalis is divided along its blood supply, and a portion is placed within the infratemporal fossa skull base defect. The remaining muscle is rotated anteriorly into its normal anatomic position for preservation of cosmesis.[92]

Large cranial base defects are closed with rotational flaps and free tissue grafts with or without overlying skin grafts. These can be harvested from the trapezius, serratus anterior, rectus abodominis, latisimus dorsi, pectoralis major, and sternocleidomastoid muscles.[93]

The latissimus dorsi, and trapezius are common pedicle flaps used for lateral skull base reconstruction. Supplied by the thoracodorsal artery and vein, the latissimus can be rotated into the infratemporal fossa, for moderate size defects. The trapezius muscle may be rotated into the subtemporal region for reconstruction of these defects. The transverse cervical artery supplies this flap, and the greatest disadvantage postoperatively is the need for neutral head positioning to facilitate blood flow through supplying vessels.

Free tissue grafts commonly come from the rectus abdominis, and latissimus dorsi. The most significant bulk of tissue is provided by a rectus abdominis flap. It is the choice for any large lateral skull base defects. The most significant issues in any vascularized free tissue graft, is quality of donor vessels and size and appropriate of recipient vessels. As discussed, the facial artery and vein are common sites for anastomosis given their proximity to most skull base defects.

MANAGEMENT OF COMPLICATIONS IN SKULL BASE SURGERY

Complication rates for skull base surgery involving the anterior and anterolateral cranial regions range from 18 to 63%,[11] with mortality rates up to 4.7%. In one study of 54 patients with malignancies of the anterior and anterolateral skull base, 10 patients (18%) experienced complications related primarily to reconstruction. This emphasizes the difficulty encountered in such procedures where the separation of the intracranial compartment and aerodigestive tracts are violated.

In general, complications can be divided into three categories. Anticipation of complications permits proactive avoidance of problems. Brain injury can be circumvented with adequate bone removal during the approach portion of an operation. In the case of anterior cranial fossa resection, removal of the supraorbital ridge allows for a low approach to the middle cranial fossa. Avoiding CSF drainage during the extradural dissection can provide a buffer for direct contact with the frontal lobes. Head extension allows for posterior movement of the frontal lobes, eliminating the need for retractors.[11]

Infection is difficult to avoid as the operative field in many craniofacial resections involves entry into the paranasal sinuses and nasopharynx. All patients undergoing anterior or anterolateral craniofacial resection receive intravenous ceftriaxone. Clindamycin is present in all irrigating solutions. Intradural tumor is removed, and the dural envelope is reconstructed (often with a pericranial free graft) before extensive sinonasal work proceeds. The cranial compartment and nasal cavity are isolated from one another with a vascularized pericranial flap. Epidural and subgaleal drains are used, and the patient remains on perioperative antibiotics. Postoperative endoscopic examinations and debridement are vital in the management of nasal hygiene, particularly if adjuvant chemoradiation is anticipated.[11]

Cerebrospinal fluid fistula and pneumocephalus are two complications that may result from inadequate skull base reconstruction. Dural banding results from a foreshortened vascularized pericranial graft, in which the brain is tethered posterosuperiorly. The brain cannot re-expand into its normal anatomic configuration. This is observed in cases where the pericranial graft is brought over rather than under the orbital ridge. Pericranial complications include infarction from venous congestion, resulting in late onset pneumocephalus (postoperative days 3 to 7), or new epidural hemorrhage. Common causes for this include placement of the flap over the supraorbital ridge, or constriction of the flap by the orbital ridge during reapproximation.

CSF fistula remains another potential complication, avoided in part by attentive skull base reconstruction, the use of sealants after closure of the dura, and then again after placement of the vascularized pericranial graft. Nasal packing completes the closure. If pnuemocephalus or CSF is noted, endoscopic exploration is the first treatment employed, allowing for focused repair of a persistent defect with abdominal fat, sealants, and hemostatic agents.[11]

Large cranial base defects are generally closed with vascularized free flaps. These must be contoured to avoid compression and tethering of the brain. The fat component of a vascularized graft is contoured to allow for normal brain expansion. This side is then placed against the brain to prevent CSF leakage and pneumocephalus.[94]

Intracranial hypotension occurs when there is a negative pressure differential between the intracranial and spinal compartments. This may occur iatrogenically because of overuse of lumbar spinal drainage. Obtaining brain relaxation by cistern dissection rather than spinal drainage can avoid this complication. If a drain is used, the diagnosis of intracranial hypotension is confirmed with an intracranial pressure monitor. If the head of bed is elevated in the setting of intracranial hypotension, the intracranial pressure will be negative. The situation is remedied by removing the lumbar drain and placing a blood patch.[94]

Cerebrovascular complications related to skull base surgery include vasospasm (rare) and venous thrombosis. In one series of 120 cases over 14 years, venous complications constituted 15% (3 out of 20) of the major complications. These can be related to congenital venous anatomy, vascular changes resulting from tumor removal, or injury to a vital draining vein during lesion resection. This complication is avoided by judiciously preserving veins during surgery, maintaining normal hydration status pre- and postoperatively, and if a vein must be taken, temporarily occluding it to determine if venous congestion or edema results. In cases where the sagittal sinus may need to be sacrificed, MR venography should be performed with subsequent catheter angiography/venography to document venous drainage.[94] In cases of sinus thrombosis following surgery, the risks and benefits of anticoagulation must be considered to prevent subsequent propagation of thrombosis.

Endoscopic Resection of Skull Base Malignancies

Advances in neuroimaging, optics, instrumentation, and surgical navigation coupled with an improved understanding of the biology of cranial base neoplasms have led to the development of transnasal endoscopic techniques for the resection of selected malignant cranial base neoplasms. Transnasal endoscopic surgery of the paranasal sinuses was originally developed for the treatment of inflammatory disease and gained widespread popularity in the 1980s. Increased surgical experience in conjunction with refinements in instrumentation and the development of new biomaterials and sealants lead to the successful application of endoscopic techniques in the repair of cranial base defects. Endoscopic techniques have been successfully used in the transnasal resection of a variety of benign sinonasal neoplasm including the inverted papilloma, juvenile nasopharyngeal angiofibroma, various benign fibro-osseous lesions, and neural tumors. Transnasal endoscopic surgery for (trans) cranial tumors began with the applications of these techniques to pituitary adenomas. The initial series of 50 patients reported in 1997 indicated improved patient outcomes, reduced length of stay, and improved patient satisfaction related to endoscopic tumor resection.[95] At the same time Banhiran and Casiano[96] and others were reporting the use of the endoscope adjunctively in anterior craniofacial resection. In the endoscopic-assisted craniofacial resection the inferior portions of the procedure including removal of the inferior nasal septum, sphenoid and frontal sinusotomies, and medial orbital exposure were performed transnasal and obviated the need for any facial incision. The frontal craniotomy was performed in the standard fashion and an en bloc removal on the anterior cranial base could be performed. Buchmann[97] reported the utility of endoscopic techniques in 78 patients with anterior skull base and paranasal sinus malignancies. In their institutional series of 78 patients with a variety of histologies, 46% had a portion of the tumor resection with the endoscope.

The next iteration of the procedure involved extending the resection superiorly with removal of the bone of the planum spenoidale posteriorly, the fovea ethmoidalis laterally, and ethmoid bone anterior to the cristae galli exposing the dura of the anterior cranial fossa. The dura can be resected and submitted for frozen section analysis and the resection can be extended as indicated. Performed in this fashion the endoscopic anterior craniofacial resection could provide an oncologic result similar to than obtained with a standard transcranial procedure.[98]

Concerns remain regarding the oncologic outcomes in endoscopic resection for transcranial skull base malignancies. Data from several centers indicate local and regional control rates similar to those obtained with conventional open procedures.[99,100] Dave[99] (2007) has reported 17 patients with malignant anterior skull base tumors treated with fully endoscopic transnasal craniofacial resection. The histology was varied in this series with 53% of patients having an olfactory neuroblastoma. With a mean follow-up of 34 months, local control for all malignant neoplasms was 94%. The observed major complication rate of 11% is less than that reported in large series of open craniofacial resection.

Studies of endoscopic cranial base resections will be limited by the same factors that are observed in studies of open procedures such as limited numbers of patients and the heterogeneity of the tumors observed in this region. Studies limited to olfactory neuroblastoma indicate no local failures in patients treated with endoscopic craniofacial resection followed by postoperative conformal 3-D radiation therapy.[101-102]

Endoscopic techniques will remain critical in the management of patients with malignant tumors of the cranial base. Endoscopic techniques have evolved from enhancing physical examination, biopsy and surveillance to having a significant role in the definitive surgical resection of malignant tumors of the anterior cranial base.

CONCLUSION

Cranial base malignancies present a challenge because of their heterogeneity and difficult anatomic locations. These complex lesions are best managed by a team of physicians including neurosurgeons, otolaryngologists, radiation oncologists, medical oncologists, plastic surgeons, and pathologists. Treatment goals include management of disease without sacrifice of patient quality of life. This may require that surgical resection be minimized in some cases, and other therapies be offered in an attempt to preserve neurologic function. As radiation therapies become more precise, and chemotherapeutic agents target more specific tumor cell receptors, surgical approaches will evolve. This is most evident with the development of advanced endoscopic techniques. As treatment regimens change, treatment efficacies must continue to improve, and patient quality of life must not be sacrificed.

REFERENCES

1. Ketcham AS, Wilkins RH, Vanburen JM, Smith RR. A combined intracranial facial approach to the paranasal sinuses. *Am J Surg.* 1963;106:698–703.
2. Lang J. *The Anterior and Middle Cranial Fossae Including the Cavernous Sinus and Orbit.* New York, NY: Raven Press; 1993.
3. Netter FH. *Volume I: Nervous System, Part I: Anatomy and Physiology.* Summit, NJ: Ciba-Geigy; 1996.
4. *Operative Skull Base Surgery.* New York, NY: Churchill Livingstone; 1997.
5. Rhoton AL. *Cranial Anatomy and Surgical Approaches.* Philadelphia, Pa: Lippincott Williams & Williams; 2003.
6. Rhoton AL Jr. The temporal bone and transtemporal approaches. *Neurosurgery.* 2000;47:S211–S265.
7. *Skull Base Surgery: Anatomy, Biology, and Technology.* Philadelphia, Pa: Lippincott Raven; 1997.
8. Lang J. *Anatomy of the Posterior Cranial Fossa.* New York, NY: Raven Press; 1993.
9. Rhoton AL, Jr. The cerebral veins. *Neurosurgery.* 2002;51:S159–S205.
10. Rhoton AL, Jr. Jugular foramen. *Neurosurgery.* 2000;47:S267–S285.
11. Origitano TC, Petruzzelli GJ, Vandevender D, Emami B. Management of malignant tumors of the anterior and anterolateral skull base. *Neurosurg Focus.* 2002;12:e7.
12. Spiro RH, Huvos AG, Strong EW. Adenoid cystic carcinoma: factors influencing survival. *Am J Surg.* 1979;138:579-583.
13. Tomich C. Adenoid cystic carcinoma In: Ellis G, PL A, Gnepp D, eds. *Surgical Pathology of the Salivary Glands.* Philadelphia, Pa: WB Saunders; 1991.

14. Barnes L, Kapadia SB, Nemzek WR, Weissman JL, Janecka IP. Biology of selected skull base tumors. In: Janecka IP, Tiedemann K, eds. *Skull Base Surgery: Anatomy, Biology, and Technology*. Philadelphia, Pa: Lippincott-Raven; 1997:263–289.

15. Durden DD, Williams DW, 3rd. Radiology of skull base neoplasms. *Otolaryngol Clin North Am*. 2001;34:1043–1064, vii.

16. Ellis ER, Million RR, Mendenhall WM, Parsons JT, Cassisi NJ. The use of radiation therapy in the management of minor salivary gland tumors. *Int J Radiat Oncol Biol Phys*. 1988;15:613–617.

17. Garden AS, Weber RS, Ang KK, Morrison WH, Matre J, Peters LJ. Postoperative radiation therapy for malignant tumors of minor salivary glands. Outcome and patterns of failure. *Cancer*. 1994;73:2563–2569.

18. Schramm VL, Jr., Imola MJ. Management of nasopharyngeal salivary gland malignancy. *Laryngoscope*. 2001;111:1533–1544.

19. Laurie SA, Licitra L. Systemic therapy in the palliative management of advanced salivary gland cancers. *J Clin Oncol*. 2006;24:2673–2678.

20. Richardson MS. Pathology of skull base tumors. *Otolaryngol Clin North Am*. 2001;34:1025–1042, vii.

21. Cotran RS, Kumar V, Robbins SL. Soft tissue tumors. In: Robbins SL, ed. *Robbins Pathologic Basis of Disease*. 5th ed. Philadelphia, Pa: Saunders;1994:1267–1268.

22. Ewend M, Castillo M, Weaver K. Meningeal sarcoma. In: Winn H, ed. *Youman's Neurological Surgery*. Philadelphia, Pa: Saunders; 2004:1141–1146.

23. Raney RB, Meza J, Anderson JR, et al. Treatment of children and adolescents with localized parameningeal sarcoma: experience of the Intergroup Rhabdomyosarcoma Study Group protocols IRS-II through -IV, 1978–1997. *Med Pediatr Oncol*. 2002;38:22–32.

24. Kveton JF, Brackmann DE, Glasscock ME, 3rd, House WF, Hitselberger WE. Chondrosarcoma of the skull base. *Otolaryngol Head Neck Surg*. 1986;94:23–32.

25. Austin-Seymour M, Munzenrider J, Goitein M, et al. Fractionated proton radiation therapy of chordoma and low-grade chondrosarcoma of the base of the skull. *J Neurosurg*. 1989;70:13–17.

26. Hassounah M, Al-Mefty O, Akhtar M, Jinkins JR, Fox JL. Primary cranial and intracranial chondrosarcoma. A survey. *Acta Neurochir (Wien)*. 1985;78:123–132.

27. Neff B, Sataloff RT, Storey L, Hawkshaw M, Spiegel JR. Chondrosarcoma of the skull base. *Laryngoscope*. 2002;112:134–139.

28. Coltrera MD, Googe PB, Harrist TJ, Hyams VJ, Schiller AL, Goodman ML. Chondrosarcoma of the temporal bone. Diagnosis and treatment of 13 cases and review of the literature. *Cancer*. 1986;58:2689–2696.

29. Rosenberg AE, Nielsen GP, Keel SB, et al. Chondrosarcoma of the base of the skull: a clinicopathologic study of 200 cases with emphasis on its distinction from chordoma. *Am J Surg Pathol*. 1999;23:1370–1378.

30. Wojno KJ, Hruban RH, Garin-Chesa P, Huvos AG. Chondroid chordomas and low-grade chondrosarcomas of the craniospinal axis. An immunohistochemical analysis of 17 cases. *Am J Surg Pathol*. 1992;16:1144–1152.

31. Evans HL, Ayala AG, Romsdahl MM. Prognostic factors in chondrosarcoma of bone: a clinicopathologic analysis with emphasis on histologic grading. *Cancer*. 1977;40:818–831.

32. Al-Mefty O, Fox JL, Rifai A, Smith RR. A combined infratemporal and posterior fossa approach for the removal of giant glomus tumors and chondrosarcomas. *Surg Neurol*. 1987;28:423–431.

33. Charabi S, Engel P, Bonding P. Myxoid tumours in the temporal bone. *J Laryngol Otol*. 1989;103:1206–1209.

34. Muthukumar N, Kondziolka D, Lunsford LD, Flickinger JC. Stereotactic radiosurgery for chordoma and chondrosarcoma: further experiences. *Int J Radiat Oncol Biol Phys*. 1998;41:387–392.

35. Debus J, Schulz-Ertner D, Schad L, et al. Stereotactic fractionated radiotherapy for chordomas and chondrosarcomas of the skull base. *Int J Radiat Oncol Biol Phys*. 2000;47:591–596.

36. Heffelfinger MJ, Dahlin DC, MacCarty CS, Beabout JW. Chordomas and cartilaginous tumors at the skull base. *Cancer*. 1973;32:410–420.

37. Forsyth PA, Cascino TL, Shaw EG, et al. Intracranial chordomas: a clinicopathological and prognostic study of 51 cases. *J Neurosurg*. 1993;78:741–747.

38. O'Connell JX, Renard LG, Liebsch NJ, Efird JT, Munzenrider JE, Rosenberg AE. Base of skull chordoma. A correlative study of histologic and clinical features of 62 cases. *Cancer*. 1994;74:2261–2267.

39. Lanzino G, Dumont AS, Lopes MB, Laws ER Jr. Skull base chordomas: overview of disease, management options, and outcome. *Neurosurg Focus*. 2001;10:e12.

40. Al-Mefty O, Borba LA. Skull base chordomas: a management challenge. *J Neurosurg.* 1997;86: 182-189.

41. Burger P, Scheithauer B. *Tumors of the Central Nervous System.* Washington, DC: American Registry of Pathology; 1994.

42. Meis JM, Giraldo AA. Chordoma. An immunohistochemical study of 20 cases. *Arch Pathol Lab Med.* 1988;112:553-556.

43. Miettinen M. Chordoma. Antibodies to epithelial membrane antigen and carcinoembryonic antigen in differential diagnosis. *Arch Pathol Lab Med.* 1984;108:891-892.

44. Laws E, Thapar K. Parasellar lesions other than pituitary adenomas. In: Powell M, Lightman S, eds. *Management of Pituitary Tumors: A Handbook.* New York, NY: Churchill-Livingstone; 1996: 175-222.

45. Hruban RH, Traganos F, Reuter VE, Huvos AG. Chordomas with malignant spindle cell components. A DNA flow cytometric and immunohistochemical study with histogenetic implications. *Am J Pathol.* 1990;137:435-447.

46. Watkins L, Khudados ES, Kaleoglu M, Revesz T, Sacares P, Crockard HA. Skull base chordomas: a review of 38 patients, 1958-88. *Br J Neurosurg.* 1993;7:241-248.

47. Benk V, Liebsch NJ, Munzenrider JE, Efird J, McManus P, Suit H. Base of skull and cervical spine chordomas in children treated by high-dose irradiation. *Int J Radiat Oncol Biol Phys.* 1995;31:577-581.

48. Hug EB, Loredo LN, Slater JD, et al. Proton radiation therapy for chordomas and chondrosarcomas of the skull base. *J Neurosurg.* 1999;91: 43243-43249.

49. Terahara A, Niemierko A, Goitein M, et al. Analysis of the relationship between tumor dose inhomogeneity and local control in patients with skull base chordoma. *Int J Radiat Oncol Biol Phys.* 1999;45:351-358.

50. Catton C, O'Sullivan B, Bell R, et al. Chordoma: long-term follow-up after radical photon irradiation. *Radiother Oncol.* 1996;41:67-72.

51. Prabhu SS, Demonte F. Treatment of skull base tumors. *Curr Opin Oncol.* 2003;15:209-212.

52. Hug EB, Slater JD. Proton radiation therapy for chordomas and chondrosarcomas of the skull base. *Neurosurg Clin North Am.* 2000;11:627-638.

53. Crockard A, Macaulay E, Plowman PN. Stereotactic radiosurgery. VI. Posterior displacement of the brainstem facilitates safer high dose radiosurgery

54. Noel G, Habrand JL, Mammar H, et al. Combination of photon and proton radiation therapy for chordomas and chondrosarcomas of the skull base: the Centre de Protontherapie D'Orsay experience. *Int J Radiat Oncol Biol Phys.* 2001;51:392-398.

55. Barnes L, Kapadia SB. The biology and pathology of selected skull base tumors. *J Neurooncol.* 1994;20:213-240.

56. Barnes L, Weber PC, Krause J, Contis L, Janecka I. Angiofibroma: a flow cytometric evaluation of 31 cases. *Skull Base Surg.* 1992;2:195-198.

57. Kapadia SB, Popek EJ, Barnes L. Pediatric otorhinolaryngic pathology: diagnosis of selected lesions. *Pathol Annu.* 1994;29 (pt 1):159-209.

58. Beham A, Beham-Schmid C, Regauer S, Aubock L, Stammberger H. Nasopharyngeal angiofibroma: true neoplasm or vascular malformation? *Adv Anat Pathol.* 2000;7:36-46.

59. Jafek BW, Krekorian EA, Kirsch WM, Wood RP. Juvenile nasopharyngeal angiofibroma: management of intracranial extension. *Head Neck Surg.* 1979;2:119-128.

60. Cummings BJ, Blend R, Keane T, et al. Primary radiation therapy for juvenile nasopharyngeal angiofibroma. *Laryngoscope.* 1984;94:1599-1605.

61. Economou TS, Abemayor E, Ward PH. Juvenile nasopharyngeal angiofibroma: an update of the UCLA experience, 1960-1985. *Laryngoscope.* 1988;98:170-175.

62. Gullane PJ, Davidson J, O'Dwyer T, Forte V. Juvenile angiofibroma: a review of the literature and a case series report. *Laryngoscope.* 1992;102: 928-933.

63. Wiatrak BJ, Koopmann CF, Turrisi AT. Radiation therapy as an alternative to surgery in the management of intracranial juvenile nasopharyngeal angiofibroma. *Int J Pediatr Otorhinolaryngol.* 1993;28:51-61.

64. Gates GA, Rice DH, Koopmann CF, Jr., Schuller DE. Flutamide-induced regression of angiofibroma. *Laryngoscope.* 1992;102:641-644.

65. Goepfert H, Cangir A, Lee YY. Chemotherapy for aggressive juvenile nasopharyngeal angiofibroma. *Arch Otolaryngol.* 1985;111:285-289.

66. Schick B, Kahle G, Hassler R, Draf W. Chemotherapy of juvenile angiofibroma—an alternative? *HNO.* 1996;44:148-152.

67. Hyams V, Batsakis J, Michaels L. *Tumors of the Upper Respiratory Tract and Ear.* Washington DC: Armed Forces Institute of Pathology; 1988.

for clival chordoma. *Br J Neurosurg.* 1999;13: 65-70.

68. Kadish S, Goodman M, Wang CC. Olfactory neuroblastoma. A clinical analysis of 17 cases. *Cancer.* 1976;37:1571-1576.

69. Biller HF, Lawson W, Sachdev VP, Som P. Esthesioneuroblastoma: surgical treatment without radiation. *Laryngoscope.* 1990;100:1199-1201.

70. Oskouian RJ, Jr., Jane JA, Sr., Dumont AS, Sheehan JM, Laurent JJ, Levine PA. Esthesioneuroblastoma: clinical presentation, radiological, and pathological features, treatment, review of the literature, and the University of Virginia experience. *Neurosurg Focus.* 2002;12:e4.

71. Jacob HE. Chemotherapy for cranial base tumors. *J Neurooncol.* 1994;20:327-335.

72. Morita A, Ebersold MJ, Olsen KD, Foote RL, Lewis JE, Quast LM. Esthesioneuroblastoma: prognosis and management. *Neurosurgery.* 1993;32:706-714; discussion 14-15.

73. Elkon D, Hightower SI, Lim ML, Cantrell RW, Constable WC. Esthesioneuroblastoma. *Cancer.* 1979; 44:1087-1094.

74. Dulguerov P, Calcaterra T. Esthesioneuroblastoma: the UCLA experience 1970-1990. *Laryngoscope.* 1992;102:843-849.

75. Foote RL, Morita A, Ebersold MJ, et al. Esthesioneuroblastoma: the role of adjuvant radiation therapy. *Int J Radiat Oncol Biol Phys.* 1993;27: 835-842.

76. Parsons JT, Mendenhall WM, Mancuso AA, Cassisi NJ, Million RR. Malignant tumors of the nasal cavity and ethmoid and sphenoid sinuses. *Int J Radiat Oncol Biol Phys.* 1988;14:11-22.

77. Goldsweig HG, Sundaresan N. Chemotherapy of recurrent esthesioneuroblastoma. Case report and review of the literature. *Am J Clin Oncol.* 1990;13:139-143.

78. Chao KS, Kaplan C, Simpson JR, et al. Esthesioneuroblastoma: the impact of treatment modality. *Head Neck.* 2001;23:749-757.

79. Polonowski JM, Brasnu D, Roux FX, Bassot V. Esthesioneuroblastoma. Complete tumor response after induction chemotherapy. *Ear Nose Throat J.* 1990;69:743-746.

80. Barnes L, Taylor SR. Carotid body paragangliomas. A clinicopathologic and DNA analysis of 13 tumors. *Arch Otolaryngol Head Neck Surg.* 1990;116:447-453.

81. Gee MS, Kliewer KE, Hinton DR. Nucleolar organizer regions in paragangliomas of the head and neck. *Arch Otolaryngol Head Neck Surg.* 1992;118:380-383.

82. Barnes L, Taylor SR. Vagal paragangliomas: a clinical, pathological, and DNA assessment. *Clin Otolaryngol Allied Sci.* 1991;16:376-382.

83. Weber PC, Patel S. Jugulotympanic paragangliomas. *Otolaryngol Clin North Am.* 2001;34: 1231-1240, x.

84. Robertson J, Brodkey J, Wang P. Glomus Jugulare Tumors. In: Winn H, ed. *Youmans Neurological Surgery.* Philadelphia, Pa: Saunders; 2004:1295-1310.

85. Gjuric M, Rudiger Wolf S, Wigand ME, Weidenbecher M. Cranial nerve and hearing function after combined-approach surgery for glomus jugulare tumors. *Ann Otol Rhinol Laryngol.* 1996;105: 949-954.

86. Green JD Jr, Brackmann DE, Nguyen CD, Arriaga MA, Telischi FF, De la Cruz A. Surgical management of previously untreated glomus jugulare tumors. *Laryngoscope.* 1994;104:917-921.

87. Gstoettner W, Matula C, Hamzavi J, Kornfehl J, Czerny C. Long-term results of different treatment modalities in 37 patients with glomus jugulare tumors. *Eur Arch Otorhinolaryngol.* 1999;256: 351-355.

88. Pollock BE, Foote RL. The evolving role of stereotactic radiosurgery for patients with skull base tumors. *J Neurooncol.* 2004;69:199-207.

89. Osguthorpe JD, Patel S. Craniofacial approaches to tumors of the anterior skull base. *Otolaryngol Clin North Am.* 2001;34:1123-1142, ix.

90. Branovan DI, Schaefer SD. Lateral craniofacial approaches to the skull base and infratemporal fossa. *Otolaryngol Clin North Am.* 2001;34: 1175-1195, x.

91. al-Mefty O, Ayoubi S, Smith RR. The petrosal approach: indications, technique, and results. *Acta Neurochir Suppl (Wien).* 1991;53:166-170.

92. Liu JK, Niazi Z, Couldwell WT. Reconstruction of the skull base after tumor resection: an overview of methods. *Neurosurg Focus.* 2002;12:e9.

93. Day TA, Davis BK. Skull base reconstruction and rehabilitation. *Otolaryngol Clin North Am.* 2001; 34:1241-1257, xi.

94. Origitano TC, Petruzzelli GJ, Leonetti JP, Vandevender D. Combined anterior and anterolateral approaches to the cranial base: complication analysis, avoidance, and management. *Neurosurgery.* 2006;58:ONS-327-336; discussion ONS-36-37.

95. Jho HD, Carrau RL. Endoscopic endonasal transsphenoidal surgery: experience with 50 patients. *J Neurosurg.* 1997;87:44-51.

96. Banhiran W, Casiano RR. Endoscopic sinus surgery for benign and malignant nasal and sinus neoplasm. *Curr Opin Otolaryngol Head Neck Surg.* 2005;13:50-54.

97. Buchmann L, Larsen C, Pollack A, Tawfik O, Sykes K, Hoover LA. Endoscopic techniques in resection of anterior skull base/paranasal sinus malignancies. *Laryngoscope.* 2006;116:1749-1754.

98. Castelnuovo PG, Belli E, Bignami M, Battaglia P, Sberze F, Tomei G. Endoscopic nasal and anterior craniotomy resection for malignant nasoethmoid tumors involving the anterior skull base. *Skull Base.* 2006;16:15-18.

99. Dave SP, Bared A, Casiano RR. Surgical outcomes and safety of transnasal endoscopic resection for anterior skull tumors. *Otolaryngol Head Neck Surg.* 2007;136:920-927.

100. Podboj J, Smid L. Endoscopic surgery with curative intent for malignant tumors of the nose and paranasal sinuses. *EJSO.* 2007;33:1081-1806.

101. Walch C, Stammberger H, Anderhuber W, et al. The minimally invasive approach to olfactory neuroblastoma: Combined endoscopic and stereotactic treatment, *Laryngoscope.* 2000;110:635-640.

102. Belli E, Castelnuovo PG, Bignami M, et al, Endoscopic nasal and anterior craniotomy resection for malignant nasoethmoidal tumors involving the anterior skull base. *Skull Base.* 2006;16:15-18.

14

Advanced Oral Cavity Cancer

Brett A. Miles
Larry L. Myers

INTRODUCTION

The oral cavity is the most common location for cancer of the upper aerodigestive tract. The management of early staged oral cavity cancer (stage I and II) is typically treated by a single modality, but the management of advanced oral cavity cancer (stage III and stage IV) is increasingly complex. It presents a wide array of challenges that require the surgeon to avoid, limit or restore the severe functional impairments to mastication, deglutition, and phonation resulting from surgical and adjunctive measures.

Squamous cell carcinoma (SCC) in the head and neck region is the sixth most prevalent neoplasm in the world.[1] Although SCC of the oral cavity is more common in developing countries, it continues to plague more developed countries.[2] In the United States, SCC of the oral cavity represents 3% to 4% of all new cancers. The American Cancer Society estimates about 30,990 new cases (20,180 in men and 10,810 in women) of oral cavity and oropharyngeal cancer will be diagnosed in the United States in 2006 with an estimated 7,430 deaths attributed to this disease.[3-7] Higher rates reported in developing countries are likely due to a combination of environmental risk factors and possible differences in the genetic profile of specific local populations.[4-9]

A literature review of SCC of the head and neck reveals that the reported overall prognosis of these malignancies remains unchanged.[10] Although loco-regional control in oral cavity cancers has improved significantly with the use of multimodality therapy, the incidence of distant failure has doubled.[11] This is especially true for advanced stage disease. Over the last 20 years, however, the number of new cases of this disease has been decreasing at a rate slightly above 1% per year. The decrease in new oral cavity cancer diagnoses is most likely secondary to more effective cancer prevention strategies. The mortality rate for oral cavity and oropharyngeal cancer has been decreasing since the late 1970s.[3,6,7,12]

This chapter discusses the pathologies, epidemiology, radiographic evaluation, management (surgery, chemotherapy, irradiation therapy), reconstruction, and prognosis of advanced malignancies arising from the oral cavity.

ANATOMY

The oral cavity is divided into seven anatomic subsites: the lips, buccal mucosa, upper and lower alveolar ridges, floor of the mouth, anterior two-thirds of the tongue, retromolar trigone, and hard palate. The anterior boundary of the oral cavity is the vermillion border of the upper and lower lips and the posterior boundary is the anterior surface of the faucial arch. The entire oral cavity is lined by stratified squamous epithelium. The epithelial lining is divided into two broad types, the masticatory epithelium and lining epithelium. The masticatory epithelium covers the surfaces involved in the processing of food, namely, the tongue, gingiva, and hard palate. The magnitude of physical forces during function dictates the degree of epithelial keratinization for any given surface within the oral cavity. The lining epithelium is nonkeratinized stratified squamous epithelium and covers the remaining surfaces of the oral cavity.

The pattern of lymphatic drainage of the oral cavity has been well established in the literature.[13-15] The presence of cervical lymph node metastasis has been repeatedly correlated with the size of the primary tumor, depth of invasion, location, and the degree of differentiation. In general, the frequency of lymph node metastasis increases with the size and depth of penetration of the lesion. Additionally, a further posterior location in the oral cavity of the primary lesion is correlated to a greater the risk of lymphatic spread to lower echelon nodal basins (levels III-IV). The lymphatic spread of oral SCC generally occurs in an orderly manner, involving first the uppermost (levels I-II), then middle (levels II-III), and finally the lower cervical lymph nodes (level IV). The pattern of lymphatic spread often follows the arterial supply of the region in which the primary tumor is located and primary and secondary echelons of lymph node drainage have been derived for each region of the oral cavity. The lip, cheek, and anterior gingiva drain to submandibular and submental lymph node basins (levels I-II) and occasionally the inferior parotid nodal basin. The posterior gingiva and palate drain to the internal jugular chain and lateral retropharyngeal nodes (levels II-IV). Lymphatic drainage for the tongue and floor of mouth includes the internal jugular, subdigastric, omohyoid, submandibular, and submental nodal basins (levels I-III). The deep lymphatic network for the oral tongue consists of anterior, lateral, and central lymphatic pathways. The anterior pathway drains the tip of the oral tongue and primarily drains to level III (or less commonly levels I-II). The lateral group drains the lateral one-third of the dorsum of the tongue from the tip to the circumvallate papillae to submandibular, and internal jugular nodal basins and occasionally the submental node basin (levels I-III). The central pathway drains the central two-thirds of the tongue. These vessels drain to the submental region (level I) or the upper cervical chain nodal

basin via the sublingual nodes (level III).[16-18] Primary lesions which approach midline often drain to bilateral nodal basins. This is especially true for lesions of the tongue and floor of mouth as there exists significant lymphatic crossover in this region.[16-20]

PATHOLOGY

Premalignant Lesions

In accordance with the concept of multi factorial cumulative insults resulting in epithelial damage eventually leading to the development of malignant lesions, a variety of premalignant lesions have been described which may predispose to the development of oral cavity SCC. These include leukoplakia, erythroplakia, smokeless tobacco keratosis, oral submucous fibrosis, and others. Continuous monitoring with clinical observation and biopsy when warranted is critical when evaluating these lesions due to the inherent risk of the lesions to develop malignant change resulting in oral cavity carcinoma.

The most common premalignant lesion of the oral cavity is leukoplakia. Oral leukoplakia is defined as a white patch or plaque that cannot be characterized clinically or pathologically as any other disease. Approximately 5 to 25% of these lesions will exhibit histopathologic evidence of epithelial dysplasia. Leukoplakia generally presents in patients older than 40 years of age and has a strong male predilection thought to be related to tobacco abuse patterns. Tobacco use is the most commonly associated risk factor for the development of leukoplakia. Other risk factors include alcohol, candidal infection/colonization, and human papilloma virus infection. The majority of leukoplakia are found on the gingiva, lip vermilion, or buccal mucosa; however, lesions of the tongue, lip vermilion, and floor of mouth account for 90% of those that exhibit dysplasia. Although the majority of oral cavity leukoplakia do not represent malignant lesions, the presence of such a lesion warrants formal biopsy. Long-standing lesions (greater than 3-6 months), and lesions of the tongue and floor of mouth are particularly concerning for malignant transformation. Small lesions should undergo excisional biopsy; however, incisional biopsy may be performed for extensive lesions not amenable to excision. In general, the more granular or exophytic the lesion appears, the greater the risk for malignant transformation. Histopathologic features of leukoplakia include hyperkeratosis, acanthosis, and inflammatory cell patterns consistent with chronic inflammation. Dysplastic changes, if present, include enlarged nuclei, prominent nucleoli, increased nuclear to cytoplasmic ratio, hyperchromatism, pleomorphism, and increased or abnormal mitotic activity.[21,22] Erythroplakia, in striking contrast to leukoplakia, are red mucosal lesions of the mucosal surfaces of the oral cavity which exhibit an extremely high rate of malignant transformation. Although these lesions are far less common relative to leukoplakia, the majority exhibit evidence of dysplasia or frank malignancy on histopathologic evaluation. These lesions should be aggressively investigated and quickly biopsied.[21,22]

Smokeless tobacco keratosis is extremely common lesion among users of smokeless tobacco and often presents as a thin, white patch or plaque located in the mucosal surface most often in direct contact with the tobacco. This lesion is clinically distinct from leukoplakia due to the low likelihood of malignant transformation in these lesions.[22-24] Because of this fact, routine biopsy of these lesions is not warranted. Smokeless tobacco keratosis ("snuff dipper's pouch") should be clinically observed at regular intervals with biopsy reserved for lesions which have undergone recent change such as ulceration or thickening, or are granular, erythematous, speckled, or verruciform in appearance.

Oral submucous fibrosis is a chronic, progressive lesion associated with betel quid chewing and is most commonly observed in India and Southeast Asia. Betel quid consist of areca nut, slaked lime, and tobacco rolled in the betel leaf. Areca nut has been reported as the main etiologic factor in this disease process. Chemicals associated with areca nut appear to interfere with the molecular processes of deposition and/or degradation of extracellular matrix molecules such as collagen leading to the development of the severe submucosal fibrosis associated with this lesion. Clinically these lesions appear as leukoplakia or keratotic mucosa with thickened, marble-like subepithelium in the area in contact with the betel quid. Oral submucous fibrosis is a chronic, debilitating disease due to the associated burning pain and severe trismus which often results from the disease. These lesions have significant malignant potential and should be monitored closely for the development of oral cavity SCC.[21,25]

Squamous Cell Carcinoma (SCC)

Squamous cell carcinoma (SCC) is the most common malignant neoplasm of the oral cavity. SCC of the oral cavity occurs most commonly in the tongue (26%) and the lip (23%). Sixteen percent (16%) of all oral cavity cancers are located in the floor of the mouth. The minor salivary glands account for an additional 11% of lesions.[3,5,12] The disease generally presents in the 5th and 6th decade of life and is more common in males.[5,26] Environmental factors play a significant role in the development of SCC of the upper aerodigestive tract. The strong association between smoking tobacco and ethanol abuse with head and neck SCC has been well documented.[4,26-29] Tobacco smoke contains numerous carcinogens including polycyclic aromatic hydrocarbons, phenol, benzopyrene, formaldehyde, and nitrosamines which contribute to carcinogenesis. In addition to the known association with malignancy, premalignant lesions of the mucous membranes, such as leukoplakia, occur more frequently in smokers than non smokers. Ethanol is also recognized that a significant synergism exists in patients who abuse tobacco and ethanol leading to reported 6 to15 fold increased risk for oral cavity malignancy.[4,26,27,29] Additional environmental risk factors such as chronic disease, smokeless tobacco, marijuana, dietary factors (fat, calcium, sodium, riboflavin, retinols), poor oral hygiene, have been reported to increase risk for the development of mucosal SCC, although the role of these risk factors is somewhat difficult to define.[4,27,30-34] Human viral infection, such as with human papilloma virus, has been implicated in many investigation related to oral SCC.[35,36] Considerable investigation within the literature continues, attempting to define genetic risk factors which play a key role in the development of this disease.[35,37-43] The development of SCC within the head and neck is the culmination of numerous environmental, genetic, and random molecular events altering programmed physiologic squamous cell apoptosis.

The diagnosis of SCC is predicated on formal biopsy of the lesion in question with histopathologic examination. The histologic features of SCC are well known and are characterized by invasive malignant epithelial cells penetrating the basement membrane of the epithelial surface which separates SCC from other dysplastic lesions such as carcinoma in situ. Malignant cells exhibit eosinophilic cytoplasm with enlarged nuclei resulting in the often described increased nuclear-cytoplasmic ratio. As in the case of epithelial dysplasia, various cellular and nuclear histopathologic features indicating altered cellular maturation are commonly observed in SCC. These include cellular/nuclear pleomorphism, increased or abnormal mitotic activity, islandlike epithelial formations (keratin pearls), dyskeratosis, loss of epithelial polarity, loss of cellular cohesiveness, and altered cellular morphology.

ADDITIONAL MALIGNANCIES OF THE ORAL CAVITY

Salivary Gland Malignancies

Malignant salivary gland neoplasms account for approximately 3% to 5% of all head and neck cancers and primary lesions of the minor salivary glands occurring within the oral cavity are relatively rare. More that 30 histologic types of epithelial tumors of the salivary glands have been described but the most common malignant neoplasms of the minor salivary glands include mucoepidermoid carcinoma, polymorphous low-grade adenocarcinoma, adenocarcinoma, and adenoid cystic carcinoma.[44-47] The palate is the most common site of minor salivary gland tumors followed by the upper lip and buccal mucosa. Approximately 50% of palate tumors are malignant. Lesions of the lower lip, floor of mouth, sublingual glands, and retromolar trigone have malignancy rates as high as 90% and generally have poor prognoses. Salivary gland malignancies of the sublingual glands and minor salivary gland carry a worse prognosis compared to their major salivary

gland counterparts.[45,46] As a general rule the treatment of malignant salivary gland tumors should be wide surgical excision and may be followed by adjuvant radiotherapy if indicated. Early stage low-grade malignant salivary gland tumors are usually curable by adequate surgical resection alone. Extensive or high-grade lesions are most effectively treated with surgical resection combined with postoperative radiation therapy. Additionally, radiotherapy is generally required in cases with positive surgical margins after resection. Elective surgical therapy of the cervical lymph nodes is generally not indicated with most salivary gland malignancies. The specific characteristics of the most common minor salivary gland tumors presenting in the oral cavity are discussed below.

Mucoepidermoid carcinoma is the most common malignant lesion of the salivary glands and may present within the oral cavity. Although most commonly occurring in the parotid gland, approximately 25% of patient with mucoepidermoid carcinoma have primary lesions involving the minor salivary glands. Mucoepidermoid carcinoma is commonly classified into low, intermediate, and high-grade variants based on histologic criteria including mitotic figures (>4/10 high-power fields), neural invasion, necrosis, intracystic components, and cellular anaplasia. In general low-grade tumors have higher percentages of mucinous cell types with high-grade variants exhibiting a large proportion of epithelial cell types on histopathologic evaluation. Survival and recurrence after therapy is reported as approximately 60% to 80% in 5 years for all lesions, influenced by tumor grade, stage, and margin status.[48,49]

Adenocarcinoma of the minor salivary gland is a rare but aggressive neoplasm. This neoplasm is an adenocarcinoma which a high-grade salivary neoplasm which has many subclass variants arising from ductal elements of the salivary gland. The palate is the most common site of origin within the oral cavity. Clinically these tumors generally present as an asymptomatic mass although other symptoms such as pain may be present. Oral cavity survival data for salivary adenocarcinoma is approximately 40% to 50% in 5 years. Cervical metastasis has been reported in approximately 10% to 20% of cases.[45,46,50] Histologically these rare tumors are aggressive, poorly differentiated adenocarcinomas which do not meet criteria for other malignant salivary gland tumors such as the invasive ductal carcinomas, acinic cell carcinoma, or adenoid cystic carcinoma.[51] The treatment for undifferentiated adenocarcinoma is surgical resection with postoperative radiotherapy with neck dissection reserved for patients who present with cervical metastatic disease. Polymorphous low-grade adenocarcinoma (PGLA) is a variant of salivary adenocarcinoma with a benign course and excellent prognosis when compared to the undifferentiated salivary adenocarcinoma. PGLA is thought to arise from intercalated ducts within the salivary unit and has been called terminal duct carcinoma although the classification of salivary gland tumors is extremely complex and PGLA has been confused with adenoid cystic carcinoma due to its propensity for perineural invasion.[47,52] The treatment of PGLA is surgical excision. Radiotherapy has not been universally accepted as beneficial for this lesion.[53,54] Overall 5-year survival data for PGLA have been reported to be greater than 95% although malignant degeneration has been reported.[47,55]

Adenoid cystic carcinoma is the most common malignant neoplasm of the minor salivary glands.[46,56] As with other minor salivary gland malignancies, the most common presenting location within the oral cavity is the palate. Adenoid cystic carcinoma is divided into three distinct types based on the histologic pattern of the tumor: cribriform, tubular, and solid. Historically, the cribriform pattern has been reported to have the most favorable prognosis with the tubular variant being somewhat intermediate and the solid variant having the worst prognosis in terms of overall survival and locoregional recurrence. In terms of prognosis, it has been noted that histologic grade may not be as important as stage upon presentation.[56,57] Adenoid cystic carcinoma is widely recognized to exhibit aggressive behavior and generally has a poor long-term prognosis when compared to other salivary gland malignancies. 10-year survival rates have been reported to range from 75% (stage I) to 15% (stage IV) depending on the stage at presentation.[56,57] Cervical metastases are rare; however, locoregional recurrences and distant metastasis often develop many years after initial therapy and 40% to 50% of patients with adenoid cystic carcinoma will eventually suffer a recurrence.[56,58,59] The most common metastatic lesion is pulmonary; however, locoregional failure is a common observation related to perineural extension and cervical and/or skull base recurrence is commonly observed. Oral cavity/oropharyngeal primary lesions have favorable recurrence-free survival, and local and distant recurrence rates when compared to primary lesions located elsewhere in the head and neck.[56] The treatment of adenoid cystic carcinoma is complete surgical excision and many authors recommend radical resections due poor outcomes with positive surgical margins.[53,56,57] Unfortunately, surgical margins are not reliable with adenoid cystic carcinoma secondary to its proclivity for perineural spread. Therefore, routine adjuvant radiotherapy is warranted in most cases. Postoperative radiotherapy has been shown to significantly decrease locoregional recurrence rates in the treatment of adenoid cystic carcinoma.[58,59]

Kaposi's Sarcoma

Kaposi's sarcoma is a malignant vascular connective tissue neoplasm associated with immunosuppression as in the case of HIV/AIDS or organ transplant recipients.[60,61] Several subtypes exist including the classical type, AIDS-related type, African cutaneous or lymphadenopathic types, and Kaposi's of immunosuppression. Kaposi's sarcoma has been repeatedly shown to be associated with human herpes viral infection (HHV-8) now described as the Kaposi's-sarcoma-associated herpes virus (KSHV).[62,63] It is believed that coinfection with HIV/KSHV leads to the development of an angiogenic inflammatory state that is responsible for the pathogenesis of Kaposi's sarcoma.[63] Definitive diagnosis is confirmed with biopsy; however, histopathologic findings vary depending on the maturity of the lesion and include vascular proliferation with dilation of thin-walled vessels, spindle cell proliferation, and mild inflammatory infiltrates at the periphery of the lesion. The more mature lesions may resemble fibrosarcoma with densely packed spindle cell populations predominating but are differentiated due to the slitlike vascular spaces containing erythrocytes and hemosiderin.

Oral cavity lesions are common among patients afflicted with Kaposi's sarcoma and appear as violaceous patches, submucosal purplish masses, or nodular/papular lesions. The disease is often multifocal;

however, and isolated oral lesions are rare. Biopsy confirmed Kaposi's sarcoma of the oral cavity should prompt systemic workup for involved areas and includes computerized tomography of the abdomen and pelvis as well as HIV testing if warranted. The clinical presentation and progression is highly variable and gastrointestinal tract, lung, and lymph node involvement are common. Treatment options depend on the extent of the tumor and growth rate, as well as the HIV viral load, and host factors such as the CD4 T-lymphocyte count and medical condition. The most effective treatment for Kaposi's sarcoma is appropriate retroviral therapy which is evident by the marked decline the disease when highly active antiretroviral therapy (HAART) became available.[63-65] Additional treatment options include interferon-alpha and systemic chemotherapy (anthracyclines, paclitaxel, vincristine, etoposide, bleomycin), intralesional chemotherapy, or radiation and should be managed by the medical oncologist. Radiation therapy usually consists of electron or proton beam external radiation with dosages usually ranging from 600 to 3000 cGy and offers excellent response rates for local control and palliation.[66,67] Surgical excision, cryotherapy, or laser ablation may be useful for symptomatic focal lesions amenable to local therapy. Targeted strategies, such as the angiogenesis inhibitors, are under investigation.[60,63-65]

Osteosarcoma/Chondrosarcoma

Malignant sarcomas of the oral cavity usually arise from the mandible or maxilla with osteosarcoma being the most common lesion. Other more rare lesions include chondrosarcoma, rhabdomyosarcoma, angiosarcoma, and liposarcoma. Osteosarcoma is a malignant mesenchymal neoplasm arising from the osseous structure of the jaws. Common presenting signs and symptoms include an expansile, firm mass with pain, paresthesia, and occasionally tooth mobility. Radiographic findings generally include a mottled, expansile osseous lesion with cortical destruction and the classic "sun ray" appearance. Periosteal thickening, extracortical bone formation and radiographic findings consistent with osteomyelitis may confuse the diagnosis. Histopathologic examination of biopsy

specimens reveals formation of osteoid matrix with a sarcomatous stroma which may appear osteoblastic, chondroblastic, or fibroblastic. Marked cellular atypia with myxoid stroma, and abnormal osseous maturation may be observed as well as increased mitotic activity, although the latter finding is rare. The treatment of osteosarcoma generally includes induction chemotherapy with most protocols including doxorubicin, vincristine, cyclophosphamide, and prednisone followed by complete surgical resection with 2 to 3-cm margins. Cervical metastasis from osteosarcoma is rare and routine neck dissection is not warranted. Radiation therapy is generally reserved for extensive lesions, positive surgical margins and palliation.[68,69] Treatment outcomes for osteosarcoma of the head and neck vary by stage but 5-year survival rates typically range from 30% to 60% with the most common failure being locoregional recurrence.[68-70]

In contrast to osteosarcoma, chondrosarcoma is an extremely rare mesenchymal tumor of the jaws. The clinical presentation of chondrosarcoma is similar to osteosarcoma and lesions are most commonly located in the anterior maxilla or posterior mandible following the embryologic progression of the cartilaginous elements of the jaws. Chondrosarcoma tends to exhibit slower growth when compared to osteosarcoma and neural invasion is a late feature in the disease. Radiographic findings are similar to osteosarcoma with expansile, lytic lesions of the mandible or maxilla with cortical destruction. Histopathologic examination of biopsy specimens reveals malignant cartilage cells within a sarcomatous stroma. Cellular pleomorphism, with nuclear atypia including multinucleate/binucleate cells, are common features with higher grade tumors showing increasing numbers of spindle cells. Fortunately, most chondrosarcomas of the jaws are low-grade, slow growing variants; however, this fact poses significant risk that the lesion may be misdiagnosed as a benign cartilaginous tumor.[71] Treatment of chondrosarcoma is generally surgical resection with 2-cm margins followed by chemotherapy protocols similar to those utilized in osteosarcoma although response rates tend to be decreased with these tumors. Elective neck dissection may be considered in high grade lesions as there is propensity for high-grade chondrosarcomas to metastasize to the cervical lymph nodes. In general treatment outcomes from chondrosarcomas of the jaws are favorable when compared to osteosarcoma.[71-73] Locoregional recurrences have been reported 10 to 20 years after initial diagnosis and patients should be followed appropriately.[71]

Mucosal Melanoma

Malignant melanoma of the oral cavity is an extremely rare but devastating disease. Mucosal melanomas comprise less than 1% of all melanoma and occur in the nasal cavity, paranasal sinuses, and less frequently the oral cavity. The most common locations for melanoma to occur within the oral cavity are the palate and gingiva of the maxilla. Other sites including the floor of mouth and tongue have been reported. Many mucosal melanomas are diagnosed at late stages and these lesions are associated with an extremely poor prognosis.[74,75] Five-year survival rates for oral mucosal melanoma have been reported at approximately 15% to 50% depending on the stage at presentation.[74-77] Locoregional recurrences and distant metastasis are common failures associated with this disease. Diagnosis is confirmed by biopsy coupled with immunohistochemical testing such as S-100 and HMB-45. Immunohistochemical evaluation is especially critical if the diagnosis of amelanotic melanoma is entertained. It should be noted that traditional cutaneous melanoma classifications such as Clark's levels and the Breslow depth have not been well correlated with prognosis in mucosal melanoma and therefore should not be utilized. The role of sentinel node biopsy or elective neck dissection in oral mucosal melanoma remains to be elucidated. Oral mucosal melanomas seem to have a greater propensity for cervical metastasis when compared to their sinonasal counterparts and therefore elective neck dissection should be considered. Abundant lymphatic tissue, variable drainage patterns, and watershed areas make treatment planning difficult in head and neck melanoma.[76,78]

There is little question that the most effective treatment for mucosal melanoma is aggressive surgical excision. Due to the aggressive behavior of this disease a 3 to 5 cm margin of surrounding tissue is generally recommended. This is especially impor-tant for deeply infiltrative lesions.[74-77] Adjuvant modalities including radiotherapy, chemotherapy or immunotherapy have offered minimal improvement in overall survival.[74,77] Radiotherapy may offer improved locoregional control, provide improved palliation, and may offer primary modality therapy for non resectable lesions.[77]

DIAGNOSTIC CONSIDERATIONS

Delayed diagnosis resulting in patients presenting with advanced stage SCC of the head and neck continues to plague physicians despite extensive attempts at increasing social awareness of this devastating disease. Numerous psychosocial factors including denial, fear, isolation, substance abuse, and advancing age have been implicated in this perplexing observation.[79] The increased complexity and additional cost associated with the treatment of these patients is well recognized. More concerning, however, are well-documented poor outcomes related to locoregional control and disease-free survival in patients who present with advanced stage SCC.[79-84] SCC of the oral cavity which presents in the advanced stage has been shown to require multimodality therapy often including surgery, radiotherapy, and chemotherapy but, although a significant improvement in locoregional control and disease-free survival has been shown, overall outcomes remain discouraging. Additionally, it is accepted that treatment outcomes of advanced stage oral cavity SCC are worse when compared to similarly staged SCC located elsewhere within the head and neck.[79,81-91,92]

Patients who present for the evaluation of a malignancy of the head and neck require a detailed history and thorough physical examination. Although the presence of advanced stage disease often makes the diagnosis obvious, recording the presence and duration of symptoms such as pain, otalgia, odyno-phagia, dysphagia, trismus, and hoarseness is important and may increase suspicion for unusual patterns of presentation which may, in turn, alter the diagnostic modalities selected during the treatment planning process. Furthermore, discussion regarding the patient's complaints may alter the treatment planning in order to provide appropriate oncologic therapy without ignoring the wishes of the patient, especially if elaborate reconstructive procedures are a consideration. The history should document risk factors such as the use of tobacco and alcohol, previous exposure to radiation, recent dietary habits, weight loss, medical comorbidities, and family history of disease.

The necessity of a complete physical examination of the patient cannot be overstated when evaluating a patient who presents with advanced SCC of the oral cavity. Physical examination, in conjunction with fiberoptic laryngoscopy, is paramount in order to document the pretreatment condition of the patient, determine the extent of primary disease, and to screen for concomitant pathology such as infection or synchronous primary malignancies. This includes examination of oral cavity, pharynx, as well as palpation of the floor of the mouth, tongue, base of the tongue, and tonsillar fossa. Examination of the dentition, alveolus, and proximity of the malignancy to the mandible or maxilla is critical to evaluate extent of disease and interpret imaging studies. Fiberoptic nasopharyngoscopy/laryngoscopy further aids in the evaluation of the primary tumor as well as offering the definitive examination of the airway which is often compromised in advanced disease. Physical examination of the neck is performed in order to record the location (levels I–VI), size, mobility, and relationship of the involved lymph node(s) to adjacent structures. The staging of the primary tumor and involved cervical lymph nodes must be documented as outlined below.

Confirming the suspected histopathologic diagnosis with biopsy is obligatory. The clinical presentation of SCC in the oral cavity may mimic numerous disease processes including immune-mediated disease, infectious disease, or other malignant processes including nonmucosal primary malignancy or metastatic lesions from primary malignancies distant from the head and neck. Biopsy of oral cavity/oral pharyngeal lesions usually can be performed in the clinical setting with local anesthesia or may be performed under anesthesia during formal panendoscopy. Palpable neck masses or large metastatic cervical lymph nodes often are amenable to fine-needle aspiration biopsy. Ultrasound-guided fine needle aspiration is often useful in obtaining a diagnosis when suspected cervical disease is difficult to localize and has been reported to have superior sensitivity and specificity when compared to traditional fine needle aspiration.[93,94] Open surgical biopsy of suspected metastatic disease generally is not indicated.

Oral SCC in the Young Patient

Although extremely rare in children, oral cavity SCC may present in unexpectedly young nonsmokers and there is some evidence that these patients suffer from aggressive disease which responds poorly to treatment.[95] Despite this evidence, other data suggest that younger age and the lack of accepted risk factors such as smoking and alcohol abuse does not appear to portend worse survival compared to older patients. Rather, survival in this group of patients tends to correlate with the stage upon presentation as with all head and neck SCC.[96-98] Genetic risk factors have been implicated but, interestingly, genetic alterations have been reported as higher in smokers suggesting that factors related to the development of oral SCC remain unclear.[38] At the current time there is insufficient evidence to support the theory that young patients who present with similarly staged oral cavity SCC have a worse prognosis than older patients. Therefore, there is currently no evidence to support dissimilar or more aggressive therapy for advanced stage oral cavity SCC in younger patients than would be provided for other patients.[99]

Oral SCC in the Elderly Patient

With the currently aging population, advanced stage oral cavity carcinoma may often present in elderly patients. Treatment planning is complicated by comorbid medical conditions, delayed healing associated with age, altered nutritional status, and often a lack of social support for these aging patients. Furthermore, isolation and depression may inhibit the acceptance of treatment in the elderly patient. There is evidence that elderly patients have a tendency to receive nonstandard treatment for head and neck SCC.[100] This may be related to patient preferences, marital status of the patient, age as an isolated factor, or quality of life concerns. Often, there is trepidation to perform surgical procedures on elderly patients with advanced disease. This may lead to alternative strategies such as chemotherapy and radiation for advanced malignancy.

The literature does not support this approach, however, and surgical therapy, including resection and flap reconstruction, is generally well tolerated in the elderly patient.[101] Additionally, studies have found no significant differences in the complication rate and quality of life aspects between surgically treated elderly and younger patients.[102,103] Aggressive therapy including surgery and radiation for advanced oral cavity SCC should not be withheld solely on the basis of age.[104] The effects of significant medical comorbidities may complicate treatment but do not appear to affect survival in elderly patients after therapy for advanced stage oral cavity cancer.[105] Therefore, elderly patients should be addressed on an individual basis when treatment planning for advanced oral cavity SCC as significant benefit may be obtained from the traditional multimodal approach.[104,106] It should be noted, however, that consideration should be made prior to enrolling elderly patients for chemotherapy, specifically those older than 70 years of age, as they may perform poorly with this modality. Discussion with the medical oncologist will allow appropriate selection of elderly patients who are candidates for chemotherapy.

Oral SCC in the African-American Patient

Several reports have illuminated the fact that the rate of development of oral cavity SCC is statistically higher among the African-American population.[5,7] Ratios exceeding 2:1 have been reported for cancers of the palate, tonsil, oropharynx, and piriform sinus, in African-American males.[7] Unfortunately, there is evidence that African American patients have poorer survival outcomes, with race as a significant independent predictor of survival, after treatment for oral SCC.[107,108] Of further concern, differences in stage upon presentation, smoking, alcohol abuse, and treatment strategies between African-American and Caucasian patients have been reported and, combined with variation of socioeconomic status, have led to significantly increased mortality in the African-

American population affected by this disease.[5,7,108] Further research is needed to determine genetic, social, and economic factors which may be contributing to these alarming findings among African-American patients with advanced oral cavity SCC.

DIAGNOSTIC IMAGING

The role of diagnostic imaging when evaluating advanced stage oral cavity SCC is well established in the literature. Imaging studies also form the backbone for screening examinations as well as follow-up on completion of therapy for head and neck malignancy. Diagnostic imaging protocols used to evaluate patients with head and neck malignancy undergo constant change, a fact driven by advances in imaging technology. Nevertheless, any imaging modality is only useful with an understanding of the sensitivity and specificity of the technique, coupled with appropriate interpretation.

Computed Tomography

The most significant radiologic advancement in the evaluation of head and neck malignancy was the development of high-resolution computed tomography (CT). Contrast CT allows for a three-dimensional evaluation of the primary tumor giving invaluable information regarding related anatomic structures and the extent of local invasion. CT is the primary imaging modality in use today for the evaluation of advanced stage head and neck malignancy.[109] In general, patients diagnosed with advanced SCC of the oral cavity should undergo contrast CT scanning of the head, neck, and chest to evaluate locoregional extent of disease and screen for pulmonary metastatic disease. CT scans of the primary lesion will provide invaluable information related to factors which alter the treatment plan such as previously unsuspected extension of disease, airway compression/compromise, vascular involvement/invasion, or mandible invasion.

The presence of mandible invasion is an important finding when treatment planning for advanced stage oral cavity SCC. When assessing candidates for mandible resection/marginal mandibulectomy CT scanning is the gold standard imaging modality. The diagnostic accuracy of CT scanning has been evaluated in the literature with a reported sensitivity and specificity approaching 90% when comparing radiologic findings with histologic confirmation of mandible invasion.[110] Unfortunately, this accuracy may vary depending on the site evaluated with the anterior mandible and mandible body being the most amenable to imaging, whereas other regions, such as the retromolar trigone, mandible ramus, and mandible condyle exhibit a greater tendency for imprecise results. The sensitivity for histologically confirmed bone invasion in these areas has been reported as low as 50% indicating that CT is potentially inaccurate depending on the region being evaluated.[111]

Computed tomography remains the imaging modality of choice when evaluating the neck for cervical metastatic disease in the patient with advanced oral cavity SCC. In the absence of palpable adenopathy, obesity, or previously radiated neck CT scanning is useful to assess the status of the cervical lymph nodes. When a large node is palpable in the neck CT scanning is useful to clarify its relationship to the anatomic structures of the neck such as the carotid artery, internal jugular vein, paraspinal muscles, and the cervical spine. Cervical CT findings may alter the staging of head and neck SCC in nearly 30% of patients who have a clinically N0 neck.[112] CT scanning allows for relatively accurate staging for advanced nodal disease (area = 45 mm^2) with accuracy approaching 80% with histologic confirmation.[113] However, as in the case with mandible invasion, CT does not possess the accuracy to evaluate nodal metastatic disease at the histologic level and it is generally accepted that the accuracy of CT in staging for cervical metastasis ranges from 60 to 80%[114-116] (Fig 14–1).

Magnetic Resonance Imaging

Magnetic resonance imaging (MRI) has been utilized in the evaluation of head and neck malignancy and it is accepted that MRI offers superior soft tissue resolution when compared to computerized tomography. Increased diagnostic accuracy in extension of

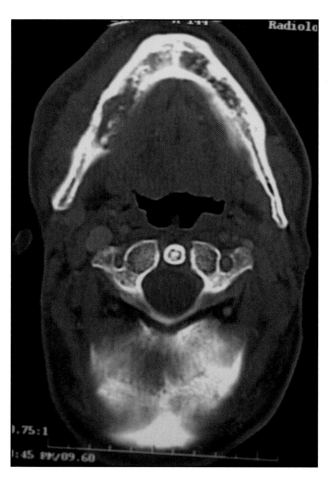

Fig 14–1. Axial CT demonstrating right mandible body erosion of lingual cortex.

soft tissue primary lesion as well as improved accuracy for cervical lymph node staging has prompted some authors to recommend routine MRI scanning for head and neck malignancy.[109,115,117]MRI offers an excellent imaging modality, with accuracy superior to conventional CT scanning, when evaluation of the extent of invasion of the primary tumor is required. Large lesions located within the tongue and floor of mouth that are subject to dental and osseous tomographic artifact are particularly amenable to MRI. MRI is especially useful in cases which exhibit perineural invasion and can improve accuracy related to extension of disease in these lesions.[118] Despite this increased accuracy, as in the case of CT, MRI offers insufficient accuracy to detect micrometastatic disease. Additionally, MRI may be overly sensitive to detect recurrent SCC as its superior resolution often leads to erroneous investigations of abnormalities located within the post therapy tissues.[117]

Traditionally, CT is regarded to be superior to MRI to evaluate malignant osseous invasion. Recent studies have challenged this traditional view and have shown superior imaging accuracy with MRI over CT in the evaluation of osseous invasion and medullary involvement.[118-121] Although CT remains the primary imaging modality utilized for patients with advanced oral cavity cancer, MRI may play an increasing role in the workup of these patients in the future.

Positron Emission Tomography

Positron emission tomography (PET) is perhaps the most dynamic field of imaging currently applied to head and neck oncology. PET is a functional imaging technique which utilizes a radiolabeled tracer, most commonly 18-FDG (18-fluoro-2-deoxyglucose), that is utilized by metabolically active cells, as is the case with active malignancy. Radiolabeled tracer is transported across the cellular membrane of metabolically active cells. Once inside the cell, tyrosine kinase phosphorylates 18-FDG which does not allow this molecule to be further metabolized or to be transported back across the cell membrane. The radioactivity of 18-FDG collides with gamma rays in an annihilation reaction which produces positrons. This form of radioactivity is detected by the PET scanner.[115] PET scanning has been shown to increase accuracy (true positives) for the detection of head and neck malignancy and is currently utilized in the detection of unknown primary tumors, post-therapy tumor surveillance, and evaluation for cervical/distant metastatic disease.[114,116,118,122-124] PET has also been utilized to determine which patients require elective neck dissection after primary radiotherapy for head and neck malignancy.[125]

The primary role of PET in the evaluation of advanced oral cavity SCC is the detection of subclinical, metastatic disease. With a known primary lesion in the advanced stage, PET offers little advantage over CT/MRI in the evaluation of the primary tumor or cervical region. PET offers inferior resolution for evaluating the extent of the primary lesion

and should be combined with CT to improve diagnostic accuracy. Small primaries or primaries in areas demonstrating physiologically increased FDG uptake may not be detected with PET. Currently, the limit of detection correlates to a resolution of approximately 5 mm.[124] Although PET offers significant promise in the evaluation of the N0 neck in early stage disease, in patients with advanced primary lesions, the status of the neck is only of prognostic significance. These patients generally benefit from formal therapy of the neck, either radiation or surgery. Furthermore, the literature regarding PET has shown shortcomings similar to CT/MRI for the detection of micrometastatic disease. Therefore, patients with advanced primary oral cavity malignancy require more aggressive evaluation of the neck including staging neck dissection and possibly (see section below), sentinel node biopsy.[118,123,124,126,127]

Traditional Radiography

Advanced imaging modalities such as CT, MRI, and PET have virtually replaced plain radiographs in the evaluation of advanced head and neck malignancies. But, there remains an adjunct role for chest radiographs and the panoramic mandible radiograph.

Chest radiographs may be obtained in the initial evaluation of advanced head and neck malignancy and a significant amount of information is obtained from a quick and inexpensive study. Given the risk factors associated with head and neck SCC, evaluation for synchronous pulmonary tumor, metastatic tumor and acute/chronic pulmonary disease remain the objectives of conventional chest radiography. Abnormal findings or suspicions lesions which are discovered may need further imaging including computed tomography of the chest. Additionally, chest radiographs remain a cost-effective screening modality post-therapy to monitor for metastatic disease.

The panoramic radiograph should be obtained in all patients undergoing evaluation for an advanced malignancy of the oral cavity. Information is obtained related to mandible osseous/cortical involvement, state of the dentition, and preoperative planning in the event a mandibulectomy/segmental resection is considered. In the event radiotherapy is planned, as is often the case with advanced stage tumors, the panoramic radiograph allows for surgical planning of dental extractions which may be required in order to proceed without subjecting the patient to increased risk for osteoradionecrosis.

Panendoscopy

The role of panendoscopy (direct laryngoscopy, esophagosopy, bronchoscopy) in the evaluation of head and neck malignancy is well established. When evaluating a patient with advanced oral cavity SCC, formal panendoscopy in the operating room affords the opportunity to thoroughly examine the patient and includes direct laryngoscopy, pharyngoscopy, esophagoscopy, or flexible or rigid bronchoscopy as indicated. Extent of the primary tumor is evaluated, particularly the relationship of the tumor to the midline, base of tongue, and mandible. Biopsies are obtained at the time of the panendoscopy if the histologic diagnosis of the malignancy is unknown.

This technique is also utilized to rule out the existence of other primary tumors in the aerodigestive tract as it has been stated that 5% to 15% of patients newly diagnosed with oral and oropharyngeal cancers will also have another primary malignancy. Patients who are post-therapy for oral cavity/oropharyngeal malignancy have an approximately 10% to 40% incidence of developing an upper aerodigestive tract malignancy of the oral cavity or oropharynx at a later time. Lung cancer is also more prevalent in this patient population.[3] For these reasons, panendoscopy is commonly utilized for post-therapy examination of patients who have completed therapy for head and neck malignancy. It should be noted, however, that the routine use of panendoscopy has been questioned in the literature as the true incidence of synchronous primary malignancy has been reported as low as 1.3% to 2.6% depending on the anatomic site.[128] Although the utility of panendoscopy may be in question for some head and neck malignancies, it is frequently helpful when evaluating the advanced stage oral cavity malignancy. Large primary tumors, especially with hypopharyngeal extension, are often difficult to evaluate clinically and panendoscopy allows for accurate evaluation of the extent of the primary lesion which is critical for surgical treatment planning. Additionally, multiple biopsies in different locations within the primary lesion may be obtained to accurately evaluate the character of the malignancy.

DECISION FACTORS IN TREATMENT PLANNING

The treatment planning of patients with advanced malignancy of the oral cavity requires an in-depth knowledge of multiple factors relating to the patient, tumor, and the planned therapy. This has led to the development of the tumor board which is an important part of the evaluation of the patient with a head and neck malignancy. Ideally, the tumor board should be composed of the head and neck surgeon, medical oncologist, radiation oncologist, histopathologist, oral surgeon or dentist, reconstructive surgeon, speech pathologist, nutritionist, and other consultants involved in the care of the patient including the cardiologist, pulmonlogist, and anesthesiologist if required. Due to the complexity of this patient population, accurate examination, diagnostic imaging, staging, histopathologic evaluation, and appropriate treatment planning, are crucial to provide acceptable management for this difficult disease.

STAGING

Currently the American Joint Committee on Cancer (AJCC) TNM staging system for oral cavity lesion is shown in Table 14-1 and Table 14-2.[12] All patients evaluated for head and neck malignancy should be staged according the AJCC system. This is the most widely utilized staging system for head and neck malignancy, including advanced oral cavity malignancy, and provides a uniform platform to develop treatment strategies and compare results. Although the AJCC staging system is the most universally applied system its shortcomings have been frequently noted in the literature. Pathologic information has been incorporated into the staging in an attempt to improve the accuracy of the traditional tumor stag-

Table 14–1. AJCC TNM Classification: Oral Cavity SCCA

Primary Tumor (T)

TX	Primary tumor cannot be assessed
T0	No evidence of primary tumor
Tis	Carcinoma in situ
T1	Tumor 2 cm or less in greatest dimension
T2	Tumor more than 2 cm but not more than 4 cm in greatest dimension
T3	Tumor more than 4 cm in greatest dimension
T4	(Lip) Tumor invades through cortical bone, inferior alveolar nerve, floor of mouth, or skin of face, that is, chin or nose
T4a	(Oral cavity) Tumor invades through cortical bone, into deep (extrinsic) muscle of tongue (genioglossus, hyoglossus, palatoglossus, and styloglossus) maxillary sinus, or skin of face
T4b	Tumor involves masticator space, pterygoid plates, or skull base and/or encases internal carotid artery

Regional Lymph Nodes (N)

NX	Regional lymph nodes cannot be assessed
N0	No regional lymph node metastasis
N1	Metastasis in a single ipsilateral lymph node, 3 cm or less in greatest dimension
N2	Metastasis in a single ipsilateral lymph node, more than 3 cm but not more than 6 cm in greatest dimension; or in bilateral or contralateral lymph nodes, none more than 6 cm in greatest dimension
N2a	Metastasis in single ipsilateral lymph node more than 3 cm but not more than 6 cm in greatest dimension
N2b	Metastasis in multiple ipsilateral lymph nodes, none more than 6 cm in greatest dimension
N2c	Metastasis in bilateral or contralateral lymph nodes, none more than 6 cm in greatest dimension
N3	Metastasis in a lymph node more than 6 cm in greatest dimension

Distant Metastasis (M)

MX	Distant metastasis cannot be assessed
M0	No distant metastasis
M1	Distant metastasis

Reproduced with permission from American Joint Committee on Cancer. *AJCC Cancer Staging Manual*, 6th ed. New York, NY: Springer; 2002:23–24.

Table 14–2. AJCC Staging System: Oral Cavity SCCA[12]

Stage Grouping			
0	Tis	N0	M0
I	T1	N0	M0
II	T2	N0	M0
III	T3	N0	M0
	T1	N1	M0
	T2	N1	M0
	T3	N1	M0
IVA	T4a	N0	M0
	T4a	N1	M0
	T1	N2	M0
	T2	N2	M0
	T3	N2	M0
IVB	Any T	N3	M0
	T4b	Any N	M0
IVC	Any T	Any N	M1

ing system.[129] Other more involved staging systems have been proposed in order to improve accuracy but none have gained general acceptance.[130-132]

Approximately 50 to 60% of patients with SCC of the oral cavity present with advanced stage (stage III and IV) disease.[84,133] Factors associated with delay in presentation include lesions located in the posterior oral cavity/oropharynx or floor of mouth lesions, elderly patients, mental disability, edentulism, and infrequent dental visits.[30] Advanced stage (stage III and stage IV) malignancies have been repeatedly investigated and shown to exhibit poor locoregional control rates after therapy with significantly decreased survival.[5,84,89,129,134-141] Additionally, the location of the primary tumor in advanced disease affects survival with increased locoregional recurrence associated with the buccal mucosa (75%), sinopalate (50%), and gingiva (100%) compared with mobile tongue (27%), and oropharynx (13%).[142] Despite recent advances in the management of these advanced stage malignancies, they remain a challenge.

FACTORS AFFECTING PROGNOSIS

Cervical Metastasis

The presence of cervical lymph node metastasis has been repeatedly cited as the most significant factor which portends decreased survival in oral cavity SCC. In addition, patients who present with cervical lymph node metastasis have increased rates of locoregional recurrence.[2,11,15,26,80,81,83,88,115,134,136,139,140,143-158] Patients with multiple cervical nodes (>2) have higher rates of locoregional recurrence than patients with one or two positive cervical lymph nodes.[159] Furthermore, cervical lymph node metastasis located at more distant levels within the neck (III/IV), or within the contralateral neck, also tend to have significantly decreased survival rates.[156] Overall 5-year survival rates when comparing patients without evidence of cervical lymph node metastasis to those with positive nodal disease have been reported as 42.8% and 17.5%, respectively.[81] Patients who present with advanced stage oral cavity SCC generally present with lymph node metastasis by definition. The presence of cervical lymph node metastasis should be considered an ominous sign and should prompt early, aggressive treatment in order to optimize outcomes.

Histologic Factors

The histopathologic evaluation of tissue is invaluable in the treatment planning of head and neck malignancy. Histopathologic grading may influence treatment decision making when deciding on appropriate principal and adjuvant therapy. Despite the fact that poorly differentiated SCCs are predictably worse in terms of prognosis when compared to well-differentiated counterparts, several distinctive histopathologic findings that deserve attention.

Tumor Thickness

The affect of tumor thickness related to prognosis has been examined by multiple investigators. In general, increased tumor size and thickness is significantly predictive of decreased survival and increases the rate of locoregional recurrence.[80,83,160] Measuring tumor thickness and pattern of invasion in patients with early oral cancer may allow for the identification of those patients with more aggressive disease.[20,80,160] Patients with tumor diameter greater than 1.5 cm or greater than 5 mm of tumor thickness may then be considered for more aggressive adjuvant therapy and elective neck dissection regardless of stage due to increased risk for cervical lymph node metastasis.[19,80,136,143,161,162] MRI scans are sufficiently accurate to determine tumor thickness of oral cavity SCC, although histologic evaluation remains the standard.[163,164] Although tumor thickness reliably predicts regional nodal metastasis and decreased survival, specific treatment strategies based on tumor thickness have yet to be evaluated due to the wide range of factors related to prognosis among patients with oral cavity SCC.[165] In the case of advanced stage oral cavity SCC (III,IV), tumor thickness is generally not a consideration in treatment planning as the depth usually exceeds 5 mm and patients generally receive aggressive surgery with neoadjuvant and/or adjuvant chemoradiotherapy.

Perineural Invasion

Perineural invasion has been associated with increased risk local recurrence and cervical metastasis and is generally thought to be an independent predictor of survival for patients with oral cavity SCC.[166-169] The involvement of large nerves, especially those associated with the skull base or cervical vertebrae, is particularly concerning; however, even small peripheral nerve involvement has been associated with decreased survival.[142,166] The presence of pathologically confirmed perineural invasion should prompt strong consideration for surgical excision followed by full-course radiotherapy to treat the primary tumor as outcomes related to locoregional recurrence are poor when this histologic finding is present.[170,171]

Positive Surgical Margins

It has long been accepted that microscopic residual tumor resulting from positive surgical margins statistically increases local recurrence and mortality when treating SCC of the head and neck.[141,168,169,172,173]

Patients treated with surgery as the primary modality exhibit significantly improved local control rates if a negative surgical margin is obtained.[174] Surgeons performing resections for advanced primary oral cavity SCC should strive for a minimum of 1-cm margin, with 2- to 3-cm margins preferred, to minimize the likelihood of positive margins.[171] Positive surgical margins either at the primary site or within the neck after neck dissection require the use of postoperative radiotherapy to improve outcomes. Two-year disease-free survival has been reported to improve from 33.6% to 75.6% in patients with positive surgical margins who received postoperative radiotherapy (= 62.5 Gy).[173] In general, advanced stage oral cavity SCC will receive postoperative radiotherapy or chemoradiotherapy regardless of margin status due to the documented locoregional control and survival benefit.

Extracapsular Invasion

Cervical lymph node metastasis which exhibit extracapsular invasion has been repeatedly evaluated in the literature and statistically decreases overall survival. The presence of nodal extracapsular invasion is also a concern for cervical recurrence after therapy.[134,144,149,166] Advanced stage oral cavity SCC often presents with extensive cervical nodal disease which increases the likelihood of extracapsular invasion. Patients with multiple lymph nodes exhibiting extracapsular invasion generally have an extremely poor prognosis.[150,175,176] Interestingly, smoking may be a statistically significant risk factor for the development of extracapsular invasion and is an independent risk factor for pathologic nodal stage as well.[29] It has been suggested, due to the significant effect regarding outcomes, that extracapsular invasion be incorporated into current staging systems.[144] This being the case, evidence of extracapsular invasion noted during histopathologic examination of cervical specimens should indicate intensive regional and systemic adjuvant therapy may be required in the treatment of oral cavity SCC.[177]

Mandible Invasion

Frequently in patients with advanced oral cavity SCC, mandible invasion is observed. Thin-section computed tomography (3 mm) of the mandible is the most common and accurate technique utilized for detection of mandible involvement with malignant disease.[110] Traditionally, invasion of the osseous structure of the mandible has been associated with aggressive malignant disease. There is some evidence, however, that mandible invasion may not be as critical of a prognostic factor as previously anticipated.[178] Despite this evidence, the evaluation of the extent of mandible invasion in advanced primary tumors of the oral cavity is extremely important for surgical treatment planning. Clinical or radiologic evidence of mandible invasion requires strong consideration for surgical mandible resection.

Although segmental en bloc resection has been the traditional technique, marginal mandibular resection has been reported to achieve comparable control rates.[179-183] Regardless of the selected technique, obtaining a negative surgical margin is critical as significant differences in survival have been reported with osseous infiltration and positive surgical margins.[169] Frozen section techniques may be utilized for osseous margins if question remains after the initial resection.[184] Advanced oral cavity SCC (T3, T4a, T4b), especially with poor histologic findings, often demonstrate an aggressive nature and reduce the utility of more conservative marginal mandibular resections.[185] Due to poor survival outcomes and the morbidity of mandible resection, the technique has been questioned for extremely advanced disease (T4a, T4b). Interestingly, the adjuvant radiation generally required in this patient population may have more of an effect on morbidity and decreased quality of life than the necessity of mandible resection.[186] Nevertheless, there exists considerable evidence that mandible resection with aggressive adjuvant chemoradiotherapy and microvascular reconstruction is beneficial for patients with advanced stage oral cavity SCC invading the mandible.[135,153,169,187-194]

Molecular/Genetic Profile of SCC

Perhaps the most promising and exciting frontier of research in head and neck SCC is genetic characterization of malignancy and host factors which may lead to novel management strategies. Recent work has led to the development of a progressive model of the development of oral SCC. Epithelial stem cells, which acquire genetic alterations due to genetic or environmental factors, form clonal regions of preneoplastic cells, which upon acquiring further genetic alterations ultimately become clonal populations of SCC.[37] Patterns of gene expression and regulation which control the progression from histologically normal tissue to primary carcinoma and eventually to nodal/distant metastasis are currently under investigation.[9,195] Although most research is currently investigating factors related to tumor biology/behavior and the prognostic significance of such factors, targeted molecular/gene therapy for SCC remains the ultimate goal. Unfortunately, large areas of epithelium within the oral cavity are subject to the same host/environmental factors which led to the development of SCC and thus the concept of field cancerization is generally accepted. Because of this regional effect, current techniques such as surgery and radiotherapy have considerable shortcomings when treating advanced stage oral cavity SCC. Chemotherapy regimens in current use are systemic by nature but are not targeted directly to the malignant cells and therefore subject the host to widespread immune suppression and multiple side effects. In the future targeted molecular/genetic techniques may significantly alter the treatment of oral cavity SCC. Due to the complexity of molecular and genetic research in this arena, a full review of the literature on this topic is beyond the scope of this chapter; however, several current areas of investigation bear mentioning. Molecular tumor markers currently undergoing investigation may be divided into four functional groups as outlined in a recent meta-analysis on the subject.[196] Given the outcomes with advanced stage oral cavity SCC research in this area is critical and may eventually offer effective molecular or genetically based therapy regardless of the stage of disease.

ENHANCEMENT OF TUMOR GROWTH: CELL CYCLE ACCELERATION AND PROLIFERATION

Investigation into the complex molecular mechanisms responsible for tumor growth is the subject of many current investigations. Tumor growth factors

such as epithelial growth factor (EGF) and its receptor EGFR, cell cyclins, telemorase, and multiple other regulatory proteins are currently under investigation. EGF/EGFR has been repeatedly found to correlate with tumor stage and prognosis in multiple recent investigations.[41,43,197-200] The high expression of EGFR in oral cavity SCC offers evidence may indicate that EGFR may serve as a suitable receptor for future targeted molecular therapies.[197] Patients with high expression of EGFR may benefit from accelerated radiation therapy schedules during adjuvant therapy.[199] High expression of EGFR coupled with p53 expression may indicate increased tumor aggressiveness, alter prognosis, and be a determinant of chemotherapy sensitivity.[198] Cell cyclins regulate cell replication and are currently being investigated related to SCC of the oral cavity.[201,202] Telomerase an RNA-dependent DNA polymerase which is an important check point in cell apoptosis is also being investigated.[203,204]

Current research indicates that SCC exhibits a high level of genetic heterogeneity, especially at advanced stages. Flow cytometric characterization of tumors to detect intratumoral genetic heterogeneity may be beneficial in the characterization of tumor growth and proliferation.[42,84,205] Tumor expression of factors such as EGFR or the multiple matrix metalloprotease complex (MMP), detected with polymerase chain reaction (PCR), may offer a distinct tumoral characterization or signature which will provide information related to prognosis, nodal metastasis, clinical screening modalities, and eventual therapeutic strategies.[206-208]

Tumor Suppression and Anti-Tumor Defense: Immune Response and Apoptosis

Multiple tumor markers related to tumor suppression and anti-tumor host defense are currently undergoing evaluation within the literature. These include transcription factors such as p53, cyclin dependent kinase inhibitors, Fas/Fas ligand, and others. p53 is a polypeptide transcription factor which controls the cell cycle by arresting cells in the G1 phase or inducing apoptosis. Mutations of p53 result in unchecked cell proliferation and replication contributing to malignancy. The presence of a p53 mutation coupled with other genetic or environmental insults has been repeatedly correlated to the development of oral SCC.[35] Concomitant infection with HPV has been evaluated extensively with relation to p53 mutation and most studies have demonstrated statistically significantly decreased survival and poor prognosis when these findings are present in oral cavity SCC.[35,36,39,209] Another factor intimately involved with the regulation of apoptosis is the Fas/Fas ligand antigen system. Binding of Fas antigen via the Fas ligand triggers apoptosis during the apoptosis cascade of the cell cycle. Tumors with positive Fas antigen status generally have better prognosis with increased response to radiation and chemotherapy, whereas those with negative Fas antigen expression demonstrate poorer prognosis.[210,211]

Defects within double-strand DNA repair genes have been implication in the formation and progression of oral cavity SCC. Alteration of these genetic repair mechanisms from environmental insults may impair the host ability to repair epithelial DNA damage playing an important role in the progression of oral SCC.[212] Other host factors related to tumor surveillance such as macrophage factors, human leukocyte antigen subtypes, and dendritic antigen presenting cells are being investigated to elucidate the role of the host response to oral cavity SCC.[140,213,214] Tumors which have large populations of dendritic cells that mediate anti-tumor T-cell responses have been correlated with good prognosis.[215-217] High levels of dendritic cells have been reported within sentinel lymph nodes as well, and surface markers of these dendritic cells may offer an additional method to identify cervical metastatic nodes.[216] Macrophage content within the primary tumor may be correlated to tumor aggressiveness.[140]

At the present time however, the biological significance of many of these immune factors remains in question and will require further investigation to provide clinically useful information.

ANGIOGENESIS

The effect of increased angiogenesis related to tumor biology and metastatic potential has been the sub-ject of much controversy in the literature. Angiogenesis is a critical process in the development and proliferation of malignancy. It is also accepted that tumor angiogenesis plays some role in the development of distant metastases. Although the theory of increased angiogenesis factor expression or micro vessel density relating to tumor behavior is attractive, there is a lack of quality controlled evidence to support the clinical utility of specific angiogenic factors at this point in time. This being stated, some interesting findings related to angiogenesis bear mentioning.

Amid the multitude of factors evaluated by investigators related to angiogenesis vascular endothelial growth factor (VEGF) remains a leading topic of current research.[215,218-221] High levels of VEGF expression have been associated with higher clinical stage and worse overall survival in oral cavity.[219] VEGF expression by malignant cells may allow tumors to escape host immune surveillance by increasing levels of dysfunctional dendritic cells.[215] VEGF may offer some promise as a tumor marker in the progression of oral cavity SCC and may offer some indication of the propensity of the primary tumor to metastasize.[218,220] Additionally, angiogenic factors such as VEGF may predict tumor response rates to chemotherapeutic agents.[221] Factors such as VEGF may increase micro vessel density which has been implicated in increased tumor aggressiveness and persistence of disease after therapy.[222]

The inducible synthase of nitric oxide (NOS) is responsible for the synthesis of nitric oxide (NO) in neutrophils and in peripheral blood mononuclear cells. High levels of NO within tumors have been implicated in angiogenesis and tumor dissemination. Enhanced expression of NOS and the subsequent production of NO as well as the molecular control mechanisms involved in this pathway are currently under investigation for their role in the development of oral cavity SCC.[223-225] Significantly higher levels of total NO have been observed in patients with advanced stage (IV) oral cavity SCC when compared to controls. This may indicate immunological responses which may affect the anti neoplastic effect of the host immune system.[223] Conversely expression of NOS and NO production may have a yet unknown role in the development of oral SCC.[225]

TUMOR INVASION AND METASTATIC POTENTIAL: ADHESION MOLECULES AND MATRIX DEGRADATION

Factors related to tumor invasion and metastatic potential are frequent subjects of the current literature regarding oral cavity SCC. These factors include cell adhesion molecules such as integrins, cadherins, and cathepsines which are integral for tumorigenesis and metastatic spread via altered cell adhesion patterns.[226-228] Decreased expression of E-cadherin has been associated with poor prognosis in oral cavity SCC and is thought to be related to tumor suppression.[227] Other factors related to lymphangiogenesis are being investigated as predictors for lymph node metastasis.[90] Further work will elucidate the role of cell adhesion molecules in the development and progression of oral cavity SCC.

Fibroblast-derived factors such as the multiple matrix metalloproteases (MMP) are expressed within head and neck SCC and continuing work to discover their role in tumorigenesis continues.[228,229] MMP are metalloenzymes involved in degradation of the extracellular matrix during remodeling.[230] Fibroblast-derived MMP have been implicated in tumor growth and invasion in head and neck carcinoma.[230,231] Novel targeted therapies which block the activity of MMP in order to halt tumor progression have been suggested; however, further work regarding the role of MMP is required before clinically acceptable therapies are developed.[229]

SURGICAL MANAGEMENT OF PRIMARY TUMOR BY SITE

Currently, it is generally accepted that advanced stage oral cavity SCC is most effectively treated with combined modality therapy including surgery, radiation, and chemotherapy.[2,5,87,89,98,135,138,139,142,158,179,181,182,186, 193,232-244] Although some stage I, II SCC of the oral cavity may be amenable to alternate strategies such as primary radiotherapy,[161] the fact remains that outcomes are improved when multimodality approach is utilized for stage III, IV oral cavity SCC. Other malignancies such as salivary gland tumors, mela-noma, and sarcoma require alternative treatment strategies in some cases and are beyond the scope of this chapter. Therefore, this chapter covers topics related to the treatment of advanced stage oral cavity SCC.

Oral Tongue SCC

The most common location for oral cavity SCC is the oral tongue. Although base of tongue lesions may remain unnoticed and therefore undiagnosed for considerable time, a surprising number of oral cavity tongue carcinoma is diagnosed at the advanced stage. T1 or T2 lesions of the oral tongue generally are safely excised through the mouth via partial glossectomy. Surgical excision should include a 1 to 2-cm margin of normal tongue mucosa as well as the deep muscle for adequate resection of the primary lesion. After frozen section analysis, the tongue may be closed primarily with polygalactin or catgut sutures. In the event significant floor of mouth mucosa was excised, a split- or full thickness skin graft may be applied to the resected area. Adjacent submandibular or sublingual salivary ducts may require rerouting or marsupialization to maintain function. Deeply infiltrative tumors with involvement of significant portions of the floor of mouth, lingual surface of the mandible, or lesions which cross midline should prompt the surgeon to consider alternate approaches such as paramedian or posterior mandible osteotomy for surgical resection[180,245] (Fig 14–2).

Tongue/Floor of Mouth SCC

For access to advanced tongue and floor of mouth lesions, we do not perform a lip split/mandibulotomy. Most, if not all, of these lesions can be accessed via the combined oral and cervical approaches. If a mandibulectomy is required for adequate surgical margins, a lip splitting procedure need not be performed in combination. If the lip split with median or paramedian mandible osteotomy is performed, then complications from this procedure may be decreased by combining the paramedian approach (including stair step) with rigid fixation of the osteotomy with titanium plates/screws.[245] Wide excision

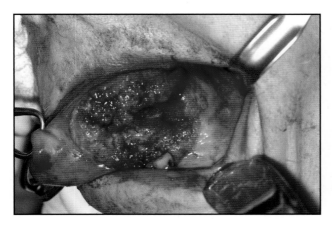

Fig 14–2. T3 SCC left oral tongue.

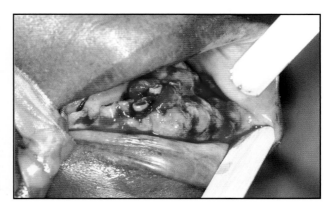

Fig 14–3. T4 SCC left floor of mouth with extension over mandible alveolus.

of the primary tumor with 1- to 2-cm margin of normal tissue is recommended. Lingual artery ligation is often required for large tongue resections. Careful attention to the location of the hypoglossal nerve is critical to preserve the function of the remainder of the tongue in order to optimize speech and swallowing outcomes. Unless malignant involvement is present, total sublingual gland resection provides minimal oncologic benefit and increases complication rates and therefore should not be performed routinely.[247]

Preoperative assessment should include panoramic radiography to examine the location of the proposed osteotomy, adjacent teeth, and mental foramina. Locoregional control and survival rates are improved with combined modality therapy of advanced SCC of the tongue and functional outcomes for this procedure are acceptable.[98,139] It should be stated that the incidence of cervical metastasis is extremely high for advanced SCC of the tongue and elective treatment of the neck is recommended (see surgical: Management of the Neck)[143] (Fig 14-3).

Retromolar Trigone SCC

SCC within the oral cavity with involvement of the retromolar trigone has been associated with poor outcomes. Overall 5-year survival rates for these lesions are near 50% and locoregional recurrence is common. Computerized tomography should be obtained for any floor of mouth lesion suspected to involve the retromolar trigone, keeping in mind the inherent inability of CT to detect invasion at the histologic level.[111] Traditionally these tumors have been managed with wide excision of the primary lesion and full thickness segmental resection of the mandible.[86] Generally, surgery consists of hemimandibulectomy with resection of the involved oropharyngeal/oral cavity structures including the floor of mouth and tongue as well as excision of the pterygoid and masseter muscles. In selected earlier stage (I, II) cases marginal mandibulectomy may be performed.[180,248] Ipsilateral neck dissection is usually performed as the reported risk of cervical metastatic disease ranges from 60% to 80% in these lesions.[180,248,249] There is a consensus within the literature that patients with advanced stage oral cavity SCC involving the retromolar trigone benefit from combined modality therapy including surgical resection, postoperative radiotherapy, and adjuvant chemotherapy[92,178,180,189,248-251] (Fig 14-4).

Mandible Invasion

Mandible invasion from oral cavity SCC has traditionally been associated with aggressive disease and significantly alters the stage of disease as indicated by the AJCC Staging System (see Tables 14-1 and 14-2). Traditional mandible segmental resection of the involved segment of the mandible remains the mainstay

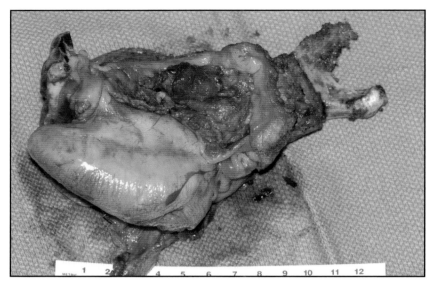

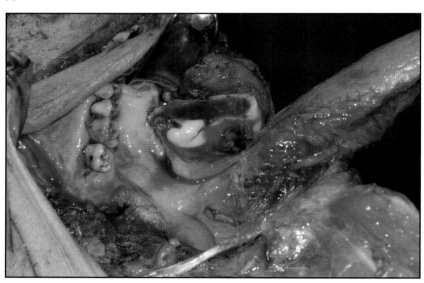

Fig 14–4. Right oral composite resection of T4 SCC right retromolar trigone. Defect following right oral composite resection.

of surgical approaches to these lesions.[182,189,252-254] Gross invasion of the mandible cortex with invasion of the marrow space or large regions of mandible involvement requires segmental resection of the tumor.[255] Primary tumors that encase the mandible making resection of the soft tissue tumor impossible without violating the surgical specimen are indica-tions for segmental resection as well. Advanced stage III and stage IV lesions often require a com-posite resection including the ipsilateral neck spec-imen. Although generally reserved for smaller T1 and T2 lesions, marginal mandibulectomy has been examined recently in the literature for more ad-vanced lesions. Results comparable to segmental resection have been reported and marginal mandibulectomy has several advantages due to maintenance of mandible continuity.[180,182,189,256,257] Accurate preoperative assessment that combines clinical examination and radiographic evaluation is critical for patient selection when considering marginal mandibular resection.[257,258] Nevertheless, larger or more deeply invading tumors in the soft tissue are more likely to invade the mandible and show the more aggressive form of tumor spread, reducing the options of a more conservative resection.[185] The ultimate goal is resection to negative margin as the status of the surgical margin is the main factor which affects prognosis for oral SCC involving the mandible[189,257] (Fig 14-5).

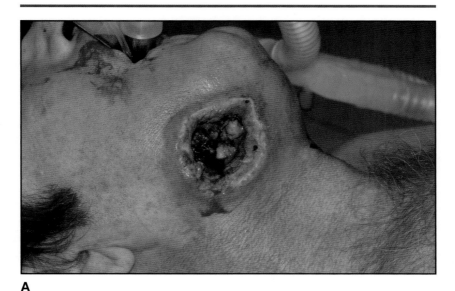

A

B

Fig 14–5. T4 SCC right floor of mouth invading through mandible and external skin. Surgical specimen: oral composite resection with external skin.

SCC of the Maxilla

Maxilla involvement is relatively uncommon for oral cavity SCC when compared to other sites. Moreover, lesions involving the maxillary alveolus or hard palate are less likely to present at advanced stage and less likely to exhibit metastatic disease when compared to other sites such as the floor of mouth or tongue.[244] Surgical management may include partial or total maxillectomy for advanced stage lesions.[259-261] Combined modality therapy including wide resection of maxillary lesions with 1- to 2-cm margins including the underlying osseous structure is recommended[262,259,260] (Fig 14-6).

Buccal Mucosal SCC

Advanced stage oral cavity SCC of the buccal mucosa is commonly regarded a highly aggressive form of oral cavity cancer, with a tendency for locoregional recurrence and poor prognosis. Involvement of muscle and salivary gland ducts have been associated with decreased survival.[263] Several investigations have reported worse stage for stage survival relative to other oral cavity sites.[175,264] Recent literature has reputed these findings, however, and the debate continues regarding the prognosis of SCC of the buccal mucosa.[265] Nonetheless, there is little doubt that advanced stage SCC of the buccal mucosa is an aggressive malignancy and outcomes

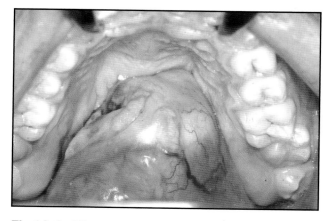

Fig 14–6. T4 mucoepidermoid carcinoma hard palate.

reported for the salvage therapy for recurrent disease are universally dismal.[162,263-265] Therefore, as with other similarly staged oral cavity SCC, combined modality therapy remains the standard of care. Ipsilateral neck dissection should be performed routinely in T3 and T4 patients, and strongly considered for tumors with greater than 5-mm thickness regardless of T status.[162] In addition, postoperative radiotherapy has been reported as effective in decreasing locoregional failure in patients with close surgical margins, tumor thickness greater than 10 mm, poorly differentiated histologic findings, or in tumors that exhibit osseous invasion and should be administered accordingly[263] (Figs 14-7 and 14-8).

SURGICAL MANAGEMENT OF THE NECK

Since the description of the radical neck dissection by Crile in 1906 there have been voluminous repots regarding the neck dissection for head and neck SCC.[266] Over the last 100 years, the continued evolution of the neck dissection has resulted in less aggressive operations with preservation of nonlymphatic structures, such as the spinal accessory nerve, internal jugular vein, and sternocleidomastoid muscle, which led to the development of the modified radical neck dissection.[267-269] Ultimately, as metastatic patterns were described and the outcomes following neck dissection were evaluated, selective neck dissection was introduced.[157,270] This allowed surgeons to tailor surgical therapy to the cervical node levels at greatest risk for metastatic disease, thereby sparing the patient from unnecessarily aggressive surgery. Further work continues to define the role of neck dissection and alternative techniques such as sentinel node biopsy are currently being evaluated for oral cavity SCC.

As noted previously, the presence of metastatic cervical lymph nodes is the most important factor in outcomes with head and neck SCC. Therefore, the treatment of the neck is critical in patients with advanced stage oral cavity malignancy. Current imaging modalities offer approximately 70% to 80% accuracy for the detection of cervical metastatic disease and it has been observed that neck dissection

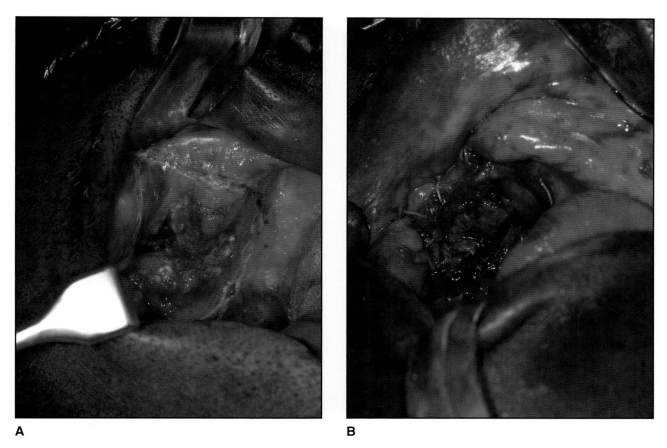

A

B

Fig 14–7. T3 SCC right buccal mucosa. Defect right buccal mucosa reconstructed with right temporalis muscle rotation flap.

offers substantially more accurate information for staging, treatment planning and surveillance.[115,129,159] The anatomic levels of the neck may be reviewed in Figure 14-1.

Despite continued debate in the literature regarding the appropriate therapy for the NO neck it is generally accepted that routine surgical dissection of the N+ neck is required for advanced stage oral cavity SCC.[113,122,81,271,10] This recommendation is in light of the fact that oral cavity SCC has an extremely high rate (60% to 80%) of clinically evident and occult cervical lymph node metastasis to levels I to III, with a moderate risk of level IV involvement.[147,156,180,248,249,272]

Traditionally, surgical management of the ipsilateral neck in advanced oral cavity SCC consists of the modified radical neck dissection including lev-els I, II, III, and IV with preservation of the spinal accessory nerve, internal jugular vein and sterno-cleidomastoid muscle.[13,147,267] T3 or T4 lesions, lesions located in the floor of mouth, or lesions approaching the midline require bilateral modified radical neck dissection due to the risk of contralateral lymph node metastasis.[13,147,267,273,274] The risk of level V cervical lymph node metastasis in oral cavity SCC is extremely low and therefore the utility of level V dissection may is questionable for many these lesions.[196,275,276] It should also be noted that the utility of dissection in the submuscular recess (level IIa), namely, the cervical nodes superior to the spinal accessory nerve, has also been questioned for oral cavity SCC as the risk of metastatic disease to this area is extremely low in the clinically negative neck. Involvement of this compartment is

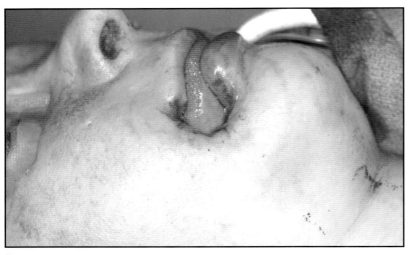

A

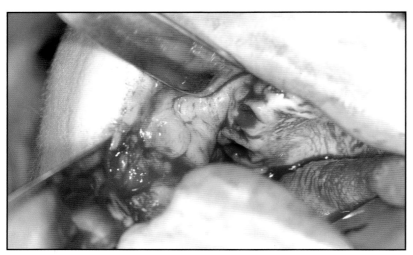

B

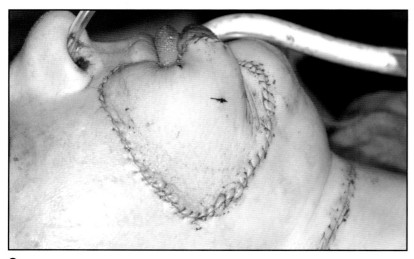

C

Fig 14–8. T4 adenoid cystic carcinoma right buccal mucosa. Intraoral view of T4 adenoid cystic carcinoma right buccal mucosa. Reconstruction of full-thickness right buccal mucosal defect with radial forearm flap.

increased if there is greater than N2 cervical disease, however, and in this case dissection of level IIa should routinely be performed.[154,268]

Recently, many investigators have reported employing a selective neck dissection, including levels I, II, and III, with similar results in terms of locoregional control and overall survival.[13,14,267,277,278] Despite the interest in selective neck dissection, many investigators recommend more aggressive cervical lymphadenectomy with advanced stage disease.[135,147,148,156,158,267,269,274,276,279-285] Further work in this area may reveal more clear indications for the type of neck dissection but at the current time the selective neck dissection (levels I–III) is the minimum surgical therapy for advanced disease, with most authors recommending modified radical neck dissection (I–IV) the operation of choice for advanced stage oral cavity SCC. Additional adjunctive radiotherapy is warranted for increased regional control of disease in the presence of cervical metastasis.[13,174]

Sentinal Node Biopsy

Recently, much interest and research has been reported regarding sentinel lymph node biopsy (SLB) for SCC of the head and neck, including the oral cavity. Although the interpretation of results is somewhat less straightforward when compared to cutaneous melanoma results, the technique has some promise for head and neck SCC. The primary advantage of the sentinel node technique is the potential to decrease the number of neck dissections performed in clinically negative necks (N0), thus reducing the associated surgical morbidity in this group of patients. The technique has been shown to be feasible and relatively accurate for the N0 neck.[286-289] A recent international conference on the subject of sentinel lymph node biopsy for mucosal head and neck cancer evaluated the literature and reported on the results of 20 institutions which performed SLB in over 370 patients with N0. The consensus panel reported an encouraging 96% negative predictive value for SLB in the clinically negative neck. Minimal requirements for the technique included the use of a radiotracer, lymphoscintigraphy, and a hand-held gamma probe for lymphatic mapping. The use of hematoxylin and eosin staining with immunohistochemistry for cytokeratin was determined to be a mandatory component of this technique. Step-sectioning of the entire node at intervals of 150 micrometers was recommended as well.[288] The consensus conference concluded that SLB for early stage (N0) oral and oropharyngeal cancer should be considered sufficiently validated although work continues to define the role of SLB in SCC of the head and neck.

In the case of advanced stage oral cavity carcinoma there is currently little role for sentinel lymph node mapping due to the propensity of this disease to present with occult or clinically evident lymph node metastasis. Additionally unpredictable patterns of lymphatic spread have been reported with advanced stage disease.[147,156,180,248,249,272] As noted previously, patients who present with advanced stage (III, IV) oral cavity SCC should undergo formal neck dissection for both staging and therapeutic reasons. In cases of recurrent disease, the previously operated or radiated neck may exhibit altered lymphatic drainage patterns and the reliability of SLB is questionable.

ADJUVANT THERAPY FOR ORAL CAVITY SCC

Radiation Therapy

As previously stated, it is generally accepted that advanced stage oral cavity SCC is most effectively treated with combined modality therapy including surgery, radiation, and chemotherapy. The benefits of radiation therapy for head and neck SCC are well known and postoperative radiotherapy is indicated for all tumors with T3 or T4 status, cervical metastasis (>N1), high-grade histologic features, perineural invasion, or close or positive margins after surgical resection.[290] Therefore, postoperative radiotherapy should be routinely employed in patients with advanced stage oral cavity SCC. [2,5,87,89,98,135,138,139,142, 158,179,181,182,186,193,232-244,291] Postoperative radiotherapy is generally administered within 6 weeks of surgery and longer delays have been associated with increased risk of cervical metastasis.[292,293] Total dosages usually range from 6000 to 6800 cGy for the primary tumor, divided into 180 to 200-cGy fractions administered

5 days per week.[85,193,280,292-295] Positive surgical margins should receive full-dose radiotherapy with a dosage of 6250 cGy for maximum benefit.[96,173,237,251,296] Dosages greater than 6600 cGy have been reported to significantly improve outcomes with oral cavity lesions demonstrating the poor response rates when compared to primary tumors of other locations within the head and neck.[190]

Preoperative radiotherapy has been recommended based on the theory of increased tumor radiosensitivity due to well-oxygenated tumor characteristics prior to surgery. Many investigations, however, have indicated that postoperative radiation offers significantly superior locoregional control when compared to preoperative regimens.[87,142,174,297,298] It should be noted, however, that investigation of preoperative protocols continues and encouraging results have been reported.[191] Further work examining the advantages, disadvantages, and outcomes of preoperative versus postoperative radiotherapy is currently in progress.

Patients who are candidates for radiation therapy should undergo routine physical examination, baseline hematocrit (>30 recommended prior to therapy), and thyroid function studies prior to radiation. Thyroid function studies should be monitored throughout the treatment period due to the risk of hypothyroidism (5–20%) when subjecting the cervical region to radiation. Dental evaluation with completion of dental work or dental extractions is required prior to radiation involving the oral cavity to minimize future risk of osteoradionecrosis.[299] Fluoride therapy should be routinely employed for dentate patients. Ophthalmologic examination is also recommended if the orbit or paranasal sinuses are to be included in the radiation field. Nutritional assessment with speech therapy consultation for evaluation of pre/postradiation swallowing function is necessary to ensure adequate nutrition during and after radiation therapy.

There are several recent advances regarding radiation therapy that have significantly impacted the ability of the radiation oncologist to deliver high-dose radiation to the target while minimizing untoward radiation damage to the surrounding tissue (ie, therapeutic ratio). Traditional radiation protocols have been modified and novel hyperfractionation protocols, which subdivide radiation fractions in order to decrease side effects with equivalent or greater total doses, have been investigated and reported with promising outcomes.[300-304] Unfortunately, the effectiveness of radiation therapy is somewhat limited by the toxic effects of the total delivered dose (approximately 7000 cGy) regardless of the protocol.[305,306] Intensity modulation techniques (IMRT or 3 DCRT) which decrease the radiation delivered to surrounding tissues while targeting the tumor have had encouraging results and are currently recommended by many investigators. These techniques utilize pretreatment three-dimensional treatment planning with computerized tomography as well as targeted linear accelerator delivery systems. Recently FDG-PET/CT guided IMRT has been evaluated.[307] These techniques, specifically in the case of oral cavity malignancy, have significant advantages for salivary gland preservation and improved functional outcomes.[301,307,308]

Brachytherapy is a radiotherapy technique which employs a radioisotope delivery system such as seeds or interstitial catheters to deliver radiation directly to the tumor bed. The primary advantage of this technique is targeted radiotherapy directly delivered to the tumor with a high therapeutic ratio due to the rapid intensity decrease in peripheral dosage associated with the inverse square law of distance. Protocols currently in use include low-dose rate (LDR) brachytherapy (40–200 cGy/hour), high-dose rate (HDR) brachytherapy (1000–1200 cGy/hr), and pulsed does rate (PDR) brachytherapy.[309] Common isotopes used for head and neck brachytherapy include I^{125} Ir^{192} Au^{198}.[309-311]

Brachytherapy has been evaluated in the literature for the treatment of oral cavity SCC either as part of multimodal therapy or as primary therapy for patients who are not candidates for surgical intervention. Locoregional control and survival data have been reported by multiple investigators which would indicate equivalent results to conventional radiation therapy while shortening treatment time and limiting radiation to surrounding tissue.[161,311-314] Total radiation dosage to the tumor bed may range as high as 8000 to 12000 cGy.[310-312]

Brachytherapy offers an attractive option for adjuvant therapy in surgical cases with positive surgical margins after resection.[313] In addition, brachytherapy combined with surgery may offer an alternate modality for recurrent oral cavity SCC when conventional multimodality therapy has failed.[310,315]

Despite the decreased delivery of radiation to surrounding tissues, complications of brachytherapy include complications associated with traditional external beam radiotherapy such as mucositis, infection, poor oral intake, and xerostomia. Of particular concern is the increased incidence of local soft tissue and bone necrosis adjacent to the radioactive implants.[309,311,313,316] Nevertheless, brachytherapy offers distinct advantages when compared to conventional external beam irradiation future investigation of treatment protocols, indications, and outcomes will define the role of brachytherapy in the management of advanced oral cavity SCC.

CONCOMITANT CHEMOTHERAPY/ CHEMORADIOTHERAPY

Chemotherapy regimens used in conjunction with radiation therapy (concomitant chemotherapy) are widely utilized in the treatment of advanced oral cavity SCC. It is widely accepted that chemotherapy as a standalone treatment for advanced oral cavity SCC is largely ineffective with high rates of locoregional recurrence and metastatic disease. When combined with radiation, however, chemotherapy may potentiate the effects of radiation and offers an excellent adjunctive therapy after surgical resection as well as a primary modality in patients who are not candidates for surgery. Several chemoradiotherapy regimens have been described including continuous radiotherapy with concomitant chemotherapy, split-course radiotherapy with concomitant chemotherapy, and alternating radiotherapy with chemotherapy.

Mucosal SCC of the oropharynx/oral cavity has been treated with several classes of chemotherapeutic agents which act to disrupt the cell cycle of rapidly dividing malignant cells. Alkylating agents act to inhibit DNA synthesis by direct cross-linking of DNA which prevents DNA replication and include cyclophosphamide, cisplatin, and carboplatin. The antimetabolites such as methotrexate and 5-fluorouracil

are competitive inhibitors of DNA synthesis by acting as purine or pyrimidine analogs. Alkaloids are compounds which disrupt the process of mitosis by preventing microtubule formation within the mitotic spindle and include the vinca alkaloids and taxanes. Topoisomerase inhibitors such as irinotecan and etoposide interfere with ordered supercoiling of the DNA structure during DNA replication. Combinations of these agents and others have been utilized in various investigation protocols for the treatment of head and neck SCC.

Traditional concomitant regimens for oral cavity SCC usually comprise cisplatin/carboplatin and 5-flurouracil-based chemotherapy with the addition of various other chemotherapeutic agents. Concomitant chemotherapy has been reported to decrease metastatic disease and increase locoregional control in multiple investigations including randomized trials.[88,139,240,241,298,317-323] Additional agents such as docetaxel, paclitaxel, and amifostine have shown promise in increasing the efficacy of current concomitant chemotherapy regimens.[192,320,324,325] Unfortunately, overall survival data from many investigations indicate equivocal results when compared to surgery and adjuvant radiotherapy.[89,323,326,327] The data are somewhat confusing due to the paucity of site-specific randomized trials related to advanced malignancy involving the oropharynx/oral cavity. There is, however, some evidence that concomitant chemotherapy may have a significant survival benefit for this patient population.[318,321,328-330] Recent investigations have shown promising results with cetuximab, a recombinant monoclonal antibody that binds specifically to the epidermal growth factor receptor (EGFR) and competitively inhibits the binding of epidermal growth factor resulting in inhibition of cell growth, induction of apoptosis, and decreased vascular endothelial growth factor production.[331-333] Radiotherapy with cetuximab has been shown to significantly prolonged progression free survival and improve locoregional control in patients with advanced head and neck SCC.[334,335] Forthcoming randomized controlled trial data are required to determine the locoregional control and survival benefit of current concomitant chemotherapeutic regimens in the treatment of advanced oral cavity SCC.

NEOADJUVANT/INDUCTION/ CHEMOTHERAPY

Neoadjuvant or induction chemotherapy refers to chemotherapy regimens administered prior to definitive multimodality therapy for malignancy. Sequential chemotherapy refers to neoadjuvant chemotherapy followed by multimodality therapy which includes additional chemotherapy as part of the treatment protocol. Purported advantages of neoadjuvant protocols include superior response rates, decreased toxicity, and valuable prognostic information as complete responders tend to have superior prognosis compared to patients with an incomplete response. Multiple investigations, generally with cisplatin based multiagent protocols, have been performed to evaluate neoadjuvant chemotherapy. Numerous investigations have reported decreased failure due to distant metastasis although with a lack of benefit when overall survival data are analyzed.[89,244,298,319,336-341] Interpretation of the results of these investigations is difficult due to design problems related to inclusion criteria, protocol differences, compliance issues, and interpretation of results.[342,343] Neoadjuvant protocols may also incur the disadvantages of delaying locoregional therapy and selecting for aggressive tumor clonogens prior to definitive therapy.

Nevertheless, several recent studies have reported increased survival benefit with sequential chemotherapy regimens in the treatment of oral cavity SCC.[342,344] The role of neoadjuvant chemotherapy in the treatment of advanced oral cavity SCC remains in question and further randomized controlled trials are needed to determine whether a significant benefit can be achieved with sequential chemotherapy protocols.

PRIMARY CHEMORADIOTHERAPY FOR ADVANCED STAGE ORAL CAVITY SCC

Modern chemoradiotherapy is an important modality in the treatment of advanced stage oropharyngeal/ oral cavity SCC. Current protocols may allow adequate therapy for advanced lesions with comparable outcomes to surgical intervention, minimize side effects, and offer a nonsurgical option to patients who are not candidates for extensive surgical resection of advanced disease. Significant work has been performed in this area to define which patient populations benefit from nonsurgical management of oropharyngeal/oral cavity mucosal malignancy. Several authors have reported acceptable results with chemoradiotherapy strategies.[241,298,317,318,321,323,345-348] Investigators have reported that a significant percentage of patients can be spared surgical resection when employing these protocols.[317,323,347,348]

Unfortunately, the currently available data regarding chemoradiotherapy for the treatment of advanced SCC of the oral cavity alone are not well established. This is largely due to the inclusion of oropharyngeal, hypopharyngeal, and various other subsites which influence the results. There is little doubt that treatment outcomes for advanced oral cavity SCC are significantly worse when compared to oropharyngeal/ hypopharyngeal SCCs of similar stage when using current chemoradiotherapy protocols as the primary treatment modality.[139,182,235,241,250,298,317,318,321,341,346,349] This fact, coupled with the extremely poor outcomes for recurrent oral cavity SCC, has prompted many investigators to recommend multimodality therapy including surgical resection for these malignancies.[139,182,235,250,318,341] Therefore, the current standard of care for advanced (stage III, IV) oral cavity SCCs is multimodality therapy including surgical resection with adjuvant therapy including chemotherapy and postoperative radiotherapy.

SURVEILLANCE

Regardless of the protocol used to treat advanced oral cavity SCC, patients who are undergoing treatment, or have completed therapy, require close clinical surveillance. Follow-up appointment intervals are determined by the risk of recurrence or synchronous lesions and to provide social and psychological support. Patients undergoing radiotherapy often experience odynophagia, dysphagia, and poor nutritional status secondary to radiation-induced mucositis as well as significant pain and occasional airway obstruction. Wound care, complications, or morbidity resulting from therapy may require more frequent clinical appointments. Periodic preventative dental evaluations are also required in patients undergoing radiation therapy.

Current practice guidelines from the American Head and Neck Society regarding the clinical surveillance of patients who have been treated for advanced oral cavity/oropharyngeal SCC are outlined below:[350]

1st year post-treatment: 1 to 3-month interval

2nd year post-treatment: 2 to 4-month interval

3rd year post-treatment: 3 to 6-month interval

4th and 5th years: 4 to 6-month interval

After 5 years: Every 12-month interval

Annual chest radiograph

Annual liver enzymes

Annual thyroid function studies in patients that received radiation to the lower neck.

Physical examination including fiberoptic laryngoscopy should be performed at each interval to assess the response to therapy as well as monitor for recurrent and/or second malignant neoplasms which occur at rate of approximately 5 to 6% in this patient population.[351,352] Computerized tomography or magnetic resonance imaging may be obtained as clinically indicated to assess the response to therapy, investigate for occult malignancy, as well as monitor the neck for cervical metastasis. Positron emission tomography (PET) offers an excellent surveillance instrument as it represents a functional imaging modality, rather than a static imaging modality as in the case of CT or MRI, and is currently recommended by many investigators.[353,354] PET has been shown to be highly effective in detecting locoregional recurrence as well as distant metastases after multimodality therapy for head and neck SCC, and a negative PET is highly reliable in the surveillance of the head and neck cancer patient. PET is not without limitations, however, and significant unreliability exists due to a high rate of false-positive results, especially if performed early after completion of therapy. For this reason, most investigators recommend a period of 8 to 12 weeks prior to obtaining PET imaging in the surveillance of head and neck SCC.[353,355]

RECURRENCE

Recurrence following therapy for oral cavity SCC is an extremely discouraging development. Significant risk of locoregional recurrence or cervical recurrence has been reported in patients with advanced stage lesions.[160,282,356,357] Patients with recurrent disease are candidates for salvage therapy such as surgery, additional chemotherapy, and brachytherapy/radiotherapy depending on the primary therapy administered. There is some evidence that surgical salvage may offer a slight outcome advantage compared to other modalities such as radiation and chemotherapy.[232,356,357] Unfortunately, despite the type of salvage therapy, survival outcomes in this patient population are somewhat dismal and have been reported to range between approximately 15 to 35% at 5 years.[85,138,141,232,233,356,358,359] Consequently, patients should be cautiously counseled regarding the morbidity of salvage therapy and the limited chance for cure prior to initiating salvage therapy for recurrent advanced stage oral cavity SCC.

SURGICAL RECONSTRUCTION OF DEFECTS

Resection of advanced oral cavity malignancy often results in extensive defects which are extremely challenging from the standpoint of surgical reconstruction. A comprehensive review of the technical aspects of surgical reconstruction of defects resulting from the resection of advanced oral cavity SCC is beyond the scope of this chapter. Several important issues related to oral cavity reconstruction after extirpative surgery are central to successful treatment outcomes and are discussed.

The goals of reconstructive surgery of the oral cavity relate to the restoration of the form and function of the oral cavity. Specifically these goals include mastication, deglutition, and speech as well as an acceptable aesthetic result. In order to achieve these goals, multispecialty reconstructive and rehabilitative efforts are paramount. This requires the expertise of the oncologic and reconstructive surgeon, oral/maxillofacial surgeon, general dentist, speech/swallowing therapist, physical therapist, and nutritionist.

Achieving the goals of reconstruction can be obtained via a variety of surgical techniques depending on the configuration of the defect. Surgical resection of advanced stage oral cavity lesions generally results in large composite defects including the tongue, floor of mouth, mandible, external skin, and/or the oropharynx/hypopharynx and discussion is limited to defects of this type.

Historically, reconstruction of large composite defects of the oral cavity relied on skin grafts, local flaps, or the early tubed cutaneous flaps. Unfortunately, functional and aesthetic outcomes with these early attempts were poor. The traditional mainstay of oral cavity reconstruction that followed was the regional and pedicled flaps, which included fasciocutaneous, myocutaneous, osteocutaneous, or myoosteocutaneous variants. Examples of regional flaps in head and neck construction include the temporalis, pectoralis major, lattisimus dorsi, trapezius, sternocleidomastoid, or deltopectoral flaps. These flaps represent an extremely dependable reconstructive option and remain in use today due to tissue availability, excellent reliability, technical simplicity, and acceptable donor site morbidity. Osseous reconstruction is possible (rib, scapula) and coupled with advances in reconstructive technology, such as titanium reconstruction plating systems, these flaps continue to be used successfully in the reconstruction of large ablative defects of the oral cavity. Regional myocutaneous rotation flaps such as the pectoralis and trapezius pedicled flaps also provide an excellent salvage option for failed microvascular free-tissue transfer procedures.[360-362] Nonetheless, significant problems including fistula, plate dehiscence/infection of hardware, and functional deficits related to both donor and recipient sites have been observed with these reconstruction techniques.[187,362]

The advent of microvascular free-tissue transfer techniques has revolutionized oral cavity reconstruction after ablative surgery for advanced malignancy. Examples of microvascular flaps utilized in the reconstruction of defects in the head and neck include the fibular, radial forearm, rectus, anterior/lateral thigh, iliac crest, scapular, and lattisimus free flaps as well as the jejunal, or gastro-omental free flaps.

Significant advantages to free-tissue transfer procedures include the ability to select the donor site which matches the requirements of the defect, large quantities of tissue availability including skin, fascia, muscle, and bone, and the possibility of sensory/motor restoration via microneurorrhaphy techniques. Another significant advantage is the ability to provide donor tissue that has not been subjected to locoregional therapy such as radiation, thus offering superior vascularity and healing potential. Reported disadvantages of microvascular techniques are the technical expertise required, donor site morbidity, and increased time and cost. The increasing prevalence and progression of microvascular techniques has negated many of these concerns, however, and these techniques have resulted in significant improvement of the quality of life of patients afflicted with advanced oral cavity malignancy requiring surgical resection.[188,363-365]

Mandible Reconstruction

Mandible reconstruction with the fibula free flap offers exceptional restoration of large mucosal, cutaneous and osseous defects coupled with an extremely reliable blood supply and reported success rates approaching 92% to 95% in experienced centers.[188,252,253,364,366,367] The superior vascularity obtained with microvascular mandible reconstruction techniques offers excellent resistance to infection and sufficient reliability if postoperative radiotherapy is planned. Another advantage is sufficient quantity/quality of bone to facilitate dental prosthetic rehabilitation with osseointegrated titanium dental implants which have been reported to statistically improve functional outcomes related to oral reconstruction.[252] Additional options for mandible reconstruction include the deep circumflex iliac crest and scapular free flap.[253] Osteomyocutaneous free-tissue transfer is currently the preferred reconstruction for large, composite mandible defects after ablative surgery for oral cavity malignancy. This is especially true if the resection is larger than 5 cm or involves the anterior symphyseal region of the mandible as complication rates are higher in this region when traditional techniques are used[187,188,252,253,364,366,368] (Figs 14-9 and 14-10).

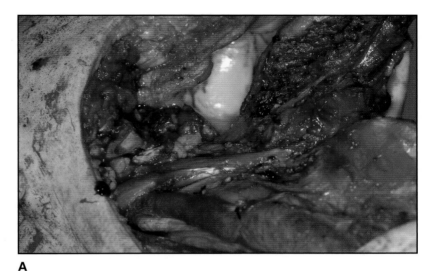

A

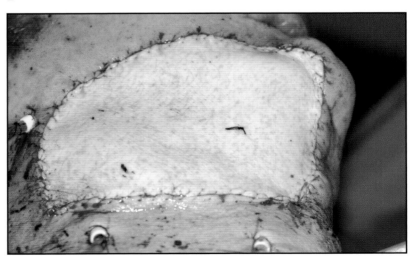

B

Fig 14–9. Right oral composite defect. Right fibula free flap (4 segments, 3 osteotomies). Flap skin of fibula used for neck and cheek reconstruction.

C

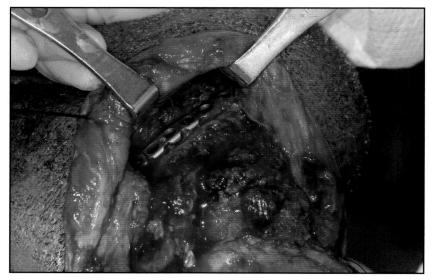

A

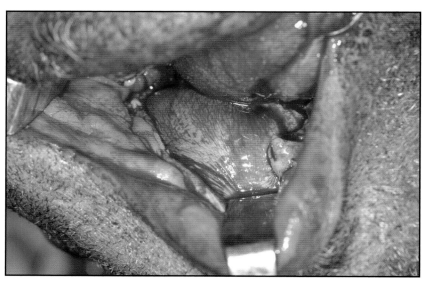

B

Fig 14–10. Right mandible defect reconstructed with fibula free flap. Right oral composite defect with flap skin used for intraoral reconstruction.

Reconstruction of the Tongue

As previously noted, the tongue is the most common primary site for oral cavity SCC. This is unfortunate as the tongue likely represents the most vital structure of the oral cavity. Multimodality therapy for advanced oral cavity tumors of the tongue often results in severe functional impairment related to speech, chewing, swallowing, and taste disturbance. There is currently no reconstructive option which offers complete restoration of the form and function of the tongue. Goals of restoration include preservation of residual function, facilitate movement by counterbalancing the remaining tongue and providing adequate bulk, use of most pliable tissue available to avoid tethering/scarring, and maintenance of sensation if possible. Local flaps and split thickness skin grafts have been utilized and have the advantages of being thin, pliable, and readily available but are generally reserved for smaller (<20-30%) defects.

Currently, most reconstructive surgeons prefer microvascular free-tissue transfer for the reconstruction of large defects of the tongue and floor of mouth. The radial forearm free flap offers an excellent option for larger defects resulting from partial glossectomy as it is reliable and thin/pliable which allows for reconstruction without compromising the function of the remaining tongue.[365,369-371] The possibility of providing sensate reconstruction is another advantage of the radial forearm flap.[372] Larger, total glossectomy defects may benefit from reconstruction with the rectus abdominus or anterior lateral thigh free flap due to the need for increased bulk which is difficult to achieve with the radial forearm flap[369,373-375] (Figs 14-11, 14-12, and 14-13).

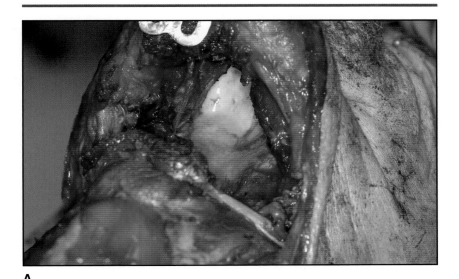

A

B

Fig 14-11. Total glossectomy defect. Total glossectomy defect reconstructed with anterolateral thigh flap.

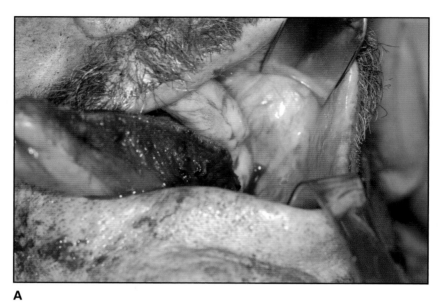

A

B

Fig 14–12. Left hemiglossectomy defect. Left hemiglossectomy defect reconstructed with radial forearm flap.

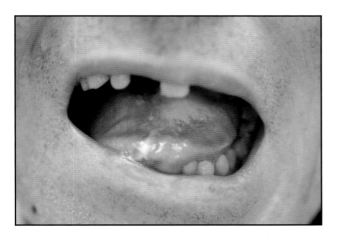

Fig 14–13. Postoperative appearance of right tongue reconstruction with forearm flap.

Maxilla/Palate Reconstruction

Surgical resection of advanced maxillary oral cavity SCC often results in defects of the hard/soft palate, nasal floor, and maxillary alveolus including the dentition. Continuity of the oral cavity and nasal cavities, and/or maxillary sinus, results in significant functional and aesthetic morbidity. Deficits in speech, chewing, swallowing, and unacceptable facial contour are common problems reported by patients after resection of advanced maxillary tumors. Traditional management of many of these defects has consisted of maxillofacial prosthesis or obturators. Prosthetics remain in use today and offer several advantages such as decreased time to rehabilitation, excellent aesthetics, reasonable function, and superior tumor surveillance as the prosthesis can be removed and the surgical bed examined directly.

Several disadvantages of prosthetic reconstruction, including maintenance/compliance issues and functional shortcomings, have led to the development of various surgical techniques used in the reconstruction of ablative defects of the maxilla. The goals of surgical reconstruction include obliteration of the ablative defect, recreation of midfacial contour, and sufficient reconstruction to allow for adequate swallowing function, phonation, and mastication with prosthetic dental rehabilitation if feasible. Advances in microvascular free-tissue transfer

technique have greatly increased the reconstructive options available to the surgeon and patient. A variety of techniques have been used in the reconstruction of large defects of the maxilla including calvarial bone grafts, iliac crest grafts, temporalis flaps, and iliac, radial forearm, scapular, and fibular microvascular tissue transfers.[376-380] The reconstructive treatment plan should follow the osseous and soft tissue contours of the defect as well as the available prosthodontic support and goals/motivation of the patient. A multidisciplinary approach including the reconstructive surgeon, oral/maxillofacial surgeon, prosthodontist/restorative dentist, and maxillofacial prosthetist is requisite to obtain optimal results.

REFERENCES

1. Chin D, Boyle GM, Porceddu S, Theile DR, Parsons PG, Coman WB. Head and neck cancer: past, present and future. *Expert Rev Anticancer Ther.* 2006;6(7):1111-1118.
2. Carvalho AL, Singh B, Spiro RH, Kowalski LP, Shah JP. Cancer of the oral cavity: a comparison between institutions in a developing and a developed nation. *Head Neck.* 2004;26(1):31-38.
3. American Cancer Society. *Cancer Facts and Figures.* 2006.
4. Llewellyn CD, Johnson NW, Warnakulasuriya KA. Risk factors for oral cancer in newly diagnosed patients aged 45 years and younger: a case-control study in Southern England. *J Oral Pathol Med.* 2004;33(9):525-532.
5. Funk GF, Karnell LH, Robinson RA, Zhen WK, Trask DK, Hoffman HT. Presentation, treatment, and outcome of oral cavity cancer: a National Cancer Data Base report. *Head Neck.* 2002;24(2):165-180.
6. Hoffman HT, Karnell LH, Funk GF, Robinson RA, Menck HR. The National Cancer Data Base report on cancer of the head and neck. *Arch Otolaryngol Head Neck Surg.* 1998;124(9):951-962.
7. Canto MT, Devesa SS. Oral cavity and pharynx cancer incidence rates in the United States, 1975-1998. *Oral Oncol.* 2002;38(6):610-617.
8. Elango JK, Gangadharan P, Sumithra S, Kuriakose MA. Trends of head and neck cancers in urban and rural India. *Asian Pac J Cancer Prev.* 2006; 7(1):108-112.

9. Kornberg LJ, Villaret D, Popp M, et al. Gene expression profiling in SCC of the oral cavity shows abnormalities in several signaling pathways. *Laryngoscope.* 2005;115(4):690–698.

10. Shah JP, Singh B. Keynote comment: why the lack of progress for oral cancer? *Lancet Oncol.* 2006; 7(5):356–357.

11. Taneja C, Allen H, Koness RJ, Radie-Keane K, Wanebo HJ. Changing patterns of failure of head and neck cancer. *Arch Otolaryngol Head Neck Surg.* 2002;128(3):324–327.

12. American Joint Committee on Cancer. *AJCC Cancer Staging Manual.* 6th ed. New York, NY: Springer; 2002:23–42.

13. Ambrosch P, Kron M, Pradier O, Steiner W. Efficacy of selective neck dissection: a review of 503 cases of elective and therapeutic treatment of the neck in SCC of the upper aerodigestive tract. *Otolaryngol Head Neck Surg.* 2001;124(2):180–187.

14. Candela FC, Kothari K, Shah JP. Patterns of cervical node metastases from squamous carcinoma of the oropharynx and hypopharynx. *Head Neck.* 1990;12(3):197–203.

15. Hughes CJ, Gallo O, Spiro RH, Shah JP. Management of occult neck metastases in oral cavity squamous carcinoma. *Am J Surg.* 1993;166(4): 380–383.

16. Mukherji SK, Armao D, Joshi VM. Cervical nodal metastases in SCC of the head and neck: what to expect. *Head Neck.* 2001;23(11):995–1005.

17. Byers RM, Wolf PF, Ballantyne AJ. Rationale for elective modified neck dissection. *Head Neck Surg.* 1988;10(3):160–167.

18. Lindberg R. Distribution of cervical lymph node metastases from SCC of the upper respiratory and digestive tracts. *Cancer.* 1972;29(6):1446–1449.

19. Fukano H, Matsuura H, Hasegawa Y, Nakamura S. Depth of invasion as a predictive factor for cervical lymph node metastasis in tongue carcinoma. *Head Neck.* 1997;19(3):205–210.

20. Hayashi T, Ito J, Taira S, Katsura K. The relationship of primary tumor thickness in carcinoma of the tongue to subsequent lymph node metastasis. *Dentomaxillofac Radiol.* 2001;30(5):242–245.

21. Gillenwater AM, Chambers MS. Diagnosis of premalignant lesions and early cancers of the oral cavity. *Tex Dent J.* 2006;123(6):512–520.

22. Neville BW, Day TA. Oral cancer and precancerous lesions. *California Cancer J Clin.* 2002;52(4): 195–215.

23. Rodu B, Cole P. Smokeless tobacco use and cancer of the upper respiratory tract. *Oral Surg Oral Med Oral Pathol Oral Radiol Endod.* 2002;93(5): 511–515.

24. Rodu B, Jansson C. Smokeless tobacco and oral cancer: a review of the risks and determinants. *Crit Rev Oral Biol Med.* 2004;15(5):252–263.

25. Ariyawardana A, Athukorala AD, Arulanandam A. Effect of betel chewing, tobacco smoking and alcohol consumption on oral submucous fibrosis: a case-control study in Sri Lanka. *J Oral Pathol Med.* 2006;35(4):197–201.

26. Chen AY, Myers JN. Cancer of the oral cavity. *Curr Probl Surg.* 2000;37(10):633–731.

27. Patel MM, Pandya AN. Relationship of oral cancer with age, sex, site distribution and habits. *Indian J Pathol Microbiol.* 2004;47(2):195–197.

28. Iype EM, Pandey M, Mathew A, Thomas G, Sebastian P, Nair MK. Oral cancer among patients under the age of 35 years. *J Postgrad Med.* 2001; 47(3):171–176.

29. Mansour OI, Snyderman CH, D'Amico F. Association between tobacco use and metastatic neck disease. *Laryngoscope.* 2003;113(1):161–166.

30. Rubright WC, Hoffman HT, Lynch CF, et al. Risk factors for advanced-stage oral cavity cancer. *Arch Otolaryngol Head Neck Surg.* 1996;122(6): 621–626.

31. Rosenquist K. Risk factors in oral and oropharyngeal SCC: a population-based case-control study in southern Sweden. *Swed Dent J Suppl.* 2005; (179):1–66.

32. Marshall JR, Boyle P. Nutrition and oral cancer. *Cancer Causes Control.* 1996;7(1):101–111.

33. Mashberg A, Boffetta P, Winkelman R, Garfinkel L. Tobacco smoking, alcohol drinking, and cancer of the oral cavity and oropharynx among U.S. veterans. *Cancer.* 1993, 15;72(4):1369–1375.

34. Zhang ZF, Morgenstern H, Spitz MR, et al. Marijuana use and increased risk of SCC of the head and neck. *Cancer Epidemiol Biomarkers Prev.* 1999;8(12):1071–1078.

35. Kozomara R, Jovic N, Magic Z, Brankovic-Magic M, Minic V. p53 mutations and human papillomavirus infection in oral SCCs: correlation with overall survival. *J Craniomaxillofac Surg.* 2005; 33(5):342–348.

36. Nemes JA, Deli L, Nemes Z, Marton IJ. Expression of p16(INK4A), p53, and Rb proteins are independent from the presence of human papillomavirus genes in oral SCC. *Oral Surg Oral Med Oral Pathol Oral Radiol Endod.* 2006;102(3):344–352.

37. Braakhuis BJ, Leemans CR, Brakenhoff RH. A genetic progression model of oral cancer: cur-

rent evidence and clinical implications. *J Oral Pathol Med.* 2004;33(6):317–322.

38. Koch WM, Lango M, Sewell D, Zahurak M, Sidransky D. Head and neck cancer in nonsmokers: a distinct clinical and molecular entity. *Laryngoscope.* 1999;109(10):1544–1551.

39. Zhang Z, Wang Y, Yao R, Li J, Lubet RA, You M. p53 Transgenic mice are highly susceptible to 4-nitroquinoline-1-oxide-induced oral cancer. *Mol Cancer Res.* 2006;4(6):401–410.

40. Myers JN, Holsinger FC, Bekele BN, et al. Targeted molecular therapy for oral cancer with epidermal growth factor receptor blockade: a preliminary report. *Arch Otolaryngol Head Neck Surg,* 2002; 128(8):875–879.

41. Werkmeister R, Brandt B, Joos U. Clinical relevance of erbB-1 and -2 oncogenes in oral carcinomas. *Oral Oncol.* 2000;36(1):100–105.

42. Gotte K, Tremmel SC, Popp S, et al. Intratumoral genomic heterogeneity in advanced head and neck cancer detected by comparative genomic hybridization. *Adv Otorhinolaryngol.* 2005;62:38–48.

43. Xia W, Lau YK, Zhang HZ, et al. Strong correlation between c-erbB-2 overexpression and overall survival of patients with oral SCC. *Clin Cancer Res.* 1997;3(1):3–9.

44. Jaber MA. Intraoral minor salivary gland tumors: a review of 75 cases in a Libyan population. *Int J Oral Maxillofac Surg.* 2006;35(2):150–154.

45. Lopes MA, Santos GC, Kowalski LP. Multivariate survival analysis of 128 cases of oral cavity minor salivary gland carcinomas. *Head Neck.* 1998; 20(8):699–706.

46. Strick MJ, Kelly C, Soames JV, McLean NR. Malignant tumours of the minor salivary glands— a 20 year review. *Br J Plast Surg.* 2004;57(7): 624–631.

47. Adornato MC, Penna K, Vinoski M. Polymorphous low-grade adenocarcinoma of the oral cavity. *N Y State Dent J.* 2000;66(5):28–32.

48. Kokemueller H, Brueggemann N, Swennen G, Eckardt A. Mucoepidermoid carcinoma of the salivary glands—clinical review of 42 cases. *Oral Oncol.* 2005;41(1):3–10.

49. Kolude B, Lawoyin JO, Akang EE. Mucoepidermoid carcinoma of the oral cavity. *J Natl Med Assoc.* 2001;93(5):178–184.

50. Spiro RH, Huvos AG, Strong EW. Adenocarcinoma of salivary origin. Clinicopathologic study of 204 patients. *Am J Surg.* 1982;144(4):423–431.

51. Batsakis JG, El-Naggar AK, Luna MA. "Adenocarcinoma, not otherwise specified": a diminishing group of salivary carcinomas. *Ann Otol Rhinol Laryngol.* 1992;101(1):102–104.

52. Lucarini JW, Sciubba JJ, Khettry U, Nasser I. Terminal duct carcinoma. Recognition of a low-grade salivary adenocarcinoma. *Arch Otolaryngol Head Neck Surg.* 1994;120(9):1010–1015.

53. Dequanter D, Andry G, Lothaire P, Larsimont D, Deraemaecker R. Wide localized excision and reconstruction for minor salivary gland tumours. *B-ENT.* 2005;1(4):187–190.

54. Castle JT, Thompson LD, Frommelt RA, Wenig BM, Kessler HP. Polymorphous low grade adenocarcinoma: a clinicopathologic study of 164 cases. *Cancer.* 1999;86(2):207–219.

55. Simpson RH, Pereira EM, Ribeiro AC, Abdulkadir A, Reis-Filho JS. Polymorphous low-grade adenocarcinoma of the salivary glands with transformation to high-grade carcinoma. *Histopathology.* 2002;41(3):250–259.

56. Khan AJ, DiGiovanna MP, Ross DA, et al. Adenoid cystic carcinoma: a retrospective clinical review. *Int J Cancer.* 2001;96(3):149–158.

57. Spiro RH, Huvos AG. Stage means more than grade in adenoid cystic carcinoma. *Am J Surg.* 1992;164(6):623–628.

58. Fordice J, Kershaw C, El-Naggar A, Goepfert H. Adenoid cystic carcinoma of the head and neck: predictors of morbidity and mortality. *Arch Otolaryngol Head Neck Surg.* 1999;125(2):149–152.

59. Garden AS, Weber RS, Morrison WH, Ang KK, Peters LJ. The influence of positive margins and nerve invasion in adenoid cystic carcinoma of the head and neck treated with surgery and radiation. *Int J Radiat Oncol Biol Phys.* 1995;32(3): 619–626.

60. Dezube BJ. Acquired immunodeficiency syndrome-related Kaposi's sarcoma: clinical features, staging, and treatment. *Semin Oncol.* 2000;27(4): 424–430.

61. Bowie SA, Jr., Bach D. Oral Kaposi's sarcoma in a non-AIDS patient. *Gen Dent.* 1999;47(4):413–415.

62. Webster-Cyriaque J, Duus K, Cooper C, Duncan M. Oral EBV and KSHV infection in HIV. *Adv Dent Res.* 2006;19(1):91–95.

63. Dezube BJ, Sullivan R, Koon HB. Emerging targets and novel strategies in the treatment of AIDS-related Kaposi's sarcoma: bidirectional translational science. *J Cell Physiol.* 2006;209(3): 659–662.

64. Aldenhoven M, Barlo NP, Sanders CJ. Therapeutic strategies for epidemic Kaposi's sarcoma. *Int J STD AIDS.* 2006;17(9):571–578.

65. Grabar S, Abraham B, Mahamat A, Del GP, Rosenthal E, Costagliola D. Differential impact of combination antiretroviral therapy in preventing Kaposi's sarcoma with and without visceral involvement. *J Clin Oncol.* 2006;24(21):3408-3414.

66. Becker G, Bottke D. Radiotherapy in the management of Kaposi's sarcoma. *Onkologie.* 2006; 29(7):329-333.

67. Yildiz F, Genc M, Akyurek S, et al. Radiotherapy in the management of Kaposi's sarcoma: comparison of 8 Gy versus 6 Gy. *J Natl Med Assoc.* 2006;98(7):1136-1139.

68. Osteogenic sarcoma of the mandible and maxilla: a Canadian review (1980-2000). *J Otolaryngol.* 2004;33(3):139-144.

69. Ogunlewe MO, Ajayi OF, Adeyemo WL, Ladeinde AL, James O. Osteogenic sarcoma of the jaw bones: a single institution experience over a 21-year period. *Oral Surg Oral Med Oral Pathol Oral Radiol Endod.* 2006;101(1):76-81.

70. Mardinger O, Givol N, Talmi YP, Taicher S. Osteosarcoma of the jaw. The Chaim Sheba Medical Center experience. *Oral Surg Oral Med Oral Pathol Oral Radiol Endod.* 2001;91(4):445-451.

71. Hackney FL, Aragon SB, Aufdemorte TB, Holt GR, Van Sickels JE. Chondrosarcoma of the jaws: clinical findings, histopathology, and treatment. *Oral Surg Oral Med Oral Pathol.* 1991;71(2): 139-143.

72. Bernasconi G, Preda L, Padula E, Baciliero U, Sammarchi L, Bellomi M. Parosteal chondrosarcoma, a very rare condition of the mandibular condyle. *Clin Imaging.* 2004;28(1):64-68.

73. Gorsky M, Epstein JB. Craniofacial osseous and chondromatous sarcomas in British Columbia—a review of 34 cases. *Oral Oncol.* 2000;36(1):27-31.

74. Cebrian Carretero JL, Chamorro PM, Montesdeoca N. Melanoma of the oral cavity. Review of the literature. *Med Oral.* 2001;6(5):371-375.

75. Tanaka N, Mimura M, Ogi K, Amagasa T. Primary malignant melanoma of the oral cavity: assessment of outcome from the clinical records of 35 patients. *Int J Oral Maxillofac Surg.* 2004;33(8): 761-765.

76. Medina JE, Ferlito A, Pellitteri PK, et al. Current management of mucosal melanoma of the head and neck. *J Surg Oncol.* 2003;83(2):116-122.

77. Mendenhall WM, Amdur RJ, Hinerman RW, Werning JW, Villaret DB, Mendenhall NP. Head and neck mucosal melanoma. *Am J Clin Oncol.* 2005; 28(6):626-630.

78. Balkissoon J, Rasgon BM, Schweitzer L. Lymphatic mapping for staging of head and neck cancer. *Semin Oncol.* 2004;31(3):382-393.

79. Stoykova M. Delayed diagnosis of cancer with emphasis on oral cavity cancers. *Folia Med (Plovdiv).* 1999;41(1):132-135.

80. Sheahan P, O'Keane C, Sheahan JN, O'Dwyer TP. Predictors of survival in early oral cancer. *Otolaryngol Head Neck Surg.* 2003;129(5): 571-576.

81. Tankere F, Camproux A, Barry B, Guedon C, Depondt J, Gehanno P. Prognostic value of lymph node involvement in oral cancers: a study of 137 cases. *Laryngoscope.* 2000;110(12):2061-2065.

82. Tankere F, Golmard JL, Barry B, Guedon C, Depondt J, Gehanno P. Prognostic value of mandibular involvement in oral cavity cancers. *Rev Laryngol Otol Rhinol (Bord).* 2002;123(1):7-12.

83. Tralongo V, Rodolico V, Luciani A, Marra G, Daniele E. Prognostic factors in oral SCC. A review of the literature. *Anticancer Res.* 1999;19(4C): 3503-3510.

84. Tytor M, Olofsson J. Prognostic factors in oral cavity carcinomas. *Acta Otolaryngol Suppl.* 1992;492:75-78.

85. Agra IM, Carvalho AL, Ulbrich FS, et al. Prognostic factors in salvage surgery for recurrent oral and oropharyngeal cancer. *Head Neck.* 2006; 28(2):107-113.

86. Airoldi M, Fazio M, Gandolfo S, et al. Combined cryosurgical, chemotherapeutic, and radiotherapeutic management of T1-4N0M0 oral cavity cancers. *Cancer.* 1985;1;56(3):424-431.

87. Al-Rajhi N, Saleem M, Al-Amro AS, et al. Stage IV oral cavity carcinoma. Is conventional radical treatment an option? *Saudi Med J.* 2002;23(9): 1095-1098.

88. Turner SL, Kalnins I, Gebski V, Tiver KW. Locally advanced (stage III and IV) head and neck cancer: Westmead Hospital experience. *Aust N Z J Surg.* 1991;61(10):744-752.

89. Umeda M, Komatsubara H, Ojima Y, et al. Lack of survival advantage in patients with advanced, resectable SCC of the oral cavity receiving induction chemotherapy with cisplatin (CDDP), docetaxel (TXT) and 5-fluorouracil (5FU). *Kobe J Med Sci.* 2004;50(5-6):189-196.

90. Yuan P, Temam S, El-Naggar A, et al. Overexpression of podoplanin in oral cancer and its association with poor clinical outcome. *Cancer.* 2006; 107(3):563-569.

91. Zelefsky MJ, Gaynor J, Kraus D, Strong EW, Shah JP, Harrison LB. Long-term subjective functional outcome of surgery plus postoperative radiotheraphy for advanced stage oral cavity and oropharyngeal carcinoma. *Am J Surg.* 1996;171(2): 258-261.

92. Carinci F, Pelucchi S, Farina A, Bonsetti G, Mastrandrea M, Calearo C. Site-dependent survival in cancer of the oral cavity. *J Craniofac Surg.* 1997; 8(5):399-403.

93. Robinson IA, Cozens NJ. Does a joint ultrasound guided cytology clinic optimize the cytological evaluation of head and neck masses? *Clin Radiol.* 1999;54(5):312-316.

94. Knappe M, Louw M, Gregor RT. Ultrasonography-guided fine-needle aspiration for the assessment of cervical metastases. *Arch Otolaryngol Head Neck Surg.* 2000;126(9):1091-1096.

95. Friedlander PL, Schantz SP, Shaha AR, Yu G, Shah JP. SCC of the tongue in young patients: a matched-pair analysis. *Head Neck.* 1998;20(5):363-368.

96. Cusumano RJ, Persky MS. SCC of the oral cavity and oropharynx in young adults. *Head Neck Surg.* 1988;10(4):229-234.

97. Hyam DM, Conway RC, Sathiyaseelan Y, et al. Tongue cancer: do patients younger than 40 do worse? *Aust Dent J.* 2003;48(1):50-54.

98. Konsulov SS. Surgical treatment of anterolateral tongue carcinoma. *Folia Med (Plovdiv).* 2005; 47(3-4):20-23.

99. Veness MJ, Morgan GJ, Sathiyaseelan Y, Gebski V. Anterior tongue cancer: age is not a predictor of outcome and should not alter treatment. *ANZ J Surg.* 2003;73(11):899-904.

100. Derks W, de L, Jr., Hordijk GJ, Winnubst JA. Reasons for non-standard treatment in elderly patients with advanced head and neck cancer. *Eur Arch Otorhinolaryngol.* 2005;262(1):21-26.

101. Ehlinger P, Fossion E, Vrielinck L. Carcinoma of the oral cavity in patients over 75 years of age. *Int J Oral Maxillofac Surg.* 1993;22(4):218-220.

102. Derks W, de L, Jr., Hordijk GJ, Winnubst JA. Elderly patients with head and neck cancer: short-term effects of surgical treatment on quality of life. *Clin Otolaryngol Allied Sci.* 2003;28(5):399-405.

103. Derks W, De LR, Winnubst J, Hordijk GJ. Elderly patients with head and neck cancer: physical, social and psychological aspects after 1 year. *Acta Otolaryngol.* 2004;124(4):509-514.

104. Derks W, de Leeuw RJ, Hordijk GJ. Elderly patients with head and neck cancer: the influence of comorbidity on choice of therapy, complication rate, and survival. *Curr Opin Otolaryngol Head Neck Surg.* 2005;13(2):92-96.

105. Piccirillo JF, Spitznagel EL Jr, Vermani N, Costas I, Schnitzler M. Comparison of comorbidity indices for patients with head and neck cancer. *Med Care.* 2004;42(5):482-486.

106. Cinamon U, Hier MP, Black MJ. Age as a prognostic factor for head and neck SCC: should older patients be treated differently? *J Otolaryngol.* 2006;35(1):8-12.

107. Moore RJ, Doherty DA, Do KA, Chamberlain RM, Khuri FR. Racial disparity in survival of patients with SCC of the oral cavity and pharynx. *Ethn Health.* 2001;6(3-4):165-177.

108. Arbes SJ, Jr., Olshan AF, Caplan DJ, Schoenbach VJ, Slade GD, Symons MJ. Factors contributing to the poorer survival of black Americans diagnosed with oral cancer (United States). *Cancer Causes Control.* 1999;10(6):513-523.

109. Mukherji SK, Castelijns J, Castillo M. SCC of the oropharynx and oral cavity: how imaging makes a difference. *Semin Ultrasound CT MR.* 1998; 19(6):463-475.

110. Mukherji SK, Isaacs DL, Creager A, Shockley W, Weissler M, Armao D. CT detection of mandibular invasion by SCC of the oral cavity. *AJR Am J Roentgenol.* 2001;177(1):237-243.

111. Lane AP, Buckmire RA, Mukherji SK, Pillsbury HC, III, Meredith SD. Use of computed tomography in the assessment of mandibular invasion in carcinoma of the retromolar trigone. *Otolaryngol Head Neck Surg.* 2000;122(5):673-677.

112. Sham JS, Cheung YK, Choy D, Chan FL, Leong L. Computed tomography evaluation of neck node metastases from nasopharyngeal carcinoma. *Int J Radiat Oncol Biol Phys.* 1993;26(5):787-792.

113. Umeda M, Nishimatsu N, Teranobu O, Shimada K. Criteria for diagnosing lymph node metastasis from SCC of the oral cavity: a study of the relationship between computed tomographic and histologic findings and outcome. *J Oral Maxillofac Surg.* 1998;56(5):585-593.

114. Myers LL, Wax MK. Positron emission tomography in the evaluation of the negative neck in patients with oral cavity cancer. *J Otolaryngol.* 1998; 27(6):342-347.

115. Krestan C, Herneth AM, Formanek M, Czerny C. Modern imaging lymph node staging of the head and neck region. *Eur J Radiol.* 2006;58(3): 360-366.

116. Bruschini P, Giorgetti A, Bruschini L, et al. Positron emission tomography (PET) in the staging of head neck cancer: comparison between PET and CT. *Acta Otorhinolaryngol Ital.* 2003;23(6): 446–453.

117. Leslie A, Fyfe E, Guest P, Goddard P, Kabala JE. Staging of SCC of the oral cavity and oropharynx: a comparison of MRI and CT in T- and N-staging. *J Comput Assist Tomogr.* 1999;23(1):43–49.

118. Maroldi R, Battaglia G, Farina D, Maculotti P, Chiesa A. Tumours of the oropharynx and oral cavity: perineural spread and bone invasion. *JBR-BTR.* 1999;82(6):294–300.

119. Bolzoni A, Cappiello J, Piazza C, et al. Diagnostic accuracy of magnetic resonance imaging in the assessment of mandibular involvement in oral-oropharyngeal SCC: a prospective study. *Arch Otolaryngol Head Neck Surg.* 2004;130(7):837–843.

120. Nallet E, Piekarski JD, Bensimon JL, Ameline E, Barry B, Gehanno P. Value of MRI and computerized tomography scanner in oro-buccopharyngeal cancers with bone invasion. *Ann Otolaryngol Chir Cervicofac.* 1999;116(5):263–269.

121. Sigal R, Zagdanski AM, Schwaab G, et al. CT and MR imaging of SCC of the tongue and floor of the mouth. *Radiographics.* 1996;16(4):787–810.

122. Stuckensen T, Kovacs AF, Adams S, Baum RP. Staging of the neck in patients with oral cavity SCCs: a prospective comparison of PET, ultrasound, CT and MRI. *J Craniomaxillofac Surg.* 2000;28(6): 319–324.

123. Stoeckli SJ, Steinert H, Pfaltz M, Schmid S. Is there a role for positron emission tomography with 18F-fluorodeoxyglucose in the initial staging of nodal negative oral and oropharyngeal SCC. *Head Neck.* 2002;24(4):345–349.

124. Stoeckli SJ, Mosna-Firlejczyk K, Goerres GW. Lymph node metastasis of SCC from an unknown primary: impact of positron emission tomography. *Eur J Nucl Med Mol Imaging.* 2003;30(3): 411–416.

125. Pellitteri PK, Ferlito A, Rinaldo A, et al. Planned neck dissection following chemoradiotherapy for advanced head and neck cancer: is it necessary for all? *Head Neck.* 2006;28(2):166–175.

126. Ng SH, Yen TC, Liao CT, et al. 18F-FDG PET and CT/MRI in oral cavity SCC: a prospective study of 124 patients with histologic correlation. *J Nucl Med.* 2005;46(7):1136–1143.

127. Wensing BM, Vogel WV, Marres HA, et al. FDG-PET in the clinically negative neck in oral SCC. *Laryngoscope.* 2006;116(5):809–813.

128. Davidson J, Gilbert R, Irish J, et al. The role of panendoscopy in the management of mucosal head and neck malignancy-a prospective evaluation. *Head Neck.* 2000;22(5):449–454.

129. Andruchow JL, Veness MJ, Morgan GJ, et al. Implications for clinical staging of metastatic cutaneous squamous carcinoma of the head and neck based on a multicenter study of treatment outcomes. *Cancer.* 2006;106(5):1078–1083.

130. Carinci F, Pelucchi S, Farina A, Calearo C. A comparison between TNM and TANIS stage grouping for predicting prognosis of oral and oropharyngeal cancer. *J Oral Maxillofac Surg.* 1998;56(7): 832–836.

131. Ghouri AF, Zamora RL, Harvey JE, Spitznagel EL Jr, Sessions DG. Epidermoid carcinoma of the oral cavity and oropharynx: validity of the current AJCC staging system and new statistical tools for the prediction of subclinical neck disease. *Otolaryngol Head Neck Surg.* 1993;108(3):225–232.

132. Howaldt HP, Kainz M, Euler B, Vorast H. Proposal for modification of the TNM staging classification for cancer of the oral cavity. DOSAK. *J Craniomaxillofac Surg.* 1999;27(5):275–288.

133. Erisen L, Basut O, Tezel I, et al. Regional epidemiological features of lip, oral cavity, and oropharyngeal cancer. *J Environ Pathol Toxicol Oncol,* 1996;15(2–4):225–229.

134. Wong RJ, Rinaldo A, Ferlito A, Shah JP. Occult cervical metastasis in head and neck cancer and its impact on therapy. *Acta Otolaryngol.* 2002; 122(1):107–114.

135. Liao CT, Chang JT, Wang HM, et al. Surgical outcome of T4a and resected T4b oral cavity cancer. *Cancer.* 2006;107(2):337–344.

136. Massano J, Regateiro FS, Januario G, Ferreira A. Oral SCC: review of prognostic and predictive factors. *Oral Surg Oral Med Oral Pathol Oral Radiol Endod.* 2006;102(1):67–76.

137. Kim JG, Sohn SK, Kim DH, et al. Phase II study of concurrent chemoradiotherapy with capecitabine and cisplatin in patients with locally advanced SCC of the head and neck. *Br J Cancer.* 2005;93(10):1117–1121.

138. Gleich LL, Ryzenman J, Gluckman JL, Wilson KM, Barrett WL, Redmond KP. Recurrent advanced (T3 or T4) head and neck SCC: is salvage possible? *Arch Otolaryngol Head Neck Surg.* 2004; 130(1):35–38.

139. Malone JP, Stephens JA, Grecula JC, Rhoades CA, Ghaheri BA, Schuller DE. Disease control, survival, and functional outcome after multimodal

treatment for advanced-stage tongue base cancer. *Head Neck.* 2004;26(7):561-572.

140. Marcus B, Arenberg D, Lee J, et al. Prognostic factors in oral cavity and oropharyngeal SCC. *Cancer.* 2004;101(12):2779-2787.

141. Shikama N, Sasaki S, Nishikawa A, et al. Risk factors for local-regional recurrence following preoperative radiation therapy and surgery for head and neck cancer (stage II-IVB). *Radiology.* 2003;228(3):789-794.

142. Brandwein-Gensler M, Teixeira MS, Lewis CM, et al. Oral SCC: histologic risk assessment, but not margin status, is strongly predictive of local disease-free and overall survival. *Am J Surg Pathol.* 2005; 29(2):167-178.

143. Veness MJ, Morgan GJ, Sathiyaseelan Y, Gebski V. Anterior tongue cancer and the incidence of cervical lymph node metastases with increasing tumour thickness: should elective treatment to the neck be standard practice in all patients? *ANZ J Surg.* 2005;75(3):101-105.

144. Woolgar JA, Rogers SN, Lowe D, Brown JS, Vaughan ED. Cervical lymph node metastasis in oral cancer: the importance of even microscopic extracapsular spread. *Oral Oncol.* 2003;39(2): 130-137.

145. Kurita H, Koike T, Narikawa JN, et al. Clinical predictors for contralateral neck lymph node metastasis from unilateral SCC in the oral cavity. *Oral Oncol.* 2004;40(9):898-903.

146. Olasoji HO. Clinical significance and surgical management of regional lymph nodes in oral cancers—a review of English literature up till July 2001. *Niger Postgrad Med J.* 2004;11(4): 279-285.

147. Chow TL, Chow TK, Chan TT, Yu NF, Fung SC, Lam SH. Contralateral neck recurrence of SCC of oral cavity and oropharynx. *J Oral Maxillofac Surg.* 2004;62(10):1225-1228.

148. Duvvuri U, Simental AA, Jr., D'Angelo G, et al. Elective neck dissection and survival in patients with SCC of the oral cavity and oropharynx. *Laryngoscope.* 2004;114(12):2228-2234.

149. Zbaren P, Nuyens M, Caversaccio M, Stauffer E. Elective neck dissection for carcinomas of the oral cavity: occult metastases, neck recurrences, and adjuvant treatment of pathologically positive necks. *Am J Surg.* 2006;191(6):756-760.

150. Greenberg JS, Fowler R, Gomez J, et al. Extent of extracapsular spread: a critical prognosticator in oral tongue cancer. *Cancer.* 2003;97(6): 1464-1470.

151. Kramer D, Durham JS, Jackson S, Brookes J. Management of the neck in N0 SCC of the oral cavity. *J Otolaryngol.* 2001;30(5):283-288.

152. Ohara K, Tatsuzaki H, Kurosaki Y, et al. Metastatic lymph-node clearance from head and neck epidermoid carcinomas following radiotherapy. *Acta Oncol.* 1999;38(2):261-266.

153. de Vicente JC, Recio OR, Pendas SL, Lopez-Arranz JS. Oral SCC of the mandibular region: a survival study. *Head Neck.* 2001;23(7):536-543.

154. Talmi YP, Hoffman HT, Horowitz Z, et al. Patterns of metastases to the upper jugular lymph nodes (the "submuscular recess"). *Head Neck.* 1998; 20(8):682-686.

155. Kowalski LP, Carvalho AL, Martins Priante AV, Magrin J. Predictive factors for distant metastasis from oral and oropharyngeal SCC. *Oral Oncol.* 2005;41(5):534-541.

156. Kowalski LP, Bagietto R, Lara JR, Santos RL, Silva JF Jr, Magrin J. Prognostic significance of the distribution of neck node metastasis from oral carcinoma. *Head Neck.* 2000;22(3):207-214.

157. Shah JP, Candela FC, Poddar AK. The patterns of cervical lymph node metastases from squamous carcinoma of the oral cavity. *Cancer.* 1990;66(1): 109-113.

158. Carvalho AL, Ikeda MK, Magrin J, Kowalski LP. Trends of oral and oropharyngeal cancer survival over five decades in 3267 patients treated in a single institution. *Oral Oncol.* 2004;40(1):71-76.

159. Hosal AS, Carrau RL, Johnson JT, Myers EN. Selective neck dissection in the management of the clinically node-negative neck. *Laryngoscope.* 2000;110(12):2037-2040.

160. Godden DR, Ribeiro NF, Hassanein K, Langton SG. Recurrent neck disease in oral cancer. *J Oral Maxillofac Surg.* 2002;60(7):748-753.

161. Ichimiya Y, Fuwa N, Kamata M, et al. Treatment results of stage I oral tongue cancer with definitive radiotherapy. *Oral Oncol.* 2005;41(5):520-525.

162. Jing J, Li L, He W, Sun G. Prognostic predictors of SCC of the buccal mucosa with negative surgical margins. *J Oral Maxillofac Surg.* 2006;64(6): 896-901.

163. Lam P, Au-Yeung KM, Cheng PW, et al. Correlating MRI and histologic tumor thickness in the assessment of oral tongue cancer. *AJR Am J Roentgenol.* 2004;182(3):803-808.

164. Preda L, Chiesa F, Calabrese L, et al. Relationship between histologic thickness of tongue carcinoma and thickness estimated from preoperative MRI. *Eur Radiol.* 2006;16(10):2242-2248.

165. Pentenero M, Gandolfo S, Carrozzo M. Importance of tumor thickness and depth of invasion in nodal involvement and prognosis of oral SCC: a review of the literature. *Head Neck.* 2005; 27(12):1080-1091.

166. Fagan JJ, Collins B, Barnes L, D'Amico F, Myers EN, Johnson JT. Perineural invasion in SCC of the head and neck. *Arch Otolaryngol Head Neck Surg.* 1998;124(6):637-640.

167. Kurtz KA, Hoffman HT, Zimmerman MB, Robinson RA. Perineural and vascular invasion in oral cavity squamous carcinoma: increased incidence on re-review of slides and by using immunohistochemical enhancement. *Arch Pathol Lab Med.* 2005;129(3):354-359.

168. Sparano A, Weinstein G, Chalian A, Yodul M, Weber R. Multivariate predictors of occult neck metastasis in early oral tongue cancer. *Otolaryngol Head Neck Surg.* 2004;131(4):472-476.

169. Garzino-Demo P, Dell'Acqua A, Dalmasso P, et al. Clinicopathological parameters and outcome of 245 patients operated for oral SCC. *J Craniomaxillofac Surg.* 2006;34(6):344-350.

170. Rahima B, Shingaki S, Nagata M, Saito C. Prognostic significance of perineural invasion in oral and oropharyngeal carcinoma. *Oral Surg Oral Med Oral Pathol Oral Radiol Endod.* 2004;97(4): 423-431.

171. McMahon J, O'Brien CJ, Pathak I, et al. Influence of condition of surgical margins on local recurrence and disease-specific survival in oral and oropharyngeal cancer. *Br J Oral Maxillofac Surg.* 2003;41(4):224-231.

172. Looser KG, Shah JP, Strong EW. The significance of "positive" margins in surgically resected epidermoid carcinomas. *Head Neck Surg.* 1978; 1(2):107-111.

173. Smeele LE, Leemans CR, Langendijk JA, et al. Positive surgical margins in neck dissection specimens in patients with head and neck SCC and the effect of radiotherapy. *Head Neck.* 2000; 22(6):559-563.

174. Hicks WL, Jr., Loree TR, Garcia RI, et al. SCC of the floor of mouth: a 20-year review. *Head Neck.* 1997;19(5):400-405.

175. Diaz EM Jr, Holsinger FC, Zuniga ER, Roberts DB, Sorensen DM. SCC of the buccal mucosa: one institution's experience with 119 previously untreated patients. *Head Neck.* 2003;25(4): 267-273.

176. Kokemueller H, Brachvogel P, Eckardt A, Hausamen JE. Neck dissection in oral cancer—

clinical review and analysis of prognostic factors. *Int J Oral Maxillofac Surg.* 2002;31(6):608-614.

177. Myers JN, Greenberg JS, Mo V, Roberts D. Extracapsular spread. A significant predictor of treatment failure in patients with SCC of the tongue. *Cancer.* 2001;92(12):3030-3036.

178. Ash CS, Nason RW, Abdoh AA, Cohen MA. Prognostic implications of mandibular invasion in oral cancer. *Head Neck.* 2000;22(8):794-798.

179. Song CS, Har-El G. Marginal mandibulectomy: Oncologic and nononcologic outcome. *Am J Otolaryngol.* 2003;24(1):61-63.

180. Petruzzelli GJ, Knight FK, Vandevender D, Clark JI, Emami B. Posterior marginal mandibulectomy in the management of cancer of the oral cavity and oropharynx. *Otolaryngol Head Neck Surg.* 2003;129(6):713-719.

181. Pathak KA, Agarwal R, Deshpande MS. Marginal mandibulectomy for lateral sulcus tumours. *Eur J Surg Oncol.* 2004;30(7):804-806.

182. Wolff D, Hassfeld S, Hofele C. Influence of marginal and segmental mandibular resection on the survival rate in patients with SCC of the inferior parts of the oral cavity. *J Craniomaxillofac Surg.* 2004;32(5):318-323.

183. Guerra MF, Campo FJ, Gias LN, Perez JS. Rim versus sagittal mandibulectomy for the treatment of SCC: two types of mandibular preservation. *Head Neck.* 2003;25(12):982-989.

184. Forrest LA, Schuller DE, Karanfilov B, Lucas JG. Update on intraoperative analysis of mandibular margins. *Am J Otolaryngol.* 1997;18(6):396-399.

185. Brown JS, Lowe D, Kalavrezos N, D'Souza J, Magennis P, Woolgar J. Patterns of invasion and routes of tumor entry into the mandible by oral SCC. *Head Neck.* 2002;24(4):370-383.

186. Van Cann EM, Dom M, Koole R, Merkx MA, Stoelinga PJ. Health related quality of life after mandibular resection for oral and oropharyngeal SCC. *Oral Oncol.* 2005;41(7):687-693.

187. Mariani PB, Kowalski LP, Magrin J. Reconstruction of large defects postmandibulectomy for oral cancer using plates and myocutaneous flaps: a long-term follow-up. *Int J Oral Maxillofac Surg.* 2006;35(5):427-432.

188. Aydin A, Emekli U, Erer M, Hafiz G. Fibula free flap for mandible reconstruction. *Kulak Burun Bogaz Ihtis Derg.* 2004;13(3-4):62-66.

189. Munoz Guerra MF, Naval GL, Campo FR, Perez JS. Marginal and segmental mandibulectomy in patients with oral cancer: a statistical analysis of 106 cases. *J Oral Maxillofac Surg.* 2003;61(11):1289-1296.

190. Dinshaw KA, Agarwal JP, Ghosh-Laskar S, Gupta T, Shrivastava SK. Radical radiotherapy in head and neck SCC: an analysis of prognostic and therapeutic factors. *Clin Oncol (R Coll Radiol).* 2006; 18(5):383-389.

191. Lindholm P, Valavaara R, Aitasalo K, et al. Preoperative hyperfractionated accelerated radiotherapy and radical surgery in advanced head and neck cancer: a prospective phase II study. *Radiother Oncol.* 2006;78(2):146-151.

192. Ozer E, Grecula JC, Agrawal A, Rhoades CA, Young DC, Schuller DE. Long-term results of a multimodal intensification regimen for previously untreated advanced resectable squamous cell cancer of the oral cavity, oropharynx, or hypopharynx. *Laryngoscope.* 2006;116(4):607-612.

193. Dinshaw KA, Agarwal JP, Laskar SG, Gupta T, Shrivastava SK, Cruz AD. Head and neck SCC: the role of post-operative adjuvant radiotherapy. *J Surg Oncol.* 2005;91(1):48-55.

194. Podrecca S, Salvatori P, Saraceno MS, et al. Review of 346 patients with free-flap reconstruction following head and neck surgery for neoplasm. *Br J Plast Surg.* 2006;59(2): 122-129.

195. Belbin TJ, Singh B, Smith RV, et al. Molecular profiling of tumor progression in head and neck cancer. *Arch Otolaryngol Head Neck Surg.* 2005; 131(1):10-18.

196. Schliephake H. Prognostic relevance of molecular markers of oral cancer—a review. *Int J Oral Maxillofac Surg.* 2003;32(3):233-245.

197. Ekberg T, Nestor M, Engstrom M, et al. Expression of EGFR, HER2, HER3, and HER4 in metastatic SCCs of the oral cavity and base of tongue. *Int J Oncol.* 2005;26(5):1177-1185.

198. Hitt R, Ciruelos E, Amador ML, et al. Prognostic value of the epidermal growth factor receptor (EGRF) and p53 in advanced head and neck SCC patients treated with induction chemotherapy. *Eur J Cancer.* 2005;41(3):453-460.

199. Smid EJ, Stoter TR, Bloemena E, et al. The importance of immunohistochemical expression of EGFr in SCC of the oral cavity treated with surgery and postoperative radiotherapy. *Int J Radiat Oncol Biol Phys.* 2006;65(5):1323-1329.

200. Xia W, Lau YK, Zhang HZ, et al. Combination of EGFR, HER-2/neu, and HER-3 is a stronger predictor for the outcome of oral SCC than any individual family members. *Clin Cancer Res.* 1999; 5(12):4164-4174.

201. Vora HH, Shah NG, Patel DD, Trivedi TI, Chikhlikar PR. Prognostic significance of biomarkers in SCC of the tongue: multivariate analysis. *J Surg Oncol.* 2003;82(1):34-50.

202. Carlos d, V, Herrero-Zapatero A, Fresno MF, Lopez-Arranz JS. Expression of cyclin D1 and Ki-67 in SCC of the oral cavity: clinicopathological and prognostic significance. *Oral Oncol.* 2002;38(3): 301-308.

203. Koscielny S, Eggeling F, Dahse R, Fiedler W. The influence of reactivation of the telomerase in tumour tissue on the prognosis of SCCs in the head and neck. *J Oral Pathol Med.* 2004;33(9): 538-542.

204. Luzar B, Poljak M, Marin IJ, Eberlinc A, Klopcic U, Gale N. Human telomerase catalytic subunit gene re-expression is an early event in oral carcinogenesis. *Histopathology.* 2004;45(1):13-19.

205. Rubio BP, Naval GL, Garcia DR, Domingo CJ, az Gonzalez FJ. Tumor DNA content as a prognostic indicator in SCC of the oral cavity and tongue base. *Head Neck.* 1998;20(3):232-239.

206. Schmalbach CE, Chepeha DB, Giordano TJ, et al. Molecular profiling and the identification of genes associated with metastatic oral cavity/pharynx SCC. *Arch Otolaryngol Head Neck Surg.* 2004; 130(3):295-302.

207. O'Donnell RK, Kupferman M, Wei SJ, et al. Gene expression signature predicts lymphatic metastasis in SCC of the oral cavity. *Oncogene.* 2005; 24(7):1244-1251.

208. Szelachowska J, Dziegiel P, Jelen-Krzeszewska J, et al. Mcm-2 protein expression predicts prognosis better than Ki-67 antigen in oral cavity squamocellular carcinoma. *Anticancer Res.* 2006;26(3B):2473-2478.

209. Lopez M, Aguirre JM, Cuevas N, et al. Use of cytological specimens for p53 gene alteration detection in oral SCC risk patients. *Clin Oncol (R Coll Radiol).* 2004;16(5):366-370.

210. Muraki Y, Tateishi A, Seta C, et al. Fas antigen expression and outcome of oral SCC. *Int J Oral Maxillofac Surg.* 2000;29(5):360-365.

211. Uno M, Otsuki T, Yata K, et al. Participation of Fas-mediated apoptotic pathway in KB, a human head and neck SCC cell line, after irradiation. *Int J Oncol.* 2002;20(3):617-622.

212. Korabiowska M, Voltmann J, Honig JF, et al. Altered expression of DNA double-strand repair genes Ku70 and Ku80 in carcinomas of the oral cavity. *Anticancer Res,* 2006;26(3A):2101-2105.

213. Reinders J, Rozemuller EH, van der WP, et al. Genes in the HLA region indicative for head and neck SCC. *Mol Immunol.* 2007;44(5):848-855.

214. Reinders J, Rozemuller EH, Otten HG, van d, V, Slootweg PJ, Tilanus MG. HLA and MICA associations with head and neck SCC. *Oral Oncol.* 2007; 43(3):232-240.

215. Kikuchi K, Kusama K, Sano M, et al. Vascular endothelial growth factor and dendritic cells in human SCC of the oral cavity. *Anticancer Res.* 2006;26(3A):1833-1848.

216. Sakakura K, Chikamatsu K, Sakurai T, et al. Infiltration of dendritic cells and NK cells into the sentinel lymph node in oral cavity cancer. *Oral Oncol.* 2005;41(1):89-96.

217. Kikuchi K, Kusama K, Taguchi K, et al. Dendritic cells in human SCC of the oral cavity. *Anticancer Res.* 2002;22(2A):545-557.

218. Jablonska E, Piotrowski L, Jablonski J, Grabowska Z. VEGF in the culture of PMN and the serum in oral cavity cancer patients. *Oral Oncol.* 2002; 38(6):605-609.

219. Kyzas PA, Stefanou D, Batistatou A, Agnantis NJ. Prognostic significance of VEGF immunohistochemical expression and tumor angiogenesis in head and neck SCC. *J Cancer Res Clin Oncol.* 2005;131(9):624-630.

220. Nakazato T, Shingaki S, Kitamura N, Saito C, Kuwano R, Tachibana M. Expression level of vascular endothelial growth factor-C and -A in cultured human oral SCC correlates respectively with lymphatic metastasis and angiogenesis when transplanted into nude mouse oral cavity. *Oncol Rep.* 2006;15(4):825-830.

221. Takagi S, Inenaga R, Oya R, Nakamura S, Ikemura K. Blood vessel density correlates with the effects of targeted intra-arterial carboplatin infusion with concurrent radiotherapy for SCCs of the oral cavity and oropharynx. *Br J Cancer.* 2006;94(11):1580-1585.

222. Ascani G, Balercia P, Messi M, et al. Angiogenesis in oral SCC. *Acta Otorhinolaryngol Ital.* 2005; 25(1):13-17.

223. Jablonska E, Puzewska W, Charkiewicz M. Effect of IL-18 on leukocyte expression of iNOS and phospho-IkB in patients with SCC of the oral cavity. *Neoplasma.* 2006;53(3):200-205.

224. Jablonska E, Puzewska W, Marcinczyk M, Grabowska Z, Jablonski J. iNOS expression and NO production by neutrophils in cancer patients. *Arch Immunol Ther Exp (Warsz).* 2005;53(2): 175-179.

225. Connelly ST, abeo-Ong M, Dekker N, Jordan RC, Schmidt BL. Increased nitric oxide levels and iNOS over-expression in oral SCC. *Oral Oncol.* 2005;41(3):261-267.

226. Thomas GJ, Nystrom ML, Marshall JF. Alphavbeta6 integrin in wound healing and cancer of the oral cavity. *J Oral Pathol Med.* 2006;35(1): 1-10.

227. Kurtz KA, Hoffman HT, Zimmerman MB, Robinson RA. Decreased E-cadherin but not beta-catenin expression is associated with vascular invasion and decreased survival in head and neck squamous carcinomas. *Otolaryngol Head Neck Surg.* 2006;134(1):142-146.

228. Munoz-Guerra MF, Marazuela EG, Fernandez-Contreras ME, Gamallo C. P-cadherin expression reduced in SCC of the oral cavity: an indicatior of poor prognosis. *Cancer.* 2005;103(5):960-969.

229. Impola U, Uitto VJ, Hietanen J, et al. Differential expression of matrilysin-1 (MMP-7), 92 kD gelatinase (MMP-9), and metalloelastase (MMP-12) in oral verrucous and squamous cell cancer. *J Pathol.* 2004;202(1):14-22.

230. de Vicente JC, Fresno MF, Villalain L, Vega JA, Hernandez VG. Expression and clinical significance of matrix metalloproteinase-2 and matrix metalloproteinase-9 in oral SCC. *Oral Oncol.* 2005;41(3):283-293.

231. Zhang W, Matrisian LM, Holmbeck K, Vick CC, Rosenthal EL. Fibroblast-derived MT1-MMP promotes tumor progression in vitro and in vivo. *BMC Cancer.* 2006;6:52.

232. Koo BS, Lim YC, Lee JS, Choi EC. Recurrence and salvage treatment of SCC of the oral cavity. *Oral Oncol.* 2006. 42(8):789-794.

233. Andry G, Hamoir M, Leemans CR. The evolving role of surgery in the management of head and neck tumors. *Curr Opin Oncol.* 2005;17(3):241-248.

234. Genden EM, Rinaldo A, Jacobson A, et al. Management of mandibular invasion: when is a marginal mandibulectomy appropriate? *Oral Oncol.* 2005; 41(8):776-782.

235. Lee KH, Veness MJ, Pearl-Larson T, Morgans GJ. Role of combined modality treatment of buccal mucosa SCC. *Aust Dent J.* 2005;50(2):108-113.

236. Arnold DJ, Goodwin WJ, Weed DT, Civantos FJ. Treatment of recurrent and advanced stage SCC of the head and neck. *Semin Radiat Oncol.* 2004;14(2):190-195.

237. Hinerman RW, Mendenhall WM, Morris CG, Amdur RJ, Werning JW, Villaret DB. Postoperative irradiation for SCC of the oral cavity: 35-year experience. *Head Neck.* 2004;26(11):984-994.

238. Palme CE, Gullane PJ, Gilbert RW. Current treatment options in SCC of the oral cavity. *Surg Oncol Clin N Am.* 2004;13(1):47-70.

239. Rashid M, Ahmad T, Sarwar SU, et al. Management of oromandibular cancers. *J Coll Physicians Surg Pak.* 2004;14(1):29-34.

240. Kovacs AF, Ghahremani MT, Stefenelli U, Bitter K. Postoperative chemotherapy with cisplatin and 5-fluorouracil in cancer of the oral cavity and the oropharynx—long-term results. *J Chemother.* 2003;15(5):495-502.

241. Licitra L, Grandi C, Guzzo M, et al. Primary chemotherapy in resectable oral cavity squamous cell cancer: a randomized controlled trial. *J Clin Oncol.* 2003;21(2):327-333.

242. Luukkaa M, Minn H, Aitasalo K, et al. Treatment of SCC of the oral cavity, oropharynx and hypopharynx—an analysis of 174 patients in southwestern Finland. *Acta Oncol.* 2003;42(7):756-762.

243. Magge KT, Myers EN, Johnson JT. Radiation following surgery for oral cancer: impact on local control. *Laryngoscope.* 2003;113(6):933-935.

244. Grau JJ, Domingo J, Blanch JL, et al. Multidisciplinary approach in advanced cancer of the oral cavity: outcome with neoadjuvant chemotherapy according to intention-to-treat local therapy. A phase II study. *Oncology.* 2002;63(4):338-345.

245. Nam W, Kim HJ, Choi EC, Kim MK, Lee EW, Cha IH. Contributing factors to mandibulotomy complications: a retrospective study. *Oral Surg Oral Med Oral Pathol Oral Radiol Endod.* 2006;101(3):e65-e70.

246. Spiro RH, Gerold FP, Shah JP, Sessions RB, Strong EW. Mandibulotomy approach to oropharyngeal tumors. *Am J Surg.* 1985;150(4):466-469.

247. Clark JR, Franklin JH, Naranjo N, Odell MJ, Gullane PJ. Sublingual gland resection in SCC of the floor of mouth: is it necessary? *Laryngoscope.* 2006;116(3):382-386.

248. Antoniades K, Lazaridis N, Vahtsevanos K, Hadjipetrou L, Antoniades V, Karakasis D. Treatment of SCC of the anterior faucial pillar-retromolar trigone. *Oral Oncol.* 2003;39(7):680-686.

249. Kowalski LP, Hashimoto I, Magrin J. End results of 114 extended "commando" operations for retromolar trigone carcinoma. *Am J Surg.* 1993;166(4):374-379.

250. Carvalho AL, Magrin J, Kowalski LP. Sites of recurrence in oral and oropharyngeal cancers according to the treatment approach. *Oral Dis.* 2003;9(3):112-118.

251. Kumar PP, Good RR, Epstein BE, Yonkers AJ, Ogren FP, Moore GF. Outcome of locally advanced stage III and IV head and neck cancer treated by surgery and postoperative external beam radiotherapy. *Laryngoscope.* 1987;97(5):615-620.

252. Teoh KH, Patel S, Hwang F, Huryn JM, Verbel D, Zlotolow IM. Prosthetic intervention in the era of microvascular reconstruction of the mandible—a retrospective analysis of functional outcome. *Int J Prosthodont.* 2005;18(1):42-54.

253. Puxeddu R, Ledda GP, Siotto P, et al. Free-flap iliac crest in mandibular reconstruction following segmental mandibulectomy for SCC of the oral cavity. *Eur Arch Otorhinolaryngol.* 2004;261(4):202-207.

254. Shaha AR. Mandibulotomy and mandibulectomy in difficult tumors of the base of the tongue and oropharynx. *Semin Surg Oncol.* 1991;7(1):25-30.

255. Shaha AR. Preoperative evaluation of the mandible in patients with carcinoma of the floor of mouth. *Head Neck.* 1991;13(5):398-402.

256. Shaha AR. Marginal mandibulectomy for carcinoma of the floor of the mouth. *J Surg Oncol.* 1992;49(2):116-119.

257. Shah JP. The role of marginal mandibulectomy in the surgical management of oral cancer. *Arch Otolaryngol Head Neck Surg.* 2002;128(5):604-605.

258. Werning JW, Byers RM, Novas MA, Roberts D. Preoperative assessment for and outcomes of mandibular conservation surgery. *Head Neck.* 2001;23(12):1024-1030.

259. Roy BC, Bahadur S, Thakar A. Partial maxillectomy for malignant neoplasms of para nasal sinuses and hard palate. *Indian J Cancer.* 2002;39(3):83-90.

260. Yucel A, Cinar C, Aydin Y, et al. Malignant tumors requiring maxillectomy. *J Craniofac Surg.* 2000;11(5):418-429.

261. Truitt TO, Gleich LL, Huntress GP, Gluckman JL. Surgical management of hard palate malignancies. *Otolaryngol Head Neck Surg.* 1999;121(5):548-552.

262. Inagi K, Takahashi H, Okamoto M, Nakayama M, Makoshi T, Nagai H. Treatment effects in patients with SCC of the oral cavity. *Acta Otolaryngol Suppl.* 2002;(547):25-29.

263. Dixit S, Vyas RK, Toparani RB, Baboo HA, Patel DD. Surgery versus surgery and postoperative radiotherapy in SCC of the buccal mucosa: a comparative study. *Ann Surg Oncol.* 1998;5(6):502-510.

264. Govett GS, Amedee RG. Carcinoma of the buccal mucosa: a 30-year analysis at the Medical Center of Louisiana at New Orleans. *J La State Med Soc.* 1997;149(6):182-185.

265. Coppen C, de Wilde PC, Pop LA, van den Hoogen FJ, Merkx MA. Treatment results of patients with a SCC of the buccal mucosa. *Oral Oncol.* 2006; 42(8):795-799.

266. Crile G. Landmark article Dec 1, 1906: Excision of cancer of the head and neck. With special reference to the plan of dissection based on one hundred and thirty-two operations. By George Crile. *JAMA.* 1987;258(22):3286-3293.

267. Brazilian Head and Neck Cancer Study Group. Results of a prospective trial on elective modified radical classical versus supraomohyoid neck dissection in the management of oral squamous carcinoma. *Am J Surg.* 1998;176(5):422-427.

268. Andersen PE, Shah JP, Cambronero E, Spiro RH. The role of comprehensive neck dissection with preservation of the spinal accessory nerve in the clinically positive neck. *Am J Surg.* 1994;168(5): 499-502.

269. Andersen PE, Cambronero E, Shaha AR, Shah JP. The extent of neck disease after regional failure during observation of the N0 neck. *Am J Surg.* 1996;172(6):689-691.

270. Mira E, Benazzo M, Rossi V, Zanoletti E. Efficacy of selective lymph node dissection in clinically negative neck. *Otolaryngol Head Neck Surg.* 2002;127(4):279-283.

271. Majoufre C, Faucher A, Laroche C, et al. Supraomohyoid neck dissection in cancer of the oral cavity. *Am J Surg.* 1999;178(1):73-77.

272. O'Brien CJ, Traynor SJ, McNeil E, McMahon JD, Chaplin JM. The use of clinical criteria alone in the management of the clinically negative neck among patients with SCC of the oral cavity and oropharynx. *Arch Otolaryngol Head Neck Surg.* 2000;126(3):360-365.

273. Koo BS, Lim YC, Lee JS, Choi EC. Management of contralateral N0 neck in oral cavity SCC. *Head Neck.* 2006;28(10):896-901.

274. Kowalski LP, Bagietto R, Lara JR, Santos RL, Tagawa EK, Santos IR. Factors influencing contralateral lymph node metastasis from oral carcinoma. *Head Neck.* 1999;21(2):104-110.

275. Hamoir M, Shah JP, Desuter G, et al. Prevalence of lymph nodes in the apex of level V: a plea against the necessity to dissect the apex of level V in mucosal head and neck cancer. *Head Neck.* 2005;27(11):963-969.

276. Brennan PA, Hoffman GR, Mackenzie N, et al. Recurrent nodal metastases in the posterior triangle: implications for treatment of the atypical tumour. *Br J Oral Maxillofac Surg.* 2006;44(2): 83-86.

277. Spiro RH, Morgan GJ, Strong EW, Shah JP. Supraomohyoid neck dissection. *Am J Surg.* 1996; 172(6):650-653.

278. Ferlito A, Rinaldo A, Silver CE, et al. Neck dissection: Then and now. *Auris Nasus Larynx.* 2006; 33(4):365-374.

279. Spiro JD, Spiro RH, Shah JP, Sessions RB, Strong EW. Critical assessment of supraomohyoid neck dissection. *Am J Surg.* 1988;156(4):286-289.

280. Franceschi D, Gupta R, Spiro RH, Shah JP. Improved survival in the treatment of squamous carcinoma of the oral tongue. *Am J Surg.* 1993; 166(4):360-365.

281. Andersen PE, Warren F, Spiro J, et al. Results of selective neck dissection in management of the node-positive neck. *Arch Otolaryngol Head Neck Surg,* 2002;128(10):1180-1184.

282. Kowalski LP. Results of salvage treatment of the neck in patients with oral cancer. *Arch Otolaryngol Head Neck Surg.* 2002;128(1):58-62.

283. Santos AB, Cernea CR, Inoue M, Ferraz AR. Selective neck dissection for node-positive necks in patients with head and neck SCC: a word of caution. *Arch Otolaryngol Head Neck Surg.* 2006; 132(1):79-81.

284. Chindavijak S. Micrometastasis and recurrent neck node in supraomohyoid neck dissection field. *J Med Assoc Thai.* 2005;88(9):1287-1292.

285. Persky MS, Lagmay VM. Treatment of the clinically negative neck in oral SCC. *Laryngoscope.* 1999;109(7 pt 1):1160-1164.

286. Taylor RJ, Wahl RL, Sharma PK, et al. Sentinel node localization in oral cavity and oropharynx squamous cell cancer. *Arch Otolaryngol Head Neck Surg,* 2001;127(8):970-974.

287. Stoeckli SJ, Pfaltz M, Steinert H, Schmid S. Histopathological features of occult metastasis detected by sentinel lymph node biopsy in oral and oropharyngeal SCC. *Laryngoscope.* 2002; 112(1):111-115.

288. Stoeckli SJ, Pfaltz M, Ross GL, et al. The second international conference on sentinel node biopsy in mucosal head and neck cancer. *Ann Surg Oncol.* 2005;12(11):919-924.

289. Mozzillo N, Chiesa F, Botti G, et al. Sentinel node biopsy in head and neck cancer. *Ann Surg Oncol.* 2001;8(9 suppl):103S-105S.

290. Robertson AG, Soutar DS, Paul J, et al. Early closure of a randomized trial: surgery and postoperative radiotherapy versus radiotherapy in the management of intra-oral tumours. *Clin Oncol (R Coll Radiol).* 1998;10(3):155-160.

291. Blackburn TK, Bakhtawar S, Brown JS, Lowe D, Vaughan ED, Rogers SN. A questionnaire survey of current UK practice for adjuvant radiotherapy following surgery for oral and oropharyngeal SCC. *Oral Oncol.* 2006;43(2):143-149.

292. Delaney G, Jacob S, Barton M. Estimation of an optimal external beam radiotherapy utilization rate for head and neck carcinoma. *Cancer.* 2005;103(11):2216-2227.

293. Langendijk JA, de Jong MA, Leemans CR, et al. Postoperative radiotherapy in SCC of the oral cavity: the importance of the overall treatment time. *Int J Radiat Oncol Biol Phys.* 2003;57(3):693-700.

294. Fein DA, Mendenhall WM, Parsons JT, et al. Carcinoma of the oral tongue: a comparison of results and complications of treatment with radiotherapy and/or surgery. *Head Neck.* 1994;16(4):358-365.

295. Fein DA, Lee WR, Amos WR, et al. Oropharyngeal carcinoma treated with radiotherapy: a 30-year experience. *Int J Radiat Oncol Biol Phys.* 1996;34(2):289-296.

296. Wazer DE, Schmidt-Ullrich R, Keisch M, Karmody CS, Koch W. The role of combined composite resection and irradiation in the management of carcinoma of the oral cavity and oropharynx. *Strahlenther Onkol.* 1989;165(1):18-22.

297. Kramer S, Gelber RD, Snow JB, et al. Combined radiation therapy and surgery in the management of advanced head and neck cancer: final report of study 73-03 of the Radiation Therapy Oncology Group. *Head Neck Surg.* 1987;10(1):19-30.

298. Leemans CR, Chiesa F, Tradati N, Snow GB. Messages from completed randomized trials in head and neck cancer. *Eur J Surg Oncol.* 1997;23(6):469-476.

299. Nemeth Z, Somogyi A, Takacsi-Nagy Z, Barabas J, Nemeth G, Szabo G. Possibilities of preventing osteoradionecrosis during complex therapy of tumors of the oral cavity. *Pathol Oncol Res.* 2000;6(1):53-58.

300. Budach W, Hehr T, Budach V, Belka C, Dietz K. A meta-analysis of hyperfractionated and accelerated radiotherapy and combined chemotherapy and radiotherapy regimens in unresected locally advanced SCC of the head and neck. *BMC Cancer.* 2006;6:28.

301. Eisbruch A, Marsh LH, Martel MK, et al. Comprehensive irradiation of head and neck cancer using conformal multisegmental fields: assessment of target coverage and noninvolved tissue sparing. *Int J Radiat Oncol Biol Phys.* 1998;41(3):559-568.

302. MacKenzie R, Balogh J, Choo R, Franssen E. Accelerated radiotherapy with delayed concomitant boost in locally advanced SCC of the head and neck. *Int J Radiat Oncol Biol Phys.* 1999;45(3):589-595.

303. O'Sullivan JM, Hollywood DP, Cody N, et al. Accelerated radiation therapy, seven fractions per week, for advanced head and neck cancer—a feasibility study. *Clin Oncol (R Coll Radiol).* 2002;14(3):236-240.

304. Schuller DE, Grecula JC, Agrawal A, et al. Multimodal intensification therapy for previously untreated advanced resectable SCC of the oral cavity, oropharynx, or hypopharynx. *Cancer.* 2002;94(12):3169-3178.

305. Poulsen MG, Denham JW, Peters LJ, et al. A randomised trial of accelerated and conventional radiotherapy for stage III and IV squamous carcinoma of the head and neck: a Trans-Tasman Radiation Oncology Group Study. *Radiother Oncol.* 2001;60(2):113-122.

306. Sanguineti G, Richetti A, Bignardi M, et al. Accelerated versus conventional fractionated postoperative radiotherapy for advanced head and neck cancer: results of a multicenter phase III study. *Int J Radiat Oncol Biol Phys.* 2005;61(3):762-771.

307. Schwartz DL, Ford EC, Rajendran J, et al. FDG-PET/CT-guided intensity modulated head and neck radiotherapy: a pilot investigation. *Head Neck.* 2005;27(6):478-487.

308. Lauve A, Morris M, Schmidt-Ullrich R, et al. Simultaneous integrated boost intensity-modulated radiotherapy for locally advanced head-and-neck SCCs: II—clinical results. *Int J Radiat Oncol Biol Phys.* 2004;60(2):374-387.

309. Mazeron JJ, Gerbaulet A, Simon JM, Hardiman C. How to optimize therapeutic ratio in brachytherapy of head and neck SCC? *Acta Oncol.* 1998;37(6):583-591.

310. Ashamalla H, Rafla S, Zaki B, Ikoro NC, Ross P. Radioactive gold grain implants in recurrent and locally advanced head-and-neck cancers. *Brachytherapy.* 2002;1(3):161-166.

311. Pernot M, Hoffstetter S, Peiffert D, et al. Role of interstitial brachytherapy in oral and oropharyngeal carcinoma: reflection of a series of 1344

patients treated at the time of initial presentation. *Otolaryngol Head Neck Surg.* 1996;115(6): 519–526.

312. Karakoyun-Celik O, Norris CM Jr, Tishler R, et al. Definitive radiotherapy with interstitial implant boost for SCC of the tongue base. *Head Neck.* 2005;27(5):353–361.

313. Lapeyre M, Bollet MA, Racadot S, et al. Postoperative brachytherapy alone and combined postoperative radiotherapy and brachytherapy boost for SCC of the oral cavity, with positive or close margins. *Head Neck.* 2004;26(3):216–223.

314. Rudoltz MS, Perkins RS, Luthmann RW, et al. High-dose-rate brachytherapy for primary carcinomas of the oral cavity and oropharynx. *Laryngoscope.* 1999;109(12):1967–1973.

315. Strnad V. Treatment of oral cavity and oropharyngeal cancer. Indications, technical aspects, and results of interstitial brachytherapy. *Strahlenther Onkol.* 2004;180(11):710–717.

316. Yoshida K, Nose T, Watanabe Y, et al. Quantitative evaluation of acute mucosal reaction to interstitial brachytherapy using color histograms. *Brachytherapy.* 2005;4(4):298–303.

317. Kubota A, Furukawa M, Komatsu M, Hanamura H, Sugiyama M. Adjuvant chemotherapy (nedaplatin/UFT) after concurrent chemoradiotherapy for locally advanced head and neck SCC [in Japanese]. *Nippon Jibiinkoka Gakkai Kaiho.* 2006;109(3):149–156.

318. Pignon JP, Bourhis J, Domenge C, Designe L. Chemotherapy added to locoregional treatment for head and neck squamous-cell carcinoma: three meta-analyses of updated individual data. MACH-NC Collaborative Group. Meta-Analysis of Chemotherapy on Head and Neck Cancer. *Lancet.* 2000; 355(9208):949–955.

319. Volling P, Schroder M. Preliminary results of a prospective randomized study of primary chemotherapy in carcinoma of the oral cavity and pharynx. *HNO.* 1995;43(2):58–64.

320. Vermorken JB. Medical treatment in head and neck cancer. *Ann Oncol.* 2005;16 (suppl 2):ii258–ii264.

321. Adelstein DJ. Recent randomized trials of chemoradiation in the management of locally advanced head and neck cancer. *Curr Opin Oncol.* 1998; 10(3):213–218.

322. Adelstein DJ, Saxton JP, Lavertu P, et al. Maximizing local control and organ preservation in stage IV squamous cell head and neck cancer with hyperfractionated radiation and concurrent chemotherapy. *J Clin Oncol.* 2002;20(5):1405–1410.

323. Adelstein DJ, Saxton JP, Rybicki LA, et al. Multiagent concurrent chemoradiotherapy for locoregionally advanced squamous cell head and neck cancer: mature results from a single institution. *J Clin Oncol.* 2006;24(7):1064–1071.

324. Abitbol A, bdel-Wahab M, Lewin A, et al. Phase II study of tolerance and efficacy of hyperfractionated radiotherapy and 5-fluorouracil, cisplatin, and paclitaxel (Taxol) in stage III and IV inoperable and/or unresectable head-and-neck SCC: A-2 protocol. *Int J Radiat Oncol Biol Phys.* 2002; 53(4):942–947.

325. Abitbol A, bdel-Wahab M, Harvey M, et al. Phase II study of tolerance and efficacy of hyperfractionated radiation therapy and 5-fluorouracil, cisplatin, and paclitaxel (taxol) and amifostine (ethyol) in head and neck SCCs: A-3 protocol. *Am J Clin Oncol.* 2005;28(5):449–455.

326. Adelstein DJ, Saxton JP, Lavertu P, et al. A phase III randomized trial comparing concurrent chemotherapy and radiotherapy with radiotherapy alone in resectable stage III and IV squamous cell head and neck cancer: preliminary results. *Head Neck.* 1997;19(7):567–575.

327. Adelstein DJ, Lavertu P, Saxton JP, et al. Mature results of a phase III randomized trial comparing concurrent chemoradiotherapy with radiation therapy alone in patients with stage III and IV SCC of the head and neck. *Cancer.* 2000;88(4): 876–883.

328. Calais G, Alfonsi M, Bardet E, et al. Randomized trial of radiation therapy versus concomitant chemotherapy and radiation therapy for advanced-stage oropharynx carcinoma. *J Natl Cancer Inst.* 1999;91(24):2081–2086.

329. Ruggeri EM, Carlini P, Pollera CF, et al. Long-term survival in locally advanced oral cavity cancer: an analysis of patients treated with neoadjuvant cisplatin-based chemotherapy followed by surgery. *Head Neck.* 2005;27(6):452–458.

330. Kovacs AF, Mose S, Bottcher HD, Bitter K. Multimodality treatment including postoperative radiation and concurrent chemotherapy with weekly docetaxel is feasible and effective in patients with oral and oropharyngeal cancer. *Strahlenther Onkol.* 2005;181(1):26–34.

331. Astsaturov I, Cohen RB, Harari P. Targeting epidermal growth factor receptor signaling in the treatment of head and neck cancer. *Expert Rev Anticancer Ther.* 2006;6(9):1179–1193.

332. Cohen EE. Role of epidermal growth factor receptor pathway-targeted therapy in patients

with recurrent and/or metastatic SCC of the head and neck. *J Clin Oncol.* 2006;24(17):2659-2665.

333. Brizel DM, Esclamado R. Concurrent chemoradiotherapy for locally advanced, nonmetastatic, squamous carcinoma of the head and neck: consensus, controversy, and conundrum. *J Clin Oncol.* 2006;24(17):2612-2617.

334. Hitt R, Martin P, Hidalgo M. Cetuximab in SCC of the head and neck. *Future Oncol.* 2006;2(4): 449-457.

335. Bonner JA, Harari PM, Giralt J, et al. Radiotherapy plus cetuximab for squamous-cell carcinoma of the head and neck. *N Engl J Med.* 2006;354(6): 567-578.

336. Okura M, Hiranuma T, Adachi T, et al. Induction chemotherapy is associated with an increase in the incidence of locoregional recurrence in patients with carcinoma of the oral cavity: results from a single institution. *Cancer.* 1998;82(5): 804-815.

337. Kirita T, Ohgi K, Shimooka H, et al. Preoperative concurrent chemoradiotherapy plus radical surgery for advanced SCC of the oral cavity: an analysis of long-term results. *Oral Oncol.* 1999; 35(6):597-606.

338. Paccagnella A, Orlando A, Marchiori C, et al. Phase III trial of initial chemotherapy in stage III or IV head and neck cancers: a study by the Gruppo di Studio sui Tumori della Testa e del Collo. *J Natl Cancer Inst.* 1994;86(4):265-272.

339. Volling P, Schroder M, Eckel H, Ebeling O, Stennert E. [Results of a prospective randomized trial with induction chemotherapy for cancer of the oral cavity and tonsils]. *HNO.* 1999;47(10): 899-906.

340. Kovacs AF, Turowski B, Ghahremani MT, Loitz M. Intraarterial chemotherapy as neoadjuvant treatment of oral cancer. *J Craniomaxillofac Surg.* 1999;27(5):302-307.

341. Kohno N, Ikari T, Kawaida M, et al. Survival results of neoadjuvant chemotherapy for advanced SCC of the head and neck. *Jpn J Clin Oncol.* 2000; 30(6):253-258.

342. Adelstein DJ, Leblanc M. Does induction chemotherapy have a role in the management of locoregionally advanced squamous cell head and neck cancer? *J Clin Oncol.* 2006;24(17): 2624-2628.

343. Klug C, Keszthelyi D, Ploder O, et al. Neoadjuvant radiochemotherapy of oral cavity and oropharyngeal cancer: evaluation of tumor response by CT differs from histopathologic response assessment in a significant fraction of patients. *Head Neck.* 2004;26(3):224-231.

344. Haddad R, Wirth L, Posner M. Emerging drugs for head and neck cancer. *Expert Opin Emerg Drugs.* 2006;11(3):461-467.

345. Adelstein DJ, Li Y, Adams GL, et al. An intergroup phase III comparison of standard radiation therapy and two schedules of concurrent chemoradiotherapy in patients with unresectable squamous cell head and neck cancer. *J Clin Oncol.* 2003; 21(1):92-98.

346. Ghi MG, Paccagnella A, D'Amanzo P, et al. Neoadjuvant docetaxel, cisplatin, 5-fluorouracil before concurrent chemoradiotherapy in locally advanced SCC of the head and neck versus concomitant chemoradiotherapy: a phase II feasibility study. *Int J Radiat Oncol Biol Phys.* 2004; 59(2):481-487.

347. Colella G, Gabriele M, Lanza A, Tartaro GP, Giorgetti G. Clinical evaluation of patients with squamous carcinoma of the oral cavity. *Minerva Stomatol.* 1999;48(7-8):319-323.

348. Lavertu P, Adelstein DJ, Saxton JP, et al. Aggressive concurrent chemoradiotherapy for squamous cell head and neck cancer: an 8-year single-institution experience. *Arch Otolaryngol Head Neck Surg.* 1999;125(2):142-148.

349. Yao M, Dornfeld KJ, Buatti JM, et al. Intensity-modulated radiation treatment for head-and-neck SCC—the University of Iowa experience. *Int J Radiat Oncol Biol Phys.* 2005;63(2):410-421.

350. American Head and Neck Society Clinical Practice Guidelines. Available at: http://www.headandneckcancer.org/clinicalresources/docs/oralcavity.php 2006.

351. Vikram B, Strong EW, Shah JP, Spiro R. Second malignant neoplasms in patients successfully treated with multimodality treatment for advanced head and neck cancer. *Head Neck Surg.* 1984;6(3):734-737.

352. Cooney TR, Poulsen MG. Is routine follow-up useful after combined-modality therapy for advanced head and neck cancer? *Arch Otolaryngol Head Neck Surg.* 1999;125(4):379-382.

353. Gourin CG, Williams HT, Seabolt WN, Herdman AV, Howington JW, Terris DJ. Utility of positron emission tomography-computed tomography in identification of residual nodal disease after chemoradiation for advanced head and neck cancer. *Laryngoscope.* 2006;116(5):705-710.

354. Menda Y, Graham MM. Update on 18F-fluorodeoxyglucose/positron emission tomography and

positron emission tomography/computed tomography imaging of squamous head and neck cancers. *Semin Nucl Med.* 2005;35(4):214–219.

355. Ryan WR, Fee WE Jr, Le QT, Pinto HA. Positron-emission tomography for surveillance of head and neck cancer. *Laryngoscope.* 2005;115(4):645–650.

356. Lin YC, Hsiao JR, Tsai ST. Salvage surgery as the primary treatment for recurrent oral SCC. *Oral Oncol.* 2004;40(2):183–189.

357. Wong LY, Wei WI, Lam LK, Yuen AP. Salvage of recurrent head and neck SCC after primary curative surgery. *Head Neck.* 2003;25(11):953–959.

358. Chone CT, Silva AR, Crespo AN, Schlupp WR. Regional tumor recurrence after supraomohyoid neck dissection. *Arch Otolaryngol Head Neck Surg.* 2003;129(1):54–58.

359. Regine WF, Valentino J, Sloan DA, et al. Postoperative radiation therapy for primary vs. recurrent SCC of the head and neck: results of a comparative analysis. *Head Neck.* 1999;21(6):554–559.

360. Ugurlu K, Ozcelik D, Huthut I, Yildiz K, Kilinc L, Bas L. Extended vertical trapezius myocutaneous flap in head and neck reconstruction as a salvage procedure. *Plast Reconstr Surg.* 2004;114(2): 339–350.

361. To EW, Tsang WM, Williams MD, Pang PC, Cheng JH, Chan AC. Reconstruction challenge—combined use of pectoralis major and gastric pull-up flaps for massive naso-oropharyngeal/oesophageal defects. *Asian J Surg.* 2002;25(4):337–340.

362. Castelli ML, Pecorari G, Succo G, Bena A, Andreis M, Sartoris A. Pectoralis major myocutaneous flap: analysis of complications in difficult patients. *Eur Arch Otorhinolaryngol.* 2001;258(10):542–545.

363. Smeele LE, Goldstein D, Tsai V, et al. Morbidity and cost differences between free flap reconstruction and pedicled flap reconstruction in oral and oropharyngeal cancer: matched control study. *J Otolaryngol.* 2006;35(2):102–107.

364. Jones NF, Vogelin E, Markowitz BL, Watson JP. Reconstruction of composite through-and-through mandibular defects with a double-skin paddle fibular osteocutaneous flap. *Plast Reconstr Surg.* 2003;112(3):758–765.

365. Smith GI, O'Brien CJ, Choy ET, Andruchow JL, Gao K. Clinical outcome and technical aspects of 263 radial forearm free flaps used in reconstruction of the oral cavity. *Br J Oral Maxillofac Surg.* 2005;43(3):199–204.

366. Shpitzer T, Gullane PJ, Neligan PC, et al. The free vascularized flap and the flap plate options: comparative results of reconstruction of lateral mandibular defects. *Laryngoscope.* 2000;110(12): 2056–2060.

367. Zenn MR, Hidalgo DA, Cordeiro PG, Shah JP, Strong EW, Kraus DH. Current role of the radial forearm free flap in mandibular reconstruction. *Plast Reconstr Surg.* 1997;99(4):1012–1017.

368. Arden RL, Rachel JD, Marks SC, Dang K. Volume-length impact of lateral jaw resections on complication rates. *Arch Otolaryngol Head Neck Surg.* 1999;125(1):68–72.

369. Cipriani R, Contedini F, Caliceti U, Cavina C. Three-dimensional reconstruction of the oral cavity using the free anterolateral thigh flap. *Plast Reconstr Surg.* 2002;109(1):53–57.

370. Shibahara T, Mohammed AF, Katakura A, Nomura T. Long-term results of free radial forearm flap used for oral reconstruction: functional and histological evaluation. *J Oral Maxillofac Surg.* 2006;64(8):1255–1260.

371. Kirn DS, Finical SJ, Kenady DE. Bilateral radial forearm free flaps for oral-cavity reconstruction. *J Reconstr Microsurg.* 1998;14(8):551–553.

372. Kuriakose MA, Loree TR, Spies A, Meyers S, Hicks WL Jr. Sensate radial forearm free flaps in tongue reconstruction. *Arch Otolaryngol Head Neck Surg.* 2001;127(12):1463–1466.

373. Pigno MA, Funk JJ. Prosthetic management of a total glossectomy defect after free flap reconstruction in an edentulous patient: a clinical report. *J Prosthet Dent.* 2003;89(2):119–122.

374. Chien CY, Su CY, Hwang CF, Chuang HC, Jeng SF, Chen YC. Ablation of advanced tongue or base of tongue cancer and reconstruction with free flap: functional outcomes. *Eur J Surg Oncol.* 2006; 32(3):353–357.

375. Huang CH, Chen HC, Huang YL, Mardini S, Feng GM. Comparison of the radial forearm flap and the thinned anterolateral thigh cutaneous flap for reconstruction of tongue defects: an evaluation of donor-site morbidity. *Plast Reconstr Surg.* 2004;114(7):1704–1710.

376. Tabata M, Kuwahara M, Shimoda T, Sugihara K, Akashi M. Reconstruction of a partial maxilla with a combination of autologous bone particles and a microtitanium mesh tray covered by a forearm flap. *J Oral Maxillofac Surg.* 2004;62(5): 638–642.

377. Yamamoto Y, Kawasmhima K, Sugihara T, Nohira K, Furuta Y, Fukuda S. Surgical management of maxillectomy defects based on the concept of buttress reconstruction. *Head Neck.* 2004;26(3): 247–256.

378. Rohner D, Tan BK, Song C, Yeow V, Hammer B. Repair of composite zygomatico-maxillary defects with free bone grafts and free vascularized tissue transfer. *J Craniomaxillofac Surg.* 2001;29(6): 337–343.

379. Urken ML, Bridger AG, Zur KB, Genden EM. The scapular osteofasciocutaneous flap: a 12-year experience. *Arch Otolaryngol Head Neck Surg.* 2001;127(7):862–869.

380. Futran ND, Mendez E. Developments in reconstruction of midface and maxilla. *Lancet Oncol.* 2006;7(3):249–258.

15

Malignant Neoplasms of the Oropharynx

Guy J. Petruzzelli

EPIDEMIOLOGY AND PATHOGENESIS OF OROPHARYNGEAL CANCER

It is estimated that there will be 8000 new cases of cancer of the oropharynx (tonsils, soft palate/uvula, tongue base, and pharyngeal walls) diagnosed in the United States accounting for 3,000 cancer deaths in 2007. Oropharyngeal cancer is twice as common in men as in women with a mean age at diagnosis of 62 years and a 60% overall 5-year survival rate with significant differences in mortality observed based on stage at presentation and race.[1-4] Statistics regarding incidence, mortality and survival data for oropharyngeal malignancies are obtained and interpreted by the SEER database of the National Cancer Institute. Cancers of the tonsil and tonsillar fossa are the most common, followed by tongue base, soft palate/uvula, and posterior pharyngeal wall. Although squamous cell carcinoma is the predominant histologic type of cancer observed in this region, minor salivary gland, melanoma, small cell carcinoma (lymphoepithelioma), and lymphoreticular malignances are also observed.[5] The precise determination of the histology is critical to the development of a comprehensive treatment program. As we will discuss, patients with squamous cell carcinoma of the oropharynx, particular the tongue base, frequently present with regional nodal metastasis and require a comprehensive multidisciplinary treatment approach.

It is now accepted that invasive oropharyngeal squamous cell carcinoma arises though a multistep process in genetically susceptible individuals exposed to the risk factors of tobacco (cigarette, pipe, cigar, and smokeless), alcohol, betel quid chewing, a diet poor in fruits and vegetables (specifically vitamin A and carotenoids), and exposure to the human papilloma virus.[6-8] Oropharyngeal carcinomas satisfy all the biologic criteria for malignancy by their ability to circumvent normal cellular growth control mechanisms, invade surrounding structures, induce a blood supply, develop self-sufficiency in proliferative signaling, and spread to secondary anatomic sites. The genetic basis for these phenotypic changes include either the activation of proto-oncogenes that stimulate cell growth and promote cell-cell dissociation and migration and/or the inactivation of tumor suppressor genes responsible for restricting these activities or initiating and promoting programmed cell death (apoptosis).

Three principal mechanisms exist for activation of proto-oncogenes. The first involves a specific deletion or point mutation in the DNA sequence. As a result, normal amounts of hyperactive proteins are produced. In the second, the copy number of a gene is increased either by chromosomal gain or amplification resulting in an overproduction of a normal protein. The final mechanism involves genetic rearrangement via translocations resulting in faulty DNA regulatory sequences leading to either overproduction of normal protein or a fusion protein that is overproduced or hyperactive. Mechanisms for inhibiting tumor suppressor genes include loss of genetic information via DNA deletions or loss of heterozygosity. Another mechanism responsible for loss of tumor suppressor gene function is the blockage in production of protein via epigenetic mechanisms such as promoter hypermethylation.[9,10]

Advances in biotechnology have led to the development of the sophisticated, specific, and high-throughput techniques necessary for these detailed investigations into the genetic aberrations associated with the development of oropharyngeal cancer. Such techniques include comparative genomic hybridization (CGH), spectral karyotyping (SKY), and fluorescence in situ hybridization (FISH).[10] Multiple studies have led to the identification of gains and losses on multiple chromosomal regions (Table 15–1).

One unique feature of oropharyngeal squamous cell carcinoma is the association with the double-stranded DNA human papilloma virus type 16 (HPV 16).[11] Using Southern blot hybridization the highest percentage of squamous cell carcinomas containing HPV-16 DNA is located in the tongue base and tonsil.[12] The molecular pathogenesis of squamous cell carcinoma results from the inactivation of tumor suppressor genes p53 and pRb by oncoproteins encoded by HPV genes E6 and E7. The mechanisms for p53 and pRb inactivation are distinct from those observed in squamous cell carci-

noma in patient with chronic exposure to tobacco and alcohol. Efforts have been directed at using the relative expression of the HPV genome as a prognostic factor in oropharyngeal squamous cell carcinoma. High levels of HPV-16 DNA and in particular with coexpression of high levels of p16 may represent a distinct subcategory of these tumors with a more favorable prognosis. The presence of HPV 16 in oropharyngeal cancers has been demonstrated repeatedly and specific causal relationship are currently being elucidated.[7,8,13-17]

The result of this multistep progression model of squamous cell carcinogenesis is the development of a clone(s) of malignant cells able to produce particular proteins that enable these cells to invade local tissues and spread to other secondary sites via the lymphatic and vascular systems. Specific examples of these molecules include autocrine growth factors (epidermal growth factor and its receptor), angiogenic factors (vascular endothelial cell growth factor), proteolytic enzymes (matrix metalloproteinase and plasminogen activator), and transcription factors (STAT family). The degree to which these molecules are produced in large measure will determine the biologic behavior (radiosensitivity, sensitivity to various cytotoxic agents, local invasiveness, nodal and systemic metastasis) of a given head and neck carcinoma. Increased understanding of the molecular events of carcinogenesis has led to the development of targeted therapies (cetuximab) that are now a part of the armamentarium of antitumor systemic therapies. [18]

Table 15–1. Chromosomal Gain and Deletions in Head and Neck Cancer

Deletion	Gain
3p	3q
5q	3q
8p	5p
9p	7p
11q	7q
13p	8q
18q	11q

ANATOMIC BOUNDARIES, SUBDIVISIONS, AND FUNCTION OF THE OROPHARYNX[19]

The oropharynx is defined as the region of the upper aerodigestive tract bounded superiorly by the plane of the plate (just inferior to the torus tuberus), anteriorly by the anterior tonsillar pillars (faucial arches) and posterior third of the tongue, posteriorly by the posterior pharyngeal wall, and inferiorly by the tip of the epiglottis. The oropharynx communicates with the nasopharynx superiorly through the pharyngeal isthmus, anteriorly with the oral cavity through the (palatine) faucial arch, and inferiorly to the hypopharynx at the valeculla. The components of the oropharynx include the faucial arches or tonsillar pillars, the tonsils and tonsillar fossa, the soft palate and uvula, the tongue posterior to the sulcus terminalis (base of the tongue) including the glossoepiglottic folds, and that portion of the posterior pharyngeal wall extending from below the palate to the plane of the tip of the epiglottis.

The roof of the oropharynx is formed by the soft palate and uvula. The fibrous scaffolding of the soft palate is the palatine aponeurosis which is firmly attached at the posterior margin of the periostium of the palatal process of the maxilla (hard palate). On the oral surface the aponeurosis is covered by the palatoglossus muscle which extends from its fibrous attachments laterally to join the tongue at approximately the junction of the oral tongue and tongue base. The muscle is covered by mucous membrane and forms the palatoglossal arch or anterior tonsillar pillar. The palatopharyngeus muscle arises from the palatine aponeurosis and divides into an anterior and posterior layer which encircles the palatoglossus and levator veli palatine and fuses laterally forming the reconstituted palatopharyngeus. The palatopharyngeus extends inferior fusing with some fibers of the superior pharyngeal constrictor; it is covered by oral mucosa and forms the posterior tonsillar pillar. The levator veli palatini muscle is enveloped by the palatopharyngeus medially and forms the bulk of the soft palate. This muscle extends from the petrous temporal skull base and extends anteriorly, medially, and inferiorly to blend into the palatine aponeurosis at the midline. Loss of function of this muscle results in eustachian tube dysfunction and serous otitis media. The longitudinal fibers of the small muscularis uvula also arise from the palatal aponeurosis and are encircled by the palatopharyngeus. This muscle has no sphinteric function and patients tolerate its resection without significant functional deficit.

Tonsillar fossa is bounded anteriorly by the palatoglossus and palatopharyngeus muscles or the anterior and posterior tonsillar pillars, respectively. The depression between these two structures is the tonsillar fossa which contains the palatine tonsil. The tonsil is bounded medially by a specialized portion of the pharyngobasilar fascia referred to as the tonsillar capsule. Lateral to the capsule is a potential space—the peritonsillar or paratonsillar space. The lateral or deep surface of the tonsillar fossa is formed principally by the superior pharyngeal constrictor. Attached to the lateral surface of the superior pharyngeal constrictor is the glossopharygeal nerve; irritation of the nerve in this region by pathology within the tonsillar fossa accounts for the afferent limb of the referred otalgia commonly observed in these patients. Lateral to the superior constrictor is the fat of the parapharyngeal space in which lies the carotid artery and vagus nerve. Resection of portions of the superior constrictor to obtain negative surgical margins on tonsillar carcinomas can be performed safely with gentle bipolar dissection and magnification.

The tongue base or pharyngeal tongue begins anteriorly at the sulcus terminals, the inverted V-shaped groove located posterior to the circumvallated papillae on the lateral aspects. The foramen cecum is the pit at the apex when the sulci converge, which gives rise to the thyroid primordium. The mucosa of the tongue extends inferiorly and continues with that of the epiglottis forming paired lateral and a single median glossoepiglottic folds. The paired recesses lateral to the median glossoepiglottic folds are the epiglottic valleculae. Lymphoid follicles located across the tongue represent the most inferior aspect of Waldeyer's ring and can give rise to lymphomas.

Posterior pharyngeal wall is the mucosal-muscle-fascial complex beginning at the pharyngeal tubercule of the occipital bone. The oropharyngeal component includes that portion overlying the second and third cervical vertebrae. The posterior pharyngeal wall is suspended from the skull base by the broad thick pharyngobasilar fascia arising in the midline and extending laterally among the petrous temporal bone anterior to the carotid canals to insert on the cartilaginous portions of the eustachian tubes extending inferiorly and laterally to form the capsule of the tonsils. The superior pharyngeal constrictor does not extend to the skull base but arises from the pharyngobasilar fascia at the level of the arch of C1. Deep to the pharyngeal constructors is the buccopharyngeal (visceral) fascia which is continuous inferiorly with the visceral fascia of the esophagus. The retropharyngeal (retrovisceral) space contains loose connective tissue and a small amount of fat which prevent friction between the posterior pharyngeal wall and the spine and allow for normal swallowing. Loss of elasticity and fibrosis of the posterior pharyngeal wall with obliteration of the retropharyngeal space is one mechanism for dysphagia associated with treatment of head and neck malignancies. Deep in the prevertebral space is the bilateral prevertebral fascia or the deep layer of the deep cervical fascia investing the paraspinal muscles. The alar division arises from the skull base, extends lateral from transverse process to transverse process of the vertebral bodies, and extends inferiorly to the second thoracic vertebrae. The prevertebral fascia is anterior to the vertebral bodies and extends from the skull base to the coccyx.

The sensory and motor innervation of the oropharynx is derived from pharyngeal plexus composed of the glossopharygeal (IX) and vagus (X) nerves. After leaving the intracranial via the jugular foramen the glossopharygeal nerve provides motor innervation to only the stylopharyngeus muscle. The general sensory fibers of IX are distributed to the oropharyngeal surface of the tongue base, tonsillar fossa, and the posterior pharyngeal wall. The remaining motor innervation of the oropharynx including the superior and middle pharyngeal constrictor and palatal muscles is the pharyngeal branch of the vagus, except for the tensor veli palatine which is innervated by a branch of the third (mandibular) division of the trigeminal nerve.

The arterial supply of the oropharynx is derived from the external carotid system. The palatine branch of the ascending pharyngeal artery supplies the superior pharyngeal constrictor, soft palate, and tonsillar fossa. The dorsal lingual branch of the lingual artery also supplies the tonsillar fossa as well as the glossal palatine arch, the posterior tongue. The ascending palatine and tonsillar branches are cervical branches of the facial artery supplying the lateral soft palate superior constrictor complex and the tonsillar fossa lateral tongue base, respectively. Finally, the lesser palatine artery is derived from the pterygopalatine (third) portion of the internal maxillary artery and supplies the soft palate and the tonsillar fossa. The arterial supply to the oropharynx is known for a well-developed system of anastomoses from both the branches of ipsilateral and bilateral external carotid artery systems. The pharyngeal plexus is the main confluence of venous tributaries from this region and drains into the internal jugular vein.

The oropharynx is the region of the head and neck with the most abundant lymphatic drainage. This principle must be considered in the preoperative clinical and radiographic evaluation of patients with oropharyngeal malignancies. The principal lymphatic drainage of the tonsillar fossa and pillars is to the upper cervical nodes in Zone II. Similarly, the tongue base will also drain into Zone II and occasionally Zone III. Like other midline structures, cancer of the tongue base frequently presents with or harbors microscopic bilateral nodal metastases (see below). The lymphatics of soft palate, uvula, and posterior pharyngeal wall also will drain into the deep retropharyngeal nodes. Located deep to the buccopharyngeal fascia and medial to the internal carotid artery at the level of C-1 these nodes cannot be palpated on physical examination and must be identified primarily on imaging. The efferent drainage of the retropharyngeal nodes is to the deep cervical nodes in level III. In patients with clinical negative or early nodal metastasis (N2a), the posterior neck (Zone V) may be spared, thus reducing the morbidity of the neck dissection (Table 15-2).

The coordinated movements of the oropharynx are crucial for maintenance of effective speech and swallowing function. In speech, simultaneous motion of the posterior pharyngeal wall and soft palate are necessity to close the nasopharyngeal isthmus. Con-

Table 15–2. Lymph Node Drainage Patterns in Oropharyngeal Carcinoma

Region	Lymphatic Drainage
Anterior Tonsillar Pillar	Level I, II, III
Posterior Tonsillar Pillar	Level II or Level V
Tonsil/Tonsillar Fossa	Level II, III
Soft Palate	Level II, III, or Retropharyngeal nodes
Base of the Tongue	Level II, III, IV
Posterior Pharyngeal Wall	Level V or Retropharyngeal nodes

traction of the superior pharyngeal construction draws the posterior pharyngeal wall anteriorly and reduces the diameter of the pharynx whereas the soft palate is elevated by the palatopharyngeus, salpingopharyngeus, and tensor veli palatine muscles. Resection or loss of elasticity of these structures will lead to hypernasal and hyperresonant speech. Coordinated motion of oropharyngeal structures is critical during the second (pharyngeal) phase of swallowing characterized by the transportation of the prepared bolus from the oral cavity to the relaxed pharyngoesophgeal segment. Specific components include (1) as in speech, elevation of the palate for complete oronasal separation; (2) posterior contraction of the tongue base and generation of the piston-like "tongue driving force"; (3) direction of the bolus laterally into the vallecula; and (4) laryngeal elevation, epiglottic closure, and dilation of the pharyngoesophageal segment to allow passage of the bolus into the relaxed upper esophagus. Failure of any of these elements to function in a coordinated fashion either from surgical or nonsurgical inventions will lead to dysphagia. Operative interventions to assist in the recovery of meaningful swallowing are occasionally helpful but close cooperation with skilled speech-language pathologists is necessary to help patients develop compensatory strategies.[20]

CRITICAL ELEMENTS OF THE HISTORY AND PHYSICAL EXAMINATION

The first step in the evaluation of a patient with a suspected oropharyngeal carcinoma is a systematic and thorough history and a comprehensive head and neck examination by an experienced head and neck surgeon.

Careful inquiry regarding specific signs or symptoms may give some indication as to the site of the primary tumor. Dysphagia, odynophagia, persistent sore throat, or a painful foreign body sensation may indicate a tonsillar or pharyngeal wall malignancy. Otalgia in the normal appearing ear can be an early finding due to referred pain from irritation of the glossopharyngeal nerve in the tonsillar fossa or lateral pharyngeal wall. Trismus is an ominous finding indicat-

ing extension of the tumor lateral to the pharyngeal envelope of the buccopharyngeal fascia, pharygobasilar fascia, and the constrictor muscles into the pterygoid muscles and the infratemporal fossa. In our experience, extension of oropharyngeal malignancies into this region indicates a poor prognosis.

The base of the tongue has a paucity of pain fibers compared to other regions of the upper aerodigestive tract; therefore, tumors in this area may grow extremely large or deeply infiltrative with relatively few symptoms. Mass effect from an exophytic tumor or hypoglossal nerve paralysis from an infiltrative malignancy can result in dysarthria indicating a lesion in the tongue base.

Many of the symptoms of oropharyngeal malignancy are mistaken for those of more benign conditions such as pharyngoesophageal reflux, posterior nasal drainage, or tonsillopharyngitis. Consequently, many patients do not present until they develop metastatic cervical adenopathy. Patients or their primary care providers may have identified an otherwise asymptomatic neck mass. Failure of the neck mass to respond to a 14-day course of oral antibiotics should prompt an evaluation by an otolaryngologist-head and neck surgeon. In our experience with 253 patients with oropharyngeal squamous cell carcinoma treated with primary surgery, only 57 (22.5%) presented with no clinical metastatic adenopathy. Patients with metastatic cervical adenopathy from upper aerodigestive tract squamous cell carcinoma are by definition in stage III or IV and the best chance for positive outcomes is achieved by avoiding any further delay in diagnosis and initiating multimodality treatment.

Patients should undergo a detailed examination of the head and neck prior to obtaining costly imaging studies. Lesions of the soft palate, uvula, and anterior tonsillar pillar may be identified by the primary care provided or oral health professional (Fig 15–1). Masses in the pharyngeal walls, tongue base, and vallecula are difficult to identify without the particular equipment of the head and neck surgeon. Mucosal surfaces of the upper aerodigestive tract should be inspected and palpated. The posterior superior lateral aspects of the tonsillar fossa, walls of the oropharynx, piriform sinuses, and the base of the tongue should be carefully examined. The tongue base, vallecula, and

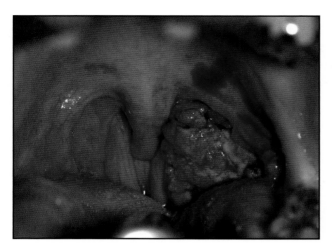

Fig 15–1. Exophytic mass of the left tonsillar fossa. Transoral biopsy revealed squamous cell carcinoma.

hypopharyngeal mucosa should be examined with a magnified angled Hopkins telescope and/or a flexible nasopharyngolaryngoscope. Areas of ulceration, induration, firmness, or erythema should be noted for biopsy. In selected individuals transoral biopsy of oropharyngeal, lesions can be performed obviating the need for routine "staging triple endoscopy."

The neck should be palpated with careful attention to the character, size, fixation, and particularly the location of any metastatic adenopathy. Primary lymphatic drainage of the tonsillar fossa and oropharyngeal wall is level II whereas that of the tongue base is level III. The cervical lymphatics are the second echelon of drainage for the soft palate and uvula. Therefore, patients with soft palatal-uvula malignancies should have their imaging studies reviewed with careful attention to the primary lymphatics in the prevertebral region. Mobility can give information regarding the relationship of the mass to the structures related to the carotid sheath. Fixation to the skin or subcutaneous tissue indicates extracapsular extension and invasion of the subdermal lymphatics.

Concurrent systemic illnesses such as coronary artery disease or diabetes should be evaluated. The severity of concurrent disease may have a significant impact on the patients overall survival in addition to potential choices for cancer treatment. Several instruments are available for measuring general

comorbidities and when collected in a systematic fashion comorbidity data have been shown to provide important prognostic information, independent of TNM staging, in cancers of the larynx, pharynx, and oral cavity.

APPROPRIATE DIAGNOSTIC OFFICE-BASED PROCEDURES

The majority of primary oropharyngeal tumors are detected in the tonsillar fossa or tongue base. Direct transoral examination and biopsy with local anesthesia are possible in the majority of cases. Palpation of the tonsils and the tongue base should be carried out in the office and if necessary under anesthesia noting areas of nodularity or induration. Despite endoscopic evaluation, some primaries may not be detected as they may be submucosal, hidden in lymphatic crypts, or have submucosally regressed. In patients with tonsil carcinoma (and as discussed later, carcinoma of the unknown primary site), we favor bilateral tonsillectomy over tonsil biopsy. Advantages of bilateral tonsillectomy include increased yield over conventional biopsy, an approximately 10% incidences of bilateral carcinomas, ease in follow-up examination, and no increased complications.[21,22]

Historically, the tongue base was evaluated with biopsies referred to as either "directed," "random," "blind," or other nonspecific terms. With the development of more sophisticated optical and laser technology these imprecise biopsy procedures have been replaced with a more selective, superficial, and wider biopsy of the tongue base and vallecula. Using this technique we have been able to identify the site of the primary tumor in greater than 90% of patients referred for the evaluation of malignant cervical adenopathy with an "unknown" primary source. Pathologic material from Waldeyer's ring should be submitted for pathologic analysis in both formalin and saline.

When a neck mass is present, fine needle aspiration (FNA) should be included in the initial evaluation. Fine-needle aspiration biopsy is the least invasive pathological test to evaluate a suspected metastatic cervical lymph node and should be attempted prior to excisional biopsy. It can be 98 to 99% accurate in the hands of an experienced cytopathologist. The procedure, performed with a 25-gauge needle, can be carried out in the office and the aspirate can be examined immediately for rapid diagnosis using alcohol-fixed and stained tissues. Conventional cytological examination on fixed slides, hematoxylin and eosin examination of centrifuges aspirates ("cell blocks"), and immunohistochemistry all can be used.

RECOMMENDED IMAGING STUDIES

The contemporary head and neck oncologist should be familiar with the modalities for both functional and anatomic imaging as reviewed in Chapter 3. Anatomic imaging (computed tomography-CT and magnetic resonance imaging-MRI) is required to precisely stage and assess the response to treatment of oropharyngeal malignancy. Pretreatment imaging complements the physical examination and is used to define the three dimensional extent of the primary tumor, determine extension into surrounding anatomic regions, characterize relationships to nearby structures, and identify clinically unrecognized metastatic adenopathy.

In the oropharynx, tumor must be differentiated from the surrounding lymphoid tissue, muscle, and fat as each of these tissues has particular imaging properties. Both CT and MRI can be used to evaluate oropharyngeal malignancies and each modality has its relative strengths and weaknesses. The greater availability, shorter image acquisition time, reduced cost, and reliable identification metastatic adenopathy make contrast-enhanced CT scans a valuable adjunct in staging oropharyngeal malignancy.[23]

Current generations of helical and multidetector CT scanners are able to acquire complete imaging datasets in a single breath-hold (20 to 30 seconds). Collimated 1.3- to 2-mm sections obtained at 1-mm intervals can be coupled with physiologic maneuvers such as puffed cheek, swallow hold, or Valsalva maneuvers, producing high-resolution images with less apposition of mucosal surfaces and greater image clarity. Software is available to produce good quality 2-dimensional sagittal and coronal reconstructions which are useful in the evaluation of patients with tumors of the tongue base or soft palate. One significant limitation to CT scanning is image degradation by dental amalgams (Fig 15–2). This can be reduced by adjusting the scan angle to avoid artifact; however, poor patient positioning can result in the loss

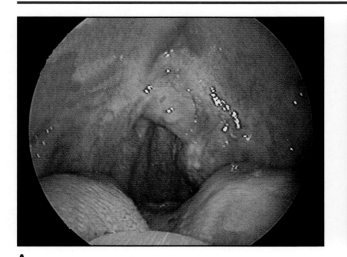

A

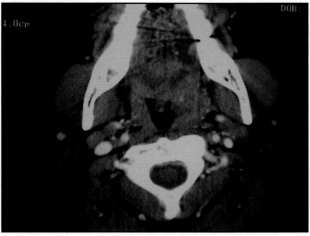

B

Fig 15–2. **A.** Endophytic squamous cell carcinoma of the tonsillar fossa. **B.** Axial contract-enhanced computed tomography scan of this patient prior to surgical excision. Note fullness and asymmetry of the tonsillar fossa.

of normal symmetry which may be confused with pathology.[24-26]

Compared to CT scanning, MRI traditionally has been associated with longer image acquisition times, increased cost, reduced availability and the inability to obtain images in the claustrophobic patient or the patient with ferromagnetic implants. The dramatic increase in the availability of MR scanners and the development of high-field strength open MRI units has increased the utilization of this imaging modality. The major advantages of MRI in the evaluation of patients with tumors of the oropharynx include superior soft tissue contrast, obtaining images in the iodine sensitive patient, and the ability to directly acquire multiplanar images (Fig 15-3).[27]

One of the recent advances in MRI is the use of dynamic contrast-enhanced imaging.[28,29] This technique leverages the biophysical properties of the enhanced metabolic activity of primary tumors or regional metastatic nodes and the local tissue reactions to the tumors. Increased enhanced of tumors is related to their increased blood flow, hypervascualtity, increased neovascular permeability, increased tissue volume, and increased overall blood volume. Briefly, initial standard spin-echo T1-weighted and fast spin-echo T2-weighted axial and sagittal localizing images are obtained before administration of contrast material. Intravenous paramagnetic contrast is delivered and axial and coronal T1-dynamic contrast-enhanced axial fast multiplanar sequences with fat saturation are acquired usually requiring 3 or 4 scanning sequences. After dynamic contrast enhanced MRI, postcontrast T1-weighted images are obtained with or without fat saturation (Fig 15-4). Specific applications of dynamic contrast-enhanced imaging have demonstrated superior identification of the margins and submucosal extension of tumors, differentiate metastatic from nonmetastatic cervical lymph nodes, and accurately predict the response of tumors to radiotherapy.[30,31]

Regardless of the imaging modality employed, several radiographic factors must be considered in the pretreatment assessment of patients with cancer of the oropharynx. Imaging must provide added data regarding the submucosal extension of the primary tumor: (a) laterally to the parapharyngeal space, (b) superior-medially to the nasopharynx, (c) posteriorly to the prevertebral muscles, and (d) anterior-medially along the palatoglossus or palatopharyngeus into the base of the tongue. With tongue base tumors

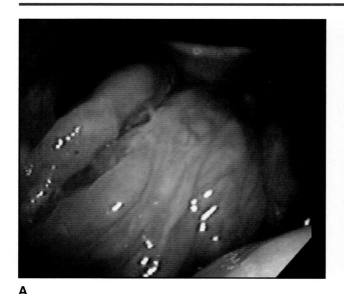

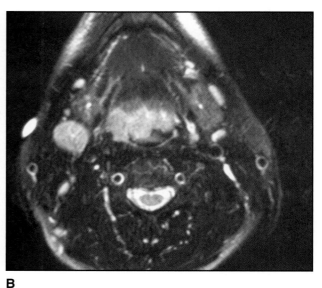

A   **B**

Fig 15–3. A. Exophytic squamous cell carcinoma of the tongue base. **B**. Contrast-enhanced axial magnetic resonance image scan of this patient prior to surgical excision. Note fullness, asymmetry, and enhancement of the tongue base tumor.

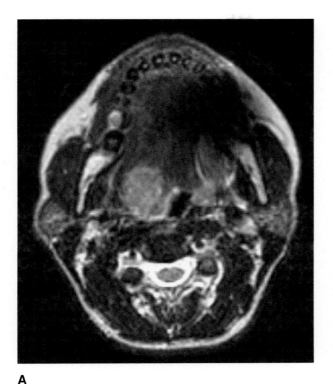 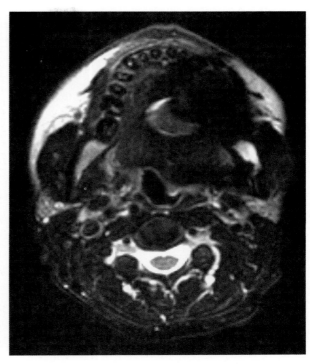

A   **B**

Fig 15–4. A. Preoperative and **B.** 1-year postoperative axial T2, fat saturation MRI scan obtained in a 49-year-old woman who underwent a transoral laser microsurgical resection of a mucoepidermoid carcinoma of the tongue base.

attention should be directed to the anterior extension of the tumor into the oral tongue and floor of the mouth and the midline or contralateral extension and involvement of one or both lingual neurovascular bundle(s). Additional information should also be available regarding bony erosion of the mandible laterally, or the skull base superiorly and medially (Fig 15–5). Finally, the cervical lymphatics should be imaged with attention to their relationship with the carotid artery and the potential for encasement of the artery by the confluence of medially extending metastatic nodes and laterally extending primary tumor.[32]

In summary, pretreatment radiographic assessment is critical to the development of a comprehensive treatment plan for the patient with oropharyngeal carcinoma. The modality (CT or MRI) used depends on the availability of imaging technology, institutional expertise, and, unfortunately, the financial circumstance of the patient (managed care restrictions, etc).

The maximum amount of useful imaging data is obtained when appropriately acquired CT and MRI images are used as complementary studies. However, the superior soft tissue detail, multiplanar imaging capabilities, and reduced distortion from dental amalgam obtained from MRI make it the preferred stand-alone study.

AJCC STAGING OF MALIGNANCY

Staging of oropharyngeal malignancy includes information obtained from a complete history and physical examination including endoscopy and CT and/or MRI imaging data. Malignant tumors of the oropharynx are staged on the basis of the size, location, and regional extension of the primary tumor. Staging of the neck and metastatic sites follow that for other sites of the upper aerodigestive tract.

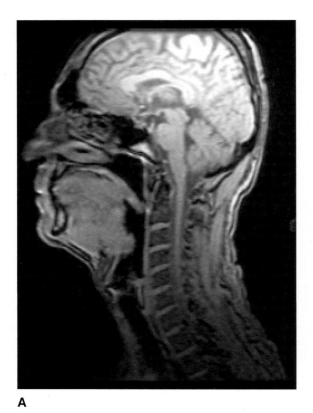

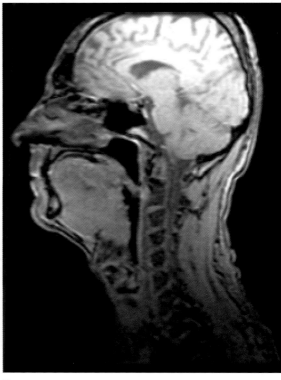

A   B

Fig 15–5. Pretreatment sagittal MRI scan obtained from a 60-year-old man prior to concurrent chemoradiation therapy for a squamous cell carcinoma of the tongue base. Images acquired in the sagittal plane demonstrate the depth of infiltration into the intrinsic muscles of the tongue and extension into the pre-epiglottic space.

Staging of the Primary Tumor

TX   Primary tumor cannot be assessed

T0   No primary tumor identified

Tis   Carcinoma in situ

T1   Primary tumor 2 cm or less in greatest dimension

T2   Primary tumor greater than 2 cm and less than 4 cm in greatest dimension

T3   Primary tumor greater than 4 cm in greatest dimension

T4a   Tumor invades the larynx, deep or extrinsic muscles of the tongue, medial pterygoid muscle, hard palate, or mandible (resectable)

T4b   Tumors invades the lateral pterygoid muscle, pterygoid plates, lateral nasopharynx, skull base, or encases carotid artery (unresectable)

NX   Regional lymph nodes cannot be assessed

N0   No regional lymph node metastasis

N1   Metastasis in a single ipsilateral lymph node 3 cm or less in greatest dimension

N2a   Metastasis in a single ipsilateral lymph node more than 3 cm but less than 6 cm in greatest dimension

N2b   Metastasis in multiple ipsilateral lymph nodes none than 6 cm in greatest dimension

N2c Metastasis in a bilateral or contralateral lymph nodes none more than 6 cm in greatest dimension

N3 Metastasis in a lymph node more than 6 cm in greatest dimension

MX Distant metastatic disease cannot be assessed

M0 No distant metastasis

M1 Distant metastasis identified

Staging

Stage I	T1	N0	M0
Stage II	T2	N0	M0
Stage III	T3	N0	M0
	T3	N1	M0
	T2	N1	M0
	T1	N1	M0
Stage IV A	T4a	N0	M0
	T4a	N1	M0
	T4a	N2	M0
	T1	N2	M0
	T2	N2	M0
	T3	N2	M0
Stage IV B	T4b	Any N	M0
	Any T	N3	M0
Stage IV C	Any T	Any N	M1

EXAMPLES OF REPRESENTATIVE HISTOPATHOLOGY

Squamous cell carcinoma remains the most common malignant neoplasm of the oropharynx. Typically, these tumors present as ulcerating exophytic masses as observed in the other regions of the head and neck. Occult squamous cell carcinomas are superficial microscopic foci of invasive squamous cell carcinomas extending into the submucosal lymphatics presenting primarily as a cystic neck mass.

The evaluation and management of this variant are discussed in detail in Chapter 20.

The normal histology of oropharynx is heterogeneous giving rise to a variety of tumor types. In general, the oropharynx is lined by stratified squamous epithelium with modifications based on regional functional requirements for lining, mastication, and specialized mucosa. Squamous cell carcinomas arise from this keratinizing squamous epithelium. Varying degrees of differentiation from well to poorly differentiated squamous cell carcinomas are observed; however, poorly differentiated carcinomas are more frequent in this region.

The relevant specialized mucosa of the oropharynx includes regional deposits of lymphoid tissue and the submucosal minor salivary glands of the tonsils, soft palate, and tongue base. Lymphoid tissue aggregates in the oropharynx are nonencapsulated and are located in a circular distribution (Waldeyer's ring) at the posterior aspect of this region. Primary extranodal head and neck lymphomas are observed in this region and present as soft, nonulcerating painless masses. Initial symptoms are related to mass effect and include muffled or "hot potato" voice or dysphagia. Minor salivary glands are located within the submucosa of the oropharyngeal mucosa. They are not encapsulated, but compound tubular glands with predominantly mucous-secreting acini and give rise to several distinct malignancies. The most common site of minor salivary gland cancer in the oropharynx is the base of the tongue. Mucoepidermoid carcinoma is the most common tumor observed in this region followed by adenoid cystic carcinoma and adenocarcinoma. Minor salivary gland carcinomas can present as an asymptomatic submucosal mass. Pain, ulceration, tongue paralysis, or fixation is all indicative of deep extension into the tongue musculature or perineural spread.[33]

TREATMENT OF OROPHARYNGEAL CANCER

The optimum treatment program for patients with cancer of the oropharynx remains to be defined. Historically, surgery and external beam radiation therapy has been the mainstay of head and neck cancer treatment. Although the use radiation therapy as single modality treatment has decreased significantly over the last 20 years, the combined use of chemotherapy with radiation has increased and the proportion of patients treated with cancer directed surgery has remained essentially stable.[34] Technical refinements in radiation oncology and the increasing application of radiosensitizing chemotherapy have led to the increased use of organ sparing chemoradiation therapy protocols. Academic medical centers remain the treatment facilities for the majority of patient with oropharyngeal malignancies, particularly those with advanced disease.

Regardless of the method(s) of treatments, several general management principles need to be emphasized. Prior to initial therapy individuals suspected of having an oropharyngeal malignancy should be carefully evaluated by a primary care physician to identify any unrecognized comorbidities, optimize the patient's current medical condition, and facilitate appropriate pretreatment subspecialty consultations. Patients with any suspicious oropharyngeal mass need a careful examination under anesthesia and generous biopsy of the primary lesion. Due to the multiple tumor types observed in this region definitive treatment should not be based on frozen section tissue examination; rather, permanent sections with appropriate immunohistochemical stains should be reviewed. Once a definitive pathologic diagnosis and imaging studies are obtained the patient should be presented at a multidisciplinary tumor conference attended by medical, radiation, dental, and surgical oncologists experienced in the treatment of these rare malignancies. Patients and their families also should have access to support from speech-language pathologists and nutritional, psychological, social, and financial support and information systems. Molecular pathology has provided significant amounts of important information regarding the biology of oropharyngeal malignancies. Unfortunately, commercially available, validated, and reproducible markers of tumor aggressiveness or metastatic potential are not yet in broad clinical use.[35]

In the remainder of this section, we discuss traditional open surgical approaches, definitive radiotherapy, concurrent chemoradiation therapy, and novel transoral laser approaches used in the management of cancer of the oropharynx.

Radiation Therapy

Radiation therapy has been employed in the treatment of oropharyngeal carcinoma as either definitive single modality therapy, concurrent with chemotherapy (chemoradiation), or as adjuvant treatment following surgical resection (with or without radiosensitizing chemotherapy, see below). Treatment guidelines are based on institutional biases, expertise of the treating providers, and retrospective analyses. It is generally assumed, although not supported by randomized trials, that early stage oropharyngeal carcinoma is treated equally well by surgery or radiation therapy.[35] The technical challenges in both radiotherapeutic and surgical management of tumors of the oropharynx further complicate issues surrounding selection of treatment. In general, radiotherapy portals must be designed with the following considerations: (1) bilateral cervical nodes should be treated in patients with tumors of middle structures (soft palate, uvula, central tongue base), (2) both the upper and lower neck are at risk for metastases even when the neck is clinically N0, and (3) the neck can be treated satisfactorily without including the larynx in the primary treatment field. This is best accomplished by dividing an upper treatment field encompassing the primary and an anterior low neck field satisfactorily shielding the larynx and reducing the dose to the spinal cord.[36]

Historically, patients with early stage oropharyngeal squamous cell carcinoma were treaded with external beam radiation therapy (EBRT) with standard fractionation regimens of 1.8 to 2 Gy/day to a total dose of 66 Gy via parallel-opposed lateral fields using 6-MV photons. Intermediate and some advanced stage tumors were treated to 72 Gy with either concomitant boost or brachytherapy techniques. Concomitant boost protocols involve treatment of the primary and neck(s) with 1.8 Gy per fraction to 54 Gy followed by a second daily boost fraction in the last 12 days of 1.2 to 1.5 Gy to a total dose of 72 Gy. Interstitial brachytherapy is used primarily for carcinoma of the tongue base. It is delivered 2 to 3 weeks following 50 to 54 Gy standard fraction EBRT and has the advantage of being able to deliver high doses of radiation to the tumor bed without exceeding the normal tolerance of surrounding tissues. Additional radiation (16 to 30 Gy) is delivered by Iridium-192 sources loaded into Silastic catheters placed into the tongue base under general anesthesia in equally spaced parallel loops. Dosimetry is based on the decay properties of the sources with either low-dose-rate or high-dose-rate calculations.[37]

Intensity modulated radiation therapy (IMRT) is an advanced form of conformal EBRT using CT (or MRI) to determine the clinical target volume (CTV) for radiotherapy planning. Traditional EBRT utilized forward planning (FP) where the planner defined the number of beams, their energies, and how they would be modulated (wedges, blocks, etc). Dose calculations would them be produced based on these calculations. Unlike conventional EBRT, IMRT uses inverse planning (IP) in which the initial step is to clinically define the treatment target then determine the appropriate beam modulation for prescribed dose. Once the target is identified planning algorithms then determine the dose distribution necessary to achieve the desired treatment. The multileaf collimator (MLC) is the computer-controlled device used to produce the beams necessary to achieve the tightly conformal dose distribution prescribed. The precise beam geometries produced by the MCL increase the precision of the dose delivery and spare the normal uninvolved tissues, thus limiting the overall toxicity of therapy.[38]

A distinct advantage of IMRT is the ability to spare the parotid gland, thus decreasing the risk of xerostomia and the attendant dental, nutritional, and communication sequelae. An initial theoretical concern was that the more conformal dosing could potentially lead to the development of more in-field and marginal recurrences. This has not been the case. Results from treatment with IMRT in all oropharyngeal subsites are encouraging, even for patients with advanced disease.[39,40]

Excellent local and regional control can be achieved for early stage and intermediate stage oropharyngeal carcinoma (T1, T2, T3- N0, and selected N1) with primary altered fractionation EBRT. Estimated 5-year local-regional control rates for stage I and II disease were 88% and 72%, respectively, in a review of 172 early stage patients in all oropharyngeal subsites from MD Anderson.[41] Similar results have been reported in tonsillar and tongue base carcinoma with EBRT and EBRT plus brachytherapy.[42,43]

Radiotherapy-based treatment regimens may also be successful in a subpopulation of advance stage patients are those with small primary tumors but advanced cervical disease (N2A or greater). Garden et al[44] retrospectively reviewed 375 patients with T1 or T2 oropharyngeal carcinoma with stage II or IV cancer based on the status of the cervical metastases treated with definitive EBRT. Patients were treated with either standard fractionation (1.8 to 2.0 Gy/d single fraction) or concomitant boost fractionation (1.8 to 2 Gy/fraction once daily to 32 Gy, followed by 1.8 to 1.5 Gy bid for final 12 fractions). Five-year local control, distant metastases, and overall survival rates were 15%, 19%, and 64%, respectively. The development of distant metastases was significantly correlated with advance cervical disease (N2B, N2C, or N3).

Unfortunately, approximately 75% of patients with oropharyngeal carcinoma will present with advanced disease either due to submucosal extension of the primary tumor or extensive cervical node metastasis. In these cases, control rates with single modality EBRT or EBRT with brachytherapy are poor with less than 50% local control at 3 years. Trismus and osteoradionecrosis are observed with greater frequency in these patients when doses exceed 70 Gy.[37,42,45,46]

Surgery with postoperative radiation therapy has been the standard treatment of these patients. In this setting, primary surgical resection of the tumor may involve segmental mandibulectomy ("Commando" or composite resection), total glossectomy or glossectomy with laryngectomy, and radical neck dissection. Morbidity from these resections is high and despite these aggressive procedures positive margins, perineural extension, and extracapsular spread of tumor (ECS) in the cervical lymph nodes predisposed these patients to local and local region failure. Extracapsular spread in particular is perhaps the single best biologic predictor of the development of distant metastases. The poor functional and oncologic results observed in these patients have led to a re-examination of the role of chemotherapy in these patients.[47,48] Combined modality treatments (chemoradiotherapy) have been used for organ preservation in patients with advanced T stage or ECS to enhance local control and prevent the development of pulmonary metastases. The treatment of advance stage oropharyngeal cancer by concurrent chemotherapy and radiation (chemoradiation) is discussed later in this chapter.

Surgery

The surgical extirpation of oropharyngeal tumors remains one of the most technically challenging procedures in head and neck oncology. Several characteristics of oropharyngeal malignancies contribute to the difficulties encountered in comprehensive surgical resection. Oropharyngeal malignancies can extend submucosal, or arise in a field of early invasive cancer or premalignanciy, making it difficult to obtain negative surgical margins on frozen section. Perineural spread and submucosal extension of oropharyngeal malignancy may be difficult to identify on preoperative imaging and physical examination, and when encountered at surgery may necessitate resection of significant tissue volume. The complex functional anatomic intricacies of the swallowing mechanism require intact motor and sensory components to function efficiently without aspiration. Even the most meticulous surgery and sophisticated reconstruction can result in some degree of swallowing impairment. Resection of large tumors of the tongue base may require laryngectomy or laryngotracheal separation to prevent life-threatening aspiration.[49]

The rich submucosal lymphatics of the oropharynx can result in metastases to bilateral cervical nodes and to nodal basins not routinely removed in standard neck dissections such as the retropharyngeal nodes. Bilateral neck dissection or neck irradiation should be considered for patients with tumor approaching the midline.

The local extension of oropharyngeal malignancy should be carefully evaluated prior to resection. Posterior and lateral extension involving the full thickness of the oropharyngeal wall may result in direct extension of tumor into the poststyloid parapharyngeal space and involvement of the carotid artery. Attempts at resection of these tumors without adequate preparation for transcervical exposure and vascular control may lead to an operative catastrophe. Laterally extending oropharyngeal tumors may "collide" with medially extending metastatic cervical nodes resulting in circumferential involvement of the carotid artery. Posterior extension and

involvement of the prevertebral muscles are associated with unacceptable high local recurrence rates. Patients resenting with trismus will often demonstrate anterior or anterior-lateral extension into pterygoid muscles or temporomandibular joint.

Transmandibular Approaches

The intact anterior mandibular arch and lateral mandibular body with its superior articulation to the skull base at the temporomandibular joint combine to form a rigid skeletal barrier to exposure of the oropharynx. Transmandibular access to the oropharynx is accomplished by segmental mandibulectomy, marginal mandibulectomy, or mandibulotomy. Segmental mandibulectomy is a resection of a portion of the mandible, which permanently or temporarily disrupts condyle to condyle continuity. Marginal mandibulectomy is a resection of either or both the alveolar process or lingual cortex of the mandible adjacent to the tumor. Native mandibular continuity is maintained with this approach. The mandibulotomy is a procedure in which the mandible is divided either anteriorly (symphyseal or parapsymphyseal mandibulotomy) or laterally (lateral mandibulotomy) to gain access to the oropharynx or posterior oral cavity. No bone is resected and the cut ends are rigidly fixed at the conclusion of the resection and reconstruction.[50]

Segmental and Marginal Mandibulectomy

The segmental mandibulectomy also known as the "Commando operation" or composite resection was introduced over 100 years ago and has remained the standard procedure for the safe 3-dimensional resection of oropharyngeal carcinoma.[51] Tumors resected with this procedure include those arising in the tonsillar fossa or tongue base with extension to the posterior body of the mandible lateral oropharyngeal wall, or the pterygoid muscles where the resection of the ramus of the mandible is necessary for exposure and complete resection of tumor. Mandibular osteotomies are usually made at the mental foramen and posteriorly below the condyle. In correctly selected patients, preservation of the native condyle can facilitate restoration and mandibular continuity with either a reconstruction bar or free tissue transfer without increasing the risk of tumor recurrence.

Preoperative imaging studies are used to determine lateral extension into the pterygoid region and invasion of mandibular bone. Radiographic evidence of enhancement of the pterygoid muscles, posterior or medial extension of tumor for the masticator space, or obliteration of the fat plane anterior to the medial pterygoid muscle are indicative of an advanced malignancy. Direct invasion of mandible bone by tumor is difficult particularly in the posterior mandible and ramus. Special software for image reconstruction and reformatting is available with current generations of CT scanners to improve visualization of the tumor mandible interface. Patients with trismus or those with radiographic evidence of mandibular ramus or pterygoid invasion generally require segmental mandibulectomy to achieve negative surgical margins.

The marginal mandibulectomy involves resection of a partial thickness rim of mandible and attached tumor arising from the gingival, ramus, or alveolar process. Originally described for oral cavity tumors involving the mandibular body and parasymphyseal region this technique has also been applied to more posterior-based tumors of the retromolar trigone. Our group has also used the posterior marginal mandibulectomy technique to facilitate resection of tonsillar and tongue base carcinomas. This involves removing the coronoid process and a portion of the anterior ramus without disarticulation of the condyle or disruption of mandibular continuity. The lateral exposure provided by posterior marginal mandibulectomy is superior to conventional transoral approach. Advantages of marginal mandibulectomy include the lack of an osteotomy and less disruption of normal intraoral structures to access the primary tumor. Reconstruction with either the radial forearm free flap or split-thickness skin graft provides excellent restoration of masticatory function.[52]

Mandibulotomy

Initial reports of the temporary division of the mandible for access to oral cavity cancers are reported in the early 19th century. However, Trotter[53] is credited with the first systematic description of a midline exposure to tumors of the oropharynx, hypopharynx, and supraglottic larynx called the median labiomandibular glossotomy. As the name indicates this procedure divided both the mandible and the tongue in the midline to gain access to the posterior oropharynx and supraglottic larynx. The mandibulotomy approach is now referred to as the mandibular "swing" indicating the lateral displacement of a single mandibular segment. The procedure has since been modified such that the soft tissue dissection extends posteriorly along the lateral floor of the mouth, thus preserving the integrity of the tongue. The resection can include the lateral oropharyngeal wall and tonsillar fossa and can be extended medially to encompass the base of tongue and vallecula as needed. The mandibulotomy approach has also been extended laterally to provide wide exposure of the more lateral structures of the parapharyngeal space, inferior infratemporal fossa, and retropharynx. The technical details of this operation including variations of the placement of the skin incisions, the orientation of the mandibular osteotomy, and the methods of osteosynthyesis have been described in detail in multiple publications.[54,55]

Limitations of this approach include the limitations in lateral displacement of the mandible and tethering associated with an intact lingual nerve. However, tumors of this region frequently extend deeply into the tongue muscles necessitating resection of the lingual nerve for oncologic control of perineural spread. Manipulation of the mandibular segment in conjunction with adjuvant radiation therapy can result in temporomandibular joint trauma and significant trismus.

Complications related to the mandibular osteotomy (nonunion, malunion, malocclusion) are uncommon but seen more frequently in the previously irradiated or edentulous patient. In correctly selected patients the mandibulotomy compares favorably to the segmental mandibulectomy in the areas of oncologic results with improved cosmesis and masticatory function.[50,56,57]

Pharyngeal Approaches

Lateral Pharyngotomy. Smaller tumors of the lateral tongue base, tonsillar region, and posterior and lateral oropharynx wall can be resected through the neck via the lateral pharyngototomy. Meticulous physical examination and preoperative imaging are necessary for the selection of patients for this procedure. Awake fiberoptic examination in the office and examination under anesthesia are complementary and both may be required to carefully assess the 3-dimensional geometry of these tumors. Medial extension of tumor into the midline tongue base, extension to the vallecula and supraglottic larynx, and inferior extension into the hypopharynx or larynx are contraindications to this procedure.[58]

The lateral pharyngotomy is preceded by an ipsilateral neck dissection, the extent of which is determined by the preoperative imaging and physical examination. In patients with lateral oropharyngeal malignancy, the minimum neck dissection should include the ipsilateral Zones II through IV. Removal of the lymph nodes facilitates exposure of the carotid sheath and the mobilization of the sternocleidomastoid muscles. The external surface of the lateral pharyngeal wall is exposed by the resection of the lateral one-third of the ipsilateral hyoid bone and the superior cornu of the thyroid cartilage and the superior mobilization of the superior laryngeal and hypoglossal nerves. Alternatively, the superior laryngeal nerve may be reflected inferiorly; however, the resulting access window between the superiorly displaced hypoglossal nerve and superior laryngeal nerves is very small. Transection of the superior laryngeal nerve and artery are frequently necessary for satisfactory exposure in the region.

The pharynx is entered by dividing the constrictor muscles at the margin of the tumor. This is best accomplished by placing the constrictor muscles under tension and palpating the tumor with a finger in the oropharynx. The tumor is resected with frozen section control and, if possible, the pharyngotomy is closed primarily with layered absorbable sutures. Pliable flaps such as the radial forearm free flap or platysma myocutaneous flap should be used, if additional tissue is needed to achieve a watertight closure avoiding bulky pedicle flaps. Infection is the most frequent complication of this procedure followed by dysphagia and laryngeal dysfunction.

Transhyoid Pharyngotomy. The transhyoid pharyngotomy involves access to the oropharynx from the midline in the vallecula. Traditionally described for tongue base and posterior pharyngeal wall tumors it has also been used for exposure of tonsillar and more laterally based oropharyngeal carcinomas.[59,60]

Like the lateral pharyngotomy the transhyoid approach is preceded by a neck dissection(s); bilat-eral neck dissections are performed for medial tongue base tumors. The hypoglossal nerves are identified and transposed superiorly, the superior surface of the hyoid is skeletonized, and the vallecula is entered at the most inferior portion at the reflection of the tongue base mucosa onto the lingual surface of the epiglottis. The tumor is resected under frozen section control and the residual tongue base is reapproximated primarily to the hyoid. As with the lateral pharyngotomy, careful anatomic staging of the tumor is required to prevent underestimation of the size of the primary. The procedure can easily be extended inferior to include the resection of supraglottic larynx. However, unrecognized anterior extension into the oral tongue may require a more extended resection with flap reconstruction not easily performed with this exposure.[61]

Transoral Resection of Oropharyngeal Cancer

Transoral laser microsurgical resection has become a part of the standard treatment armamentarium for glottis and supraglottic carcinomas. Recent technical advances in instrumentation and the use of the operating microscope have enabled the safe resection of many of the oropharyngeal malignancies traditionally resected with open approaches.[62] Carcinoma of the tonsil, tonsillar fossa, and lateral and posterior oropharyngeal walls can be approached transorally provided the tumors do not extend laterally into the parapharyngeal space and are not fixed to the deep layer of the deep cervical fascia. The use of the operating microscope provides improved visualization of the lateral borders of the tonsillar fossa allowing for en bloc resection of tonsillar cancers including the superior pharyngeal constrictor as a deep margin.

Resection of tongue base carcinoma with transoral laser microsurgery was first reported by Steiner and Ambrosch.[62] These techniques are attractive in that they can be performed without any form of pharyngotomy, thus limiting the potential for postoperative infection. The surgical defects heal by secondary intention, thus no reconstructive flaps or grafts are needed and operative time and complications are reduced. Postoperatively patients are able to swallow within 7 days and in selected cases the resection can be performed without a tracheotomy.[62] The neck is treated in the standard fashion with neck dissection as indicated. A significant advantage is that all adjuvant treatment options remain in place and patients are able to initiate postoperative radiotherapy or chemoradiotherapy earlier. As patients with positive margins are at greater risk for local recurrence aggressive early reresection is necessary.[63]

Several groups have begun to describe their oncologic and functional results with transoral laser microsurgery for oropharyngeal and tongue base malignancies, including the application of surgical robotics.[64] High rates of local control and functional organ preservation are reported. Satisfactory exposure of tongue base malignancies can be very difficult in patients with trismus and/or intact dentition.[65-67] Our own experience with transoral laser microsurgery for tongue base carcinomas has been favorable. We have treated 91 patients with primary oropharyngeal squamous cell carcinoma by transoral laser microsurgical resection with postoperative EBRT (Fig 15-6). Chemotherapy with EBRT was offered

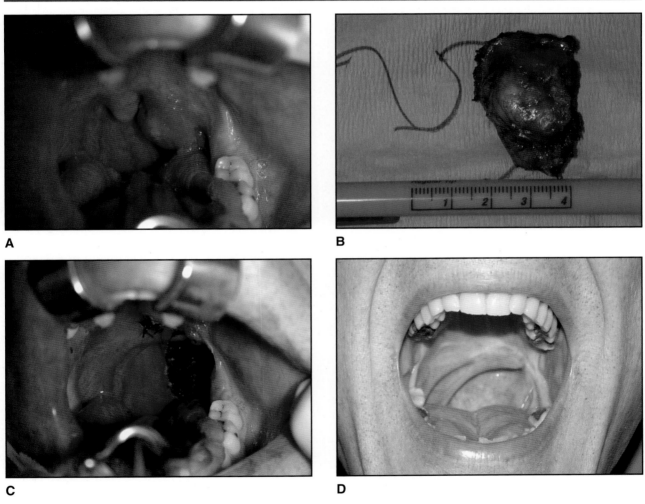

Fig 15–6. Surgically treated squamous cell carcinoma of the tonsillar fossa. **A.** Tumor identified within tonsillar fossa. **B.** En bloc surgical specimen including anterior and posterior tonsillar pillars and portion of pharyngeal constrictor muscle at the deep margin. **C.** The remnant of the uvula is used for primary reconstruction of the oropharyngeal defect with restoration of soft palatal function and prevention of velopharyngeal insufficiency. **D.** One-year postoperative appearance of oropharyngeal reconstruction.

to patients with positive surgical margins, multiple nodes involved, or the presence of extracapsular spread in the cervical lymphatics. Local regional control at 3 years is 88% with no patients requiring permanent gastrostomy or tracheotomy tubes. Specialized instrumentation, advanced training in transoral laser surgery, and patience are necessary to perform comprehensive oncologically sound transoral laser resections of oropharyngeal malignancy.

Surgery is rarely offered as single modality therapy for patients with oropharyngeal carcinoma due to the propensity for metastatic disease and the difficulties in obtaining widely negative margins. Galati et al[68] reported 84 patients treated with primary surgery for tonsil cancer treated at the University of Pittsburgh. Twenty-four of those patients had surgery for stage I disease with a 90% overall survival. However, patients treated with primary surgical therapy most often receive adjuvant EBRT or chemo-radiation due to advanced neck disease or questionable margins. Laccourreye et al[69] have reported an alternative treatment program consisting of induction chemotherapy followed by neck dissection and transoral lateral oropharyngectomy. Indications for postoperative EBRT are positive surgical margins, perineural or lymphovascular invasion, and positive nodes in the neck. This treatment program has provided excellent local control with very acceptable functional outcomes.

Several groups have advocated primary treatment of the neck with limited neck dissection prior to definitive nonsurgical management of the primary tumor. Advantages of this treatment program are (a) patients are spared the functional sequelae of oropharyngeal surgery, (b) the morbidity of neck dissection is low and is accomplished at the same anesthesia as the staging endoscopy, gastrostomy tube placement, and dental extractions, (c) a salvage procedure in a previously radiated field can be avoided, and (d) the collection of large amount of clinical material for molecular pathologic investigation including assessment of extracapsular spread. 2 and 3-year locoregional control rates as high as 95% and 88%, respectively, have been reported.[70,71]

Prospective studies comparing oncologic and functional outcomes of surgery compared to nonsurgical therapies are lacking. Soo et al[72] reviewed 119 patients (oropharynx $n = 23$) with stage III and IV HNSCC randomized to surgery with postoperative

radiation or concurrent ion EBRT with 2 cycles of cisplatin and 5-FU (days 1 and 28). No differences in survival were identified and the overall organ preservation rate or avoidance of surgery was 45% at 5 years. This study did not address functional outcomes.

Chemotherapy and Chemoradiation

Despite advances in surgical techniques and the widespread use of microvascular free-tissue transfer to reconstruct defects in the oropharynx high surgical morbidity remains high. Altered fractionation and IRMT are useful techniques that improve local and regional control but do not prevent the development of distant metastases. The desire to improve functional and oncologic outcomes led to investigations into the uses of chemotherapy and radiation therapy.[73-75]

Chemotherapy has been used in the treatment of oropharyngeal carcinoma as either induction (neoadjuvant) treatment prior to definitive local-regional therapy or concurrently with EBRT as defintive therapy (chemoradiation) or postoperatively (adjuvant chemoradiation). Historically, chemotherapy was used preoperatively in patients with oropharyngeal squamous cell carcinoma. Single agent methotrexate or bleomycin were standard regimens prior to the first reported success of cisplatin in a phase II study. The Head and Neck Contracts Program was the first prospective multi-institutional study aimed at determining the optimum sequencing of radiation therapy, chemotherapy, and surgery in patients with advanced HNSCC. Patients were randomized to receive either (1) surgery followed by EBRT (standard therapy), (2) induction chemotherapy (cisplatin and bleomycin) followed by surgery and postoperative EBRT, or (3) induction chemotherapy (cisplatin and bleomycin) followed by surgery, postoperative EBRT, and monthly maintenance chemotherapy for 6 months with single agent cisplatin. There were no differences in either overall or disease-free survival in any of the treatment groups; however, distant metastases were reduced in patients receiving maintenance chemotherapy.[76]

The biological foundation for the observed responses to the concurrent administration of cytotoxic chemotherapy and EBRT were described by

Steel and Peckham in 1979.[77] In their "spatial cooperation" paradigm, EBRT acts locally and chemotherapy acts distantly to reduce the likelihood of tumor recurrence; thus, the two modalities work independently without additive toxicities. The second component of the model is the in-field cooperation observed during the simultaneous administration of radiosensitizing chemotherapy with EBRT. The administration of chemotherapy concurrently with EBRT could potentially overcome the resistance of tumor cells to radiation. Chemotherapeutic drugs have been shown to increase the cytotoxic activity of EBRT by several mechanisms including increasing radiation damage, inhibiting repair of radiation-induced DNA damage, stabilizing tumors cells in the most radiosensitive part of the cell cycle, blocking pathways responsible for radioresistance, and prevention of tumor repopulation.[78] Review of the Meta-Analysis of Chemotherapy in Head and Neck Cancer (MACH-HN) database indicates a consistently observed 8% overall survival benefit observed for patients treated with platinum regimens and concurrent EBRT. Local tissue toxicities remain the limiting factor in concurrent use of chemotherapy with EBRT.[79,80]

Multiple trials have been reported comparing various treatments for patients with oropharyngeal carcinoma (Table 15–3). One of the difficulties observed is the heterogeneity in patient populations under study and the inclusion of patients with multiple subsites in the analysis.

In the multi-institutional randomized ORO-93-01 trial, patients with oropharyngeal carcinoma were randomized to conventional radiotherapy, concurrent chemotherapy with EBRT, or hyperfractionated radiotherapy. There were no differences in any endpoint between EBRT regimens; however, disease-free survival was significantly improved in patients treated with chemoradiation.[81] In another phase III trial, Denis reported the results of the French Head and Neck Oncology and Radiotherapy Group randomized oropharynx trial comparing standard fraction EBRT to concurrent carboplatin, 5-flourouracil, and EBRT. The addition of chemotherapy significantly improved both locoregional control and overall survival at 3 years.[82,83] Similar results were demonstrated in the German Cancer Society 95-06 trial using 5-FU and mitomycin and hyperfractionated

accelerated EBRT.[84] The addition of cisplatin to hyperfractionated EBRT also has been tested in a prospective fashion. Patients treated with 2 cycles of weekly cisplatin during weeks 1 and 5 of hyperfractionated EBRT showed significantly improved locoregional control and distant disease-free survival but no difference in overall survival. Acute toxicity was greater in the chemoradiation arm but late toxicities were comparable.[85,86]

Multiple phase II trials have been reported assessing various combinations of concurrent chemotherapy with EBRT. The majority of these studies involved patients with multiple sites in the head and neck including the oropharynx. The Radiation Therapy Oncology Group 97-03 Trial (RTOG 97-03) assessed standard fraction EBRT with one of three chemotherapy protocols. Patients were randomized to receive either cisplatin and 5-FU during the last 10 days of radiation, hydroxyurea and 5-FU with each fraction of EBRT, or paclitaxel and cisplatin weekly during EBRT. Tolerance was 92% in arm 1, 79% in arm 2, and 83% in arm 3. Estimated 2-year disease-free and overall survival rates were 38.2% and 57.4% for arm 1, 48.6% and 69.4% for arm 2, and 51.3% and 66.6% for arm 3.[87] Similar results were obtained in other multi-institution single arm phase II trials.[47,88-90] The feasibility of adding cisplatin to hyperfractionated EBRT was evaluated in the RTOG 99-14 trial. Tolerance was 86% with estimated 2-year overall survival and disease-free rates of 71.6% and 53.5%, respectively.[91,92] Single agent taxane-based concurrent chemotherapy (docetaxel) with EBRT was evaluated in 68 patients with oropharyngeal carcinoma. Calias et al[93] reported good compliance and 64% local control at 3 years in patients receiving weekly docetaxel with standard fraction EBRT.

Several groups have begun to study the role of induction chemotherapy in the management of advanced oropharyngeal cancer.[94,95] For several years, investigators at the University of Chicago have been using an intensive regimen of taxane-based chemotherapy (paclitaxel, fluorouracil, and hydroxyurea) with twice daily EBRT administered over 5 consecutive days every other week. These authors consistently report local control of up to 90% and 3-year survival rates of 60%. The addition of induction chemotherapy with carboplatin and paclitaxel has resulted in improved over-

Table 15–3. Primary Nonsurgical Management of Oropharyngeal Cancer

Investigators				
Phase III				
Denis (GORTEC)	Stage III & IV oropharynx (n = 226)	EBRT 70 Gy 2 Gy/day qd	EBRT 70 Gy 2 Gy/day qd Carbo + 5-FU days (1, 22, 43)	Improved LRC (47% vs 66%) & OS (31% vs 51%) at 3 yrs (p = 0.02)
Olmi (ORO 93-01)	Stage III & IV oropharynx (n = 192)	EBRT 70 Gy 2 Gy qd or Hfx-EBRT 1.6 Gy bid	EBRT 70 Gy 2 Gy/day qd Carbo + 5-FU days (1, 22, 43)	Improved DFS (23% vs 42%) ND in OS
Huguenin	Stage III & IV Multisite (n = 224) (oropharynx n = 59)	Hfx-EBRT 1.2 Gy bid	Hfx-EBRT 1.2 Gy bid + 2 cycles CDDP weeks 1, 5	Improved LRC and DFS
Budach (German Cancer Society 95-06)	Stage III & IV Multisite (n = 384) (oropharynx n = 119)	A-Hfx-EBRT	A-Hfx-EBRT + 5-FU+Mito-C week 1, 6	Improved LRS and OS
Bonner	Stage III & IV Multisite (n = 424) (oropharynx n = 253)	EBRT 70 Gy 2 Gy qd or Hfx-EBRT 1.2 Gy bid or A-Hfx-EBRT	EBRT + weekly cetuximab	Improved median OS (49 to 29 mo) Improved PFS
Phase II				
Garden (RTOG 97-03)	Stage III & IV Multisite (n = 241) (oropharynx n = 51)		EBRT 70 Gy 2 Gy qd + Arm A CDDP + 5-FU Arm B Hydroxyurea + 5-FU Arm C Paclitaxel + CDDP	ND is 2 yr DFS and OS
Ang (RTOG 99-14)	Stage III & IV Multisite (n = 84) (oropharynx n = 50)		Hfx-EBRT 72 Gy + CDDP (days 1 and 22)	Tolerance 86% 2 yr OS 71.6%, DFS 53.5%
Nguyen	Stage III & IV oropharynx (n = 48)		EBRT 70 Gy 1.8 to 2 Gy qd CDDP + 5-FU (days 1 and 22)	3 yr OS 52%
Calias (GORTEC-9802)	Stage III & IV oropharynx (n = 68)		EBRT 70 Gy 2 Gy qd + weekly docetaxel	3 yr OS 47 % and LRC 64%

5-FU, 5-flourouracil; A-Hfx-EBRT; accelerated hyperfractionated radiation therapy aka concomitant boost 1.8 to 2 Gy/day single fraction followed by 1.8 to 1.5 Gy bid for last 10 to 12 fractions to total dose of 76 Gy; carbo, carboplatin; CDDP, cisplatin; DSF, disease-free survival; EBRT, external beam radiation therapy 2 Gy/day single fraction; Hfx-EBRT, hyperfractionated external beam radiotherapy 1.4 to 1.5 Gy bid with 4 to 6 hours interfraction interval; LRC, locoregional control; ND, no difference; OS, overall survival; qd, once daily fractionation; PFS, progression-free survival.

all survival, progression-free survival, and functional organ preservation.[96-99] Two multi-institutional phase II trials have examined induction chemotherapy followed by definitive concurrent chemotherapy with EBRT in oropharyngeal carcinoma. The Eastern Cooperative Oncology Group Study E2399 evaluated a taxane-based regimen and the Southwest Oncology Group investigated a cisplatin-based protocol. Both studies ad-ministered two cycles of induction chemotherapy (paclitaxel and carboplatin or cisplatin and 5-FU) and concurrent chemotherapy with standard fraction EBRT. In the ECOG trial patients received weekly paclitaxel whereas in the SWOG trials patients received cisplatin on days 1, 22, and 43. Overall survival at 3 years was similar, 64% in the SWOG trail and 78% in the ECOG trial.[100,101]

Activation of the epidermal growth factor receptor (EGFR) is central to the progression of HNSCC. Overexpression of this receptor is correlated with outcome in oropharyngeal carcinoma. Cetuximab is a monoclonal antibody directed against the ligand-binding region of the EGFR and is one of a number of small-molecule targeted chemotherapeutic agents under investigation in the treatment of HNSCC. The addition of cetuximab to EBRT was evaluated in a phase III trial and with a median follow-up of 54 months demonstrated significantly improved locoregional control, and progression free and overall survival.[102] Combinations of cetuximab with standard chemotherapy and various EBRT regimens are currently under investigation.

Finally, single agent cisplatin has been administered with concurrent EBRT postoperatively in patients with extracapsular extension of tumor in the cervical nodes, positive margins, multiple nodes involved, or other high-risk pathologic features. In two phase III studies the addition of cisplatin was shown to significant reduce locoregional recurrence rates. In both studies acute toxicity was higher in the chemoradiation group. The increase in survival in the chemoradiation group observed in the European trial (EROTC 22931) was not demonstrated in the US study (RTOG 9501).[103,104]

Concurrent administration of chemotherapy with EBRT should be done in the context of a dedicated multidisciplinary head and neck cancer team. Pretreatment assessment should focus on prevention of avoidable complications and include comprehensive dental and nutritional assessments and interventions such as tooth extractions and gastrostomy tube placement. The frequency of grade 3 or 4 acute toxicities ranges from 40% to 80% with significant nutritional and functional sequelae. Close follow-up with appropriate use of supportive measures is critical. Psychosocial, family, and financial assistance are frequently required while patients are under treatment.

Management of Recurrence or Persistence

Patients with oropharyngeal carcinoma are treated more often with EBRT or chemotherapy plus EBRT than with primary surgery. Consequently, surgeons are being called on more frequently to evaluate patients following definitive nonsurgical care.[105,106] Surgery for recurrent or persistent disease ("salvage surgery"), although technically challenging, has value. Surgery in this context has several possible roles. First, there is a subpopulation of patients with localized recurrent or persistent disease who can be cured by surgery; these are primarily patients with localized residual disease in previously unoperated cervical lymphatics or low-volume persistent primary tumor. Second, there are patients in whom cure may not be possible, but who can derive significant palliation from the resection of painful, ulcerating residual necrotic tumor. Finally, there are the unfortunate patients in whom the only benefit to surgery is palliation of an obstructed airway or to provide enteral access.[107,108]

Several areas of controversy remain in the management of the cervical lymphatics following definitive nonsurgical treatment of advanced oropharyngeal malignancy. Historically, patients treated with single modality EBRT for oropharyngeal carcinoma have benefited from planned neck dissections. This remains the recommendation for most patients with N2 and all patents with N3 disease.[109-111]

It is clear that in patients with early stage neck disease (N0 or N1) there is no benefit to neck dissection following chemotherapy with EBRT.[112] Similarly, it is clear that patients with N3 or bulky multilevel N2 disease may benefit from neck dissection. Up to 50% of patients will have viable tumor demonstrated pathologically in neck dissection specimens and neck dissection has been shown to reduce local regional recurrence in these patients.[113-115] Selective neck dissection has been shown to be an oncologically sound alternative in this setting, thus reducing operative morbidity.[116] A more controversial area is the management of the patient with initially N2 disease rendered clinically N0 by therapy.[117,118] Careful post-treatment radiologic assessments with contrast-enhanced CT scans or CT/PET scans may obviate the need for surgery in patients without clinical or radiographic evidence of residual tumor.[119,120]

Persistent disease after therapy may remain in the primary site or in the cervical lymphatics. Such disease is likely biologically aggressive and will be difficult to control.[121-123] If the neck has not been treated surgically aggressive node dissection is indicated but the overall survival is poor.[124,125] Reirradiation and additional systematic therapy are possible and may improve locoregional control; however, patients remain vulnerable to the development of distant metastases. Patients with recurrence in the neck following surgery and adjuvant therapy are, in general, not candidates for aggressive local therapy. Failure to respond at the primary is an ominous finding. Salvage surgery is formidable given the difficulties associated with identifying gross tumor margins in a heavily pretreated field. Likewise, frozen section analysis of margins is hampered by the effects of EBRT and chemotherapy. Overall survival in this population is approximately 25%.[126-128]

Post-treatment Surveillance

Despite the success of initial treatment patients with HNSCC remain at an increased lifetime risk of 3% to 6% per year for the development of second primary tumors.[129-131] These patients should be followed by multiple providers with complementary expertise in the context of the multidisciplinary head and neck tumor clinic. The absence of a reliable serum marker for HNSCC and the lack of objective data analyzing surveillance practices have led to the development of clinical practice guidelines based on close clinical follow-up.[132,133] Practice guidelines for follow-up and surveillance have been developed by the national Comprehensive Cancer Center Network[134] and the American Head and Neck Society.[135,136] Both organizations favor serial physical examinations, yearly chest x-ray, and minimal routine laboratory testing over planned endoscopy and routine PET or CT scans. Aggressive planned post-treatment endoscopy and rebiopsy may identify patients with early resectable persistent disease. Although attractive, such a protocol is resource intensive and not likely cost effective or sustainable in the present health care economy.[137]

SUMMARY

The management of patients with advanced head and neck cancer, particularly in a region as complex as the oropharynx, should be done by a dedicated multidisciplinary treatment team. Careful anatomic staging, organ-sparing surgical approaches, technical refinement in the delivery of EBRT, innovative fractionation schedules, and the concurrent use of radiosensitizing chemotherapy all contribute to the observed increased in locoregional control and increased overall survival. With the increased use of these intensive multimodality therapies more patients with oropharyngeal carcinoma are being cured with greater frequency than in prior years. Despite these successes, a standard treatment programs has yet to be widely accepted. In order to make a truly informed decision, patients should have access to data regarding their institution's and provider's experiences with all forms of treatment. As local and locoregional control rates are similar for non-surgical and surgical therapies, quality of life issues and functional organ preservation need to become a significant portion of the conversation regarding treatment selection. The treatment program offered must take into consideration the patient's comorbidities and personal wishes as well as the histology, site, local extension, and metastatic spread of the tumor. The treatment team must also provide an honest representation of their institutional abilities, costs, complication rates, experience, and overall abilities to comprehensively care for patients with complex head and neck malignancies. Institutions must also provide state of the art diagnostic radiology and functional imaging facilities, high-quality radiation oncology platform, access to current chemotherapeutic agents, and comprehensive surgical facilities for staging and definitive management. The additional support in speech-language pathology, oncologic dentistry, social services, financial support, and cancer advocacy must also be on site and available to patients.

Outcomes data should be collected prospectively and not be limited to the traditional indices of overall and disease-specific survival, local control, and patterns of failure. Assessment and collection of quality of life data should also be part of the routine follow-up.[138,139] Important economic measures such as cost of therapy, time lost from work, loss of or change in insurance status, and the impact of complications on the cost of treatment should also be quantified.[140,141] Finally, patients with oropharyngeal carcinoma should be educated about their rare malignancy and actively encouraged to participate in the decision-making process. They should be encouraged to participate in clinical trials that stress the acquisition of new knowledge that advances our understanding of the biology and treatments of their cancers.

REFERENCES

1. Liao C, Chang JT, Wang H, et al. Survival in squamous cell carcinoma of the oral cavity. *Cancer.* 2007;110:564-571.
2. Canto MT, Devesa SS. Oral cavity and pharynx cancer incidence rates in the United States. 1975-1998. *Oral Oncol.* 2002;38:610-617.
3. Genden EM, Ferlito A, Scully C, Shaha AR, Higgins K, Rinaldo A. Current management of tonsillar cancer. *Oral Oncol* .2003; 39:337-342.
4. Carvalho AL, Ikeda MK, Margrin J, Kowalski LP. Trends of oral and oropharyngeal cancer survival over five decades in 3267 patients treated in a single institution. *Oral Oncol.* 2004;40:71-76.
5. Carvalho AL, Nishimoto IN, Califano JA, Kowalski, LP. Trends in incidence and prognosis for head and neck cancer in the United States: a site-specific analysis of the SEER database. *Int J Cancer.* 2005:114: 806-816.
6. Forastiere A, Koch W, Trotti A, Sidransky D. Head and neck cancer. *N Engl J Med* 2001;345: 1890-1900.
7. Vokes EE, Weichselbaum RR, Lippman SM, Hong WK. Head and neck cancer. *N Engl J Med.* 1993;328:184-194.
8. Perez-Ordonez B, Beauchemin M, Jordan RCK. Molecular biology of squamous cell carcinoma of the head and neck. *J Clin Pathol.* 2006;59, 445-453.
9. Croce CM. Oncogenes and cancer. *N Engl J Med.* 2008;358:502-511
10. Tsantoulis PK, Kastrinakis NG, Tourvas AD, Laskaris G, Gorgoulis VG. Advances in the biology of oral cancer. *Oral Oncol.* 2007;43;523-534.
11. Paz IB, Cook N, Odom-Maryon T, Xie Y, Wilczynski, SP. Human papillomavirus (HPV) in head and neck cancer. *Cancer.* 1997;79:595-604.
12. Syrjanen S. HPV infections and tonsillar carcinoma. *J Clin Pathol.* 2004;57:449-455.
13. Hoffmann M, Lohrey C, Hunziker A, Kahn T, Schwarz E. Human papillomavirus type 16 E6 and E7 genotypes in head-and-neck carcinomas. *Oral Oncol.* 2004;40:520-524.
14. Gillison M. HPV-associated head and neck cancer is a distinct epidemiologic, clinical and molecular entity. *Semin Oncol.* 2004;31:744-754.
15. Weinberger PM, Yu Z, Haffty BG, et al. Molecular classification identifies a subset of human papillomavirus-associated oropharyngeal cancers with favorable prognosis. *J Clin Oncology.* 2006;24: 736-747.
16. Van Houten VMM, Snijders PFJ, Van den Brekel MWM, et al. Biological evidence that human papilloma viruses are etiologically involved in a subgroup of head and neck squamous cell carcinomas. *Int J Cancer.* 2001;93:232-235.
17. D'Souza G, Kreimer AR, Viscidi R, et al. Case-controlled study of human papillomavirus and oropharyngeal cancer. *N Engl J Med.* 2007;356: 1944-1956.
18. Howell GMS, Grandis JR. Molecular mediators of metastasis in head and neck squamous cell carcinoma. *Head Neck.* 2005;27:710-717.
19. Hollinshead WH. *Anatomy for Surgeons*, 3rd ed. Philadelphia, Pa: Harper and Row; 1982.
20. McConnell FMS, Cerenko D, Mendelsohn MS. Manoflourographic analysis of swallowing. *Otolaryngol Clin North Am.* 1988;21:625-635.
21. Ambrosch P, Kron M, Freudenberg LS. Clinical staging of oropharyngeal carcinoma. *Cancer.* 1998;8:1613-1620.
22. Koch WM, Bhatti N, Williams MF et al. Oncologic rationale for bilateral tonsillectomy in head and neck squamous cell carcinoma of unknown primary source. *Otolaryngol Head Neck Surg.* 2001;124:331-333.
23. Mukherji SK, Pillsbury HR, Castillo M. Imaging squamous cell carcinomas of the upper areodigestive tract: what clinicians need to know. *Radiology.* 1997;205:629-646.
24. Muraki AS, Mancuso AA, Harnsberger HR, Johnson LP, Meads GB. CT of the oropharynx, tongue base, and floor of mouth: normal anatomy and range of variations, and applications in staging carcinoma. *Radiology.* 1983;148:725-731.

25. Sigal R, Zagdanski AM, Schwaab G, et al. CT and MR imaging of squamous cell carcinoma of the tongue and floor of mouth. *Radiographics.* 1996;16:787–810.

26. McCabe KJ, Rubinstein DR. Advances in head and neck imaging. *Otolaryngol Clin North Am.* 2005; 38:307–319.

27. Lufkin RB, Wortham DG, Dietrich RB, et al. Tongue and oropharynx: findings on MR imaging. *Radiology.* 1986;161:69–75.

28. Noworolski SM, Fischbein NJ., Kaplan MJ, et al. Challenges in dynamic contrast-enhanced MR imaging of cervical lymph nodes to detect metastatic disease. *J Magn Reson Imag.* 2003;17: 455–462.

29. Escott EJ, Rao VM, Ko WD, Guitierrez JE. Comparison of dynamic contrast-enhanced gradient-echo and spin-echo sequences in MR of head and neck neoplasms. *J Neuroradiol.* 1997;18:1411–1419.

30. Hoskin PJ, Saunders MI, Goodchild K, Powell MEB, Taylor NJ, Baddeley H. Dynamic contrast enhanced magnetic resonance scanning as a predictor of response to accelerated radiotherapy for advanced head and neck cancer. *Br J Radiol.* 1999;72: 1093–1098.

31. Tomura N, Omachi D, Sakuma I, et al. Dynamic contrast-enhanced magnetic resonance imaging in radiotherapeutic efficacy in the head and neck tumors. *Am J Otolaryngol.* 2005;26:163–167.

32. Ahmad A, Branstetter BF. CT versus MRI: Still a tough decision. *Otolaryngol Clin North Am.* 2008;41:1–22.

33. deVries EJ, Johnson JT, Myers EN, Mandell-Brown M. Base of tongue salivary tumors. *Head Neck Surg.* 1987;9:329–331.

34. Chen A, Schrag N, Hao Y, Stewart A, Ward E. Changes in treatment of advanced oropharyngeal cancer. *Laryngoscope.* 2007:117:16–21.

35. Kies MS, Ang KA, Clayman GL. Cancer of the oropharynx. In: Myers EN, Seun JY, Myers JN, Hanna EYN, eds. *Cancer of the Head and Neck.* 4th ed. Philadelphia, Pa: Saunders; 2003: 321–332.

36. Mendenhall WM, Amdur RJ, Palta JR. Head and neck cancer. In: Levitt SH, ed. *Technical Basis of Radiation Therapy.* Berlin: Springer; 2006: 454–484.

37. Fein DA, Lee WR, Amos WR, et al. Oropharyngeal carcinoma treated with radiotherapy a 30-year experience. *Int J Radiat Oncol Biol Phys.* 1996; 34:289–296.

38. Lee N, Puri DR, Blanco AI, Chao C. Intensity-modulated radiation therapy in head and neck cancers: an update. *Head Neck.* 2007;29:387–400.

39. Narayan S. The use of intensity-modulated radiation therapy in the treatment of oropharyngeal carcinoma. *Curr Opin Otolaryngol Head Neck Surg.* 2005;13:226–232.

40. Schwartz M, Vuong T, Ballivy O, Parker W, Patrocinio H. Accelerated radiotherapy with simultaneous integrated boost fractionation and intensity-modulated radiotherapy for advanced head and neck cancer. *Otolaryngol Head Neck Surg.* 2007;136:549–555.

41. Selek U, Garden AS, Morrison WH. El-Naggar AK, Rosenthal DI, Ang KK. Radiation therapy for early carcinoma of the oropharynx. *Int J Radiation Oncology Biol Phys.* 2004;59:743–751.

42. Chen J, Pappas L, Moeller JH, et al. Treatment of oropharyngeal squamous cell carcinoma with external beam radiation combined with interstitial brachytherapy. *Head Neck.* 2007;29: 362–369.

43. Mendenhall WM, Amdur RJ, Stringer SP, Villaret DP, Cassisi NJ. Radiation therapy for squamous cell carcinoma of the tonsillar region: a preferred alternative to surgery? *J Clin Oncol.* 2000;18: 2219–2225.

44. Garden AS, Asper JA, Morrison WH, et al. Is concurrent chemoradiation the treatment of choice for all patients with stage III or IV head and neck carcinoma? *Cancer.* 2004;100:1171–1178.

45. Horwitz, EM, Frazier AJ, Martinez AA. Excellent functional outcome in patients with squamous cell carcinoma of the base of tongue treated with external irradiation and interstitial iodine-125 boost. *Cancer.* 1996;78:948–957.

46. Mazeron JJ, Noel G, Simon JM. Head and neck brachytherapy. *Semin Rad Oncol* 2002;12:95–108.

47. Nguyen NP, Vos P, Smith HJ, et al. Concurrent chemoradiation for locally advanced oropharyngeal cancer. *Am J Otolaryngol.* 2007;28:3–8.

48. Seiwert TY, Salama JK, Vokes EE. The chemoradiation paradigm in head and neck cancer. *Nature Clin Pract Oncol.* 2007;4:156–171.

49. Petruzzelli GJ, Vandevender D. Reconstruction of the tongue base. *Oper Tech Otolaryn Head Neck Surg.* 2000;11:158–165.

50. Christopoulos E, Carrau R, Segas J, Johnson JT, Myers EN, Wagner RL Transmandibular approaches to oral cavity and oropharynx. *Arch Otolaryngol Head Neck Surg.* 1992;118:1164–1167.

51. Martin H, Tollefsen HR, Gerold FP. Median labio-mandibular glossotomy *Am J Surg.* 1961;102: 753–759.

52. Petruzzelli GJ, Knight FK, Vandevender D, et al. Posterior marginal mandibulectomy in the management of cancer of the oral cavity and oropharynx. *Otolaryngol Head Neck Surg.* 2003;129: 713–719.

53. Trotter W. Operations for malignant disease of the pharynx. *Br J Surg.* 1929;16:485–495.

54. Sullivan PK, Fabian R, Driscoll D. Mandibular osteotomies for tumor extirpation: the advantages of rigid fixation. *Laryngoscope.* 1992;102: 73–80.

55. Dubner S, Spiro RH. Median mandibulotomy: a critical assessment. *Head Neck.* 1991;13:389–393.

56. Spiro RH, Gerold FP, Strong EW. Mandibular "swing" approach for oral and oropharyngeal tumors. *Head Neck Surg.* 1981;3:371–378.

57. Dai T, Hao S, Chang K, Pan W, Yeh H, Tsang N. Complications of mandibulotomy: midline versus paramidline. *Otolaryngol Head Neck Surg.* 2003; 128:137–141.

58. Nasri S, Oh Y, Calcterra TC. Transpharyngeal approach to base of tongue tumors: a comparative study. *Laryngoscope.* 1996;106:945–950.

59. Agrawal A, Wenig BL. Resection of cancer of the tongue base and tonsil via the transhyoid approach. *Laryngoscope.* 2000;110:1802–1806.

60. Civantos F, Wenig BL. Transhyoid resection of tongue base and tonsil tumors. *Otolaryngol Head Neck Surg.* 1994;111:59–62.

61. Weber PC, Johnson, JT, Myers EN. The suprahyoid approach for squamous cell carcinoma of the base of the tongue. *Laryngoscope.* 1992;102: 637–640.

62. Steiner W, Ambrosch P. *Endoscopic Laser Surgery of the Upper Aerodigestive Tract.* Stuttgart: Thieme; 2000.

63. Jackel MC, Ambrosch P, Martin A, Steiner W. Impact of re-resection for inadequate margins on the prognosis of upper aerodigestive tract cancer treated by laser microsurgery. *Laryngoscope.* 2007;117:350–356.

64. O'Malley BW, Weinstein GS, Snyder W, Hockstein NG. Transoral robotic surgery (TORS) for base of tongue neoplasms. *Laryngoscope.* 2006;116: 1465–1472.

65. Grant DG, Salassa JR, Hinni ML, Pearson BW, Perry WC. Carcinoma of the tongue base treated by transoral laser microsurgery, Part one: untreated tumors, a prospective analysis of oncologic and functional outcomes. *Laryngoscope.* 2006;116: 2150–2155.

66. Kutter J, Land F, Monnier P, Pasche P. Transoral laser surgery for pharyngeal and pharyngolaryngeal carcinomas. *Arch Otolaryngol Head Neck Surg.* 2007;133:139–144.

67. Holsinger FC, McWhorter AJ, Menard M, Garcia D, Laccourreye O. Transoral lateral oropharyngectomy for squamous cell carcinoma of the tonsillar region. *Arch Otolaryngol Head Neck Surg.* 2005;131:583–591.

68. Galati LT, Myers EN, Johnson JT. Primary surgery as treatment for early squamous cell carcinoma of the tonsil. *Head Neck.* 2000;22:294–296.

69. Laccourreye O, Hans S, Menard M., Garcia D, Brasnu D, Holsinger FC. Transoral lateral oropharyngectomy for squamous cell carcinoma of the tonsillar region. *Arch Otolaryngol Head Neck Surg.* 2005;131:592–599.

70. Cupino A, Axelrod R, P-Rani A, et al. Neck dissection followed by chemoradiotherapy for stage IV (N+) oropharynx cancer. *Otolaryngol Head Neck Surg.* 2007;137:416–421.

71. Poulsen M, Porceddu SV, Kingsley PA, Tripcony L, Coman W. Locally advanced tonsillar squamous cell carcinoma: treatment approach revisited. *Laryngoscope.* 2007;117: 45–50.

72. Soo KC, Tan EH, Wee J, et al. Surgery and adjuvant radiotherapy vs concurrent chemoradiotherapy in stage III/IV non-metastatic squamous cell head and neck cancer: a randomized comparison. *Br J Cancer.* 2005;93:279–286.

73. Preuss SF, Quante G, Semrau R, Mueller RP, Klussmann JP, Guntinas-Lichius O. An analysis of surgical complications, morbidity and cost calculation in patients undergoing multimodal treatment for operable oropharyngeal carcinoma. *Laryngoscope.* 2007;117:101–105.

74. Sandaram K, Schwartz J, Har-El G, Lucente F. Carcinoma of the oropharynx: factors affecting outcome. *Laryngoscope.* 2005;115:1536–1542.

75. Brizel DM, Esclamado R. Concurrent chemoradiotherapy for locally advanced, nonmetastatic, squamous carcinoma of the head and neck: consensus, controversy, and conundrum. *J Clin Oncol.* 2006;24:2612–2617.

76. Wolf G, Rittes R, Fee WF, et al Adjuvant chemotherapy for advanced head and neck squamous carcinoma. The final report of the Head and Neck Contracts Program. *Cancer.* 1987;60:301–311.

77. Steel GG, Peckham M.J. Exploitable mechanisms in combined radiotherapy-chemotherapy: the concept of additivity. *Int J Radiat Oncol Biol Phys.* 1979;5:85-91.

78. Seiwert TY, Salama JK, Vokes EE. The concurrent chemoradiation paradigm general principles. *Nature Clin Prac Oncol.* 2007;4:86-100.

79. Pignon JP, Bourhis J, Domenge C, Designe L. Chemotherapy added to locoregional treatment for head and neck squamous-cell carcinoma: three meta-analyses of updated individual data. *Lancet.* 2000;355:949-955.

80. Bourhis J, Le Maitre A, Baujat B, Audry H, Pignon, JP. Individual patients' data meta-analyses in head and neck cancer. *Curr Opin Oncol.* 2007;19: 188-194.

81. Olmi P, Crispino S, Fallai C, et al. Locoregionally advanced carcinoma of the oropharynx: conventional radiotherapy vs accelerated hyperfractionated radiotherapy vs concomitant radiotherapy and chemotherapy—a multicenter randomized trial. *Int J Radiation Oncology Biol Phys.* 2003;55:78-92.

82. Denis F, Garaud P, Bardet E, et al. Late toxicity results of the GORTEC 94-01 randomized trial comparing radiotherapy with concomitant radiochemotherapy for advanced-stage oropharynx carcinoma: comparison of LENT/SOMA RTOG/ EORTC and NCI-CTC scoring systems. *Int J Radiat Oncol Biol Phys.* 2003;55:93-98.

83. Denis F, Garaud P, Bardet E, et al. Final results of the 94-01 French Head and Neck Oncology and Radiotherapy Group randomized trial comparing radiotherapy alone with concomitant radiochemotherapy in advanced-stage oropharynx carcinoma. *J Clin Oncol.* 2004;22:69-76.

84. Budach V, Stuschke W, Budach W, et al. Hyperfractionated accelerated chemoradiation with concurrent fluorouracil-mitomycin is more effective than dose-escalated hyperfractionated accelerated radiation therapy alone in locally advanced head and neck cancer: final results of the Radiotherapy Cooperative Clinical Trials Group of the German Cancer Society 95-06 prospective randomized trial. *J Clin Oncol.* 2005;23:1125-1135.

85. Calais G, Alfonsi M, Bardet E, et al. Randomized trial of radiation therapy versus comcomitant chemotherapy and radiation therapy for advanced stage oropharyngeal carcinoma. *J Natl Cancer Inst.* 1999;91:2081-2086.

86. Bourhis J, Calais G, Lapeyre M, et al. Concomitant radiochemotherapy or accelerated radiotherapy: Analysis of two randomized trials of the French Head and Neck Oncology Group (GORTEC). *Sem Oncol.* 2004;31:822-826.

87. Garden AS, Harris J, Vokes EE, et al. Preliminary results of radiation therapy oncology group 97-03: a randomized phase II trial of concurrent radiation and chemotherapy for advanced squamous cell carcinomas of the head and neck. *J Clin Oncol.* 2004;22:2856-2864.

88. Devlin J, Sherman E. Combined modality treatment of squamous cell cancer of the head and neck. *Clin Adv Hematol Oncol.* 2005;3:373-382.

89. Allal AS, Nicoucar K, Mach N, Dulguerov P. Quality of life in patients with oropharynx carcinomas: assessment after accelerated radiotherapy with or without chemotherapy versus radical surgery and postoperative radiotherapy. *Head Neck.* 2003;25:833-840.

90. Mowry SE, Ho A, LoTempio M.M, Sadeghi A, Blackwell KE, Wang MB. Quality of life in advanced oropharyngeal carcinoma after chemoradiation versus surgery and radiation. *Laryngoscope.* 2006;116:1589-1593.

91. Ang KK, Harris J, Garden AS, et al. Concomitant boost radiation plus concurrent cisplatin for advanced head and neck carcinomas: Radiation Therapy Oncology Group phase II trial 99-14. *J Clin Oncol.* 2005;23:3008-3015.

92. Huguenin P, Beer KT, Allal A, et al. Concomitant cisplatin significantly improves locoregional control in advanced head and neck cancers treated with hyperfractionated radiotherapy. *J Clin Oncol.* 2004;22:4613-4621.

93. Calais G, Bardet E, Sire, C, et al. Radiotherpy with concomitant weekly docetaxel for stages III/IV oropharynsx carcinoma. Results of the 98-02 GORTEC phase II trial. *Int J Radiat Oncol Biol Phys.* 2004;58:161-166.

94. Argiris A, Jayaram P, Pichardo D. Revisiting induction chemotherapy for head and neck cancer. *Oncologist.* 2005;19:759-770.

95. Posner MR. Paradigm shift in the treatment of head and neck cancer: the role of neoadjuvant chemotherapy. *Oncologist.* 2005;10, 11-19.

96. Vokes EE, Stenson K, Rosen FR, et al. Weekly carboplatin and paclitaxel followed by concomitant paclitaxel, fluorouracil, and hydroxyurea chemoradiotherapy: curative and organ-preserving therapy for advanced head and neck cancer. *J Clin Oncol.* 2003;21:320-326.

97. Cohen EEW, Lingen MW, Vokes EE. The expanding role of systemic therapy in head and neck cancer. *J Clin Oncol.* 2004;22:1743-1752.

98. Kies MS, Haraf DJ, Rosen F. Concomitant infusional paclitaxel and fluorouracil, oral hydroxyurea, and hyperfractionated radiation for locally advanced squamous head and neck cancer. *J Clin Oncol.* 2001;19:1961-1969.

99. Argiris A, Haraf DJ, Kies MS, Vokes EE. Intensive concurrent chemoradiotherapy for head and neck cancer with 5-flourouracil- and hydroxyurea-based regimens: revering a pattern of failure. *Oncologist.* 2003: 8:350-360.

100. Urba SG, Mool J, Giri PGS, et al. Organ preservation for advanced resectable cancer of the base of tongue and hypopharynx: a Southwest Oncology Group trial. *J Clin Oncol.* 2005;23, 88-95.

101. Cmelak AJ, Li S, Goldwasser MA, et al. Phase II trial of chemoradiation for organ preservation in resectable stage III or IV squamous cell carcinomas of the larynx or oropharynx: results of Eastern Cooperative Oncology Group study E2399. *J Clin Oncol.* 2007;25:3971-3977.

102. Bonner JA Harari PM, Giralt J. Radiotherapy plus cetuximab for squamous-cell carcinoma of the head and neck. *N Eng J Med.* 2006;354:567-578.

103. Cooper JS, Pajak TF, Forastier AA, et al. Postoperative concurrent radiotherapy and chemotherapy for high-risk squamous-cell carcinoma of the head and neck. *N Eng J Med.* 2004;350:1937-1944.

104. Bernier J, Domenge C, Ozsahin M, et al. Postoperative irradiation with or without concomitant chemotherapy for locally advanced head and neck cancer. *N Eng J Med.* 2004;350:1945-1952.

105. Wang SJ, Wang MB, Yip H, Calcaterra TC. Combined radiotherapy with planned neck dissection for small head and neck cancers with advanced cervical metastases. *Laryngoscope.* 2000;110: 1794-1797.

106. Grant DG., Salassa, JR, Hinni ML, Pearson BW, Perry WC. Carcinoma of the tongue base treated by transoral laser microsurgery, Part two: persistent, recurrent and second primary tumors. *Laryngoscope.* 2006;116:2156-2161.

107. Morton RP, Hay KD, MaCann A. On completion of curative treatment of head and neck cancer: why follow up? *Curr Opon Otolaryngol Head Neck Surg.* 2004;12:142-146.

108. Ridge JA. Surgical treatment of recurrent and metastatic head and neck cancer. *American Society of Clinical Oncology—2007 Educational Book.* 2007;7;344-347.

109. Clayman GL, Johnson CJ, Morrison W, Ginsberg L, Lippman SM. The role of neck dissection after chemoradiotherapy for oropharyngeal cancer with advanced nodal disease. *Arch Otolarygol Head Neck Surg.* 2001;127:135-139.

110. Brizel DM, Prosnitz RG, Hunter S, et al. Necessity for adjuvant neck dissection in setting of concurrent chemoradiation for advanced head-and-neck cancer. *Int J Radiat Oncol Biol Phys.* 2004;58: 1418-1423.

111. Goguen LA, Posner MR, Tishler MR, et al. Examining the need for neck dissection in the era of chemoradiation therapy for advanced head and neck cancer. *Arch Otolaryngol Head Neck Surg.* 2006;132:526-531.

112. Corry J, Smith JG, Peters LJ, The concept of a planned neck dissection is obsolete. *Cancer J.* 2001;7:472-474.

113. Lavertu P, Adelstein DJ, Saxton JP. et al. Management of the neck in a randomized trial comparing concurrent chemotherapy and radiotherapy with radiotherapy alone in resectable stage III and IV squamous cell head and neck cancer. *Head Neck.* 1997;19:559-566.

114. Stenson KM, Haraf DJ, Pelzer H, et al. The role of cervical lymphadenectomy after aggressive concomitant chemoradiotherapy. *Arch Otolaryngol Head Neck Surg.* 2000;126:950-956.

115. Mendenhall WM, Villaret, DB, Amdur RJ, Hinerman RW, Mancuso AA. Planned neck dissection after definitive radiotherapy for squamous cell carcinoma of the head and neck. *Head Neck.* 2002;24:1012-1018.

116. Robbins KT, Ferlito A, Suarez C, et al. Is there a role for selective neck dissection after chemoradiation for head and neck cancer? *J Am Col Surg.* 2004;199: 913-915.

117. Kutler DI, Patel SG, Shah JP. The role of neck dissection following definitive chemoradiation. *Oncology.* 2004;18:993-1008.

118. Yao M, Hoffman HF, Chang K, et al. Is planned neck dissection necessary for head and neck cancer after intensity-modulated radiotheraphy? *Int J Radiat Oncol Biol Phys.* 2007;68:707-713.

119. Liauw SL, Mancuso AA, Amdur RJ, et al. Postradiotherapy neck dissection for lymph node-positive head and neck cancer: the use of computed tomography to manage the neck. *J Clin Oncol.* 2006;24:1421-1428.

120. Agarwal V, Branstetter BF, Johnson JT. Indications for PET/CT in the head and neck. *Otolaryngol Clin North Am.* 2008;41:23-50.

121. Schwartz GJ, Mehta RH, Wenig GL. Salvage treatment for recurrent squamous cell carcinoma of then oral cavity. *Head Neck.* 2000;22:34-41.

122. Mahanta SR, Mendenhall WM, Stringer S, et al. Salvage treatment for neck recurrence after irradiation alone for head and neck squamous cell carcinoma with clinically positive neck nodes. *Head Neck.* 1999;21:591–594.

123. Krol BJ, Righi PD, Paydarfar JA. Factors related to outcome of salvage therapy for isolated cervical recurrence of squamous cell carcinoma in the previously treated neck: a multi-institutional study. *Otolaryngol Head Neck Surg.* 2000;123: 368–376.

124. Kowalski LP. Results of salvage treatment of the neck in patients with oral cancer; *Arch Otolaryngol Head Neck Surg.* 2002;128:58–62.

125. Richey LM., Shores CG, George J, et al. The effectiveness of salvage surgery after the failure of primary concomitant chemoradiation in head and neck cancer. *Otolaryngol Head Neck Surg.* 2007;136:98–103.

126. Wutzl A, Ploder O, Kermer C, Millesi W, Ewers R, Klug C. Mortality and causes of death after multimodality treatment for advanced oral and oropharyngeal cancer. *J Oral Maxillofac Surg.* 2007;65:255–260.

127. Langendijk JA, Kasperts N, Leemans CR. A phase II study of primary reirradiation in squamous cell carcinoma of the head and neck. *Radiother Oncol.* 2006;78:306–312.

128. Wong SJ, Machtay M, Li Y. Locally recurrent, previously irradiated head and neck cancer: concurrent re-irradiation and chemotherapy, or chemotherapy alone? *J Clin Oncol.* 2006;24: 2653–2658.

129. Day GL, Blot WJ. Second primary tumors in patients with oral cancer. *Cancer.* 10:14–19.

130. Jones AS, Morar P, Phillips DE, et al. Second primary tumors in patients with head and neck squamous cell carcinoma. *Cancer.* 1995;75: 1343–1353.

131. Cooper JS, Pajak TF, Rubin P, et al. Second primary malignancies in patients who have head and neck cancer: incidence, effect on survival and implications based on the RTOG experience. *Int J Radiat Oncol Biol Phys.* 1989;17:449–456.

132. Gillenwater AM. Head and neck cancer: what to do after successful treatment. *American Society of Clinical Oncology—2005 Educational Book.* 2005;5:416–421.

133. Sherman EJ. Head and Neck Cancer: surveillance after definitive treatment. *American Society of Clinical Oncology—2005 Education Book.* 2005;5:466–471.

134. National Comprehensive Cancer Center Network: Head and Neck Cancers, 2005. http://nccn.org/professionals/physiciangls/PDF/head-and-neck.pdf

135. American Head and Neck Society: American Head and Neck Society Clinical Resources. http://www.ahns.info/clinicalresources/guidelines.php

136. Paniello RC, Virgo KS, Johnson MH, et al. Practice patterns and clinical guidelines for post-treatment follow-up of head and neck cancers. A comparison of 2 professional societies. *Arch Otolaryngol Head Neck Surg.* 1999;125:309–313.

137. Yom SS, Machtay M, Biel MA, et al. Survival impact of planned restaging and early surgical salvage following definitive chemoradiation for locally advanced squamous cell carcinomas of the oropharynx and hypopharynx. *Am J Clinl Oncol.* 2005;28:385–392.

138. Baumann I, Seibolt M, Zalaman I, Dietz K, Maassen M, Plinkert, P. Quality of life in patients with oropharyngeal carcinoma after primary surgery and postoperative irradiation. *J Otolaryngol.* 2006;35:332–337.

139. Borggreven PA, Verdonck-de Leeuw IM, Muller MJ, et al. Quality of life and functional status in patients with cancer of the oral cavity and oropharynx: pretreatment values of a prospective study. *Eur Arch Otorhinolaryngol.* 2007; 264:651–657.

140. Vartanian JG, Carvalho AL, Toyota J, Kowalski ISG, Kowalski LP. Socioeconomic effects of and risk factors for diability in long-term survivort of head and neck cancer. *Arch Otolaryngol Head Neck Surg.* 2006;132:32–35.

141. Lang KK, Menzin J, Earle CC, Jacobson J, Hsu MA. The economic costs of squamous cell cancer of the head and neck. *Arch Otolaryngol Head Neck Surg.* 2005:131:21–26.

16

Early Cancer of the Larynx

Edward M. Stafford

Tarik Y. Farrag

Ralph P. Tufano

INTRODUCTION

Epidemiology

Cancer of the larynx comprises approximately 0.8% of all human malignancies,[1] and represents 26% of head and neck cancers.[2] There will be an estimated 11,300 new cases of larynx cancer (8,960 men and 2,340 women) in the United States for 2007. Cancer of the larynx has a peak incidence in the sixth decade of life. Men are more commonly affected than women, with recent studies reporting a ratio of 4-5:1.[1,3-5] The estimated number of deaths from larynx cancer in 2007 will approximate 3,650, compared to 4,000 in 2001. This slight decrease might imply an improvement in early diagnosis as well as improved methods in the management of larynx cancer; however, the 5-year survival rate was 66% in 1975, 66% in 1986, and 65% in 2002, which essentially has remained unchanged in the last 25 years.[1]

Anatomy

Although laryngeal cancer is relatively less frequent compared to other human malignancies, such as cancer of the breast, stomach, and lung, its clinical impact is undeniable.[1] Any treatment of laryngeal cancer has a profound impact on phonation, swal-lowing, breathing and the protection of the airway due to the anatomic location and function of the larynx. The social consequences of treatment, including adverse effects on quality of life, mental health and socioeconomic status, can be profound.[3,4]

A thorough understanding of the relevant anatomy and potential patterns of tumor extension are essential for today's head and neck surgeon, given the variety of surgical and nonsurgical options available to treat malignancies of the larynx. For the assessment and treatment of laryngeal cancer, it is useful to divide the larynx into three subsites: the supraglottis, the glottis, and the subglottis. Embryonic development of these subsites establishes distinct lymphatic drainage patterns and, thus, markedly different clinical behavior of cancers in each subsite. The glottis includes the paired true vocal folds. The supraglottis includes that portion of the larynx above the glottis; whereas the subglottis begins 5 mm below the free margin of the vocal folds and extends to the inferior border of the cricoid cartilage. The substance of the larynx is composed of a bony and cartilaginous framework, fibroelastic ligaments, and muscles. In various combinations, they form several distinct spaces that permit or inhibit the spread of tumor in various directions.

The cartilaginous and bony framework is primarily composed of the thyroid cartilage, the cricoid cartilage, the epiglottis, the hyoid bone, and the arytenoids. Through their work with whole organ sections, Kirchner and Tucker advanced the knowledge of the fibroelastic ligaments that traverse the larynx. First, the conus elasticus spans from each vocal fold to the cricoid cartilage, attaches posteriorly to the arytenoids, and condenses medially to form the vocal ligament. It attaches anteriorly to the thyroid cartilage at Broyle's ligament, otherwise known as the anterior commisure tendon. This area is devoid of perichondrium. Next, the conus elasticus condenses into the cricothyroid ligament, which lies only on the central portion of the cricoid and does not cover the cricoid circumferentially. In addition, the thyrohyoid membrane drapes the entire circumference of the thyroid cartilage and proceeds upward to the hyoid bone. The quadrangular membrane spans from the superior portion of the arytenoids to the lateral portion of the epiglottis at its superior extent and from the inferior portion of the arytenoids to the petiole of the epiglottis at its inferior extent. Finally, the hyoepiglottic ligament, as described by Zeitels and Kirchner, spans from the hyoid bone to the epiglottis.

The cartilaginous/bony framework and fibroelastic tissue condensations described above define the spaces of the larynx. The pre-epiglottic space, filled with fat and traversed by lymphatics, is bound superiorly by the vallecular mucosa and hyoid bone, anteriorly by the thyrohyoid membrane and thyroid cartilage, posteriorly by the epiglottis, and posterolaterally by the superior portions of the paraglottic space. The paraglottic space, occupied by the thyroarytenoid muscle, ventricle, and saccule, is bound superomedially by the quadrangular membrane, inferomedially by the conus elasticus, superiorly by the aryepiglottic fold, inferiorly by the cricoid cartilage, anteriorly by the preepiglottic space and thyroid cartilage, and posterolaterally by the mucosa of the medial aspect of the piriform sinus. The paraglottic space traverses from the supraglottis to the subglottis with no connective tissue barrier.

The intrinsic muscles of the larynx control the movement of the true vocal folds. All but the cricothyroid muscle are innervated by the ipsilateral recurrent laryngeal nerve, a branch of the vagus nerve. This includes the posterior cricoarytenoid muscle, the only abductor of the vocal fold. All muscles except for the cricothyroid move the arytenoid cartilage in relation to the rest of the laryngeal framework to produce vocal fold adduction or abduction. The cricothyroid muscle produces tension and elongation of the vocal folds by rocking the thyroid cartilage on the cricoid and is innervated by the ipsilateral superior laryngeal nerve, which also carries the sensory afferent fibers of the larynx above the glottis. In general, both motor and sensory innervations of the larynx are strictly lateralized; that is, there is no cross-innervation. The interarytenoid muscle may be an exception to this.

Etiology

The etiology of laryngeal cancer is generally multifactorial. Tobacco smoking and alcohol intake have a strong synergistic effect in the pathogenesis of squamous cell cancer. After cessation of smoking, the risk gradually declines, and there is almost no excess risk found after 20 years. Interestingly, a multiplicative effect has also been found for tobacco smoking and alcohol consumption.[6-13] Habitual consumption of a tea known as "mate" is associated with an increased risk of developing cancer of the larynx.[11,13] In addition, there are several reports that support the hypothesis that a low-fat diet high in antioxidants may interfere with carcinogenesis, and suggest that dietary intervention could be a means of improving survival in laryngeal cancer.[9,10] Other risk factors have been reported, such as gastroesophageal reflux disease,[14-18] dietary factors,[14-18] and exposure to asbestos, ionizing radiation, wood dust, and nitrogen mustard.[19-21] Finally, cancer of the larynx has also been reported in individuals who have never smoked or consumed alcohol.[22,23]

Pathology

Squamous cell cancer, representing 97.4% of laryngeal malignancies, is the most common histologic type. The remainder of laryngeal cancer histologic subtypes represent less than 3%.[2]

The great majority of malignant laryngeal tumors arise from the surface epithelium and therefore are SCC (squamous cell cancer) or one of its variants such as spindle cell or verrucous carcinoma.

Sarcomas, adenocarcinomas, neuroendocrine tumors, and other unusual neoplasms comprise the remainder of malignant laryngeal cancers. More than 50% of laryngeal SCCs present as localized disease, 25% present with regional metastasis, and 15% are first seen at an advanced stage with or without distant metastasis.[24,25]

Epithelial Cancers (Table 16–1)

Most laryngeal SCCs result from prolonged exposure to recognized carcinogens. Some of these changes are associated with keratosis.[26] The severity of dysplasia is described as mild, moderate, or severe, depending on the extent of involvement of the surface epithelium. In general, the degree of dysplasia correlates with the likelihood of transformation to invasive carcinoma.[27,28] At best, the gross appearance of a lesion of the mucosal surface is an inconsistent indicator of malignant potential. The term leukoplakia describes a white lesion, usually appearing as such because of keratinization. It is strongly suggested that dysplasia leads to CIS (carcinoma in situ), which then leads to invasive carcinoma, as the CIS is usually surrounded by dysplasia. Carcinoma in situ is a full-thickness mucosal epithelial dysplastic change without basement membrane invasion.

Tumor thickness and the depth of tumor invasion are strongly correlated with cervical lymph nodes metastasis. In addition, the degree of cellular differentiation appears to correlate with the probability of cervical metastasis and survival, although the degree of cellular differentiation is not considered the most significant factor upon grading the tumor.[29,30]

Spread

Local Spread

Supraglottis. Supraglottic carcinomas arise most commonly from the epiglottis and less frequently from the false vocal folds and aryepiglottic folds. They can be exophytic, ulcerative, or endophytic.[31,32] The substance of the epiglottis is often destroyed by tumors on its surface.[34,35] Early supraglottic carcinomas are initially confined to the pre-epiglottic space

by the ligamentous boundaries of that compartment. Once those barriers are invaded, however, tumor growth occurs more rapidly.[33,34] Modern imaging modalities, especially magnetic resonance imaging (MRI), have greatly improved the ability to recognize tumor extension into the pre-epiglottic space and base of tongue. Assessing the pre-epiglottic space and the anterior thyroid lamina is of paramount importance for those patients who may be candidates for either transoral laser microsurgery or open conservation laryngeal surgery. This is not always a straightforward endeavor, as patchy ossification in the laryngeal framework may present an ambiguous radiologic and clinical picture. Typically, however, healthy, nonossified cartilage provides a fairly resistant natural barrier to cancer invasion. Finally, the quandrangular membrane within the aryepiglottic fold plays an important role in diverting the leading edge of tumors.

Supraglottic carcinomas frequently metastasize to the cervical lymph nodes due to the rich lymphatic drainage.[36,37-40] The incidence of patients demonstrating clinically positive lymph nodes at the time of diagnosis is 23% to 50% for supraglottic carcinoma of all stages.[32,41-45] If a neck dissection is performed, a substantial number of those patients with clinically negative necks are found to have histologically identifiable disease. If left untreated, this progresses to gross disease.[37,38] In supraglottic cancers, the probability of cervical metastasis and of delayed contralateral metastasis increases in direct proportion to the size of the primary (ie, the T stage).[31,46,47] This trend may not be predictive for patients who have been previously irradiated.[5]

When there are clinically positive cervical nodes measuring 2 cm or more in diameter, the incidence of contralateral neck metastasis may exceed 40%.[48] The epiglottis is particularly prone to produce bilateral metastasis. Even early stage lesions may produce contralateral metastasis in more than 20%.[47]

Glottis. Glottic carcinomas are the most common type of laryngeal cancer in the United States. Two-thirds are confined to the vocal folds. Tumors arise most commonly on the anterior two-thirds of the vocal fold, whereas a small percentage are isolated to the anterior commissure. The posterior commissure is rarely affected.[49]

Table 16–1. Staging*

Tumor stage	Characteristics
Supraglottis	
T1	Tumor limited to one subsite of supraglottis with normal vocal fold mobility
T2	Tumor invades mucosa of more than one adjacent subsite of supraglottis or glottis or region outside the supraglottis (eg, mucosa of base of tongue, vallecula, medial wall of piriform sinus) without fixation of the larynx
T3	Tumor limited to larynx with vocal fold fixation or invades any of the following: postcricoid area, pre-epiglottic tissues, or minor thyroid erosion (inner cortex)
T4	Tumor invades through the thyroid cartilage, or extends into soft tissues of the neck, thyroid, or esophagus
	T4a: Resectable (eg, tumor invades trachea, soft tissues of neck, strap muscles, thyroid, or esophagus)
	T4b: Unresectable (eg, tumor invades prevertebral space, encases carotid artery, or invades mediastinal structures)
Glottis	
T1	Tumor limited to vocal fold(s) (may involve anterior or posterior commissure) with normal mobility
	T1a: Tumor limited to one vocal fold
	T1b: Tumor involves both vocal folds
T2	Tumor extends to supraglottis or subglottis, or with impaired vocal fold mobility
T3	Tumor limited to the larynx with vocal fold fixation, or invades paraglottic space, or minor thyroid cartilage erosion (inner cortex)
T4	Tumor invades through the thyroid cartilage or to other tissues beyond the larynx (eg, trachea, soft tissues of neck including thyroid, pharynx)
	T4a: Resectable, see above
	T4b: Unresectable, see above
Subglottis	
T1	Tumor limited to the subglottis
T2	Tumor extends to vocal fold(s) with normal or impaired mobility
T3	Tumor limited to larynx with vocal fold fixation
T4	Tumor invades through cricoid or thyroid cartilage or extends to other tissues beyond the larynx (eg, trachea, soft tissues of neck including thyroid,esophagus)
	T4a: Resectable. Tumor invades criciod or thyroid cartilage or invades tissues beyond the larynx (eg, trachea, soft tissues of neck, strap muscles, thyroid, or esophagus)
	T4b: Unresectable. Tumor invades prevertebral space, encases carotid artery, or invades mediastinum

*Changes that are now included in the 6th edition of the American Joint Committee on Cancer. *Cancer Staging Manual*, by Greene F, et al. New York; Springer-Verlag, 2002:47–57.

Source: Modified from American Joint Committee on Cancer. *Manual for Staging of Cancer.* 5th ed. Philadelphia, Pa: Lippincott Williams & Wilkins, 1998:45–55.

The relatively poor lymphatic drainage of the true vocal folds (except near the posterior commissure) makes early metastasis uncommon. In addition, the conus elasticus and thyroglottic ligament tend to divert vocal fold lesions at the free margin from continuing into the underlying vocalis muscle and paraglottic space. Likewise, the anterior commissure ligament (Broyle's ligament) serves as a barrier to cancer spread outside the level of the glottis.[50] If Broyle's ligament becomes invaded with carcinoma, cartilage penetration becomes more likely.[51] This event is even more prevalent in the presence of thyroid cartilage ossification.[52,53]

When caudal extension does occur, extralaryngeal spread may occur into the anterior neck either into the soft tissue or to the delphian lymph node.[54] Of note, one centimeter of subglottic extension anteriorly or 4 to 5 mm of subglottic extension posteriorly puts the border of the tumor to the upper margin of the cricoid, which potentially limits options for conservation laryngeal surgery. In addition, when vocal ligament and thyroarytenoid muscle involvement occur, paraglottic space and thyroid cartilage involvement become more likely. Finally, the neck and thyroid gland may ultimately become involved with more aggressive lesions.

Subglottis. Subglottic cancers are generally unusual, comprising 1% to 8% of all laryngeal cancers.[49] They are mostly poorly differentiated and frequently demonstrate an infiltrative growth pattern. They involve the cricoid cartilage early because there is no intervening muscle layer. The incidence of cervical metastasis from subglottic cancer is reported to be 20% to 30%. The actual incidence, however, may be significantly higher due to primary spread to prelaryngeal and pretracheal nodal basins.[55,56]

Lymphatic Spread

The primary lymphatic drainage of the supraglottic larynx is to the jugulodigastric nodes. The submandibular area is rarely involved, and there is only a small risk for nodal involvement along the spinal accessory nerve. The incidence of clinically positive nodes is 55% at the time of diagnosis. Bilateral nodal metastasis at diagnosis occurs in up to 16%.[36] In addition, elective neck dissection demonstrates pathologically positive nodes in 16% of cases, whereas observation of initially node-negative necks eventually identifies the appearance of positive nodes in 33% of cases.[57,58] Of note, these numbers tend to be very low in previously irradiated cancers.[5] Extension of the primary tumor to the piriform sinus, vallecula, and base of the tongue increases the risk for lymph node metastases.

For glottic carcinoma, the incidence of clinically positive lymph nodes at diagnosis is negligible for T1 lesions and 1.7% for T2 lesions.[59] The incidence of cervical metastases rises to 20 to 30% for T3 and T4 tumors. Supraglottic spread is associated with metastasis to the jugulodigastric nodes. Anterior commissure and anterior subglottic invasion are associated with involvement of the delphian node.

Other Cancers. Verrucous carcinoma is also of squamous origin and occurs in the oral cavity, larynx, esophagus, sinonasal tract and on the genitalia.[24,60] Some investigators consider it a separate entity[61]; however, others believe it to be a variant of well-differentiated SCC.[62]

Diagnosing verrucous carcinoma is difficult, even when the clinical index of suspicion is high. Even though these lesions often destroy cartilage, they do not tend to metastasize, and aggressiveness is characterized by local invasion. The diagnosis is largely a clinical one, achieved most effectively by a pathologist and surgeon acting in concert. The typical verrucous carcinoma is slow-growing but relentless, appears exophytic and warty, is broad-based at its interface with the mucosa, and is either tan or white. The surface often is necrotic and infected, and the associated inflammation of adjacent tissues frequently is remarkable. This tendency to cause inflammation can erroneously influence treatment planning.[63,64]

Although squamous cell carcinoma is regarded as a radiosensitive cancer, verrucous carcinoma is regarded as radioresistant.[65] In addition, the literature suggests a potential for radiation-induced dedifferentiation of these rumors into anaplastic cancer, which may occur in 7 to 30% of verrucous carcinomas.[41,60,65,66-71] Partial laryngeal surgery generally is considered the preferred strategy for verrucous larynx cancers.[72]

Recent diagnostic techniques, such as immunohistochemical analysis, allow elucidation of more unusual laryngeal malignancies, such as neuroendocrine carcinomas.[73-75] Surgical management of neuroendocrine carcinomas does not typically enhance survival.[75,76] Despite this, for other laryngeal tumors of neuroendocrine origin, such as paragangliomas and carcinoid tumors, surgical management is the preferred treatment.[77]

Other rare tumors reported to arise in the larynx include cartilaginous malignancies,[78] plasmacytomas, sarcomas, malignant fibrous histiocytomas, adenocarcinomas, melanomas, granular cell tumors, and primary lymphomas.[77-82]

PRETREATMENT EVALUATION

The preoperative workup of a patient suspected of having laryngeal cancer should serve to confirm the diagnosis through biopsy, map the extent of the lesion, and search for synchronous lesions, and/or metastatic disease. When mapping the extent of the lesion, it is of paramount importance to focus the evaluation on findings that may indicate a worse prognosis such as anterior commissure involvement, or findings that may rule in or rule out certain laryngeal preservation procedures.

Office Examination

The preoperative evaluation starts at the initial office visit. A thorough history and physical examination should be obtained. During the physical exam, the lateral and medial compartments of the neck should be palpated carefully. Extension of the cancer through the laryngeal cartilage can sometimes be palpated. Laryngeal cancers with involvement of the subglottis may present with a Delphian node or paratracheal nodal disease. Loss of the normal crepitus palpated on moving the larynx back and forth may indicate extension of the tumor into the postcricoid area. The base of tongue should be palpated to evaluate for superior extension.

Indirect mirror laryngoscopy is an invaluable tool to visualize the larynx in the office. The majority of patients can be examined via this method. Limitations include an inability to visualize the sub-glottis, and limited visualization of the anterior commissure. In addition, a rigid 90-degree laryngoscope, and a flexible fiberoptic laryngoscope are available to examine the larynx. By adding a stroboscopic light source, one can evaluate the mucosal wave of the true vocal folds, which can provide information regarding the depth of invasion of a glottic carcinoma. Also, with the addition of a camera to the fiberoptic laryngoscope, one can document photographically or videographically the extent of the lesion. The rigid endoscope provides a larger, brighter picture, but patients tend to gag more often, and the larynx is not in physiologic position when examined. The flexible laryngoscope provides a more physiologic view of the larynx, and one can navigate beyond obstructing lesions to obtain a more distal view, including a view of the proximal subglottis.

Radiographic Imaging

Preoperative imaging often supplements the findings of the physical examination and can indicate subclinical involvement of the various spaces of the larynx. CT and MRI of the neck are both useful in this regard. Both can show invasion of the laryngeal framework by SCC. In addition, MRI can demonstrate involvement of the pre-epiglottic space and/or the paraglottic space that is not evident on physical exam. Radiographic delineation of the primary lesion is of critical importance when organ preservation modalities are employed for treatment, as IMRT techniques rely on precise anatomic details to inform the treatment protocols. In addition, several radiographic modalities, including CT, MRI, PET-CT, and ultrasound are employed in the search for regional and distant metastatic disease. PET-CT technology in particular has revolutionized the workup of distant metastatic disease. More traditional modalities utilized in a metastatic workup include a chest radiograph, liver function studies, and a CT of the chest, abdomen, and pelvis as indicated.[83-85]

Direct Laryngoscopy and Biopsy

The above studies are not a substitute for operative assessment of the tumor with panendoscopy. Flexible or rigid esophagoscopy is performed to evaluate for synchronous primaries. A direct laryngoscopy or a suspension microlaryngoscopy is also performed to map the tumor more accurately and assess fixation of the arytenoids(s). The Dedo and Holinger laryngoscopes are used most often. The Holinger laryngoscope is of particular utility in laryngeal carcinoma, as it provides excellent visualization of the anterior larynx and allows the examiner to maneuver around a larynx crowded with tumor. The Dedo laryngoscope is wider and allows the use of multiple instruments at the same time. It is more often utilized in suspension laryngoscopy, allowing the surgeon to have both hands free for instrumentation. While mapping the tumor, it is important to document the anterior extent of tumor, anterior commissure involvement, involvement of the false vocal folds, ventricles, postcricoid area, hypopharyngeal mucosa, and mucosa of the arytenoids. Rigid telescopes can be used as an adjunct to examine extension of disease into the subglottis. All partial laryngeal procedures require at least one fully mobile and sensate cricoarytenoid complex; therefore, this should be a focus of the laryngoscopy. Arytenoid fixation indicates involvement of the cricoarytenoid joint, or extralaryngeal spread with tumor, and may preclude conservation laryngeal surgery. True vocal fold fixation is not the same as arytenoid fixation as vocal folds may be fixed due to the bulk of the tumor or due to paraglottic space involvement, neither of which affect arytenoid mobility. Fiberoptic laryngoscopy and palpation of the vocal process of each arytenoid during operative laryngoscopy are the best ways to assess arytenoid mobility.[86,87]

TREATMENT METHODS

Endoscopic Management of Early Larynx Cancer

The transoral laser microscopic approaches for surgically treating squamous cell carcinoma of the larynx have improved significantly over the past 20 years with improvements in endoscopic instrumentation and laser technology. Advantages over primary radiotherapy or conservation laryngeal surgery include an abbreviated treatment time, potentially only requiring an outpatient surgical procedure. In addition, with transoral laser approaches, primary control is often attainable without necessitating the use of adjuvant radiotherapy. Early reports using transoral laser techniques validated the approach as oncologically sound.[88] More recent reports demonstrate that both transoral laser microsurgery and primary radiotherapy provide roughly equivalent oncologic control. In their review of the existing literature comparing radiotherapy and transoral laser excision of early glottic cancers, Back and Sood reported a range of local control rates for early glottic cancer treated with radiotherapy between 85% to 94% for T1 lesions and 68% to 80% for T2 lesions, whereas transoral excisions offer local control rates of 83% to 93% for T1 lesions and 73% to 89% for T2 lesions.[89] Overall survival rates are similarly comparable. In addition, cost benefit analyses argue toward a transoral laser microsurgical approach. Myers and others demonstrated transoral laser surgery for T1 glottic lesions to be a cost-effective option compared to conservation laryngeal surgery and radiotherapy.[90] In a later report from the same group, Smith and others demonstrated equivalent quality of life outcomes and functional results when comparing patients treated with endoscopic excision versus radiotherapy, but with the radiated patients experiencing increased number of work hours missed, as well as increased costs related to travel.[91] Finally, though it has traditionally been accepted that vocal quality is superior after radiotherapy compared to transoral laser microsurgery for early glottic carcinomas, recent reports have brought this into question. Brandenburg compared vocal quality in patients with T1 glottic carcinoma who received radiotherapy or transoral laser microsurgery with a 63 month follow-up period. His findings demonstrated that whereas postsurgical patients tended to have a more breathy voice, and postradiotherapy patients have a harsher, raspy voice, vocal quality after laser cordotomy was comparable to voice quality after radiotherapy.[92]

Treatment of Midcord T1 Lesions

Indications. These lesions are among the most readily accessible via a transoral endoscopic approach.

Any lesion arising from the free edge of a mobile vocal fold is amenable to this approach.

Contraindications. Unfavorable anatomy, including those patients with trismus or retrognathia, preventing adequate exposure for visualization and instrumentation.

Pearls for Technique. For lesions of the midfold without evidence of vocal fold movement impairment or anterior commissure involvement, the transoral approach is fairly straightforward. A microflap technique, whereby a tissue plane is developed along the superficial lamina propria of the vocal fold, may be employed to assess the depth of invasion in these lesions. Unlike the resection of a benign lesion, the microflap in this case is resected, but the approach may afford superior visualization of the depth of invasion and increased preservation of the vocal ligament. For larger lesions of the vocal fold, the CO_2 laser may aid in finesse control of the depth of dissection as well as hemostasis.

Cordectomy

Indications. The European Laryngological Society has developed a classification scheme addressing endoscopic excisions of vocal fold lesions, including those for endoscopic cordectomy.[93] Using this classification, Gallo and others reviewed 151 patients treated with early glottic carcinoma treated with endoscopic laser surgery and stratified patients based on stage, advocating a specific type of cordectomy.

Endoscopic Cordectomy

Classification by European Laryngological Society

Subepithelial cordectomy:	Type I
Subligmental cordectomy:	Type II
Transmuscular cordectomy:	Type III
Total or complete cordectomy:	Type IV
Extended cordectomy encompassing:	
contralateral vocal fold	Type Va

arytenoids	Type Vb
ventricular fold	Type Vc
subglottis	Type Vd

Indications. See Table 16–2.

Contraindications. Although several series have demonstrated adverse outcomes in patients managed with transoral laser excisions who have anterior commissure involvement,[95] other large series show no difference in local control rates when comparing those patients with or without anterior commissure involvement.[96,97] These controversies in the literature underscore the importance of thoroughly evaluating the anterior commissure via preoperative videostroboscopy, preoperative imaging including CT and/or MRI to rule out thyroid cartilage invasion if there is any question of anterior commissure involvement, as well as the necessary endoscopic equipment requirements to ensure complete evaluation of the lesion prior to excision.

Table 16–2. Gallo et al[94] Indication by Stage for Laser Resection

T Stage	Type of Cordectomy	Indication
T in situ	Type I Type II Type III	Depending on the extension of the involved area and the results of preoperative investigation (eg, videostroboscopy)
T1a	Type III	Small (0.5–0.7 mm) superficial tumor involving middle third of TVF
T1a	Type IV	Tumor size >0.7 mm and/or deep infiltrative pattern and/or anterior commissure involvement
T1b	Type Va	Involvement of the anterior commissure in a horseshoe pattern
	Bilateral cordectomy	Multifocal cancer

Pearls for Technique. One of the long held principles of oncologic resection is Halstead's principle of en bloc resection. For the surgeon employing transoral laser techniques, it is often not possible, nor is it advisable to always attempt en bloc resection. A general principle of transoral laser techniques is that the initial incisions made with the laser are used to facilitate exposure of the tumor extent. This may include incisions through tumor, with additional laser cuts used to complete the resection with negative margins.

Endoscopic Supraglottic Laryngectomy (CO₂ laser)

Indications. Lesions that are small and accessible are the most obvious candidates for endoscopic excision for cure, including lesions of the suprahyoid epiglottis and aryepiglottic folds. Infrahyoid epiglottic lesions and false vocal fold lesions may be more challenging to resect because of their tangential orientation to the distal end of the laryngoscope.[98]

Contraindications. As with open supraglottic laryngectomy, depending on the extent of resection, patients undergoing endoscopic laser resections are likewise at risk for postoperative aspiration. An assessment of preoperative pulmonary function as well as the involvement of a speech-language pathologist to assist in swallowing rehabilitation is essential in these patients. In general, however, recovery of swallowing function in the patients who undergo endoscopic supraglottic laryngectomy is often faster than those undergoing an open approach.

Pearls for Technique. As with glottic malignancies, en bloc resection is not essential to maintain the oncologic integrity of resection. In particular, lesions of the epiglottis may be divided by going directly through the tumor, facilitating the resection at the lateral margin. Instrumentation is particularly important when attempting endoscopic excision of supraglottic carcinomas. A variety of endoscope designs are available, including bivalved supraglottoscopes which augment the area exposed for both visualization and instrumentation.

Endoscopic Extended Resections (CO₂ laser)

Indications. The oncologic feasibility of CO₂ laser treatment of supraglottic carcinoma for T1 and T2 lesions is well established. For more extensive resections, the use of transoral laser excisions may be permissible for select patients. In their series of 124 patients treated with CO₂ laser excisions of supraglottic carcinomas, Motta and others stratified their patients into three categories based on T status (T1–3).[99] For T3 patients, they demonstrated an acceptable 5-year local control rate of 77%. In this series, however, they stressed appropriate preoperative screening of these patients considering only those with limited pre-epiglottic space involvement.

Contraindications. Extensive pre-epiglottic space involvement.

Pearls for Technique. Pre-epiglottic space involvement may be underestimated by standard imaging modalities necessitating restaging based on operative findings or on final pathology. This is particularly relevant for tumors involving the laryngeal surface of the infrahyoid epiglottis. Davis and others, in their series of 46 endoscopic supraglottic laryngectomies staged as T2 preoperatively, found that 18 (39%) were upstaged based on pre-epiglottic space invasion noted on final pathology. Of note, in their series, all patients were offered planned postoperative radiation, with a 97% rate of primary control.[100] Clearly, a thorough preoperative evaluation, including a CT to rule out cartilage invasion, is essential in those patients who are candidates for endoscopic extended resections.

Open Management of Early Glottic Cancer

Open management of glottic and supraglottic malignancies provide a time tested, oncologically sound modality for the head and neck surgeon. The spectrum of these procedures range from, in increasing level of complexity, laryngofissure with cordectomy and reconstruction, vertical partial laryngectomy, open supraglottic laryngectomy, and supracricoid laryngectomy. Of paramount importance in determining whether a patient is a candidate for organ preservation surgery is the preoperative physical examination, including fiberoptic laryngoscopy. Arytenoid mobility must be carefully assessed, as arytenoid immobility secondary to cricoarytenoid joint involvement or extralaryngeal spread is a contraindication to organ preservation surgery. CT and MRI imaging modalities may aid in determining the extent of pre-epiglottic space and extralaryngeal involvement. Finally, detailed endoscopy under anesthesia using microscopic and/or endoscopic assistance to evaluate the subglottis is essential.

Cordectomy with Reconstruction

Indications. This approach is ideal for T1 glottic lesions that would otherwise be amenable to transoral laser microsurgical excision in patients with unfavorable anatomy. This includes patients with trismus or retrognathia, in whom adequate visualization of the entire larynx, particularly at the anterior commissure, is not possible.

Contraindications. More extensive lesions involving the contralateral vocal fold.

Pearls for Technique. The main advantage of this approach is the excellent visualization afforded by the laryngofissure. A tracheotomy is generally necessary. For simple cordectomy, healing by secondary intention is an acceptable initial strategy; however, patients are often left with a breathy voice. Reconstruction strategies range from medialization procedures employing autologous or alloplastic materials to local strap muscle flaps to augment the neocord. Injection medialization procedures in the setting of cordectomies are often suboptimal secondary to postoperative scarring and fibrosis.[101] Alloplastic implant medialization techniques provide more consistent voice restoration. Finally, operative reconstruction based on the strap muscles to augment the neocord have shown some efficacy in voice restoration, with both open and endoscopic cordectomies.[102] Imbrication laryngoplasty may be utilized when minimal tumor involvement of the vocal fold permits resection without violation of the false fold and underlying

cartilage. A horizontal strip of thyroid cartilage can then be removed allowing imbrication of the false fold to the glottic level.[103]

Vertical Partial Laryngectomy

Indications. Vertical partial laryngectomy (VPL) is most commonly used to treat T1 lesions of the vocal fold and select T2 lesions. Local recurrence rates after vertical hemilaryngectomy for glottic carcinoma range from 0% to 11% for T1 lesions, 4% to 26% for T2 lesions, and up to 46% for T3 lesions.[104] Excellent oncologic control is generally obtained for T1 glottic carcinomas involving the mobile membranous vocal fold. Decreased oncologic control is evident with anterior commissure involvement, extension beyond the glottis or impaired vocal fold mobility. T2 lesions with impaired vocal fold mobility may have differing degrees of thyroarytenoid invasion within the paraglottic space, explaining decreased oncologic control with VPL. Similarly, subglottic extension of T2 lesions may portend cricoid cartilage invasion, and extension into the supraglottis via the ventricle may increase the risk of thyroid cartilage invasion.[105] These factors may result in the understaging of select "T2" lesions, explaining the higher local failure rates when VPL is employed.

Contraindications. T3 lesions without cricoarytenoid joint involvement are better addressed with a supracricoid laryngectomy.

Pearls for Technique. All vertical partial laryngectomies involve a laryngofissure into the thyroid cartilage and paraglottic space. The placement of the thyrotomy depends on the position of the tumor determined by endoscopy. In the standard vertical partial laryngectomy, the resection extends from the anterior commissure to include the full extent of the membranous vocal fold and intrinsic musculature of the larynx to the vocal process of the arytenoid. The superior and inferior margins of resection are from the false vocal fold to 5 mm below the level of the true fold.[106] A variety of extensions to the basic vertical hemilaryngectomy have been described, including the frontolateral vertical hemilaryngectomy, posterolateral vertical hemilaryngectomy and extended vertical laryngectomy.[104] Of note, when performing a vertical partial laryngectomy, it is advisable to tack the petiole of the epiglottis back into position with a 2-0 Vicryl suture so that the epiglottis will not prolapse posteriorly postoperatively. In addition, after the resection, the anterior commissure of the contralateral side should be sutured to the thyroid lamina to recreate tension of the vocal fold. As was described for cordectomy with laryngofissure, a variety of reconstructive techniques have been employed to facilitate voice restoration.

Open Supraglottic Laryngectomy

Indications. T1 and T2 lesions of the supraglottic larynx. Excellent local control has been reported for T1 and T2 lesions with open supraglottic laryngectomy. T1 local control rates range from 90% to 100%, whereas T2 local control rates range from 85% to 100%. The data on local control rates for more extensive lesions are less consistent, with T3 control rates ranging from 0% to 75% and T4 control rates of 0% to 67%.[107-110]

This discrepancy in the literature may be a result of failure to appreciate extension of the glottic level via paraglottic spread.

Contraindications. Glottic level involvement, invasion of the cricoid or thyroid cartilage, involvement of the tongue base to within 1 cm of the circumvallate papillae, involvement of the deep muscles of the tongue base.

Pearls for Technique. The open supraglottic laryngectomy is defined by both the extent of the resection and the reconstruction. The typical supraglottic laryngectomy preserves both true vocal folds, both arytenoids, the tongue base, and the hyoid bone. Pre-epiglottic space involvement necessitates resection of the hyoid, which can otherwise be left intact. While resecting the hyoid, it is critical to preserve the superior laryngeal neurovascular pedicle, as successful swallowing rehabilitation is dependent on this. The reconstruction varies among surgeons. The approach of the senior author (R.P.T) reconstructs the neolarynx in a fashion analogous to the reconstruction described for supracricoid laryngectomy. Three separate, submucosal, interrupted 1-Vicryl sutures are looped around the remaining thyroid cartilage and inserted into the tongue base. In cases where the hyoid is preserved, the suture is looped around the hyoid as well. This creates an impaction of the tongue base, with or without the hyoid bone, onto the remaining thyroid cartilage.

Supracricoid Laryngectomy

Indications. T1b, T2, T3, and select T4 supraglottic carcinomas with decreased vocal fold motion or fixation, pre-epiglottic space invasion, glottic level involvement at the anterior commissure or ventricle, and limited thyroid cartilage invasion without frank extralaryngeal spread. Excellent local control and actuarial 5-year survival have been reported for both early glottic lesions (T1b-T2) and more advanced lesions.[112] Chevalier and others reported a 5-year actuarial survival of 84.7% and local control rates of 97.3% in 112 patients with either vocal fold fixation or impaired motion on presentation.[113]

Contraindications. Fixation of the arytenoid secondary to cricoarytenoid joint fixation, extrinsic laryngeal muscle involvement or recurrent laryngeal nerve involvement, subglottic extension to the level beyond 1 cm, or direct invasion of the cricoid, posterior commissure involvement, extralaryngeal spread, or extension to the outer perichondrium of the thyroid cartilage.

Pearls for Technique. The supracricoid laryngectomy is likewise defined by both the extent of the resection and reconstruction. The surgical excision is en bloc and includes both true vocal folds, both false vocal folds, both paraglottic spaces, ± epiglottis, the entire thyroid cartilage, and may include one partial or full arytenoid resection. Some key surgical points include:

1. The disarticulation of the cricothyroid joint is of critical importance and should be performed carefully to avoid recurrent laryngeal nerve damage.
2. The cricothyroid membrane should be incised along the superior border of the cricoid cartilage and the subglottic region should be inspected to rule out subglottic extension of the tumor.

3. The arytenoid cartilage (or posterior arytenoid mucosa if the arytenoid is resected) must be gently pulled forward so it will remain in proper positioning postoperatively. This is achieved by placing a 4-0 Vicryl just above the vocal process or into the arytenoid mucosa and secured anteriorly with an air knot.

4. The reconstruction is predicated upon impacting the hyoid bone and tongue base ± the epiglottis to the cricoid cartilage using three symmetric 1-vicryl submucosal sutures.

5. The tracheotomy should be placed in the incision line, but the superior skin flap should be closed to the strap muscles to separate the tracheostoma from the remainder of the neck contents.

Radiation Therapy for Early Larynx Cancer

Part of the multidisciplinary evaluation of the patient with glottic carcinoma includes an assessment by a radiation oncologist. Early glottic malignancies are notable for low incidence of occult nodal metastasis, and as such, single modality treatment with curative radiotherapy is an acceptable option for many patients. Radiotherapy has several advantages, including its noninvasive nature, acceptable voice outcome, and excellent local control rates. For early stage lesions, functional outcomes are generally good, with most patients experiencing only self-limited symptoms of mucositis, xerostomia, dysphagia, odynophagia, and local soft tissue reactions. Vocal quality has been demonstrated to change after radiotherapy, but most patients demonstrate near-normal phonation after 1 year. Harrison et al[114] prospectively examined patients treated with early glottic cancer through computer-assisted voice analysis and determined that the majority of irradiated patients with early glottic cancer demonstrated a decrease in breathiness and increased strain after primary radiotherapy, but enjoyed normal phonation 9 months after treatment.

Primary radiotherapy of glottic carcinoma results in excellent local control rates. In his review of patients treated with primary radiotherapy for T1 glottic carcinoma among series from a single institution, Lee[115] reported local control rates between 81% to 93%. Local control rates for T2 glottic lesions

ranged from 65% to 78%. Prognostic factors, such as involvement of the anterior commissure, tumor bulk, and the technical aspects of radiation biology have been evaluated in the literature. In several series, patients with involvement of the anterior commissure who were treated with primary radiotherapy fared worse in terms of local control, particularly for T1 lesions.[116,117] In a published 30-year experience of T1 glottic cancers treated with primary radiotherapy, Reddy et al[118] examined the effects of tumor bulk, T-stage, anterior-commissure involvement, treatment duration and fraction size on local control. Although anterior commissure involvement was not prognostic in this series, tumor bulk proved to be a significant prognostic factor on multivariate analysis, as patients with bulky tumors had lower local control and disease-free survival rates and shorter duration to recurrence than those with small tumors. Finally, technical aspects of radiotherapy, including total dose, fraction size, and overall time have been demonstrated to be significant prognostic factors for local control of T2 but not T1 carcinomas.[116]

Primary radiotherapy of early supraglottic malignancies likewise results in excellent local control rates. In contrast to glottic level malignancies, supraglottic carcinomas have extensive lymphatic networks bilaterally, resulting in a high incidence of occult jugulodigastric nodal metastasis at diagnosis. Local control after radiotherapy for early stage supraglottic carcinoma ranges from 88% to 100% for T1 lesions and 65% to 89% for T2 lesions.[119-124] Because of the concern for regional nodal metastasis, the treatment volume for carcinoma of the supraglottis includes both the primary lesion and the regional nodal basin.[125] The specifics of the radiation techniques vary per series, and ranges from single fractionated once daily treatments to twice daily hyperfractionation and accelerated hyperfractional schedules.

Surgical Salvage of Early Larynx Cancer

Although total laryngectomy has traditionally been standard of care for surgical salvage of radiation failure in laryngeal cancer, transoral laser microsurgical and open conservation laryngeal surgery approaches are gaining acceptance for select patients who present with recurrence. Steiner and others have advocated transoral laser microsurgery as a surgical modality in the salvage setting for patients with recurrent glottic carcinoma after radiation. In their series of 34 patients with early and advanced recurrent glottic carcinoma after full-course radiotherapy, they demonstrated a 71% cure rate with one or more laser procedures, with only one patient requiring total laryngectomy (because of chondroradionecrosis).[126]

Conservation laryngeal surgical approaches have also been used in the salvage setting with success. In their 20-year review of the MD Anderson experience of treating radiation failures with salvage surgery, Holsinger and others used well-established contraindications for conservation laryngeal surgery approaches including arytenoid fixation, extensive pre-epiglottic space invasion, subglottic extension, and extralaryngeal spread to exclude patients who were inappropriate candidates.[127] For those patients who were good candidates, a conservation laryngeal surgical approach instead of total laryngectomy did not cause a demonstrable change in locoregional control or disease-free survival. Other groups have reported similar results. In their review of 15 patients treated with supracricoid partial laryngectomy for surgical salvage, Spriano and others reported excellent long-term oncologic control.[128] Laccourreye et al[129] demonstrated a 75% long-term larynx preservation rate with 100% local control for patients initially treated with supracricoid laryngectomy after failed radiotherapy. With regard to open versus endolaryngeal approaches for surgical salvage, Motamed et al[130] investigated this question in the literature. In their metaanalysis of all published literature on surgical salvage in laryngeal cancer, they found a preponderance of literature to support the role of conservation laryngeal surgery in the treatment of recurrent localized disease after radiotherapy. They furthermore exhibited a modest benefit of open versus endolaryngeal approaches in overall local control.

Complications in the postoperative setting are higher in those patients who have previously received radiation therapy. In radiation-naïve patients, SCPL can be performed with low morbidity and mortality. In one of the largest series published of radiation-naïve patients undergoing SCPL, Naudo and others demonstrated a 1% mortality and 12% local complication rate.[131] Previously radiated patients seem to fare worse, however. In a series of 23 patients managed with supracricoid laryngectomy for surgical salvage over a 14-year period, Makeieff et al[132] found that whereas 17 of 23 experienced rapid functional recovery of swallowing, a significant percentage, (17.4%) developed long-term swallowing impairments, with two patient dying from aspiration complications. Several series have demonstrated markedly increased early and late complication rates in previously radiated patients. In their series, Laccourreye had a major complication rate of 42%.[129] Spriano et al[128] described a similarly high major complication rate in previously radiated patients. A later published series by the same group demonstrated that swallowing problems postoperatively were the most common challenge in the previously radiated patient.[133] Likewise, in their metanalysis of the literature, Marioni[134] and others found prolonged dysphagia and aspiration to be more common in radiated patients, with aspiration pneumonia and neolaryngeal edema to be the most frequent reported postoperative complications overall. Several groups have advocated early gastrostomy tube placement in this regard.[135]

Management of the Neck in Early Larynx Cancer

Factors influencing the management of the neck in early glottic cancer include the TNM staging of the primary lesion, subsite of the larynx involved, and the modality chosen to treat the primary lesion. As discussed previously, early stage lesions of the glottic larynx have low rates of regional lymph node metastasis because of the relative paucity of lymphatic drainage from this area. For early stage lesions of the glottis in the N0 neck, close observation is an acceptable management strategy. The supraglottic larynx, in contrast, has an extensive bilateral network of lymphatics along the jugulodigastric nodal basin. Lutz and other colleagues at the University of Pittsburgh,[136] in a retrospective review of 202 patients with supraglottic squamous cell carcinoma treated with surgery or combined therapy, demonstrated a locoregional failure rate of 23%. In those treatment failures, 83% occurred in the neck with 90% of neck failures occurring in the undissected, contralateral side. A later report by the same group confirmed a cervical recurrence reduction from 20% to 9% by performing routine bilateral neck dissections in these patients.[137] In their most recent report advocating routine bilateral neck dissections in all patients with T2 to T4 lesions and select patients with T1 lesions, this approach demonstrated a further risk reduction of cervical recurrence rate to 7.8%.[138] These data representing such a significant risk reduction in locoregional failure in the neck provide a compelling argument to advocate routine bilateral neck dissection in the management of supraglottic cancer. Steiner and others, in their 24-year series of patients treated with transoral laser resection of supraglottic carcinomas, determined that management of the neck, either by neck dissection or postoperative radiotherapy is advisable.[139] Observation of the neck in those patients with select T1 lesions treated with primary transoral laser mircrosurgery may be an acceptable management strategy in the N0 neck, although this remains controversial in the literature.

Management strategies of the neck in patients undergoing salvage laryngeal surgery for recurrent/persistent laryngeal cancer are highly variable. Yao and others, because of the risk of occult disease, advocate bilateral neck dissections for T3 and T4 recurrent glottic lesions, and bilateral neck dissections for all recurrent supraglottic lesions.[140] In our institution, patients undergoing salvage total or supracricoid laryngectomy for laryngeal cancer recurrence/persistence after primary radiotherapy are staged by a preoperative CT scan. In those patients staged N0, the neck is managed expectantly. We have previously reported no increased risk of recurrence in these patients with long-term follow-up.[141] The addition of PET-CT in both the preoperative staging and postoperative surveillance period could potentially aid the head and neck surgeon in assessing the risk of occult disease and treating the neck appropriately in these settings.

REFERENCES

1. Jemal A, Siegel R, Ward E, Murray T, Xu J, Thun MJ. Cancer statistics, 2007. *CA Cancer J Clin.* 2007; 57(1):43–66.

2. Davies L, Welch HG. Epidemiology of head and neck cancer in the United States. *Otolaryngol Head Neck Surg.* 2006;135(3):451–457.

3. Farrag TY, Koch WM, Cummings CW, et al. Supracricoid laryngectomy outcomes: the Johns Hopkins experience. *Laryngoscope.* 2007;117(1): 129–132.

4. Farrag TY, Lin FR, Cummings CW, et al. Importance of routine evaluation of the thyroid gland prior to open partial laryngectomy. *Arch Otolaryngol Head Neck Surg.* 2006;132(10):1047–1051.

5. Farrag TY, Lin FR, Cummings CW, et al. Neck management in patients undergoing postradiotherapy salvage laryngeal surgery for recurrent/persistent laryngeal cancer. *Laryngoscope.* 2006;116(10): 1864–1866.

6. Lewin F, Norell SE, Johansson H, et al. Smoking tobacco, oral snuff, and alcohol in the etiology of squamous cell carcinoma of the head and neck: a population-based case-referent study in Sweden. *Cancer.* 1998;82(7):1367–1375.

7. Maier H, Dietz A, Gewelke U, Heller WD, Weidauer H. Tobacco and alcohol and the risk of head and neck cancer. *Clin Inves.* 1992;70(3–4): 320–327.

8. Maier H, Tisch M, Conradt C, Potschke-Langer M. Alcohol drinking and cancer of the upper aerodigestive tract in women (abstract). *Dtsch Med Wochenschr.* 1999;124(28–29):851–854.

9. Russo A, Crosignani P, Berrino F. Tobacco smoking, alcohol drinking and dietary factors as determinants of new primaries among male laryngeal cancer patients: a case-cohort study. *Tumori.* 1996;82(6):519–525.

10. Crosignani P, Russo A, Tagliabue G, Berrino F. Tobacco and diet as determinants of survival in male laryngeal cancer patients. *Int J Cancer.* 1996;65(3):308–313.

11. De Stefani E, Correa P, Oreggia F, et al. Risk factors for laryngeal cancer. *Cancer.* 1987;60(12): 3087–3091.

12. Freudenheim JL, Graham S, Byers TE, et al. Diet, smoking, and alcohol in cancer of the larynx: a case-control study. *Nutr Cancer.* 1992;17(1): 33–45.

13. Goldenberg D, Lee J, Koch WM, et al. Habitual risk factors for head and neck cancer. *Otolaryngol Head Neck Surg.* 2004;131(6):986–993.

14. Galli J, Cammarota G, Volante M, De Corso E, Almadori G, Paludetti G. Laryngeal carcinoma and laryngo-pharyngeal reflux disease. *Acta Otorhinolaryngol Ital.* 2006;26(5):260–263.

15. Mercante G, Bacciu A, Ferri T, Bacciu S. Gastro-esophageal reflux as a possible co-promoting factor in the development of the squamous-cell carcinoma of the oral cavity, of the larynx and of the pharynx. *Acta Otorhinolaryngol Belg.* 2003; 57(2):113-117.

16. Galli J, Cammarota G, Calo L, et al. The role of acid and alkaline reflux in laryngeal squamous cell carcinoma. *Laryngoscope.* 2002;112(10):1861-1865.

17. Chen MY, Ott DJ, Casolo BJ, Moghazy KM, Koufman JA. Correlation of laryngeal and pharyngeal carcinomas and 24-hour pH monitoring of the esophagus and pharynx. *Otolaryngol Head Neck Surg.* 1998;119(5):460-462.

18. Galli J, Frenguelli A, Calo L, Agostino S, Cianci R, Cammarota G. Role of gastroesophageal reflux in precancerous conditions and in squamous cell carcinoma of the larynx: our experience. *Acta Otorhinolaryngol Ital.* 2001;21(6):350-355.

19. Kurozumi S, Harada Y, Sugimoto Y, et al. Airway malignancy in poisonous gas workers. *J Laryngol Otol.* 1977;91:217-225.

20. Morgan R, Shettigara P, Occupational asbestos exposure, smoking, and laryngeal carcinoma. *Ann N Y Acad Sci.* 1976;271:308-310.

21. Goolden A. Radiation cancer of the pharynx. *Br Med J.* 1951;2:1110-1112.

22. Wight R, Paleri V, Arullendran P. Current theories for the development of nonsmoking and non-drinking laryngeal carcinoma. *Curr Opin Otolaryngol Head Neck Surg.* 2003;11(2):73-77.

23. Leon X, Rinaldo A, Saffiotti U, Ferlito A. Laryngeal cancer in non-smoking and nondrinking patients. *Acta Otolaryngol.* 2004;124(6):664-669.

24. Luna MA, Tortoledo ME. Verrucous carcinoma. In: Gnepp DR, ed. *Pathology of the Head and Neck.* New York, NY: Churchill Livingstone; 1988:497.

25. Mansel RH, Vemeersch H. *Panendoscopies for second primaries in head and neck cancer.* Presented at: American Laryngological Society Meeting; May 1981; Vancouver, BC.

26. Crissman J, Laryngeal keratosis preceding laryngeal carcinoma. *Arch Otolaryngol.* 1982;108:445-448.

27. Sllamniku B, Bauer W, Painter C, et al. The transformation of laryngeal keratosis into invasive carcinoma. *Am J Otolaryngol.* 1989;10:42-54.

28. Hojslet PE, Nielsen VM, Palvio D. Premalignant lesions of the larynx. *Acta Otolaryngol.* 1989; 107;150-155.

29. Kashima H. The characteristics of laryngeal cancer correlating with cervical lymph node metas-tasis. In: Albert F, Bryce D, eds. *Workshops from the Centennial Conference on Laryngeal Cancer.* East Norwalk, Conn: Appleton-Century-Crofts; 1976:855.

30. Spiro RH, Alfonso AE, Parr HW, Strong EW. Cervical node metastases for epidermal carcinoma: a critical assessment of current staging. *Am J Surg.* 1974;562-567.

31. McGavran MH, Bauer WC, Ogura HJ. The incidence of cervical lymph node metastases from epidennoid carcinoma of the larynx and their relationship to certain characteristics of the primary tumor. *Cancer.* 1961;14:55-66.

32. Kirchner JA, Comog JL Jr, Holmes RE. Transglottic cancer: its growth and spread within the larynx. *Arch Otolaryngol.* 1974;99:247-251.

33. Micheau C, Luboinski B, Sancho H, et al. Modes of invasion of cancer of the larynx; a statistical, histological and radioclinical analysis of 120 cases. *Cancer.* 1976;38:346-360.

34. Kirchner JA. One hundred laryngeal cancer studies by serial section. *Ann Otol Rhinol Laryngol.* 1969;78:689-709.

35. Olofsson J, Lord IJ, van Nostrand AW. Vocal cord fixation in laryngeal carcinoma. *Acta Otolaryngol (Stockh).* 1973;75:496-510.

36. Lindberg R. Distribution of cervical lymph node metastases from squamous cell carcinoma of upper respiratory and digestive tracts. *Cancer.* 1972;29:1446-1449.

37. Ogura J, Biller H, Wette R. Elective neck dissection for pharyngeal and laryngeal cancers. *Ann Otol Laryngol.* 1971;60:646-650.

38. Putney FJ. Elective versus delayed neck dissection in cancer of the larynx. *Surg Gynecol Opstet.* 1961;112:736-742.

39. Fletcher GH. Elective irradiation of subclinical disease in cancers of the head and neck. *Cancer.* 1972;29:1450-1454.

40. Levendag P, Vikram B. The problem of neck relapse in early-stage supraglottic cancer—results of different treatment modalities for the clinically negative neck. *Int J Radial Oncol Biol Phys.* 1987; 13:1621-1624.

41. Kirchner JA, Owen JR. Five hundred cancers of the larynx and pyriform sinus. *Laryngoscope.* 1977,87:1288-1303.

42. Ogura JH, Sessions DG, Specter GJ. Conservation surgery for epidermoid carcinoma of the supraglottic larynx. *Laryngoscope.* 1975;85:1808-1815.

43. Fayos JV. Carcinoma of the endolarynx: results of irradiation. *Cancer.* 1975;35:1525-1532.

44. Hansen HS. Supraglottic carcinoma of the aryepiglottis fold. *Laryngoscope.* 1975;85:1667-1681.

45. Shah J, Tollefsen H. Epidermoid carcinoma of the supraglottic larynx. *Am J Surg.* 1974;128:494-499.

46. Ogura JH, Spector GJ, Sessions DG. Conservation surgery for carcinoma of the marginal area. *Laryngoscope.* 1975;85:1801-1807.

47. Biller HF, Davis WH, Ogura JH. Delayed contralateral cervical metastasis with laryngeal and laryngopharyngeal cancers. *Laryngoscope.* 1971;81: 1499-1502.

48. Som ML. Conservation surgery for carcinoma of the supraglottis. *J Laryngol Otol.* 1970;84:655-678.

49. Lawson W, Biller H, Suen J. Cancer of the larynx. In: Myers G, Suen J, eds. *Cancer of the Head and Neck.* 2nd ed. New York, NY: Churchill Livingstone;1989:533.

50. Kirchner JA. Staging as seen in serial sections. *Laryngoscope.* 1975;85:1816-1821.

51. Fischer JJ. Anterior commissure cancer. In: Alberti P, Bryce D, eds. *Workshops from the Centennial Conference on Laryngeal Cancer.* East Norwalk, Conn: Appleton-Century-Crofts; 1976:679.

52. Jesse RH, Lindberg RD, Horiot JC. Vocal cord cancer with anterior commissure extension; choice of treatment. *Am J Surg.* 1971;122:437-439.

53. Sessions D, Ogura, J, Fried M- Laryngeal carcinoma involving anterior commissure and subglottis. In: Alberti P, Bryce D, eds. *Workshops from the Centennial Conference on Laryngeal Cancer.* East Norwalk, Conn: Appleton-Century-Crofts; 1976: 674-678.

54. Olofsson J, van Nostrand AWP. Growth and spread of laryngeal and hypopharyngeal carcinoma with reflections on the effect of preoperative irradiation; 139 cases studied by whole organ serial sectioning. *Acta Otolaryngol Suppl (Stockh).* 1973; 308:1-84.

55. Stell P. The subglottic space. In: Alberti P, Bryce D, eds. *Workshops from the Centennial Conference on Laryngeal Cancer.* East Norwalk, Conn: Appleton-Century-Crofts; 1976:682.

56. Harrison DE. The pathology and management of subglottic cancer. *Ann Otol Rhinol Laryngol.* 1971;80:6-12.

57. Fletcher GH. Elective irradiation of subclinical disease in cancers of the head and neck. *Cancer.* 1972;29:1450-1454.

58. Ogura JH, Biller HF, Wette R. Elective neck dissection for pharyngeal and laryngeal cancers: an evaluation. *Ann Otol Rhinol Laryngol.* 1971;80; 646-650.

59. Mendenhall WM, Parsons IT, Stringer SP, et al. T1-T2 vocal cord carcinoma; a basis for comparing the results of radiotherapy and surgery. *Head Neck Surg.* 1988;10:373-377.

60. Biller HF, Ogura JH, Bauer WC. Verrucous cancer of the larynx. *Laryngoscope.* 1971;81:1323-1329.

61. Abramson AL, Brandsma J, Steinberg B, et al. Verrucous carcinoma of the larynx; possible human papillomavirus etiology. *Acta Otolaryngol (Stockh).* 1985;111:709-715.

62. Glanz H, Kleinsasser O. Verrucous carcinoma of me larynx—a misnomer. *Arch Otorhinolaryngol.* 1987;244:108-111.

63. Medina JE, Dichtel W, Luna MA. Verrucous-squamous carcinomas of the oral cavity. A clinicopathologic study of 104 cases. *Arch Otolaryngol.* 1984;110:437-440.

64. Vidyasagar MS, Fernandes DJ, Kasturi D, et al. Radiotherapy and verrucous carcinoma of the oral cavity. A study of 107 cases. *Acta Oncol.* 1992;31: 43-47.

65. Kraus FT, Perezmesa C. Verrucous carcinoma: clinical and pathological study of 105 cases involving oral cavity, larynx, and genitalia. *Cancer.* 1966;19: 26-38.

66. Fonts EA, Greenlaw RH, Rush BF, et al. Verrucous squamous cell carcinoma of the oral cavity. *Cancer.* 1969;23:152-160.

67. Perez CA, Kraus FT, Evans JC, et al. Anaplastic transformation in verrucous carcinoma of the oral cavity after radiation therapy. *Radiology.* 1966; 26:108-115.

68. Elliot GB, Macdougall JA, Elliot JD. Problems of verrucous squamous carcinoma. *Ann Surg.* 1973;177:21-29.

69. Hagen P, Lyons GD, Haindel C. Verrucous carcinoma of the larynx: role of human papillomavirus, radiation and surgery. *Laryngoscope.* 1993;103: 253-257.

70. Demian SD, Bushkin FL, Echevarria RA. Perineural invasion and anaplastic transformation of verrucous carcinoma. *Cancer.* 1973;32:395-401.

71. Tharp ME 2nd, Shidnia H. Radiotherapy in the treatment of verrucous carcinoma of the head and neck. *Laryngoscope.* 1995;105:391-396.

72. Burns HP, van Nostrand AW, Bryce DP. Verrucous carcinoma of the larynx; management by radiotherapy and surgery. *Ann Otol Rhinol Laryngol.* 1976;85:538-543.

73. Hong W O'Donoghue G, Sheetz S. Sequential response patterns to chemotherapy and radiotherapy in head and neck cancer. In: Wagener D,

Bligham G, Sweets V, et al, eds. *Primary Chemotherapy in Cancer Medicine,* Vol 201. New York, NY: Alan R. Liss; 1985:191.

74. Myerowitz R, Barnes EL, Myers E. Small cell anaplastic (oat cell) carcinoma of the larynx. *Laryngoscope.* 1978;88:1697-1702.

75. Gould VE, Linnoila RI, Memoli VA, Warren W. Neuroendocrine components of the bronchopulinonary tract. *Lab Invest.* 1983;49:519-537.

76. Mullins JD, Newman RK, Coltman CA Jr. Primary oat cell carcinoma of the larynx. *Cancer.* 1979; 43:711-717.

77. Goldman NC, Hood CI, Singleton GG. Carcinoid of the larynx. *Arch Otolaryngol.* 1969;90:64-67.

78. Huizenga C, Balogh K. Cartilaginous tumors of the larynx. *Cancer.* 1970;36:201-210.

79. Blitzer A, Lawson W, Biller H. Malignant fibrous histiocytoma of the head and neck. *Laryngoscope.* 1977;87:1479-1499.

80. Maniglia AJ, Xue JW. Plasmacytoma of the larynx. *Laryngoscope.* 1983;93:741-744.

81. Booth JB, Osborn DA. Granular cell myoblastoma of the larynx. *Acta Otolaryngol.* 1970;70:279-293.

82. Anderson HA, Maisel RH, Cantrell RW. Isolated laryngeal lymphoma. *Laryngoscope.* 1976;86: 1251-1257.

83. Mancuso AA. Imaging in patients with head and neck cancer. In; Million RR, Cassisi NJ, eds. *Management of Head and Neck Cancer: A Multidisciplinary Approach.* 2nd ed. Philadelphia, Pa: JB Lippincott Co; 1994:43-59.

84. McLaughlin MP, Mendenhall WM, Mancuso AA, et al. Retropharyngeal adenopathy as a predictor of outcome in squamous cell carcinoma of the head and neck. *Head Neck.* 1995;17:190-198.

85. Mancuso AA. Hanafee WN. *Computed Tomography and Magnetic Resonance Imagine of the Head and Neck.* 2nd ed. Baltimore, Md: Williams & Wilkins; 1985.

86. Verdonck-de Leeuw IM, Hilgers FJM, Keus RB, et al. Multidimensional assessment of voice characteristics after radiotherapy for early glottic cancer. *Laryngoscope.* 1999;109:241-248.

87. Benninger MS, Gillen J, Thieme P, et al. Factors associated with recurrence and voice quality following radiation therapy for Tl and T2 glottic carcinomas. *Laryngoscope.* 1994;104:294-298.

88. Casiano RR, Cooper JD, Lundy DS, et al. Laser cordectomy for T1 glottic carcinoma: a 10-year experience and videostroboscopic findings. *Otolaryngol Head Neck Surg.* 1991;104:831-837.

89. Back G, Sood S. The management of early laryngeal cancer: options for patients and therapists. *Curr Opin Otolaryngol Head Neck Surg.* 2005; 13:85-91.

90. Myers EN, Wagner RL, Johnson JT. Microlaryngoscopic surgery for T1 glottic lesions: a cost-effective option. *Ann Otol Rhinol Laryngol.* 1994;103:28-30.

91. Smith JC, Johnson JT, Cognetti DM, et al. Quality of life, functional outcome and costs of early glottic cancer. *Laryngoscope.* 2003;113:68-76.

92. Brandenburg JH. Laser cordotomy versus radiotherapy: an objective cost analysis. *Ann Otol Rhinol Laryngol.* 2001;110:312-318.

93. Remacle M, Eckel HE, Antonelli A, et al. Endoscopic cordectomy: a proposal for a classification by the working committee: European Laryngological Society. *Eur Arch Otorhinolaryngol.* 2000;257:227-231.

94. Gallo A, de Vincentiis M, Manciooco V, et al. CO_2 laser cordectomy for early-stage glottic carcinoma: a long term follow-up of 156 cases. *Laryngoscope.* 2002;12:370-374.

95. Chen MF, Chang JT, Tsang NM, et al. Radiotherapy of early-stage glottic cancer: analysis of factors affecting prognosis. *Ann Otol Rhinol Laryngol.* 2003;112:904-911.

96. Zeitels SM, Hillman RE, Franco RA, et al. Voice and treatment outcome from phonosurgical management of early glottic cancer. *Ann Otol Rhinol Laryngol Suppl.* 2002;190:3-20.

97. Steiner W, Ambrosch P, Rodel RM, et al. Impact of anterior commissure involvement on local control of early glottic carcinoma treated by laser microresection. *Laryngoscope.* 2004;114;1485-1491.

98. Zeitels SM. Surgical management of early supraglottic cancer. *Otolaryngol Clin North Am.* 1997;30:59-78.

99. Motta G, Esposito E, Testa D, et al. CO_2 laser treatment of supraglottic cancer. *Head Neck.* 2004; 26:442-446.

100. Davis RK, Kriskovich MD, Galloway EB, et al. Endoscopic supraglottic laryngectomy with post-operative irradiation. *Ann Otol Rhinol Laryngol.* 2004;113:132-138.

101. Hsiung MW, Woo P, Minasian A, et al. Fat augmentation for glottic insufficiency. *Laryngoscope.* 2000;110:1026-1033.

102. Su CY, Chuang HC, Tsai SS, Chiu JF. Bipedicled strap muscle transposition for focal fold defect after laser cordectomy in early glottic cancer patients. *Laryngoscope.* 2005;115:528-533.

103. Liu C, Ward PH, Pleet L. Imbrication reconstruction following partial laryngectomy. *Ann Otol Rhinol Laryngol.* 1986;95:567-571.

104. Tufano RP, Laccourreye O, Rassekh C et al. Conservation laryngeal surgery. In: *Cummings' Otolaryngology-Head and Neck Surgery.* 4th ed. Philadelphia, Pa: Elsevier Mosby; 2005:2357-2358.

105. Mohr RM, Quenelle J, Shumrick DA. Verticofrontolateral laryngectomy (hemilaryngectomy). *Arch Otolaryngol.* 1983;109:384-395.

106. Shah H. A view of partial laryngectomy in the treatment of laryngeal cancer. *J Laryngol Otol.* 1987;101:143-154.

107. Lee NK, Goepfert H, Wendt CD. Supraglottic laryngectomy for intermediate stage cancer: UT MD Anderson Cancer Center experience with combined therapy. *Laryngoscope.* 1990;100: 831-836.

108. Burstein FD, Calcaterra TC. Supraglottic laryngectomy: series report and analysis of results. *Laryngoscope.* 1985; 95:833-836.

109. Alonso Regules JE, Blasiak J, de Vilaseca BA. End results of partial horizontal (functional) laryngectomy in Uruguay. *Can J Otolaryngol.* 1975;4: 397-399.

110. Spaulding CA, Constable WC, Levine PA, et al. Partial laryngectomy and radiotherapy for supraglottic cancer: a conservative approach. *Ann Otol Rhinol Laryngol.* 1988;98:125-129.

111. Herranz-Gonzales J, Gavilan J, Martinez-Vidal J, et al. Supraglottic laryngectomy: functional and oncologic results. *Ann Otol Rhinol Laryngol.* 1996;105:18-22.

112. Laccourreye O, Muscatello L, Laccourreye L, et al. Supracricoid partial laryngectomy with cricohyoidoepiglottopexy for "early" glottic carcinoma classified as T1-T2N0 invading the anterior commissure. *Am J Otolaryngol.* 1997;18:385-390.

113. Chevalier D, Laccourreye O, Brasnu D, et al. Cricohyoidoepiglottopexy for glottic carcinoma with fixation or impaired motion of the true vocal cord: 5-year oncologic results with 112 patients. *Ann Otol Rhinol Laryngol.* 1997;106:364-369.

114. Harrison LB, Solomon B, Miller S, et al. Prospective computer-assisted voice analysis for patients with early stage glottic cancer: a preliminary report of the functional result of laryngeal irradiation. *Int J Radiat Oncol Biol Phys.* 1990;19:123-127.

115. Lee DJ. Definitive radiotherapy for squamous cell carcinoma of the larynx. *Otolaryngol Clin North Am.* 2002;35:1013-1033.

116. Le QT, Fu KK, Kroll S, et al. Influence of fraction size, total dose and overall time on local control of T1-T2 glottic carcinoma. *Int J Radiat Oncol Biol Phys.* 1997;39:115-126.

117. Nozaki M, Furata M, Murakami Y, et al. Radiation therapy for T1 glottic cancer: involvement of the anterior commissure. *Anticancer Res.* 2000;20: 1121-1124.

118. Reddy SP, Hong RL, Naqda S, et al. Effect of tumor bulk on local control and survival of patients with T1 glottic cancer: a 30-year experience. *Int J Radiat Oncol Biol Phys.* 2007; [Epub ahead of print].

119. Ghossein NA, Bataini JP, Ennuyer A, et al. Local control and site of failure in radically irradiated supraglottic laryngeal cancer. *Radiology.* 1974; 112:187-192.

120. Wall TJ, Peters LJ, Brown BW, et al. Relationship between lymph node status and primary tumor control probability in tumors of the supraglottic larynx. *Int J Radiat Oncol Biol Phys.* 1985;11: 1895-1902.

121. Wang CC, Montgomery WW. Deciding on optimal management of supraglottic carcinoma. *Oncology.* 1991;5:41-46.

122. Nakfoor BM, Spiro IJ, Wang CC, et al. Results of accelerated radiotherapy for supraglottic carcinoma: a Massachusetts General Hospital and Massachusetts Eye and Ear Infirmary experience. *Head Neck.* 1998;20:379-384.

123. Sykes AJ, Slevin NJ, Gupta NK, et al. 331 cases of clinically node-negative supraglottic carcinoma of the larynx: a study of modest size fixed field radiotherapy approach. *Int J Radiat Oncol Biol Phys.* 2000;46:1109-1115.

124. Hinerman RW, Mendenhall WM, Amdur, et al. Carcinoma of the supraglottic larynx: treatment results with radiotherapy alone or with planned neck dissection. *Head Neck.* 2002;24:456-467.

125. Kumar P. Radiation therapy for the larynx and hypopharyx. In: *Cummings Otolaryngology and Head and Neck Surgery.* 4th ed. Philadelphia, Pa: Elsevier Mosby; 2005:2401-2419.

126. Steiner W, Vogt P, Ambrosch P, et al. Transoral carbon dioxide laser microsurgery for recurrent glottic carcinoma after radiotherapy. *Head Neck.* 2004;26:477-484.

127. Holsinger FC, Funk E, Roberts DB, et al. Conservation laryngeal surgery versus total laryngectomy for radiation failure in laryngeal cancer. *Head Neck.* 2006;28:779-784.

128. Spriano G, Pellini R, Romano G, et al. Supracricoid partial laryngectomy as salvage surgery after radiation failure. *Head Neck*. 2002;24:759-765.

129. Laccourreye O, Weinstein G, Naudo P. et al. Supracricoid partial laryngectomy after failed laryngeal radiation therapy. *Laryngoscope*. 1996;106:495-498.

130. Motamed M, Laccourreye O, Bradley BJ. Salvage conservation laryngeal surgery after irradiation failure for early laryngeal cancer. *Laryngoscope*. 2006;116:45145-45155.

131. Naudo P, Laccourreye O, Weinstein G, et al. Functional outcome and prognosis factors after supracricoid partial laryngectomy with cricohyoidopexy. *Ann Otol Rhinol Laryngol*. 1997;106:291-295.

132. Makeiff M, Venegoni D, Mercante G, et al. Supracricoid partial laryngectomies after failure of radiation therapy. *Laryngoscope*. 2005;115:353-357.

133. Pellini R, Manciocco V, Spriano G. Functional outcome of supracricoid partial laryngectomy with cricohyoidopexy. *Arch Otolaryngol Head Neck Surg*. 2006;132:1221-1225.

134. Marioni G, Marchese-Ragona R, Pastore A, et al. The role of supracricoid laryngectomy for glottic carcinoma recurrence after radiotherapy failure: a critical review. *Acta Oto-Laryngologica*. 2006;126:1245-1251.

135. Clark J, Morgan G, Veness M. Salvage with supracricoid partial laryngectomy after radiation failure. *ANZ J Surg*. 2005;75:958-962.

136. Lutz CK, Johnson JT Wagner RL, et al. Supraglottic carcinoma: patterns of recurrence. *Ann Otol Rhinol Laryngol*. 1990;99:12-17.

137. Weber PC, Johnson JT, Myers EN. The impact of bilateral neck dissection on pattern of recurrence and survival in supraglottic carcinoma. *Arch Otolaryngol Head Neck Surg*. 1994;120:703-706.

138. Chiu RJ, Myers EN, Johnson JT. Efficacy of routine bilateral neck dissection in the management of supraglottic cancer. *Otolaryngol Head Neck Surg*. 2004;131:485-488.

139. Iro H, Waldfahrer F, Altendorf-Hofmann A, et al. Transoral laser surgery of supraglottic cancer: follow-up of 141 patients. *Arch Otolaryngol Head Neck Surg*. 1998;124:1245-1250.

140. Yao M, Roebuck JC, Holsinger FC, et al. Elective neck dissection during salvage laryngectomy. *Am J Otolaryngol*. 2005;26:388-392.

141. Farrag TY, Lin FR, Cummings CW, et al. Neck management in patients undergoing postradiotherapy salvage laryngeal surgery for recurrent/persistent laryngeal cancer. *Laryngoscope*. 2006;116:1864-1866.

17

Management of Advanced Laryngeal Cancer

Umamaheswar Duvvuri
Robert L. Ferris

INTRODUCTION

Laryngeal cancer accounts for approximately 1.5% of all cancers in the United States. Heavy tobacco and alcohol consumption are known to be etiologic factors and contribute to the development of squamous cell carcinoma (SCCa). The risk of developing laryngeal cancer increases with increasing exposure to tobacco and may decrease with the time after cessation. The effect of combined alcohol and tobacco use seems to be synergistic. A small fraction of these tumors harbor oncogenic HPV subtypes, but much less commonly than oropharyngeal tumors.[1]

An understanding of laryngeal anatomy and physiology is essential to allow the clinician to understand how the cancer affects laryngeal function. In addition one needs to consider the presenting symptoms and how the treatment paradigms (surgical or nonsurgical) can affect patient outcomes and quality of life. Thus, the extent of tumor within the larynx influences the choice of treatment modalities.

The larynx is generally divided into 3 regions, namely, the supraglottis, glottis, and subglottis. The supraglottis extends from the tip of the epiglottis to the superior surface of the vocal folds. The glottis begins in the ventricle, at the superior surface of the

vocal folds, and extends inferiorly to 5 mm below the vocal folds. The subglottic region starts below the true vocal fold and extends to the inferior edge of the cricoid cartilage.

The major histology in laryngeal cancer is squamous cell carcinoma (~95%). Other more rare pathologies include adenocarcinoma, mucoepidermoid carcinoma, adenoid cystic carcinoma, neuroendocrine tumors, lymphoma, melanoma, and mesenchymal tumors, such as sarcomas, leiomyosarcomas, and hemangiosarcomas.

Cancer of the glottis is three-fold more common than cancer of the supraglottis or the subglottis. For the purposes of this chapter, we focus on carcinomas arising in the supraglottis and glottis, because advanced subglottic carcinoma tends to arise from the inferior glottis in many cases and as such can be treated in the same fashion as advanced glottic carcinoma.

An understanding of the lymphatic drainage of the larynx is essential for the diagnosis and treatment of regional metastases. The patterns of lymphatic drainage from the larynx are predictable and have been well studied. Carcinomas arising from the true vocal folds generally do not metastasize to cervical nodes. This has been attributed to the relative paucity of lymphatic channels in the region of the true vocal folds. The lymphatic drainage becomes progressively richer above and below the glottis necessitating routine treatment of the neck in supraglottic cancer.[2,3] The lymphatic channels from the supraglottis drain into the upper, mid, and lower jugular nodes. The lymphatic channels from the subglottis drain to the mid and lower jugular nodes, the prelaryngeal (Delphian) nodes, and also the paratracheal nodes.

For the purposes of this chapter, advanced laryngeal cancer is defined on the basis of the primary tumor. That is, T3 and T4 lesions are considered advanced tumors. The management of the cervical nodal basins are discussed separately at the end of the chapter.

CLINICAL PRESENTATION, DIAGNOSIS, AND MANAGEMENT

The most common presenting symptoms of patients with advanced glottic cancer include hoarseness, otalgia, and dyspnea. Localized pain as a result of invasion of local tissues by the tumor is also possible. The most common presenting symptoms of advanced supraglottic cancer are the sore throat, dysphagia, and odynophagia in addition to the symptoms listed above. Advanced disease can also present with systemic symptoms such as weight loss, malaise, aspiration, and foul odor from necrotic tumor.

Unilateral referred otalgia results from involvement of the ipsilateral vagus nerve and Arnold's nerve. Sore throat, dysphagia, and odynophagia result from the mass effect of the tumor and muscular infiltration. Dysphagia is a complicated phenomenon that can result from decreased mobility of the supraglottic larynx with deglutition and/or decreased sensation of the supraglottic larynx.

DIAGNOSTIC EVALUATION

The diagnostic evaluation of any patient with suspected laryngeal cancer begins with a thorough history and physical examination.[4] The detailed history should not only seek to address the above stated

symptoms, but should also ascertain information about general physical health, in particular, the cardiopulmonary status of the patient. Any evidence of dyspnea at rest or on exertion should be elicited. The inability of a patient to sleep at night or lay in a supine position is an indicator of impending respiratory distress and warrants consideration of an emergency tracheotomy. The exercise tolerance of the patient can provide valuable information about the cardiopulmonary reserve of this group of patients who tend to be heavy smokers and drinkers. A detailed social history should be obtained with special attention to the amount, duration, and timing of alcohol consumption. The timing of the last consumption of alcohol should be documented in order to provide appropriate preoperative prophylaxis for the patient against withdrawal.

The physical examination should consist of the complete head and neck examination.[4] Particular attention should be given to palpation of the cervical nodal basins. Flexible fiberoptic laryngoscopy should be performed on all patients with suspected laryngeal cancer. Flexible laryngoscopy allows for a comfortable and detailed examination with the opportunity for photo documentation. This method is superior to mirror laryngoscopy which may not provide an adequate view, and does not allow for photography.

Flexible laryngoscopy should be used to evaluate the mucosal surfaces of the nasopharynx, oropharynx, supraglottic (including both surfaces of the epiglottis), glottic, and infraglottic larynx. The tumor involved structures, mobility of the vocal folds and the caliber of the airway should be assessed. If necessary, the vocal folds can be anesthetized with 4% topical lidocaine applied per orum with an Abrams cannula and the fiberoptic endoscope can be passed into the subglottis to visualize the trachea and the carina.

In patients with dysphagia, a fiberoptic endoscopic evaluation of swallowing (FEES) can be performed in the office setting. This serves two functions, (1) it provides the patient and physician with an objective assessment of the extent of dysphagia and/or aspiration and (2) it establishes a baseline that can be used to monitor swallowing function after treatment (surgical or nonsurgical).

The identification of baseline function is of particular importance when treating patients with conservation (partial) laryngeal surgery or with chemoirradiation protocols (which are associated with some degree of aspiration) .

Laboratory Evaluation

Laryngeal cancer patients may be malnourished, dehydrated, or anemic. Therefore, routine laboratory tests should include a complete blood count and electrolyte studies. Quantitation of liver associated enzymes, renal function, and liver function is also important. If the liver enzymes or serum alkaline phosphatase are elevated further workup for metastatic disease are indicated. The measurement of serum albumin and prealbumin levels are also important to establish a baseline for nutritional status which correlates with surgical complication rates.[5]

Imaging Studies

The goal of radiologic evaluation of patients with suspected laryngeal cancer is to establish the extent of disease within the larynx and neck. These studies facilitate surgical planning and establish the existence of distant metastases. The favored imaging modality varies between computed tomography (CT) or magnetic resonance imaging (MRI) based on institutional experience and availability. At a minimum, a chest radiograph and a contrast-enhanced CT scan of the neck should be performed, the latter using contiguous 3- to 5-mm slice intervals (Fig 17–1). A chest radiograph with two views or CT scan should be used to screen for pulmonary metastases. The sensitivity of chest radiography in detecting pulmonary metastases is approximately 60%.[6] If the chest radiograph demonstrates suspicious lesions a dedicated chest CT scan is mandatory.

CT scanning is a frequently used modality for the evaluation of the laryngeal primary and the cervical nodal basins, which has a high sensitivity for determining pre-epiglottic and paraglottic space involvement (values range from 95–100%), thus defining AJCC T3 disease. Contrast-enhanced CT is highly specific for pre-epiglottic space involvement (90–93%), but not very specific (~50%) for ruling out paraglottic space involvement.[7,8]

Magnetic resonance imaging (MRI) is another useful modality that may assess tumor-adjacent structures and evaluate cartilage invasion by the primary tumor. T1, T2-weighted, and postcontrast sequences at 3-mm slice thickness should be routinely obtained. Zbaren et al have determined the sensitivity of MRI scans to be 94%, specificity to be 74% with a negative predictive value of 96% in determining thyroid cartilage invasion.[8] The low specificity has been attributed to technical factors such as motion artifacts from swallowing and respiration and the inflammation that often accompanies the primary tumor. MRI is useful for evaluating transglottic and paraglottic extension of tumor. The role of MRI scanning in the evaluation of the neck for nodal disease remains debatable, but most experts agree that involvement of great vessels is better determined using MRI scans.

Contrast-enhanced CT scans are very useful for detecting clinically occult nodal metastases in the neck, and were found in one study to be slightly better than MRI scans.[9] In a more recent study, King et al found that CT and MRI were comparable in predicting extracapsular spread in the node positive neck.[10]

Positron emission tomography (PET) scanning is a relatively new modality that is gaining popularity because it provides functional information in addition to the anatomic localization of axial scans. The most common radioisotope used in clinical PET imaging is fluoro-deoxyglucose (FDG). The unique role of PET appears to be the detection of distant metastases and assessing tumor response to nonsurgical therapy. Recent studies have shown that PET scans have a high sensitivity in detecting local recurrence after radiotherapy for laryngeal cancer (92%), but with a specificity of 62%. When serial scans are employed the sensitivity and specificity are increased to 97% and 82%, respectively.[11] Recently, PET scans are being combined with coregistered CT scans to provide a fusion PET/CT image. The PET/CT images are superior to PET or CT alone.[12] Gordin et al demonstrated the superiority of fused PET/CT scans, and that PET/CT scans altered treatment course in 59% of patients.[13]

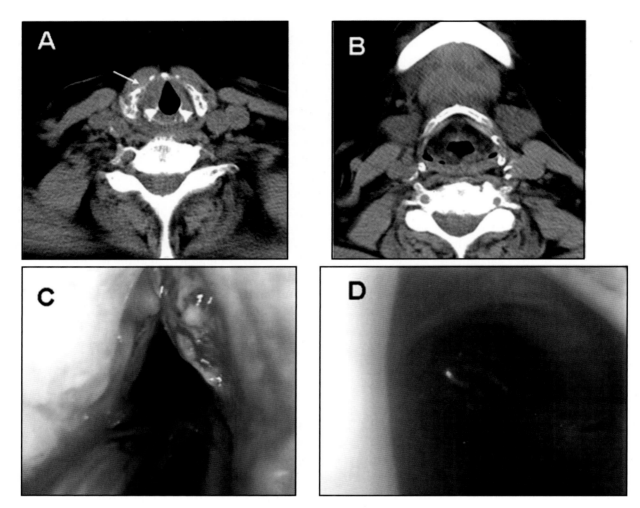

Fig 17–1. Advanced glottic cancer (T3) with paraglottic space involvement. **(A)** shows an axial CT scan demonstrating paraglottic space involvement (*arrow*). **(B)** shows another image with no supraglottic involvement. **(C)** shows the endoscopic image illustrating anterior commissure involvement. **(D)** is an endoscopic view of the subglottic area which is free of tumor.

In summary, any of these imaging modalities can be used with good accuracy to stage both the primary tumor and cervical nodal basins. The optimal choice is dependent on the comfort level of the clinicians and radiologist and the logistics of obtaining the scans.

Operative Staging

Despite the technologic advances in imaging the diagnosis of cancer is only made on histologic eval-

uation. Every suspected laryngeal cancer patient must undergo an operative endoscopy providing the possibility of detailed photo documentation of disease. Intraoperative consultation from the pathologist may be considered if the head and neck surgeon is concerned about an unusual histology.

A direct laryngoscopy with careful evaluation of the supraglottic mucosa, the arytenoid and interarytenoid mucosa, the piriform sinus, and the postcricoid region should be performed. Directed biopsies should be obtained from involved sites. Esophagoscopy, either flexible or rigid, should be performed to exclude other esophageal pathology. Tracheobronschoscopy may be performed to exclude pulmonary pathology. Photographic documentation of the primary tumor is useful (1) to establish a baseline and (2) to communicate with other physicians when multidisciplinary care involving medical and radiation oncologists in contemplated.

NONSURGICAL OPTIONS FOR THE MANAGEMENT OF ADVANCED LARYNGEAL CANCER

The concept of nonsurgical management of advanced laryngeal cancer was popularized by the Veterans Administration Trial. In this landmark paper, 332 patients were randomized to treatment with surgery and postoperative irradiation or induction chemotherapy with either cisplatin or 5-FU for 2 to 3 cycles and concomitant irradiation if there was response.[14] Those patients who did not respond underwent total laryngectomy. These data demonstrated that whereas the survival was equivalent in both arms (~68%), 64% of patients who underwent induction chemotherapy were able to preserve their larynges. There were more local recurrences, but less distant metastases in the induction chemotherapy arm. One major criticism of this study was the exclusion of a radiation therapy only arm.

To address this issue, the RTOG 91-11 trial was conducted.[15] This randomized, prospective trial accrued 547 patients, distributed into 3 arms, (1) induction chemotherapy followed by irradiation, or salvage laryngectomy, (2) concurrent chemotherapy with irradiation, or (3) irradiation alone. Patients with T1 disease, or extensive T4 disease (thyroid cartilage invasion or >1 cm of tongue base involvement) were excluded. Concurrent chemotherapy with irradiation yielded the best local control rate of 78% versus 61% for induction therapy or 56% for irradiation alone. The rate of anatomic laryngeal preservation was 88% in the concurrent therapy arm, 75% in the arm with induction therapy, and 70% for the radiation-only arm. Overall survival was similar in all arms, but disease-free survival was improved in both chemotherapy arms.

Weber et al classified the complications and the need for salvage surgery in the patients enrolled in the RTOG 91-11 trial.[16] Overall, 25% of patients in the RTOG 91-11 trial required a total laryngectomy, the major cause being disease recurrence or progression. The rates of total laryngectomy were 28%, 16%, and 31% for the three arms, respectively ($p = 0.002$). The major and minor complication rates ranged from 52 to 59%, and did not vary between the arms. The incidence of pharyngocutaneous fistula ranged from 15 to 30%, the highest rate being observed in the concurrent treatment group. Approximately 5% of patients required a total laryngectomy for aspiration or chondronecrosis without evidence of tumor persistence.

The data of the RTOG 91-11 have clearly shown that concomitant chemotherapy (cisplatin at 100 mg/m^2) with irradiation (70 Gy delivered over 7 weeks) and induction chemotherapy are superior to irradiation alone. Overall survival was comparable between the three arms. Based on this study and other data, it is possible to extrapolate that concomitant therapy likely yields comparable survival to primary surgical treatment with postoperative irradiation.

However, the data regarding quality of life and laryngeal function are still unclear. The outcomes with regard to swallowing were significantly worse in the concomitant therapy arm in RTOG 91-11 when compared to the other groups, at 1 year post-treatment. This difference appeared resolved at 2 years post-treatment, but long-term follow-up was not reported, despite 3.8-year follow-up available for laryngeal preservation endpoint. In addition, 15% of patients treated with concurrent chemoradiotherapy suffered from dysphagia 2 years after treatment, suggesting that late radiation toxicities may be augmented by concomitant chemotherapy. There were no significant differences in voice function between the 3 groups, regardless of duration of follow-up.

Even though the RTOG 91-11 trial has effectively refuted the utility of induction chemotherapy followed by irradiation, Fung et al have attempted to use sequential induction chemotherapy with concomitant chemoradiation for patients who responded to the initial induction protocol.[17] Induction chemotherapy followed by concomitant chemoradiation can yield acceptable laryngeal preservation, both anatomically and functionally. However, the voice related quality of life outcomes were significantly worse in the treated patients when compared to normative controls. Although it is generally accepted that vocal quality is best preserved with nonsurgical treatment, in those successfully treated, the acute and late toxicities, as well as prolonged treatment and costs compel additional efforts to reduce side effects while maintaining high locoregional control rates. Ultimately, as the latter endpoint is successfully achieved using surgical or nonsurgical methods, the real benefical effect of chemotherapy on overall survival may reside in its potential to reduce distant metastases.[15] However, Hoffman et al[18] have reported that survival of laryngeal cancer patients between 1994 to 1996 has decreased when compared with patients treated between 1985 to 1993. The reason(s) for this alarming trend remain unknown.

The issue with nonsurgical management of laryngeal cancer is whether there is an added benefit to chemoirradiation protocols, as all patients are still at risk for salvage TL to achieve comparable overall survival. It is also important to remember that some of the patients who were enrolled in the RTOG 91-11 trial may have been candidates for partial laryngeal surgery (either open or endoscopic) and may have avoided a total laryngectomy in the hands of a skilled head and neck surgeon.

SURGICAL MANAGEMENT OF ADVANCED LARYNGEAL CANCER

A comprehensive knowledge of the anatomy and accurate staging of the disease dictate the choice of appropriate surgical therapy for patients with advanced laryngeal cancer. It is worthy to note that the AJCC staging system does not in and of itself provide enough information to plan surgical therapy. It is of paramount importance that the head and neck surgeon be skilled in conservation techniques and examine the larynx both visually and with palpation (with a suction tip or microlaryngoscopy instruments). It is crucial to perform a staging endoscopy with angled telescopes[4,19] prior to the commencement of surgical therapy, if the patient has not had a recent staging endoscopy, or if the endoscopy was performed by another surgeon.

The mainstay of surgical therapy for large volume disease with involvement of cartilage or tongue base is total laryngectomy. This operation involves the surgical extirpation of the entire laryngeal framework and surrounding soft tissues. The first documentation of a laryngectomy for laryngeal cancer is attributed to Billroth in 1873. The technique was further refined over the later part of the 19th century. The main indications for a total laryngectomy in a patient with advanced laryngeal cancer are given in Table 17-1.

Operative Technique

The patient is prepared and draped for surgery with a horizontal shoulder roll in place, after the administration of general endotracheal anesthesia. An apron-type incision extending in a curvilinear fashion between both mastoid tips, and lying within a natural skin crease above the clavicles is made and carried through the platysma muscle. Subplatysmal flaps are raised to a level above the hyoid bone and to the clavicle. Unilateral or bilateral cervical lymphadenectomy is performed if indicated. The strap muscles are divided low in the neck. Both carotid sheaths are dissected and the laryngeal complex is freed from the attachment to the medial carotid sheath. This is known as the outer tunnel. The thy-

Table 17-1. Indications for Total Laryngectomy

Advanced disease with thyroid or cricoid cartilage invasion
Spread of disease to involve greater than 10 mm of subglottic mucosa anteriorly or 1 cm posteriorly
Laryngeal tumor causing airway obstruction with air hunger
Poor general physical health, or decreased pulmonary reserve
Involvement of the interaytenoid mucosa or bilateral arytenoid involvement
Failures of nonsurgical therapy or failure after partial laryngeal surgery
Advanced neck disease with invasion of the laryngeal framework or strap muscle invasion.

roid isthmus is divided and the trachea is freed from attachments to the thyroid lobes. It is sometimes necessary to remove one or both thyroid lobes when extralaryngeal spread of disease is noted. Para-tracheal lymph node dissection is essential when subglottic extension of tumor is appreciated.

Next, the hyoid bone is skeletonized and the superior laryngeal pedicles (superior laryngeal nerve and artery) are identified and divided. At the lateral aspect of the hyoid bone, care should be taken to visualize and preserve the hypoglossal nerves. The lateral attachments of the larynx (the constrictor muscles) are divided. A tracheotomy is performed, taking care to ensure that the tracheal incision is not close to the inferior margin of the tumor. The transoral endotracheal tube is replaced with an armored endotracheal tube placed directly into the tracheostomy. This tube should be readily accessible to the surgeon. In general 1 cm of tracheal margin should be resected. The aerodigestive tract is then entered superiorly, in the vallecula, just above the hyoid bone.

Mucosal incisions are made in a superior-to-inferior fashion under direct visualization. The surgeon should ensure that an adequate mucosal margin is resected. The piriform sinus mucosa should be preserved as much as possible, particularly on the uninvolved side. At this point, the tracheal incision is extended to completely transect the trachea and demonstrate the cervical esophagus. The superior and inferior portions of the dissection are connected to release the laryngectomy specimen. Intraoperative pathologic consultation using frozen section analysis should be obtained to ensure adequate tumor resection.

The resulting pharyngeal defect is closed with long-lasting suture material (usually 3–0 Vicryl suture) and inverted suturing technique. The lower skin flap is sutured to the most superior tracheal ring to provide an epithelium-lined tract. The wound is closed over suction drains.

Complications

The complications associated with a total laryngectomy can be classified as either early or delayed. Early complications (within 2 weeks of surgery) include hematoma formation, wound dehiscence, and pharyngocutaneous fistula formation. Hematoma formation generally requires re-exploration and identification of the bleeding source. Wound dehiscence occurs when wound healing is compromised. This is commonly due to increased tension in wound closure, pre-existing medical conditions such as diabetes, malnutrition, or hypothyroidism, which commonly occurs postchemoirradiation or irradiation alone. The rate of pharyngocutaneous fistula has been reported to be as low as 4% in primary laryngectomies.[20] The data regarding fistula formation rates in the RTOG 91-11 study are reported elsewhere in this chapter for comparison.

Late complications (2 weeks after surgery) include pharyngocutaneous fistula formation, hypothyroidism, hypoparathyroidism, stomal stenosis, and pharynoesophageal stenosis. Late fistula formation is also potentiated by preoperative irradiation or chemoradiation. Hypothyroidism results commonly from surgical removal of the thyroid gland when extralaryngeal disease is present. Hypothyroidism can also be caused by irradiation of level 6. Hypoparathyroidism usually results from a transient disruption of the blood supply to the parathyroid glands after dissection of level 6. However, this dissection is more difficult after chemoradiation protocols and high rates of parathyroid injury may occur in cases of salvage surgery.

Tracheostomal stenosis is a distressing complication that requires reoperation to establish a sufficient airway. The incidence of stomal stenosis can be reduced with meticulous closure of the stoma with a plastic-type repair to break the suture line.[21] A gradual dilation strategy can be employed if the stenosis is not critical.

Pharyngoesophageal stenosis is another relatively common problem that results in dysphagia especially to solids, often after adjuvant chemoradiation therapy. The treatment consists of endoscopy to rule out a neoplastic source of stenosis and sequential dilation to a minimum size of 36 Fr.

Outcome

The total laryngectomy provides good functional outcomes. Speech is rehabilitated with a primary or delayed tracheoesophageal puncture (TEP) and eventually with the BlomSinger prosthesis. Most patients are able to sustain their caloric needs with a completely oral diet, and the catheter inserted through the TEP may be used to immediate postoperative nutrition. Minimal care is necessary to maintain the tracheostoma. Regular saline irrigation and lavage of the trachea is necessary for the first few weeks after surgery. Patients are able to discontinue use of the laryngectomy tube soon afterward, and some surgeons do not use laryngectomy tubes at all.

Total laryngectomy with postoperative irradiation yields a local control rate of 93%.[14] Overall survival after laryngectomy and adjuvant irradiation can be quoted at 68% based on the VA trial. Recent data from a European cooperative trial indicate that, in high-risk tumors, chemoirradiation after surgery with curative intent may improve overall survival from 40% to 53 %.[22] These data were supported in a similar trial conducted in the United States, where a distinct disease-free survival advantage was demonstrated.[23] It is likely that with further refinements in adjuvant therapy, survival may be improved after definitive surgical resection. The irreplaceable contribution of chemotherapy to reduction in rates of distant metastases supports its use in those at high risk, that is, advanced disease and extranodal extension of disease.

ORGAN PRESERVATION (PARTIAL) LARYNGEAL SURGERY

The initial "organ preservation" techniques were contemplated and executed before the advent of nonsurgical techniques. Billroth is credited with performing the first partial laryngeal surgery, a laryngofissure with endolaryngeal tumor removal, in 1873. This patient suffered from tumor recurrence and was the recipient of the first total laryngectomy later that year. Conservation surgical procedures aim to achieve local tumor control (through complete excision) while preserving as much normal architecture as possible. This can be accomplished with either open surgical techniques or via endoscopic resection. Table 17–2 lists indications and contraindications for partial laryngeal surgery.

Table 17–2. Partial Laryngeal Surgery

Indications	Contraindications
Tumor limited to one subunit of the larynx	Cricoid cartilage involvement
Limited subglottic extension	Involvement of the interarytenoid mucosa
Ability to preserve at least one functional arytenoids	Poor general health/ pulmonary reserve
	Extralaryngeal spread of tumor

Open partial laryngeal surgeries can be broadly classified into two types, those which use vertical incisions in the larynx (vertical partial) and those which use horizontal incisions (horizontal partial laryngectomies). Very few patients with advanced laryngeal cancer are candidates for vertical partial laryngectomies; as such we do not discuss variants of this operation in the present chapter. There are two major variations of horizontal partial laryngectomies, the supraglottic and supracricoid laryngectomies.

Principles of Partial Laryngeal Surgery

Obtain complete tumor resection: Local control through total tumor resection with negative margins is the key principle of organ preservation surgery. This requires careful preoperative evaluation and preparation by both the patient and surgeon to convert to a total laryngectomy if tumor spread is encountered.

Accurately assess tumor extent: In order to avoid potential pitfalls in the operative plan, the surgeon should accurate assess the three-dimensional topology of the tumor both clinically and radiographically. The integrity of the laryngeal complex cannot be preserved if structural support is lost, or if mucosa that is necessary for reconstruction is resected.

Preserve the structural integrity of the laryngeal complex: The structural support of the airway is established by the integrity of the cricoid ring. If tumor resection necessitates excision of the cricoid cartilage, partial laryngeal surgery is generally not possible. Direct invasion of the cricoid cartilage or mucosal extension greater than 1 mm anteriorly or posteriorly are contraindications to conservation surgery. Similarly, the hyoid bone provides superior support element. Supracricoid laryngectomy is not feasible if the hyoid bone is involved, or if it has to be resected secondary to extensive tongue base involvement.

The cricoarytenoid unit is the fundamental unit of the larynx: The cricoarytenoid unit consists of the cricoid cartilage with the arytenoid cartilages, associated musculature, and the superior and recurrent laryngeal nerves necessary to innervate that unit. Preservation of these structures is vital for the maintenance of function of the laryngeal remnant.

Normal mucosa can be sacrificed to obtain optimal reconstruction: In the case of the supracricoid laryngectomy, one normal vocal fold may need to be removed so that the reconstruction can be accomplished. This may appear to be counterproductive; but reconstruction with the preserved arytenoids provides a superior result. It is often necessary to remove normal contralateral mucosa in the supraglottic laryngectomy, in order to achieve closure of the laryngeal remnant.

Indications for Supracricoid Laryngectomy

Advanced tumors at the glottic level are often amenable to organ preservation surgery with a supracricoid laryngectomy (SCL) with cricohyoido-epiglotopexy (CHEP), or for transglottic tumors with epiglottic involvement, cricohyoiopexy (CHP). The SCL with CHEP consists of resection of the true and false vocal folds bilaterally, the thyroid cartilage, and up to one functional arytenoid unit. The remain-

ing arytenoid(s) is tilted anteriorly to create a neoglottis. The goal of this operation is to provide the patient with glottic phonation without the need for a permanent tracheostomy.

The SCL procedure (with CHEP or CHP reconstruction) has been used mainly for T2 and T3 tumors, although selected T4 tumors (those with limited inner lamina involvement) can be resected with this technique (Fig 17-2). Once again, significant subglottic extension (10-15 mm), requiring resection of the cricoid cartilage is a contraindication.[24] Tumors that require excision of the hyoid bone cannot be resected with this approach. Furthermore, large T4 tumors with extralaryngeal spread, requiring excision of the strap muscles should not be treated with this operation. The creation of a neoglottis and the concomitant disruption of normal laryngeal anatomy invariably leads to some extent of penetration and aspiration of food material. The patient must have sufficient pulmonary reserve to withstand the pulmonary effects of aspiration. This is usually evaluated preoperatively by obtaining a careful history. Another simple method is to have the patient walk 2 flights of stairs. A patient who is able to accomplish this without significant dyspnea should be able to tolerate the postoperative sequelae. Pulmonary function tests usually are not necessary.

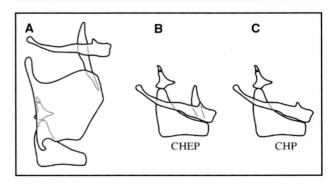

Fig 17-2. The reconstructive options available after supracricoid laryngectomy. (**A**) shows a cartoon of the normal laryngeal framework. (**B**) shows the result after cricohyoidoepiglotopexy (CHEP) and (**C**) shows the result after cricohyoidopexy (CHP). Note the absent epiglottis in (C); however, the cartilaginous reconstruction is relatively unaltered.

Surgical Technique

An apron incision extending between the mastoid tips, in line with the site of the planned tracheostomy is performed. Subplatysmal flaps are raised to the clavicle and superiorly, 2 cm above the hyoid bone. The strap muscles, sternothyroid, and sternohyoid, are individually divided from medial to lateral at the superior aspect of the thyroid cartilage. It is absolutely crucial to identify and preserve the superior laryngeal nerves. The constrictor muscles are incised sharply along the entire length of the thyroid cartilage bilaterally. The piriform sinuses are dissected away from the thyroid cartilage, particularly on the uninvolved side. Sharp dissection is used to disarticulate both cricoarytenoid joints, while taking care to preserve the recurrent laryngeal nerves. The isthmus of the thyroid gland is divided and blunt finger dissection is used to mobilize the thoracic trachea to the level of the carina. It is important to only dissect along the anterior surface of the trachea, thereby maintaining the blood supply that runs laterally. A cricothyrotomy is performed and the airway is established by passing an endotracheal tube through the cricothyrotomy. The endolarynx is entered via a transepiglottic laryngotomy at the petiole. This incision is oriented inferiorly and anteriorly to preserve as much epiglottis as possible.

Mucosal incisions in the endolarynx are then performed, first on the nontumor side, by incising the false vocal folds vertically just anterior to the arytenoid cartilage. This incision is carried through the vocal process of the ipsilateral arytenoid. This incision is then connected with the cricothyrotomy, by dividing the cricothyroid mucle. The larynx is then cracked open like a book (with a pivot along the contralateral thyroid cartilage attachements). The mucosal incisions are then completed along the tumor bearing side of the larynx under full visualization. The posterior and interarytenoid mucosa should be preserved bilaterally. Frozen section evaluation is routinely performed to ensure adequate tumor removal.

The reconstruction begins with forward rotation and suspension of both arytenoids. This is accomplished by placing a suture (4-0 Vicryl) from the superior portion of the arytenoids to the mid-anterior cricoid. This tilts the arytenoids forward and creates a neoglottis. Three submucosal sutures that pass from the cricoid, through the epiglottis and around the hyoid bone and tongue base are used to close the larynx. These sutures are placed with one in the exact midline and the other 2 sutures placed 1 cm apart from the midline on either side. The cricothyrotomy is converted to a tracheostomy, through the tracheal ring brought up to the level of the skin incision. The sutures are tied securely. The incision is closed over suction drains after the tracheostomy site is appropriately excluded from the remainder of the surgical wound. A nasogastric tube is placed for enteral access, or a gastrostomy tube may be used if the patient has previously received irradiation.

Complications and Outcomes

Temporary postoperative dysphagia is an expected sequalae of this operation. However, this resolves with time and aggressive swallowing therapy. The nasogastric tube is usually removed between 1 to 3 weeks postoperatively. Prolonged tracheostomy is another infrequent complication. This is often potentiated by chronic aspiration. Once again, aggressive swallowing therapy provided by trained speech pathologists can help to avert this complication. Dependence on enteral feeding tubes and tracheotomy tubes is prolonged by prior chemoirradiation.

Hyoid bone necrosis and laryngeal stenosis (possibly due to inappropriate impaction of the cricoid cartilage onto the hyoid bone) have been reported. The laryngeal stenosis can be managed with the placement of a laryngeal stent, or with revision of the CHEP is this is the cause. Oncologic control for selected T3 and T4 tumors can be as high as 90%.

SUPRACRICOID LARYNGECTOMY WITH CRICOHYOIDOPEXY

Tumors with significant supraglottic involvement are best treated with a SCL and a CHP. In this operation, the epiglottis is removed and a more complete supraglottic resection can be accomplished. Supraglottic tumors that are not amenable to resection via a supraglottic laryngectomy, because of extension to the glottis, limited vocal fold mobility or limited thyroid carilage invasion often can be resected with a SCL and CHP reconstruction. This operation is an extension of the SCL described earlier in this chapter, which incorporates excision of the epiglottis and pre-epiglottic space. Contraindications to this procedure are the same as those for SCL with CHEP, and include significant subglottic involvement, involvement of the interarytenoid mucosa, and pharyngeal involvement.

Surgical Technique

The steps of this operation are identical to those involved in a SCL with CHEP. The point in the operation where these procedures diverge occurs when the superior cuts into the areodigestive tract are made. Unlike the SCL with CHEP, when a transverse thyrotomy is performed through the pre-epiglottic space preserving the epiglottis, in the SCL with CHP the epiglottis is removed. This is performed in the following fashion, first, the cricothyrotomy is performed and the airway is secured. The superior portions of the sternohyoid and sternothyroid strap muscles are elevated from the thyrohyoid membrane. The medial portion of the hyoid bone is skeletonized from below with electrocautery. The aerodigestive tract is entered in the midline, just inferior to the hyoid bone. The epiglottis is then delivered and grasped with an Allis clamp. Scissors are then used to incise the mucosa medial to the entry point of the superior laryngeal nerve on the uninvolved side of the larynx. This frees the pre-epiglottic soft tissues on that side. The mucosal incisions are then carried inferiorly through the false and true vocal folds, as in the SCL with CHEP. Care is taken to stay anterior to the piriform sinus mucosa thereby preserving the piriform sinuses. The laryngeal portion of the excision is identical to the SCL with CHEP.

The reconstruction is performed with 3 interrupted 1-0 Vicryl sutures using a 65-mm atraumatic needle, placed in the midline and 1 cm apart. These submucosal sutures are passed around the cricoid to the hyoid and tongue base. The resection of the epiglottis obviates the need for reapproximation of the vallecula.[25]

Complications and Outcomes

The complications for this procedure are identical to those encountered with SCL and CHEP. However, the persistence of dysphagia and aspiration may be pronounced with the absence of the epiglottis. The base of tongue provides the sole mechanism for glottic protection. This problem is also exacerbated when one arytenoid is resected. The rate of functional laryngectomy for intractable aspiration in these patients ranges from 0 to 11%.

Laccourreye et al[25] have reported the oncologic outcomes of 19 patients with gross pathologic invasion of the pre-epiglottic treated with SCL with CHP. The local control rate was 94%.

Indications for Supraglottic Laryngectomy

Most authors advocate the use of the supraglottic laryngectomy (SGL) for the management of T1 and T2 lesions of the supraglottic larynx. Historically, T3 and T4 have demonstrated recurrence rates as high as 45% (in larger series). The supraglottic laryngectomy should be employed in highly selected cases of advanced laryngeal cancer. Extension of tumor below the false fold or impaired vocal fold mobility are contraindications to SGL.

Technique of Supraglottic Laryngectomy

The details of the surgical technique have been described in several standard texts. We review the key surgical steps of this operation for the purposes of the current discussion.

The operation starts with the administration of general endotracheal anesthesia. The patient is prepared and draped in the standard fashion. A tracheotomy is performed. An apron incision in line with the planned tracheotomy incision is carried down through the platysma. Subplatysmal flaps are raised as for a total laryngectomy. Bilateral modified neck dissections are generally warranted with this procedure (see section on management of the neck). The main trunk of both superior laryngeal nerves should be preserved. The fascia between the strap muscles is divided in the midline. The isthmus of the thyroid gland is divided and ligated. The strap muscles are divided at the level of the superior border of the thyroid cartilage. The constrictor muscles are sharply incised along the thyroid cartilage laterally to the top of the superior cornua. The superior edge of the thyroid cartilage is scored with a knife, and the periosteum is elevated off the thyroid cartilage. The external thyroid cartilage perichondrium is elevated halfway down the cartilage from the superior edge to allow for the transverse thyrotomy to be made just above the anterior commissure. The uninvolved piriform sinus is then freed from the thyroid cartilage. As most T3 tumors will demonstrate most laterality, the uninvolved mucosa is dissected. A tracheostomy is performed. A transverse thyrotomy is then performed.

There are two scenarios that must now be accounted for: (1) the tumor involves resection of the hyoid bone and portion of the tongue base or (2) the tumor involves resection of one arytenoid or portion of the piriform sinus.

Resection of the base of tongue: Enter inferiorly through the transverse thyrotomy. The hyoid bone is not skeletonized. Mucosal incisions of the tongue base are made above the hyoid bone, with direct visualization from below. An adequate margin of tissue (~1.5 cm) should also be resected. The resection should preserve at least 1 cm of tongue base posterior to the circumvallate papillae to allow for adequate function postoperatively.

Resection of arytenoids or piriform sinus: If the hyoid bone is to be resected, it is skeletonized and the lateral cornu is dissected free. The internal thyroid perichondrium is freed on the uninvolved side. The endolarynx is entered via the transverse thyrotomy. Mucosal incisions are made anterior to the uninvolved arytenoids and through the false fold. The incision is then carried through to the involved piriform sinus and the ipsilateral vocal fold.

The reconstruction requires repositioning of the anterior commisure. The goal of the reconstruction is to provide mucosal closure, and reposition the central tongue base over the laryngeal inlet to protect the glottis. This is usually accomplished by passing submucosal sutures through the remnant of the thyroid cartilage and around the tongue base and hyoid bone (if present). The strap muscles are reapproximated to the suprahyoid musculature. The skin flaps are closed, with care taken to separate the tracheostomy, over suction drains.

Complications and Outcomes

The complications encountered after supraglottic laryngectomy include pharyngocutaneous fistula formation, failure to decannulate, tracheocutaneous fistula formation, and persistent dysphagia sometimes associated with aspiration pneumonia. The reported incidence of pharyngocutaneous fistula can be as high as 12%. This can be treated by establishing a fistula tract with the use of a drain; and maintaining the patient without an oral diet until the fistula resolves. Sometimes it may be necessary to use vascularized tissue to close the defect. Up to 6% of patients may not be decannulated, prior chemoirradition therapy increases the risk of tracheotomy tube dependence.

TRANSORAL LASER MICROSURGERY FOR THE MANAGEMENT OF ADVANCED DISEASE

Transoral laser microsurgery (TLM) has been popularized by Steiner and colleagues for the treatment of advanced laryngeal disease in Europe. This technique has not garnered as much enthusiasm in the United States for the management of advanced disease, even though many centers routinely advocate its use in the management of T1 and T2 lesions. Its role as a salvage surgery option after nonsurgical therapy is also not well established. This chapter briefly describes the philosophy and tenets of TLM surgery and summarize the existing with regard to outcomes and complications. The technical details of TLM surgery are described elsewhere.

Principles of Transoral Laser Microsurgery

One of the fundamental underpinnings of modern oncologic surgery is the Halstedian concept of en bloc tumor removal. Although this concept was proposed by Halsted to improve on the treatment of advanced breast cancer, he advocated its role in the management of all soft tissue tumors. In the modern era, we are increasingly advocating more conservative surgery, mainly because the outcomes are not significantly different.

One of the fundamental tenets of TLM surgery is piecemeal resection of the tumor. This method violates the principle of en bloc resection. The tumor is removed in a piecemeal fashion and submitted for pathologic evaluation. Careful orientation of the small tissue pieces is necessary and with appropriate reresection, as guided by pathologic frozen section analysis, excellent tumor clearance is possible. In theory, this approach mimics the microdermographic surgery described by Mohs.

The use of the carbon dioxide laser has been shown to coagulate lymphatic vessels in an animal model.[26] These vessels stay sealed for up to 10 days. This allows the surgeon to incise the tumor and assess the depth of invasion, allowing for a tailored operation.

Indications for TLM

Although several European studies have demonstrated the feasibility of endoscopic resection for advanced laryngeal cancers, this is a technically challenging operation. This operation is not advocated as the first surgical option in most US centers. Nonetheless, in experienced hands it is possible to treat selected T3 and T4 cancers with endoscopic resection.

Tumor extension is the primary criterion by which candidacy for endoscopic resection should be judged. Tumors that extend into the soft tissues of the neck and are in close proximity to the great vessels should not be resected endoscopically. Advanced cancers requiring reconstruction are not generally amenable to TLM resection.

Adequate exposure is of paramount importance. The ability to exposure the tumor transorally is determined by the 3 Ts. First, trismus impairs visualization of laryngeal anatomy. Second, the patient must be able to tilt the head for suspension laryngoscopy. The presence of significant cervical spine disease or cervical spine surgery significantly impairs visualization. Third, the presence of carious teeth and significant retrognathia will impair tumor exposure.

Surgical Technique

The patient is induced for general anesthesia and intubated with an armored laser-safe endotracheal tube. The patient is prepared for laser surgery in the appropriate fashion with protective eye covering, moistened towels, and so forth. The tumor is exposed with a suspension laryngoscopy. The operating microscope with a CO_2 laser is brought into the field. Tumor dissection is initiated by bisecting the tumor. This allows the surgeon to judge the depth of invasion and establish the deep plane of dissection. The laser is used to incise the tissues and remove the tumor in a piecemeal fashion. Electrocautery or surgical clips may be necessary to control bleeding. Sometimes it is necessary to divide the tumor into arbitrary "subunits." As each subunit is resected, the surgeon should re-evaluate the exposure and residual tumor (Fig 17–3).

During the dissection it is important to maintain orientation of the specimen, to know what has been resected and what remains. It is also important to orient the specimen with inking, preferably in the operating room for the pathologist. The laser is used in a cutting mode to accurately dissect and incise tissues, as opposed to an ablation mode that vaporizes the tissue. This allows for precise dissection and yields a tangible specimen that can be processed for histologic evaluation. The pathologist plays an important role in ensuring a successful outcome with TLM. Often, the tissue specimen is small and the establishing proper orientation may be difficult. The pathologist should be made aware of the inherent challenges and appropriate care must be exercised by the pathologist to ensure that the sections are adequate and generate meaningful information.

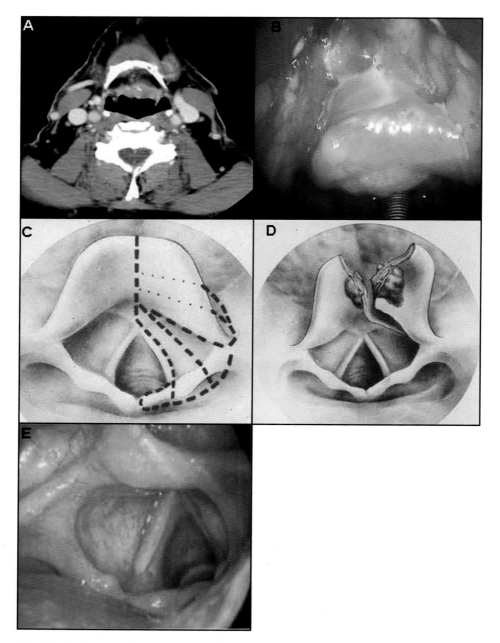

Fig 17–3. Transoral resection of a large supraglottic tumor. (**A**) shows an endo-scopic view of a large tumor centered at the epiglottis. (**B**) shows an axial CT scan demonstrating the tumor. (**C**) shows the subunit concept of resection as marked with the dashed lines. (**D**) shows the intial incision through the tumor mass. (**E**) shows the postoperative result after healing.

Complications and Outcomes

The obvious minor complications of TLM include, chipped teeth, mucosal lacerations from laryngoscopy, and minor burns to uninvolved mucosa from stray laser beams. The more devastating complications associated with TLM are related to airway compromise. These include hemorrhage (perioperative or postoperative), vascular injury, and tongue contusion resulting in swelling.[27] Transient hypoglossal or lingual nerve weakness is also possible; this is the result of a compression injury from the laryngoscope.

Steiner coworkers[28] have reported good results with TLM resection of advanced laryngeal cancer. The recurrence-free survival rates were 74% for stage III and 45% for stage IV disease. However, because of the need for reresection(s) and the technical complexity, the authors advocated careful selection of advanced lesions. Many of these patients will require adjuvant therapy with irradiation alone or concurrent chemoradiotherapy. Pradier et al have suggested that outcomes are improved after TLM for advanced cancers in patients with a hemoglobin level greater than 13.5 g/dL.[29]

MANAGEMENT OF THE CERVICAL NODAL BASINS

The management of the neck is dependent on accurate staging of the cervical nodes. Cervical nodes with evidence of metastatic disease should be treated with the same modality as the primary tumor. If the primary tumor is treated with surgery then cervical lymphadenectomy should be performed. However, if the primary tumor is treated with concurrent chemoradiation then the neck(s) should be included in the treatment field. There is controversy regarding the management of the neck (in cases of advanced disease, N2 and N3), after chemoradiotherapy. Some authors advocate for routine neck dissection 6 to 10 weeks after the completion of therapy to eradicate any residual disease, as residual tumor cells have been found in 15% to 35% of neck dissection specimens after the completion of chemoradiotherapy.[30,31] Other authors advocate for radiographic evaluation of the neck with PET/CT

scans after the completion of therapy and reserve surgery for those patients who demonstrate persistent disease based on radiographic evaluation.[32] Brkovich et al have found that PET has a negative predictive value of 91.7%, suggesting that PET scans aid in identifying those patients at low risk for harboring metastatic deposits in the lymph nodes after chemoirradiation.[32] We believe that routine neck dissections can be safely deferred in patients who do not have evidence of disease on PET/CT evaluation after the completion of therapy, although this approach is associated with a finite rate of false negative and false positive cases.

More controversy exists regarding the management of the clinically node negative neck. It is well known that T3 glottic tumors have a 15% incidence of occult neck metastasis. This rate is higher for T4 glottic tumors. However, supraglottic tumors have a much higher rate (30%) of occult neck metastasis, probably because of the rich lymphatic drainage of the supraglottis. Furthermore, these tumors have a 16% incidence of bilateral metastasis at the time of diagnosis, and therefore require treatment of both heminecks.

As stated previously, the sensitivity and specificity of CT scans for the diagnosis of cervical metastases is about 70%, using a criterion of 1 cm for abnormal nodal size. This suggests that 30% of necks will be understaged. As there is no definitive evidence to suggest that elective lymphadenectomy improves survival, one might advocate a "wait and see" policy for patients with glottic tumors and no cervical disease. However, recent data from randomized trials show that adjuvant chemoradiotherapy improves disease control and possibly survival in patients with stage III and IV disease. Therefore, we advocate elective lymphadenectomy in patients with advanced laryngeal cancer, as it adds little morbidity and can help to refine adjuvant therapy protocols.

Post-treatment Follow-Up

The head and neck surgeon is often faced with the challenge of dealing with tumor recurrence or persistence despite therapy. In the modern era of increasing nonsurgical therapy, the head and neck surgeon will frequently perform salvage surgery. In the RTOG

91-11 trial, up to 16% of patients required laryngectomy after concurrent chemoradiotherapy. For this reason, it is crucially important that an experienced head and neck surgeon be involved in the initial management and care of every laryngeal cancer patient, even if the primary modality is nonsurgical. This is also important because the complications of chemoradiotherapy: dysphagia, aspiration, and tracheotomy dependence are all usually managed by the otolaryngologist/head and neck surgeon.

Routine surveillance must be performed by the head and neck surgeon at 4- to 6-week intervals for the first year after treatment. This can be extended to every 8 to 12 weeks for the second year. The number of visits can be reduced if the patient remains free of disease. The detection of recurrence can be particularly difficult in the previously treated patient. Significant fibrosis and swelling resulting from chemoradiotherapy can impair visualization of the aerodigestive tract by indirect laryngoscopy. The interpretation of PET/CT scans is also more difficult after treatment. For this reason, biopsies should be obtained of any suspicious lesion.

Salvage Surgery

The gold standard of surgical therapy for recurrent disease is considered to be total laryngectomy. This technique has been described above. Total laryngectomy in the context of prior nonsurgical therapy is complicated by a high rate of mucocutaneous fistula (as high as 30% in the RTOG trial). Some experts advocate the use of vascularized tissue from a nonirradiated portion of the body to reconstruct the pharyngeal defect. The options include pedicled pectoralis muscle flaps or free tissue transfer. Salvage total laryngectomy is also performed for nonfunctional larynges after organ preservation protocols.

More recently, the role of conservation laryngeal surgery in the management of radiotherapy failures of T1 and T2 tumors has been studied.[33] In a retrospective study, it was determined that the majority of patients who recurred after definitive irradiation were treated with total laryngectomy (68%). However, those that were treated with conservation surgeries (either open or endoscopic) had comparable oncologic control rates (88% for total and 84% for conservation). This studied focused on the outcomes of patients with early stage disease at initial presentation. Christiansen et al found that advanced, recurrent tumors could be treated with TLM and boost irradiation.[34] The majority of these tumors were laryngeal, but this study included oral cavity, oropharyngeal, and hypopharyngeal tumors. The locoregional control rate was 48%, with a 50% laryngeal preservation rate. The overall 5-year survival rate was 21%. These data indicate that although recurrent disease can be treated in the context of salvage surgery, the survival for patients who fail the primary treatment modality is generally poor.

CONCLUSION

The treatment of a patient with suspected advanced laryngeal cancer begins with a through diagnosis and evaluation. After establishing a histologic diagnosis and appropriate staging, the treatment decision(s) should be made by a multidisciplinary team consisting of a head and neck surgeon, a medical oncologist, and a radiation oncologist at the minimum. A thorough discussion of the treatment alternatives should allow the patient to make the most informed decision. Total laryngectomy is most appropriate for patients who have advanced disease that has already compromised the laryngeal airway or swallowing function, either due to cartilage invasion or functional defect resulting in aspiration or airway obstruction. The role of concurrent chemoradiotherapy has been well characterized by the RTOG 91-11 trial. However, the long-term impact on quality of life and laryngeal function remains unclear. Similarly, although a certain subgroup of patients will clearly benefit from conservation laryngeal surgery, this subgroup has not been clearly defined. Future directions include the development of selection criteria, either clinical or molecular, to predict and individualize therapy based on the likelihood of success with acceptable functional outcomes.

Good surgical judgment and careful preoperative evaluation and counseling will help both the patient and surgeon to obtain the best possible outcomes.

REFERENCES

1. Ferris RL, Martinez I, Sirianni N, et al. Human papillomavirus-16 associated squamous cell carcinoma of the head and neck (SCCHN): a natural disease model provides insights into viral carcinogenesis. *Eur J Cancer.* 2005;41:807–815.

2. Chiu RJ, Myers EN, Johnson JT. Efficacy of routine bilateral neck dissection in the management of supraglottic cancer. *Otolaryngol Head Neck Surg.* 2004;131:485–488.

3. Lutz CK, Johnson JT, Wagner RL, et al. Supraglottic carcinoma: patterns of recurrence. *Ann Otol Rhinol Laryngol.* 1990;99:12–27.

4. Thedki AA, Ferris RL. Diagnostic assessment of laryngeal cancer. *Otolaryngol Clin North Am.* 2002;35:953–969.

5. van Bokhorst-de van der Schueren MA, van Leeuwen PA, Sauerwein HP, et al. Assessment of malnutrition parameters in head and neck cancer and their relation to postoperative complications. *Head Neck.* 1997;19:419–425.

6. Feuerstein IM, Jicha DL, Pass HI, et al. Pulmonary metastases: MR imaging with surgical correlation—a prospective study. *Radiology.* 1992;182:123–129.

7. Becker AM, Gourin CG, Terris DJ. Delaying postoperative radiotherapy in advanced laryngeal cancer. *Otolaryngol Head Neck Surg.* 2005;133:998–999.

8. Zbaren P, Becker M, Lang H. Pretherapeutic staging of laryngeal carcinoma. Clinical findings, computed tomography, and magnetic resonance imaging compared with histopathology. *Cancer.* 1996;77:1263–1273.

9. Curtin HD, Ishwaran H, Mancuso AA, et al. Comparison of CT and MR imaging in staging of neck metastases. *Radiology.* 1998;207:123–130.

10. King AD, Tse GM, Yuen EH, et al. Comparison of CT and MR imaging for the detection of extranodal neoplastic spread in metastatic neck nodes. *Eur J Radiol.* 2004;52:264–270.

11. Terhaard CH, Bongers V, van Rijk PP, et al. F-18-fluoro-deoxy-glucose positron-emission tomography scanning in detection of local recurrence after radiotherapy for laryngeal/ pharyngeal cancer. *Head Neck.* 2001;23:933–941.

12. Branstetter BFt, Blodgett TM, Zimmer LA, et al. Head and neck malignancy: is PET/CT more accurate than PET or CT alone? *Radiology.* 2005;235:580–586.

13. Gordin A, Daitzchman M, Doweck I, et al. Fluorodeoxyglucose-positron emission tomography/ computed tomography imaging in patients with carcinoma of the larynx: diagnostic accuracy and impact on clinical management. *Laryngoscope.* 2006;116:273–278.

14. Induction chemotherapy plus radiation compared with surgery plus radiation in patients with advanced laryngeal cancer. The Department of Veterans Affairs Laryngeal Cancer Study Group. *N Engl J Med.* 1991;324:1685–1690.

15. Forastiere AA, Goepfert H, Maor M, et al. Concurrent chemotherapy and radiotherapy for organ preservation in advanced laryngeal cancer. *N Engl J Med.* 2003;349:2091–2098.

16. Weber RS, Berkey BA, Forastiere A, et al. Outcome of salvage total laryngectomy following organ preservation therapy: the Radiation Therapy Oncology Group trial 91-11. *Arch Otolaryngol Head Neck Surg.* 2003;129:44–49.

17. Fung K, Lyden TH, Lee J, et al. Voice and swallowing outcomes of an organ-preservation trial for advanced laryngeal cancer. *Int J Radiat Oncol Biol Phys.* 2005;63:1395–1399.

18. Hoffman HT, Porter K, Karnell LH, et al. Laryngeal cancer in the United States: changes in demographics, patterns of care, and survival. *Laryngoscope.* 2006;116:1–13.

19. Ferris RL, Simental A. Endoscopic surgery for early glottic carcinoma. *Op Tech Otolaryngol.* 2003;14:3–11.

20. McCombe AW, Jones AS. Radiotherapy and complications of laryngectomy. *J Laryngol Otol.* 1993;107:130–132.

21. Wax MK, Touma BJ, Ramadan HH. Tracheostomal stenosis after laryngectomy: incidence and predisposing factors. *Otolaryngol Head Neck Surg.* 1995;113:242–247.

22. Bernier J, Domenge C, Ozsahin M, et al. Postoperative irradiation with or without concomitant chemotherapy for locally advanced head and neck cancer. *N Engl J Med.* 2004;350:1945–1952.

23. Cooper JS, Pajak TF, Forastiere AA, et al. Postoperative concurrent radiotherapy and chemotherapy for high-risk squamous-cell carcinoma of the head and neck. *N Engl J Med.* 2004;350:1937–1944.

24. Sparano A, Chernock R, Feldman M, et al. Extending the inferior limits of supracricoid partial laryngectomy: a clinicopathological correlation. *Laryngoscope.* 2005;115:297–300.

25. Laccourreye O, Brasnu D, Merite-Drancy A, et al. Cricohyoidopexy in selected infrahyoid epiglottic carcinomas presenting with pathological pre-epiglottic space invasion. *Arch Otolaryngol Head Neck Surg.* 1993;119:881–886.

26. Werner JA, Lippert BM, Schunke M, et al. Animal experiment studies of laser effects on lymphatic vessels. A contribution to the discussion of laser surgery segmental resection of carcinomas. *Laryngorhinootologie.* 1995;74:748–755.

27. Vilaseca-Gonzalez I, Bernal-Sprekelsen M, Blanch-Alejandro JL, et al. Complications in transoral CO_2 laser surgery for carcinoma of the larynx and hypopharynx. *Head Neck.* 2003;25:382–388.

28. Iro H, Waldfahrer F, Altendorf-Hofmann A, et al. Transoral laser surgery of supraglottic cancer: follow-up of 141 patients. *Arch Otolaryngol Head Neck Surg.* 1998;124:1245–1250.

29. Pradier O, Christiansen H, Schmidberger H, et al. Adjuvant radiotherapy after transoral laser microsurgery for advanced squamous carcinoma of the head and neck. *Int J Radiat Oncol Biol Phys.* 2005;63:1368–1377.

30. Pellitteri PK, Ferlito A, Rinaldo A, et al. Planned neck dissection following chemoradiotherapy for advanced head and neck cancer: is it necessary for all? *Head Neck.* 2006;28:166–175.

31. Stenson KM, Huo D, Blair E, et al. Planned post-chemoradiation neck dissection: significance of radiation dose. *Laryngoscope.* 2006;116:33–36.

32. Brkovich VS, Miller FR, Karnad AB, et al. The role of positron emission tomography scans in the management of the N-positive neck in head and neck squamous cell carcinoma after chemoradiotherapy. *Laryngoscope.* 2006;116:855–858.

33. Holsinger FC, Funk E, Roberts DB, et al. Conservation laryngeal surgery versus total laryngectomy for radiation failure in laryngeal cancer. *Head Neck.* 2006;28:779–784.

34. Christiansen H, Hermann RM, Martin A, et al. Long-term follow-up after transoral laser microsurgery and adjuvant radiotherapy for advanced recurrent squamous cell carcinoma of the head and neck. *Int J Radiat Oncol Biol Phys.* 2006;65:1067–1074.

18

Hypopharyngeal Cancer

Amit Agrawal
Joshua D. Waltonen

INTRODUCTION

Malignant neoplasms arising in the hypopharynx are uncommon head and neck tumors. Hypopharyngeal carcinomas are less frequently identified compared to laryngeal and oral cavity/oropharyngeal malignancies. Unfortunately, patients with hypopharyngeal carcinoma commonly present with advanced stage disease. The abundance of submucosal lymphatics in this region predispose to both submucosal tumor spread and metastasis to the cervical lymph nodes. Traditionally, the surgical treatment of hypopharyngeal carcinoma requires total laryngectomy, whereas aggressive nonsurgical treatment protocols aimed at laryngeal preservation place patients at risk for permanent dysphagia due to pharyngeal esophageal stricture.

This chapter reviews the current evaluation and therapeutic options for patients with hypopharyngeal carcinoma. Surgical and nonsurgical treatment options are discussed. Management of and strategies for reducing treatment-related toxicities are presented.

DEFINITIONS OF UNIQUE TERMS

A. *Piriform sinus*—One of the three subsites of the hypopharynx. "Piriform" (also spelled "pyriform") means "pear-shaped." This area is also known as the piriform fossa or the piriform recess. On both sides of the hypopharynx, the piriform sinuses form inverted pyramids, which lie between the larynx and the thyroid cartilage. The piriform sinuses provide a pathway for food boluses to pass around the larynx and into the esophagus. This is the most common subsite for hypopharyngeal cancers.

B. *Posterior pharyngeal wall*—The second of the subsites of the hypopharynx. This region forms the posterior aspect of the hypopharynx, extending from the hyoid bone superiorly to the esophageal inlet inferiorly.

C. *Postcricoid region*—The third subsite of the hypopharynx. This refers to the mucosa posterior to the arytenoids and overlying the cricoid cartilage.

D. *Paraglottic space*—Medial to the piriform sinus, this space extends from the conus elasticus to the quadrangular membrane. Invasion of this space by hypopharyngeal tumors is common, and may preclude the use of conservation laryngeal surgery for hypopharyngeal cancer.

EPIDEMIOLOGY

Hypopharynx carcinomas account for about 6.5% of squamous cell carcinomas of the upper aerodigestive tract. The incidence of hypopharyngeal cancer in the United States is about 2,500 cases per year, or 1 per 100,000 per year. The most common subsite of hypopharyngeal cancer is the piriform sinus, followed by the posterior pharyngeal wall, and then the postcricoid region. Squamous cell carcinoma makes up the vast majority (>95%) of malignant lesions involving this region.[1,2]

Hypopharyngeal cancer is diagnosed at an average age of 60 years. There is a strong male preponderance in piriform sinus and posterior pharyngeal wall lesions, whereas postcricoid lesions have a slight female predominance. From the years 1975 to 2001, the incidence of hypopharyngeal cancer actually fell by 35%, and thus total mortality dropped accordingly. Unfortunately, none of the decrease in mortality can be attributed to improval in survival, as this disease still carries a poor prognosis.[3,4]

Risk factors for hypopharyngeal cancer include those common to other upper aerodigestive tract tumors, including chronic tobacco and alcohol use.[5] These agents are thought to act synergistically in carcinogenesis. Prior radiation exposure is implicated in some hypopharyngeal cancers. Plummer-Vinson syndrome (iron deficiency, esophageal webs) is present in 4 to 6% of cases of postcricoid cancer. Workers in the following industries have been shown to be at higher risk for pharyngeal cancer: asbestos, textiles, leather, paint, and welding. The association between human papillomavirus and head and neck cancer is under investigation.[6] Finally, the association of chronic laryngopharyngeal reflux in the etiology of head and neck cancer is being evaluated.[7]

ANATOMIC BOUNDARIES

The pharynx consists of the nasopharynx, oropharynx, and hypopharynx. The anatomic limits of the hypopharynx have been defined as the hyoid bone superiorly and the lower border of the cricoid cartilage inferiorly. There is an intimate relationship with the larynx, as the medial border of the hypopharynx consists of the aryepiglottic folds and the lateral borders are formed by the thyrohyoid membrane and lamina of the thyroid cartilage. The remaining lateral border consists of the inferior pharyngeal constrictor muscle.

Within the hypopharynx are three subsites. First, the bilateral piriform sinuses extend from the aryepiglottic folds medially to the inner surface of the thyroid cartilage laterally. They are shaped like inverted pyramids, with the apices at the level of the inferior border of the cricopharyngeus muscle. These are continuous with the esophagus inferiorly. The second subsite, the posterior pharyngeal wall, extends the length of the hypopharynx, bound posteriorly by the prevertebral fascia. Laterally, the posterior pharyngeal wall merges with the piriform sinuses. The third subsite, the postcricoid region, includes the mucosa posterior to the larynx, extending from the arytenoid cartilages to the inferior border of the cricoid cartilage.[8]

The hypopharynx is associated with a rich bilateral network of lymphatic drainage. The first echelon of lymphatic drainage includes the jugulodigastric, upper and mid-jugular nodes, as well as retropharyngeal nodes. For inferior tumors, drainage also occurs to the lower jugular chain and paratracheal nodes. The high frequency of cervical metastatic disease in hypopharyngeal cancer can be partially attributed to this abundant submucosal lymphatic vasculature. These lymphatics are readily involved by hypopharyngeal tumors by the time they are diagnosed.[9]

CRITICAL ELEMENTS OF HISTORY AND PHYSICAL

Symptoms of hypopharyngeal tumors are often vague and insidious, with diagnosis at an advanced stage common. Patients with early-stage disease may present with common symptoms of dysphagia, globus sensation, and odynophagia. Otalgia is also a frequent complaint, thought to be mediated by referred pain through Jacobson's nerve, a branch of the glossopharyngeal nerve, or Arnold's nerve, which shares a common origin with the superior laryngeal nerve off the vagus nerve. Hemoptysis, hoarseness, weight loss, and airway symptoms may also be among presenting symptoms, particularly for more locally advanced tumors. Clinically evident cervical lymph node metastases are common. In about 25% of cases, a mass in the neck is the initial presenting symptom. Occasionally, a neck metastasis with an occult primary tumor is later found to originate in the hypopharynx.

When taking an initial history, the patient's overall health status and functional capacity should be carefully assessed. Patients with hypopharyngeal cancer frequently have multiple comorbidities, including pulmonary and cardiovascular disease. Malnutrition and alcoholism associated with significant weight loss and functional debility are common, and their presence may significantly impact patients' ability to tolerate aggressive treatment and thus alter therapeutic planning.

Physical examination must include an assessment of the overall health and nutritional status of the patient in addition to complete head and neck examination. Assessment of the neck for cervical adenopathy is critical. Also, the larynx should be palpated by the examiner and moved side-to-side; tumors that involve the postcricoid or posterior pharyngeal wall areas may prevent laryngeal mobility and result in loss of the normal laryngeal crepitus. Extralaryngeal extension is occasionally noted on palpation of the thyroid lamina and may even present as a paramedian neck mass or fullness.

Evaluation of the hypopharynx itself can be challenging via physical examination alone. Indirect mirror laryngoscopy may demonstrate a mass or granular lesion in the hypopharynx although the primary tumor may not be easily visualized, particularly for more distal hypopharyngeal tumors. When an obvious tumor is not apparent, more subtle signs may be present, including asymmetric effacement of the piriform sinus and/or pooling of saliva. Paraglottic space involvement may be accompanied by submucosal fullness of the false vocal fold within the endolarynx. Vocal fold paralysis is indicative of invasion of the posterior cricoarytenoid muscle, the paraglottic space, or, more rarely, the cricoarytenoid joint. Airway obstruction is possible with large, bulky disease. Hypopharyngeal cancer has a propensity for deep extension and submucosal spread; thus, the examiner should be cognizant that more extensive disease often exists than is readily appreciated during office examination.

APPROPRIATE DIAGNOSTIC OFFICE-BASED PROCEDURES

Flexible fiberoptic laryngoscopy can be performed in the office with topical anesthesia. This may offer more comprehensive evaluation of the hypopharynx and larynx than indirect mirror laryngoscopy, especially among patients with unfavorable anatomy or hyperactive gag reflex. It is often difficult even with flexible fiberoptic laryngoscopy to adequately assess the inferior or distal hypopharynx. Having a patient "puff out their cheeks," however, may allow adequate insufflation and expansion of the hypopharyngeal walls, thus improving the view through the laryngoscope. In certain circumstances, biopsy of a hypopharyngeal mass may be performed in the office through appropriate flexible endoscopes.[10]

Fine-needle aspiration biopsy (FNAB), when adequately performed and evaluated by experienced personnel, is a valuable tool. FNAB has proven extremely useful in diagnosing metastatic lymphadenopathy, whether for initial clinical staging, therapeutic planning, or diagnosis of recurrent disease. This technique allows cytopathologic confirmation of squamous cell carcinoma in patients with cervical neck metastases without resorting to biopsy in the operating room. The accuracy of FNAB in diagnosing malignancy is over 95%.[11]

Transnasal esophagoscopy (TNE) can be performed in the office under topical anesthesia. TNE has been shown to be useful in evaluating patients with dysphagia, for biopsy of hypopharyngeal or esophageal lesions, and for ruling out second primary tumors of the esophagus.[12] Monitoring of patients following treatment for recurrences or stenoses of the pharynx also can be performed via TNE. Although no prospective comparative studies exist, TNE may supplant rigid esophagoscopy under general anesthesia for these indications in the future.

RECOMMENDED IMAGING STUDIES

Imaging of patients with hypopharyngeal tumors plays a critical role in clinical staging and treatment planning. Due to the propensity of hypopharyngeal tumors for deep extension, cartilaginous involvement, and submucosal spread, evaluation of the extent of such tumors using imaging modalities such as computed tomography (CT) or magnetic resonance imaging (MRI) is improved substantially over endoscopic assessment alone.[13] Nonpalpable cervical metastases can often be identified via adjunctive imaging. The importance of detection of synchronous primary tumors and distant metastases is well documented.[14]

Computed tomography (CT) scan of the neck with intravenous contrast currently is the most commonly ordered imaging study for hypopharyngeal cancers. This test can characterize the primary tumor and help define the status of regional lymph nodes. Magnetic resonance imaging (MRI) is also used for these purposes, although it is lengthier, more expensive, and subject to motion artifact. MRI, however, tends to be more accurate in defining soft tissue extent than CT. This is especially important in patients in whom surgical therapy with a laryngeal conservation procedure is considered.[13] Otherwise, there usually is not an indication to obtain both studies.

Imaging of the lungs is essential to search for distant metastasis or second primary tumors, which are not uncommon in patients with hypopharyngeal cancer. Traditional anterior-posterior and lateral chest radiographs (CXR) have long been utilized for these purposes. Many physicians perform CXR at the initial time of diagnosis and on an annual basis following treatment for screening or surveillance purposes.[15]

Recent studies have demonstrated increased sensitivity of chest CT for detecting synchronous lung tumors over that of CXR. In fact, many investigators advocate routine use of chest CT in screening of head and neck cancer patients.[16,17] Chest CT can be obtained at the same time as the neck CT, and adds about 30 seconds to the exam.

Positron emission tomography (PET), often fused with a CT scan (PET-CT), is advocated by some as a sensitive means of detecting synchronous primary tumors[18] as well as locoregional and distant metastases, all of which are not uncommon phenomena in patients diagnosed with hypopharyngeal malignancy. It is also finding utility in detection of occult primary tumors,[19] which are not uncommonly found to be located within the hypopharynx. PET is currently undergoing evaluation for post-treatment surveillance in patients treated for head and neck cancer.[20] The actual sensitivity, specificity, and practical utility of PET and PET-CT for these purposes is undefined, however, and currently remains under active investigation.

The utility of barium esophagography to characterize hypopharyngeal tumors is limited. On occasion, esophagram performed for symptoms of dysphagia will detect filling defects in the hypopharynx, leading to the diagnosis of hypopharyngeal cancer. Esophagography can occasionally demonstrate extension of the disease inferiorly into the cervical esophagus, and may carry utility in situations when endoscopy is not easily accomplished. It seems intuitive that other methods including direct endoscopy or CT/MR imaging would be more sensitive than esophagography in this regard, although no formal comparisons have been made in the literature. Barium swallow has some utility in detecting second primary tumors of the esophagus, although the sensitivity of esophagography remains questionable.[21]

It should be emphasized that physical examination, office endoscopic procedures, and imaging are supplements to direct laryngopharyngoscopy and esophagoscopy under general anesthesia, which remain essential for evaluation of hypopharyngeal tumors. Only at this time can the true inferior extent of a mucosal lesion be determined. In addition, relationship between adjacent structures, such as the larynx, the cervical esophagus, and the oropharynx, are better clarified with this examination. Panendoscopy (which adds rigid or flexible esophagoscopy and bronchoscopy to laryngopharyngoscopy) has long assumed a traditional role in an effort to detect synchronous primary tumors of the upper aerodigestive tract, esophagus, or tracheobronchial tree.[22,23] The true utility of this procedure as well as whether other methods of evaluation such as detailed imaging serve as effective adjuncts or even should supplant traditional endoscopy remains a subject of debate.

AMERICAN JOINT COMMITTEE ON CANCER (AJCC) STAGING OF HYPOPHARYNGEAL CANCER

Current staging criteria for hypopharyngeal malignancies have been defined as follows: the primary tumor is staged both anatomically on size and functionally by impairment of vocal fold motion. Cervical lymphatics are staged like other mucosal subsites in the head and neck, with the exception of the nasopharynx.[24]

Primary Tumor

Tis   Carcinoma in situ

T1   Tumor limited to one subsite of hypopharynx and 2 cm or less in greatest dimension

T2   Tumor invades more than one subsite of hypopharynx or an adjacent site, or measures more than 2 cm but not more than 4 cm in greatest diameter without fixation of hemilarynx

T3   Tumor more than 4 cm in greatest dimension or with fixation of hemilarynx

T4a   Tumor invades thyroid/cricoid cartilage, hyoid bone, thyroid gland, esophagus, or central compartment soft tissue

T4b   Tumor invades prevertebral fascia, encases carotid artery, or involves mediastinal structures

Regional Lymph Nodes

NX   Regional lymph nodes cannot be assessed

N0   No regional lymph node metastasis

N1   Metastasis in a single ipsilateral lymph node 3 cm or less in greatest dimension

N2   Metastasis in a single ipsilateral lymph node, more than 3 cm but not more than 6 cm in greatest dimension; or in multiple ipsilateral lymph nodes, none more than 6 cm in greatest dimension; or in bilateral or contralateral lymph nodes, none more than 6 cm in greatest dimension

N2a   Metastasis in a single ipsilateral lymph node more than 3 cm but not more than 6 cm in greatest dimension

N2b   Metastasis in multiple ipsilateral lymph nodes, none more than 6 cm in greatest dimension

N2c   Metastasis in bilateral or contralateral lymph nodes, none more than 6 cm in greatest dimension

N3   Metastasis in a lymph node more than 6 cm in greatest dimension

Distant Metastases

MX   Distant metastasis cannot be assessed

M0   No distant metastasis

M1   Distant metastasis

Stage Grouping

Stage 0   Tis N0 M0

Stage I   T1 N0 M0

Stage II   T2 N0 M0

Stage III   T3 N0 M0
            T1 N1 M0
            T2 N1 M0
            T3 N1 M0

Stage IVA   T4a N0 M0
            T4a N1 M0
            T1 N2 M0
            T2 N2 M0
            T3 N2 M0
            T4a N2 M0

Stage IVB   T4b Any N M0
            Any T N3 M0

Stage IVC   Any T Any N M1

HISTOPATHOLOGY

Over 95% of hypopharyngeal malignancies are squamous cell carcinomas.[1] Variants of squamous cell carcinoma, such as spindle cell squamous carcinoma, verrucous carcinoma, basaloid squamous cell carcinoma, and undifferentiated carcinoma have been reported.[25,26] Less commonly reported histologies include adenocarcinoma (0.5%), lymphoma (0.5%), and adenoid cystic carcinoma (0.3%).[1] Other histologies are exceedingly rare; reports in the literature describe minor salivary gland tumors (mucoepidermoid carcinoma), sarcomas (eg, chondrosarcomas, synovial sarcomas, and leimyosarcomas), and metastases from other sites (eg, breast cancer).

IDENTIFICATION OF CRITICAL DECISION POINTS

Patients with hypopharyngeal malignancies usually will be recommended for multimodal treatment due to advanced stage presentation and aggressive behavior, whether primary surgical or nonsurgical protocols are employed. Deciding optimal therapy for patients with hypopharyngeal malignancy requires careful consideration of several key decision points which ultimately impact selected therapy. Critical concepts necessarily include consideration of modalities of therapy which achieve goals including maximization of chances of cure, effective palliation of symptoms, tolerability of therapy, and functional outcome. In patients selected for surgical therapy, this should include considerations of whether laryngeal preservation or conservation laryngeal procedures might be feasibly incorporated into surgical plans. Treatment decision necessarily includes incorporation of patient preference with regards to anticipated functional outcome, particularly swallowing, voice, and airway.

Locally Advanced Disease

There is little debate that for locally advanced hypopharyngeal malignancy with gross cartilage involvement and/or extralaryngeal extension that surgery involving laryngopharyngectomy as a component of multimodal therapy is preferred over nonsurgical treatment alone in order to optimize chances for both locoregional disease control as well as effective symptom palliation provided that patient is an acceptable surgical risk. In such cases, it is imperative for the surgeon to assess whether these tumors

fall into the category of resectable disease. Tumors involving the posterior pharyngeal wall or manifesting with extralaryngeal extension require specific mention.

Posterior Pharyngeal Wall Lesions

Tumors involving the posterior pharyngeal wall must be assessed with regard to their relation to the prevertebral space and possible invasion of the prevertebral fascia/musculature. Involvement of the prevertebral fascia is associated with dismal rates of cure, regardless of therapeutic modality employed. At the time of diagnostic endoscopy, fixation of tumors to the prevertebral region upon palpation should raise concern regarding possible invasion of tumors beyond the prevertebral space. Preoperative modalities including constrast-enhanced MRI and CT are useful studies to assess for disruption of the normal tissue planes or evidence of bony erosion in this region (Fig 18–1A and 18–1B). For example, preservation of the retropharyngeal fat plane between the tumor and the prevertebral compartment on T1-weighted MRI images has been found to carry a high negative predictive probability of 98% for absence of prevertebral space fixation found at the time of surgical exploration.[27] Although the negative predictive value of both CT and MRI are generally quite high for predicting absence of prevertebral involvement,[27,28] these modalities have also been criticized for lacking set criteria which accurately determine this parameter with adequate sensitivity and specificity.[28,29] Ultimately, it must be emphasized that definitive judgment in this regard requires that this region be assessed via early exploration of the prevertebral space during surgery and confirmed with frozen section biopsy if necessary (Fig 18-2).

Extralaryngeal Disease

Extralaryngeal extension is a common feature of locally advanced hypopharygeal malignancy. In some cases, direct disease extension into the neck occurs as a consequence of disease extending around the posterior border of the thyroid cartilage ala and may present as a neck mass that may be confused with metastatic adenopathy. Imaging techniques such as

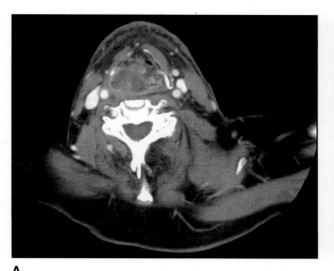

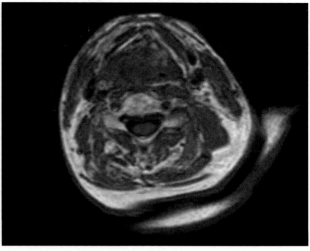

A   **B**

Fig 18–1. CT and MR imaging of a locally advanced right piriform sinus and posterior pharyngeal wall carcinoma. This tumor extensively occupies the visceral pharyngeal space. Note, there is attenuation and loss of the normal prevertebral fat plane seen on both the CT (**A**) as well as T1-weighted MR (**B**) imaging, particularly along the right side, raising concern about the possibility of prevertebral space involvement. Presence of this finding, however, is not specific and assessment of actual involvement of this region requires surgical determination (Fig 18–2).

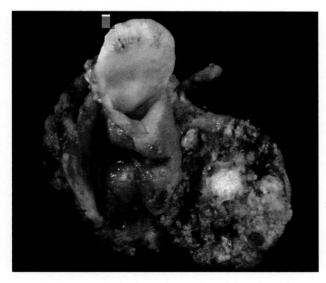

Fig 18–2. Locally advanced right piriform sinus and posterior wall carcinoma. Resected specimen from patient described in Figure 18–1. For this particular patient, the prevertebral space was explored early during surgery and found to be uninvolved. Resection was achieved with negative margins.

CT of the neck or PET-CT are often helpful adjuncts in assessing primary and regional disease extent (Figs 18-3 and 18-4). It is critical to recognize this possibility as such disease extension may be intimately associated with adjacent carotid sheath structures (Figs 18-3 and 18-5), and, as such, the surgeon must be prepared to encounter and address this possibility including intraoperative availability of vascular surgery consultation.

Circumferential Disease Extent

Preoperative assessment of extent of circumferential disease involvement becomes an important surgical consideration with regard to re-establishing the swallowing conduit at the time of disease resection. In selected cases, primary closure may be accomplished while maintaining adequate diameter of the reconstructed neopharynx. As established criteria have not been defined, this requires individualized determination by the surgeon on a case by case basis.

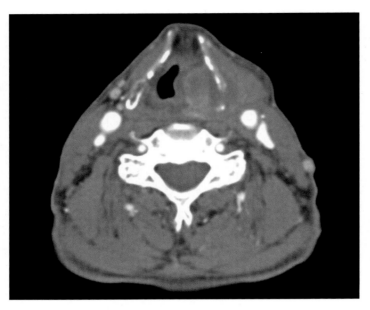

Fig 18–3. Left piriform sinus carcinoma with extralarygeal extension. This patient initially presented with hoarseness and a left-sided paramedian neck mass, however, was otherwise asymptomatic. Office endoscopy revealed left vocal fold fixation and only mild submucosal fullness along the left arytenoid and false vocal fold without obviously apparent granular tissue. CT imaging above for this patient demonstrated a left piriform sinus tumor with paraglottic space involvement and extralaryngeal extension around the posterior border of the thyroid cartilage ala into the soft tissues of the neck. Note the disease proximity to the left carotid sheath structures.

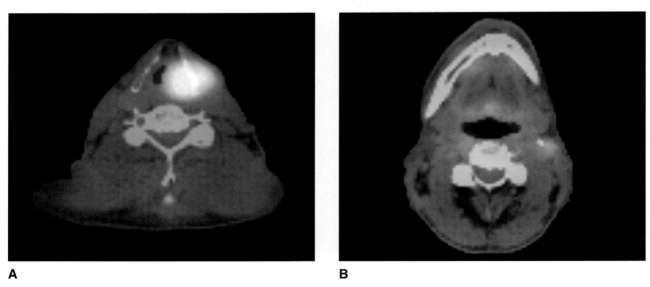

A   B

Fig 18–4. PET-CT imaging of left piriform sinus carcinoma. **A.** This PET-CT (patient previously described in Fig 18–2) demonstrates dramatic [18F]-FDG uptake of the primary tumor. **B.** Focal abnormal uptake of [18F]-FDG in a small, nonpalpable, metastatic left level 2 lymph node in the same patient.

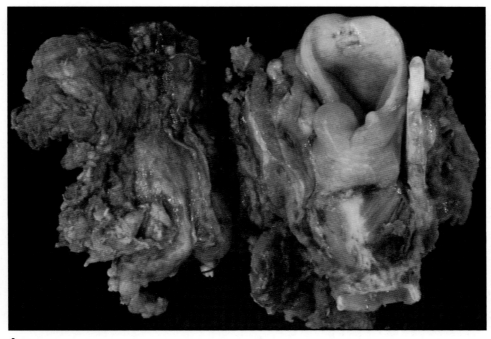

A

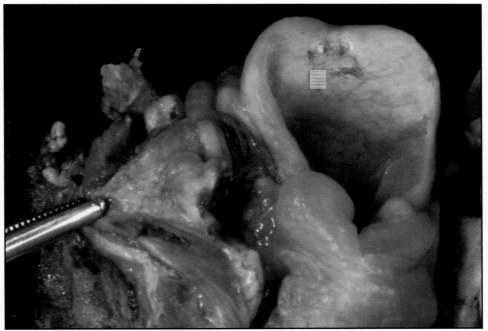

B

Fig 18–5. Resected left piriform carcinoma. **A.** Specimen (from patient described in Fig 18–3) resected en bloc with attached neck contents due to the significant extralaryngeal disease extension with proximity to carotid sheath structures. Although vascular surgery service was available on standby for this procedure, the carotid artery was able to be preserved in situ. **B.** Close-up view of this resected specimen demonstrates an endophytic tumor along the left piriform sinus. *continues*

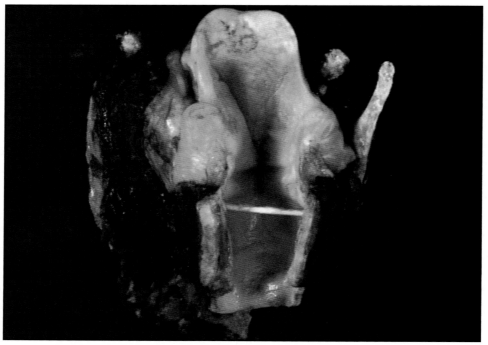

C

Fig 18–5. *continued* **C.** Note other than mild fullness and asymmetry along the left aryepiglottic fold, arytenoid, and false vocal fold, the otherwise relatively normal appearance of the endolaryngeal surface despite previously noted extensive paraglottic space involvement with vocal fold fixation and extralaryngeal extension (Fig 18–3).

Many surgeons prefer at least a 4-cm wide strip of remaining pharynx to allow for primary repair. In cases where a remaining strip of pharynx exists but is inadequate for primary repair, this will require flap augmentation via a variety of reconstructive methods involving either regional flaps or free tissue transfer. Although no prospective comparative studies exist comparing regional flap versus free tissue transfer for this specific purpose, both appear to be reliable methods to reconstruct partial pharyngeal defects. Although regional myocutaneous flap reconstruction of total circumferential defects has been reported with reasonable success in some series,[30] in cases requiring total (or near total) circumferential resection of the laryngopharynx, reconstruction of the neopharynx and cervical esophagus

is preferred via microvascular free tissue transfer techniques utilizing either enteric jejunal free flap or other tubed cutaneous free flaps.[31]

Inferior Disease Extent

Determination of the extent of inferior disease involvement when contemplating surgical therapy particularly when disease is identified involving the distal piriform apex/esophageal inlet carries specific relevance, and careful intraoperative assessment at the time of diagnostic endoscopy remains critical in assessing this parameter. Hypopharyngeal malignancy is notorious for submucosal disease extension, which must be accounted for when achieving adequate surgical margins. Tumors of the cervical esophagus frequently extend superiorly to involve the hypopharynx, and this situation must be recognized. In cases where proximal esophageal involvement occurs and adequate resection or reconstruction cannot be accomplished via transcervical route, this will require conversion to total laryngopharyngoesophagectomy with gastric pull-up procedures in order to achieve an acceptable oncologic result and/or predictable functional outcome. Such possibility must be planned for in advance to allow for intraoperative availability and involvement of other surgical disciplines.

Management of the Larynx

Decision-making with regard to management of the larynx remains an important yet controversial topic in patients in whom surgical therapy is contemplated, particularly in cases where disease extent either does not directly involve the larynx, or involvement of the larynx is limited to the point where laryngeal conservation resection procedures can be considered. Careful assessment of the larynx during endoscopy is crucial in determining the degree of laryngeal involvement which typically occurs as a consequence of either direct extension into the paraglottic space and/or mucosal extension. Fullness or firmness of the false vocal fold region can be indicative of this finding (see Fig 18–5). Information gained from preoperative CT (see Fig 18–3) or MRI[13] is often helpful in assessing this region as well. In patients where disease extent causes vocal fold fixation suggesting significant paraglottic (or cricoarytenoid involvement), involves the postcricoid region, involves the distal hypopharynx/piriform apex, or extensively involves the posterior pharyngeal wall, few would argue that surgical removal of the entire larynx is preferred for both oncologic and functional reasons. For less extensive lesions, the issue at hand is not whether such disease can be resected in an effective oncologic manner, but rather whether the postoperative functional outcome can be reliably predicted. For the uncommon situation of small, limited tumors involving the lateral pharynx, resection via lateral pharyngotomy with laryngeal preservation is feasible with reasonable functional and oncologic results.[32]

For the uncommon situation of limited tumors involving the posterior pharyngeal wall, resection via transhyoid approach may be feasible. For limited tumors involving the superior hypopharynx or marginal region, the postoperative outcome with partial laryngopharyngectomy often yields reasonable functional recovery in appropriately selected patients with adequate pulmonary reserve. Despite some variability, several series have reported that partial laryngopharygeal resection procedures are not only feasible from a disease control perspective, but also are compatible with swallowing recovery in a high proportion of patients, along with ability to maintain voice and uncommon need for permanent tracheostomy.[33-35] In cases of partial laryngopharyngectomy, flap reconstruction may be required to achieve adequate wound closure with reasonable functional outcome.[34,36]

It is important to bear in mind that when adequate tumor removal requires more extended laryngopharygeal resection, a greater degree of unpredictability with regard to postoperative functional outcome results, particularly with regard to swallowing recovery. Due to such concerns in these patients, the safest predictable outcome is likely achieved by total laryngectomy with flap reconstruction if necessary. In patients in whom functional concerns are overriding and total laryngectomy is not an acceptable option, it is appropriate to enter into discussions with regard to nonsurgical organ preservation approaches to treating such tumors.

ANALYSIS OF VARIOUS TREATMENT OPTIONS

Surgical Therapy

Conventional treatment for hypopharyngeal carcinoma typically has involved surgery followed by postoperative adjuvant radiotherapy in these patients, the large majority of whom present with advanced disease. The use of adjuvant radiotherapy following surgery is associated with reduced locoregional disease recurrence and improved survival.[37] In several large series, overall survival for hypopharyngeal carcinoma treated with surgery and planned post-operative radiation reveals 5-year overall survival rates reported in the range of 20% to 40%.[37-39] Furthermore, although local and regional disease recurrence continue to remain a significant challenge, the eventual emergence of distant metastases or second primary tumors has developed as a major obstacle to long-term survival for a substantial proportion of patients treated for hypopharyngeal carcinoma.[40,41]

Laryngeal Conservation

Several series assessing partial laryngopharyngectomy have shown that rates of local disease control are acceptable when laryngeal conservation measures are employed in an attempt to maintain aspects of laryngeal function. Local disease control rates of 80 to 90% are reported with partial laryngopharyngectomy procedures and are noted to be comparable to historical rates of local disease control when more extended procedures are performed.[33,34,42]

Minimally invasive endoscopic resection of hypopharyngeal malignancy has been also been reported in a limited number of series typically reporting endoscopic management of such tumors with planned adjunctive radiotherapy or chemoradiotherapy. In experienced centers, long-term local disease control rates of nearly 90% with high rates of laryngeal preservation have been reported.[43,44] Although endoscopic management is commonly reported for management of selected glottic and supraglottic malignancies, it must be emphasized that endoscopic resection of hypopharyngeal cancer has not been evaluated in sufficient prospective format to recommend its routine use for this disease site. As such, endoscopic treatment of hypopharyngeal malignancies should be left to surgeons highly experienced in the endoscopic management of upper aerodigestive tract malignancies.

Postoperative Adjunctive Chemoradiotherapy

Recently reported data from two large separate randomized prospective trials carried out by the Radiation Therapy Oncology/Head and Neck Intergroup and the European Organization for Research and Treatment of Cancer (EORTC) support the use of adjunctive platinum-based chemotherapy along with radiotherapy in the postoperative setting in patients defined as having high risk or advanced head and neck malignancy.[45,46]

Although "high-risk"/advanced disease groups differed somewhat between the two trials (Intergroup: positive margins, multiple positive nodes, or extracapsular spread[46]; EORTC: T3, T4 disease, N2 or greater, extracapsular spread, lymphovascular invasion, perineural invasion, positive margins[45]), both studies demonstrated improved locoregional disease control and improved disease-specific survival associated with patient cohorts receiving adjuvant chemoradiotherapy versus adjuvant radiotherapy alone. Results of the EORTC trial also revealed improved overall survival in the adjuvant chemotherapy group.[45] As such, surgical schema to treat patients with hypopharyngeal carcinoma most of whom likely fall into a high-risk/advanced category will likely incorporate increasing use of adjuvant concomitant chemoradiation in the postoperative setting.

Intensified Therapy Regimens

Through a series of phase II pilot studies conducted over the past 12 years, the use of intensified regimens to treat advanced head and neck malignancies including hypopharyngeal tumors has been explored at our own institution.[47] Recently, we reported long-term 5-year overall survival of 56% in a subset of 34 patients with advanced hypopharyngeal carcinoma who underwent intensified combination therapy consisting of preoperative accelerated chemoradiation (cis-platinum), surgery with intraoperative radiotherapy, followed by postoperative chemoradiation with multiagent systemic chemotherapy (cis-platinum, paclitaxel). Long-term locoregional disease control in this series was also favorable (91%). The primary hindrance to the delivery of such therapy, however, remains the specialized and complex nature of the treatment regimen as well as substantial resources required to provide adequate multidisciplinary support for patients undergoing such treatment. Even with such measures in place at our own institution, we found that overall protocol compliance was approximately 62%, underscoring the need to further explore methods to improve patient tolerance of complex therapy regimens.

Nonsurgical Organ Preservation— Induction Chemotherapy

The success seen with sequential nonsurgical regimens involving induction chemotherapy and radiation therapy for advanced laryngeal malignancy demonstrating feasibility of preservation of the laryngeal organ without compromise of survival has led to its application in other head and neck disease sites including the hypopharynx. The European Organization for Research and Treatment of Cancer Head and Neck Cancer Cooperative Group reported the important results of their randomized prospective study assessing induction chemotherapy followed by definitive radiotherapy in patients with advanced hypopharyngeal carcinoma comparing this group with a second group randomized to undergo standard surgery (laryngopharyngectomy) and postoperative radiation therapy.[48] Although overall long-term survival in both groups was poor (5-year survival 35% and 30% for surgery and nonsurgical groups, respectively), no compromise in survival was seen the nonsurgical group compared to the immediate surgery group. Although laryngeal preservation was clearly feasible in a subset of patients, the overall rate of long-term laryngeal preservation was low (35%) in patients who were initially randomized to receive nonsurgical therapy.

Nonsurgical Organ Preservation— Concomitant Chemoradiotherapy

Concomitant chemoradiotherapy holds the theoretical advantage of administering systemic treatment while also potentiating the antitumor effects of radiotherapy via radiosensitization. Encouraging randomized prospective study data reveal significant improvement in both locoregional disease control as well as rate of laryngeal preservation associated with use of concomitant chemoradiation schema over sequential schema (or radiation alone) for treatment of advanced laryngeal malignancy.[49] Given the desire

to achieve similar results for other disease sites, the use of concomitant chemoradiation as primary treatment for advanced head and neck malignancy including hypopharyngeal sites has been increasingly described. Although large prospective comparative experience assessing concomitant chemoradiation with other modalities for this specific disease subsite are presently lacking, data from several reported series would appear to indicate benefit from a locoregional disease control perspective with regard to use of concomitant chemoradiation for the treatment of advanced head and neck malignancy.[50,51]

Nonsurgical Organ Preservation— RADPLAT

The use of intra-arterial chemotherapy to provide selective antitumor effect via infusion of effective antineoplastic platinum-based therapy in relative proximity to tumor blood supply in conjunction with concomitant radiotherapy (RADPLAT) has been increasingly reported in the treatment of advanced head and neck malignancy.[52,53] Locoregional disease control rates achieved by such treatment have been encouraging, with initial locoregional complete response observed in 70 to 80% of patients. Although the specialized and labor-intensive nature of this type of treatment has hindered its widespread adoption, recent data published by the Radiation Therapy Oncology Group have reported the feasibility of carrying out such treatment across a multi-institutional setting citing encouraging rates of overall treatment compliance and initial disease response.[54] The data from these phase II trials have been encouraging; however, it should also be noted that results from recent randomized study has brought into question the relative value of intra-arterial delivery of chemotherapy over standard methods involving traditional intravenous route delivery of chemotherapy.[55]

Functional Outcome—Surgical Therapy

Surgical therapy for hypopharyngeal malignancy in which the entire larynx is removed results in the predictable outcome of permanent loss of natural voice as well as creation of permanent stoma for respiration. Swallowing recovery in the majority of patients in whom either the pharynx is repaired primarily or in whom flap augmentation is required is usually quite good, with very few patients requiring long-term enteral nutrition once adequate healing has occurred. Vocal rehabilitation via tracheoesophageal methods allows for effective speech acquisition in a substantial majority of subjects. In patients requiring circumferential reconstruction with either tubed cutaneous or jejunal free flaps, postoperative stricture formation occurs in about 15 to 20% of patients.[56] Speech acquisition via tracheoesophageal methods is achievable in a significant proportion of patients requiring circumferential reconstruction, although poorer results occur in patients having undergone enteric flap reconstruction compared to tubed cutaneous free flaps.[56]

Several series examining functional outcome following partial laryngopharyngectomy report reasonable rates of swallowing recovery even when flap reconstruction is required for closure. The rate of permanent tracheostomy following partial laryngopharyngectomy is also extremely low in these series.[33-36] Similarly, the few existing series reporting results following endoscopic resection of hypopharyngeal tumors also report excellent rates of maintenance of voice and swallowing, again with uncommon need for adjunctive tracheostomy.[43,44]

Functional Outcome— Chemoradiotherapy

Obvious goals of nonsurgical organ preservation strategies stem from the desire to achieve disease control while attempting to preserve the structure, and indirectly function, of the laryngopharyngeal region. Randomized study examining the use of sequential chemotherapy followed by radiation in the treatment of advanced hypopharyngeal malignancy have clearly revealed the feasibility of preservation of the larynx in a minority yet significant percentage of patients without compromise in overall survival. Nonetheless, it must be noted that despite apparent feasibility of these goals, the overall rates of laryngeal preservation with such treatment remains quite low (35%) and patients should thus

be made aware of this.[48] Consequently, as more aggressive nonsurgical schema have been employed in an attempt to improve on these results, it also has become increasingly clear that the toxicity and significant morbidity associated with such treatment, as well as long-term effects including potential outcome of a preserved yet dysfunctional laryngopharyngeal organ, are substantially increased as well.[57] As such, the need for adjunctive measures including feeding tubes or tracheostomy by a substantial proportion of patients undergoing aggressive nonsurgical therapy, the high rate of complications and morbidity associated with surgical salvage of failed chemoradiotherapy, and the reliable predictability of functional outcome as well as effective palliation of symptoms associated with primary surgical therapy continue to remain compelling arguments for proponents of primary surgery in the management of hypopharyngeal malignancies.

Surgical Versus Nonsurgical Treatment: Quality of Life (QOL) Comparisons

Similar to other disease sites, controversy continues over whether primary consideration should be given to surgical versus nonsurgical methods for treatment of hypopharyngeal malignancy. In the absence of a proven clear survival advantage of surgical versus nonsurgical regimens, it has become important for clinicians to become familiar with issues involving quality of life when evaluating available treatment options. The advent of several validated quality of life instrument measures over the past decade have allowed for direct comparison of patient groups, including those having undergone surgical therapy versus those having undergone nonsurgical therapy for advanced head and neck cancer. One might assume that compared to surgery, successful treatment of advanced head and neck cancer with nonsurgical methods might result in a more satisfactory outcome from a quality of life perspective, particularly when centered around the issue of presence or absence of the larynx. Interestingly, however, retrospective analyses in recent years examining QOL measures following treatment for advanced head and neck malignancy of several disease sites, including larynx and pharynx, have revealed that when comparing surgical versus nonsurgical groups, overall measures of QOL actually appear similar between groups.[58,59] Furthermore, although these studies reveal some differences favoring either the surgical or nonsurgical groups among individual QOL domain scores, scores involving speech and swallowing measures also appear to be similar between surgical and nonsurgical groups despite the frequent absence of the larynx in a substantial proportion of patients in the surgical groups.[58,59] It is postulated that surgical efforts at functional preservation including conservation surgery, surgical reconstruction, and rehabilitative strategies to restore speech serve to positively impact long-term health-related QOL measures. On the other hand, nonsurgical treatment regimens, which necessarily have become more intensive and hence toxic, carry greater degree of negative impact with regard to quality of life, thus achieving similar overall health-related quality of life measures between surgical and nonsurgical groups.[58]

COMPLICATIONS OF THERAPY

General

For all surgical approaches, patients should be counseled about general complications of surgery including bleeding, infection, wound healing problems, as well as complications relating to general anesthesia. Given the frequent presence of other comorbidities in patients with head and neck malignancies, cardiopulmonary complications following surgery are not uncommon events. Most patients undergoing primary surgery for hypopharyngeal malignancy will typically undergo neck dissection given the high rate of nodal involvement associated with this disease subsite. As such, morbidities relating to neck dissection, including cranial nerve injury, should be discussed.

Fistula

As with any external approach to the pharynx and larynx, there is risk of development of pharyngocutaneous fistula in the postoperative period. Higher rates of fistula formation are seen in patients under-

going laryngectomy for hypopharyngeal malignancy (ie, extended laryngectomy).[60,61] Salivary fistula occur in 15% to over 30% of patients undergoing laryngopharyngectomy,[61-63] the incidence of which relates to multiple factors, including extent of resection (partial vs circumferential) and prior therapy. Several studies have demonstrated high rates of postsurgical complication rates, including fistula formation (up to 30%), following laryngectomy in patients having received prior radiation or chemoradiation therapy.[62-64] Gastric pull-up procedures are effective in the reconstruction of total laryngopharyngoesophagectomy defects[65] but also are associated with significant complications including fistulous/anastomotic leakage, as well as pulmonary complications, including chylothorax, pneumothorax, and pneumonia.

Stricture

Pharyngoesophageal stricture can be a significant cause for post-treatment dysphagia following either surgical or nonsurgical treatment for hypopharyngeal malignancy. Stricture rates up to 20% are reported in patients undergoing laryngectomy, with significantly higher rates for individuals undergoing surgery for hypopharyngeal primary tumors versus surgery for glottic tumors.[66]

Patients undergoing primary chemoradiation as part of organ-preserving protocols for head and neck malignancy also carry significant risk of pharyngoesophageal stricture formation, which occurs in 20% of patients with even higher risk of stricture formation occurring in patients treated for primary hypopharyngeal tumors.[67] In some patients, development of complete stricture is possible as a consequence of chemoradiation therapy. This is postulated to occur as a consequence of confluent circumferential mucositis, which results in ulceration and subsequent adhesion of opposing mucosal surfaces within the hypopharynx or cervical esophagus. In addition, mucosa damaged or replaced by tumor infiltration may heal by secondary intention with subsequent wound contracture.[68]

Although partial strictures can often be managed adequately with anterograde endoscopic dilation,[68] similar management of patients with complete stenoses can be more challenging given the significant risk for pharyngoesophageal perforation when an obvious lumen is absent. In cases with complete obstruction, successful endoscopic management has been reported in situations where separable adhesions exist (rather than mature fibrous stricture),[69] or utilizing a combination of retrograde endoscopic approaches (through an existing gastrostomy) and anterograde approaches.[68] In situations, however, where endoscopic management is not feasible, surgical measures including laryngopharyngectomy with flap reconstruction may be required for patients who desire the ability to swallow, although this results in the obvious outcome of a permanent breathing stoma as well as loss of natural voice.

Dysphagia/Aspiration

Surgery

In patients undergoing surgical therapy for hypopharyngeal malignancy, which includes total laryngectomy, swallowing recovery is typically straightforward, with adequate function reasonably expected for most patients when stricture is absent. Even when flap reconstruction is required to reconstruct substantial partial or circumferential pharyngeal defects, adequate oral intake is achieved in 90% of patients when the larynx is removed.[70] In patients undergoing partial pharyngectomy or partial laryngopharyngectomy in which the entire larynx or a portion of the larynx is preserved, functional deficits pertaining to swallowing function are more commonly expected. Although best results in some series have demonstrated eventual adequate functional recovery in 80% to 90% of patients undergoing partial laryngopharyngectomy,[34,35] the rate of significant dysphagia is very high in the immediate postoperative period, with recovery typically observed occurring over a period of several weeks or even months.[35] These patients not uncommonly require temporary use of adjunctive nasogastric or gastric feeding tubes, although the possibility of long-term need of such devices also exists and should be reviewed as a possibility. Although voicing ability is typically preserved in patients undergoing partial laryngopharyngectomy, not infrequently there are alter-ations of speech including hoarse or breathy voice quality, which depend in part on the extent of laryngeal resection.

Nonsurgical Therapy

With increasing use of protocols utilizing radiation therapy with concomitant chemotherapy in an effort to improve disease control and achieve organ preservation, a significant proportion of patients undergoing intensive chemoradiation for advanced head and neck malignancy experience significant dysphagia and/or aspiration as a consequence of laryngopharyngeal dysfunction. Analysis of swallowing function via videofluoroscopy following intensive chemoradiation therapy reveal effects including delayed swallow initiation, incoordination in the timing of the swallowing reflex, and incomplete cricopharyngeal relaxation.[71] These events contribute to rates of aspiration reported as high as 65% in post-therapy studies, with development of pneumonia requiring hospitalization in a substantial proportion of these patients.[71,72] Although improvement occurs over the first 12 months,[73] long-term post-treatment dysphagia requiring substantial diet alteration has been documented in up to 40% of patients having undergone intensive chemoradiotherapy.[74] Rates ranging from 20 to 39% of patients undergoing concomitant chemoradiation for advanced head and neck malignancy require long-term or permanent gastrostomy tube feeding as a consequence of persistent swallowing problems despite documented disease control.[72,75,76]

Other Complications of Radiation and Chemotherapy

Other treatment-related side-effects and complications associated with radiation therapy of the head and neck are well documented.[77] These may occur in the settings of primary treatment with or without chemotherapy or in postsurgical adjuvant therapy. During treatment, patients may experience variable degrees of acute effects, such as mucositis, xerostomia, edema, and skin reactions which can range from mild to severe. Severe (grade 3–4) mucositis with standard radiotherapy treatment alone occurs in about 30% of patients with rates increasing to 56% in patients undergoing altered fractionation schema.[78] Addition of chemotherapy characteristically exacerbates the side effects of radiotherapy, particularly mucositis, and creates significant risks of additional side effects including neutropenia, anemia, and nausea.[49] Such side effects, which are not infrequently severe, carry potential for causing significant treatment interruption.

Although there is typical improvement of many acute effects of radiotherapy over time, some effects persist or become manifest as late toxicities of radiotherapy, many of which are often permanent. Permanent xerostomia is very common following head and neck radiotherapy, although it is hoped that newer more conformal methods of delivery of radiation such as intensity modulated radiation therapy (IMRT) will positively impact this variable.[79,80] The effects of long-term xerostomia are significant and can worsen dysphagia and result in multiple dental caries. Radionecrosis of laryngeal cartilages and the mandible are other known complications of radiotherapy. Eventual thyroid dysfunction is extremely common in the head and neck cancer population following radiotherapy, with published rates of hypothyroidism occurring in 12 to 67% of patients during long-term follow-up.[81,82]

SUMMARY

Hypopharyngeal carcinoma remains one of the most challenging malignancies of the upper aerodigestive tract to treat due to its typical advanced stage at diagnosis, propensity for aggressive locoregional extent, distant metastases, and functionally critical anatomic location. This disease pattern has led to the development of aggressive surgical as well as nonsurgical combined modality treatment regimens. Nonsurgical schema have clearly demonstrated the feasibility of preservation of the laryngopharynx without compromise in survival, although rates of disease control and organ preservation remain low. Nonsurgical regimens thus have evolved into increased utilization of intensive concomitant chemoradiation schema in an effort to improve both rates of disease control and organ preservation, however, are also associated with high rates of significant toxicity and long-term morbidity particularly with respect to swallowing function. Contemporary surgical advances have allowed for the application of effective organ-preserving surgical strategies including partial laryngopharyngectomy and even endoscopic resection with acceptable functional outcome as well as comparable levels of disease control compared to more radical surgical options in appropriately selected patients. For locally advanced or recurrent tumors, however, more extensive surgery including total laryngectomy with partial or total pharyngectomy is still required. Despite its extent, this procedure reliably achieves immediate oncologic impact, effective symptom palliation including swallowing recovery, as well as potential for vocal rehabilitation via tracheoesophageal speech for most patients. Given the similarity in survival as well as overall quality of life measures associated with very different available surgical and nonsurgical treatment options, individual patient preference must be taken into account when providing counseling regarding recommended therapy.

REFERENCES

1. Carvalho AL, Nishimoto IN, Califano JA, Kowalski LP. Trends in incidence and prognosis for head and neck cancer in the United States: a site-specific analysis of the SEER database. *Int J Cancer*. 2005; 114(5):806–816.
2. Canto MT, Devesa SS. Oral cavity and pharynx cancer incidence rates in the United States, 1975-1998. *Oral Oncol*. 2002;38(6):610–617.
3. Davies L, Welch HG. Epidemiology of head and neck cancer in the United States. *Otolaryngol Head Neck Surg*. 2006;135(3):451–457.
4. Krespi YP, Atiyah RA. Hypopharyngeal carcinoma. *Otolaryngol Clin North Am*. 1985;18(3):469–477.
5. Blot WJ, McLaughlin JK, Winn DM. Smoking and drinking in relation to oral and pharyngeal cancer. *Cancer Res*. 1988;48(11):3282–3287.
6. Mineta H, Ogino T, Amano HM, et al. Human papilloma virus (HPV) type 16 and 18 detected in head and neck squamous cell carcinoma. *Anticancer Res*. 1998;18(6B):4765–4768.

7. Ward PH, Hanson DG. Reflux as an etiological factor of carcinoma of the laryngopharynx. *Laryngoscope*. 1998;8:1195-1199.

8. Janfaza P, Fabian R. Pharynx. In: Janfaza P, Nadol JB, Galla RJ, et al, eds. *Surgical Anatomy of the Head and Neck*. Philadelphia, Pa. Lippincott Williams & Wilkins; 2000: 367-392.

9. Candela FC, Kothari K, Shah JP. Patterns of cervical node metastases from squamous carcinoma of the oropharynx and hypopharynx. *Head Neck*. 1990; 12(3):197-203.

10. Woo P. Office-based laryngeal procedures. *Otolaryngol Clin North Am*. 2006;39(1):111-133.

11. Amedee RG, Dhurandhar NR. Fine-needle aspiration biopsy. *Laryngoscope*. 2001;111(9):1551-1557.

12. Postma GN, Bach KK, Belafsky PC, Koufman JA. The role of transnasal esophagoscopy in head and neck oncology. *Laryngoscope*. 2002;112(12): 2242-2243.

13. Zbaren P, Becker M, Lang H. Pretherapeutic staging of hypopharyngeal carcinoma. Clinical findings, computed tomography, and magnetic resonance imaging compared with histopathologic evaluation. *Arch Otolaryngol Head Neck Surg*. 1997;123(9): 908-913.

14. Schwartz LH, Ozsahin M, Zhang GN, et al. Synchronous and metachronous head and neck carcinomas. *Cancer*. 1994;74(7):1933-1938.

15. Loh KS, Brown DH, Baker JT, Gilbert RW, Gullane PJ, Irish JC. A rational approach to pulmonary screening in newly diagnosed head and neck cancer. *Head Neck*. 2005;27(11):990-994.

16. de Bree R, Deurloo EE, Snow GB, Leemans CR. Screening for distant metastases in patients with head and neck cancer. *Laryngoscope*. 2000;110 (3 Pt 1):397-401.

17. Houghton DJ, Hughes ML, Garvey C, Beasley NJ, Hamilton JW, Gerlinger I, Jones AS. Role of chest CT scanning in the management of patients presenting with head and neck cancer. *Head Neck*. 1998;20(7):614-618.

18. Wax MK, Myers LL, Gabalski EC, Husain S, Gona JM, Nabi H. Positron emission tomography in the evaluation of synchronous lung lesions in patients with untreated head and neck cancer. *Arch Otolaryngol Head Neck Surg*. 2002;128(6):703-707.

19. Jungehulsing M, Scheidhauer K, Damm M. 2[F]-fluoro-2-deoxy-D-glucose positron emission tomography is a sensitive tool for the detection of occult primary cancer (carcinoma of unknown primary syndrome) with head and neck lymph node manifestation. *Otolaryngol Head Neck Surg*. 2000; 123(3):294-301.

20. Ryan WR, Fee WE Jr, Le QT, Pinto HA. Positron-emission tomography for surveillance of head and neck cancer. *Laryngoscope*. 2005;115(4):645-650.

21. Grossman TW. The incidence and diagnosis of secondary esophageal carcinoma in the head and neck cancer patient. *Laryngoscope*. 1989; 99(10 pt 1): 1052-1056.

22. Haughey BH, Gates GA, Arfken CL, Harvey J. Meta-analysis of second malignant tumors in head and neck cancer: the case for an endoscopic screening protocol. *Ann Otol Rhinol Laryngol*. 1992;101 (2 pt 1):105-112.

23. Stoeckli SJ, Zimmermann R, Schmid S. Role of routine panendoscopy in cancer of the upper aerodigestive tract. *Otolaryngol Head Neck Surg*. 2001; 124(2):208-212.

24. *American Joint Committee on Cancer Staging Manual*. 6th ed. New York, NY: Springer-Verlag; 2002.

25. Wenig BM. Neoplasms of the larynx and hypopharynx. In: Wenig BM, ed. *Atlas of Head and Neck Pathology*. Philadelphia, Pa. WB Saunders; 1993:227-265.

26. Helliwell TR. Evidence-based pathology: squamous carcinoma of the hypopharynx. *J Clin Pathol*. 2003;56(2):81-85.

27. Hsu WC, Loevner LA, Karpati R, et al. Accuracy of magnetic resonance imaging in predicting absence of fixation of head and neck cancer to the prevertebral space. *Head Neck*. 2005;27(2):95-100.

28. Righi PD, Kelley DJ, Ernst R. Evaluation of prevertebral muscle invasion by squamous cell carcinoma. Can computed tomography replace open neck exploration? *Arch Otolaryngol Head Neck Surg*. 1996;122(6):660-663.

29. Loevner LA, Ott IL, Yousem DM, et al. Neoplastic fixation to the prevertebral compartment by squamous cell carcinoma of the head and neck. *AJR Am J Roentgenol*. 1998;170(5):1389-1394.

30. Jegoux F, Ferron C, Malard O, Espitalier F, Beauvillain de Montreuil C. Reconstruction of circumferential pharyngolaryngectomy using a 'horseshoe-shaped' pectoralis major myocutaneous flap. *J Laryngol Otol*. 2007;121(5):483-488.

31. Lewin JS, Barringer DA, May AH, et al. Functional outcomes after circumferential pharyngoesophageal reconstruction. *Laryngoscope*. 2005;115(7): 1266-1271.

32. Holsinger FC, Motamed M, Garcia D, Brasnu D, Menard M, Laccourreye O. Resection of selected

invasive squamous cell carcinoma of the pyriform sinus by means of the lateral pharyngotomy approach: the partial lateral pharyngectomy. *Head Neck*. 2006;28(8):705-711.

33. Ogura JH, Marks JE, Freeman RB. Results of conservation surgery for cancers of the supraglottis and pyriform sinus. *Laryngoscope*. 1980;90(4):591-600.

34. Plouin-Gaudon I, Lengele B, Desuter G, et al. Conservation laryngeal surgery for selected pyriform sinus cancer. *Eur J Surg Oncol*. 2004;30(10):1123-1130.

35. Laccourreye O, Ishoo E, de Mones E, Garcia D, Kania R, Hans S. Supracricoid hemilaryngopharyngectomy in patients with invasive squamous cell carcinoma of the pyriform sinus. Part I: technique, complications, and long-term functional outcome. *Ann Otol Rhinol Laryngol*. 2005;114(1 pt 1):25-34.

36. Schuller DE, Mountain RE, Nicholson RE, Bier-Laning CM, Powers B, Repasky M. One-stage reconstruction of partial laryngopharyngeal defects. *Laryngoscope*. 1997;107(2):247-253.

37. Sewnaik A, Hoorweg JJ, Knegt PP, Wieringa MH, van der Beek JM, Kerrebijn JD. Treatment of hypopharyngeal carcinoma: analysis of nationwide study in the Netherlands over a 10-year period. *Clin Otolaryngol*. 2005;30(1):52-57.

38. Pingree TF, Davis RK, Reichman O, Derrick L. Treatment of hypopharyngeal carcinoma: a 10-year review of 1,362 cases. *Laryngoscope*. 1987;97(8 pt 1):901-904.

39. Kraus DH, Zelefsky MJ, Brock HA, Huo J, Harrison LB, Shah JP. Combined surgery and radiation therapy for squamous cell carcinoma of the hypopharynx. *Otolaryngol Head Neck Surg*. 1997;116(6 pt 1):637-641.

40. Spector JG, Sessions DG, Haughey BH, Chao KS, Simpson J, El Mofty S, Perez CA. Delayed regional metastases, distant metastases, and second primary malignancies in squamous cell carcinomas of the larynx and hypopharynx. *Laryngoscope*. 2001;111(6):1079-1087.

41. Garavello W, Ciardo A, Spreafico R, Gaini RM. Risk factors for distant metastases in head and neck squamous cell carcinoma. *Arch Otolaryngol Head Neck Surg*. 2006;132(7):762-766.

42. Kania R, Hans S, Garcia D, Brasnu D, De Mones E, Laccourreye O. Supracricoid hemilaryngopharyngectomy in patients with invasive squamous cell carcinoma of the pyriform sinus. Part II: incidence and consequences of local recurrence. *Ann Otol Rhinol Laryngol*. 2005;114(2):95-104.

43. Steiner W, Ambrosch P, Hess CF, Kron M. Organ preservation by transoral laser microsurgery in piriform sinus carcinoma. *Otolaryngol Head Neck Surg*. 2001;124(1):58-67.

44. Rudert HH, Hoft S. Transoral carbon-dioxide laser resection of hypopharyngeal carcinoma. *Eur Arch Otorhinolaryngol*. 2003;260(4):198-206.

45. Bernier J, Domenge C, Ozsahin M, et al. European Organization for Research and Treatment of Cancer Trial 22931. Postoperative irradiation with or without concomitant chemotherapy for locally advanced head and neck cancer. *N Engl J Med*. 2004;350(19):1945-1952.

46. Cooper JS, Pajak TF, Forastiere AA, et al. Radiation Therapy Oncology Group 9501/Intergroup. Postoperative concurrent radiotherapy and chemotherapy for high-risk squamous-cell carcinoma of the head and neck. *N Engl J Med*. 2004;350(19):1937-1944.

47. Ozer E, Grecula JC, Agrawal A, Rhoades CA, Schuller DE. Intensification regimen for advanced-stage resectable hypopharyngeal carcinoma. *Arch Otolaryngol Head Neck Surg*. 2006;132(4):385-389.

48. Lefebvre JL, Chevalier D, Luboinski B, Kirkpatrick A, Collette L, Sahmoud T. Larynx preservation in pyriform sinus cancer: preliminary results of a European Organization for Research and Treatment of Cancer phase III trial. EORTC Head and Neck Cancer Cooperative Group. *J Natl Cancer Inst*. 1996;88(13):890-899.

49. Forastiere AA, Goepfert H, Maor M, et al. Concurrent chemotherapy and radiotherapy for organ preservation in advanced laryngeal cancer. *N Engl J Med*. 2003;349(22):2091-2098.

50. Adelstein DJ, Li Y, Adams GL, et al. An intergroup phase III comparison of standard radiation therapy and two schedules of concurrent chemoradiotherapy in patients with unresectable squamous cell head and neck cancer. *J Clin Oncol*. 2003;21(1):92-98.

51. Wendt TG, Grabenbauer GG, Rodel CM, et al. Simultaneous radiochemotherapy versus radiotherapy alone in advanced head and neck cancer: a randomized multicenter study. *J Clin Oncol*. 1998;16(4):1318-1324.

52. Robbins KT, Kumar P, Regine WF, et al. Efficacy of targeted supradose cisplatin and concomitant radiation therapy for advanced head and neck cancer: the Memphis experience. *Int J Radiat Oncol Biol Phys*. 1997;38(2):263-271.

53. Balm AJ, Rasch CR, Schornagel JH, et al. High-dose superselective intra-arterial cisplatin and concomitant radiation (RADPLAT) for advanced head and neck cancer. *Head Neck.* 2004;26(6):485–493.

54. Robbins KT, Kumar P, Harris J, et al. Supradose intra-arterial cisplatin and concurrent radiation therapy for the treatment of stage IV head and neck squamous cell carcinoma is feasible and efficacious in a multi-institutional setting: results of Radiation Therapy Oncology Group Trial 9615. *J Clin Oncol.* 2005;23(7):1447–1454.

55. Rasch CR, Balm AJ, Schornagel JH, et al. *Intra-arterial versus intravenous chemoradiation for advanced head and neck cancer, early results of a multi-institutional trial.* Plenary Session abstract presentation, 48th Annual Meeting of the American Society for Therapeutic Radiology and Oncology, Philadelphia, Pa; November, 2006.

56. Yu P, Lewin JS, Reece GP, Robb GL. Comparison of clinical and functional outcomes and hospital costs following pharyngoesophageal reconstruction with the anterolateral thigh free flap versus the jejunal flap. *Plast Reconstr Surg.* 2006;117(3):968–974.

57. Hanna E, Alexiou M, Morgan J, et al. Intensive chemoradiotherapy as a primary treatment for organ preservation in patients with advanced cancer of the head and neck: efficacy, toxic effects, and limitations. *Arch Otolaryngol Head Neck Surg.* 2004;130(7):861–867.

58. El-Deiry M, Funk GF, Nalwa S, et al. Long-term quality of life for surgical and nonsurgical treatment of head and neck cancer. *Arch Otolaryngol Head Neck Surg.* 2005;131(10):879–885.

59. Hanna E, Sherman A, Cash D, Adams D, Vural E, Fan CY, Suen JY. Quality of life for patients following total laryngectomy vs. chemoradiation for laryngeal preservation. *Arch Otolaryngol Head Neck Surg.* 2004;130(7):875–879.

60. Morton RP, Mehanna H, Hall FT, McIvor NP. Prediction of pharyngocutaneous fistulas after laryngectomy. *Otolaryngol Head Neck Surg.* 2007;136 (4 suppl):S46–S49.

61. Herranz J, Sarandeses A, Fernandez MF, Barro CV, Vidal JM, Gavilan J. Complications after total laryngectomy in nonradiated laryngeal and hypopharyngeal carcinomas. *Otolaryngol Head Neck Surg.* 2000;122(6):892–898.

62. Galli J, De Corso E, Volante M, Almadori G, Paludetti G. Postlaryngectomy pharyngocutaneous fistula: incidence, predisposing factors, and therapy. *Otolaryngol Head Neck Surg.* 2005;133(5):689–694.

63. Clark JR, de Almeida J, Gilbert R, et al. Primary and salvage (hypo)pharyngectomy: analysis and outcome. *Head Neck.* 2006;28(8):671–677.

64. Weber RS, Berkey BA, Forastiere A, et al. Outcome of salvage total laryngectomy following organ preservation therapy: the Radiation Therapy Oncology Group trial 91-11. *Arch Otolaryngol Head Neck Surg.* 2003;129(1):44–49.

65. Triboulet JP, Mariette C, Chevalier D, Amrouni H. Surgical management of carcinoma of the hypopharynx and cervical esophagus: analysis of 209 cases. *Arch Surg.* 2001;136(10):1164–1170.

66. Kaplan JN, Dobie RA, Cummings CW. The incidence of hypopharyngeal stenosis after surgery for laryngeal cancer. *Otolaryngol Head Neck Surg.* 1981;89(6):956–959.

67. Lee WT, Akst LM, Adelstein DJ, et al. Risk factors for hypopharyngeal/upper esophageal stricture formation after concurrent chemoradiation. *Head Neck.* 2006;28(9):808–812.

68. Sullivan CA, Jaklitsch MT, Haddad R, et al. Endoscopic management of hypopharyngeal stenosis after organ sparing therapy for head and neck cancer. *Laryngoscope.* 2004;114(11):1924–1931.

69. Franzmann EJ, Lundy DS, Abitbol AA, Goodwin WJ. Complete hypopharyngeal obstruction by mucosal adhesions: a complication of intensive chemoradiation for advanced head and neck cancer. *Head Neck.* 2006;28(8):663–670.

70. Lewin JS, Barringer DA, May AH, et al. Functional outcomes after laryngopharyngectomy with anterolateral thigh flap reconstruction. *Head Neck.* 2006;28(2):142–149.

71. Eisbruch A, Lyden T, Bradford CR, et al. Objective assessment of swallowing dysfunction and aspiration after radiation concurrent with chemotherapy for head-and-neck cancer. *Int J Radiat Oncol Biol Phys.* 2002;53(1):23–28.

72. Nguyen NP, Moltz CC, Frank C, et al. Dysphagia following chemoradiation for locally advanced head and neck cancer. *Ann Oncol.* 2004;15(3):383–388.

73. Rademaker AW, Vonesh EF, Logemann JA, et al. Eating ability in head and neck cancer patients after treatment with chemoradiation: a 12-month follow-up study accounting for dropout. *Head Neck.* 2003;25(12):1034–1041.

74. Hanna E, Alexiou M, Morgan J, et al. Intensive chemoradiotherapy as a primary treatment for organ preservation in patients with advanced can-

cer of the head and neck: efficacy, toxic effects, and limitations. *Arch Otolaryngol Head Neck Surg.* 2004;130(7):861–867.

75. van den Broek GB, Balm AJ, van den Brekel MW, Hauptmann M, Schornagel JH, Rasch CR. Relationship between clinical factors and the incidence of toxicity after intra-arterial chemoradiation for head and neck cancer. *Radiother Oncol.* 2006;81(2): 143–150.

76. Garden AS, Harris J, Vokes E, et al. *Results of Radiation Therapy Oncology Group 97-03: a randomized phase II trial of concurrent radiation and chemotherapy for advanced squamous cell carcinomas of the head and neck: long-term results and late toxicities.* Abstracts of the RTOG Presentations at the 48th Meeting of ASTRO, November 5–9, 2006, Philadelphia, Pa.

77. Trotti A. Toxicity in head and neck cancer: a review of trends and issues. *Int J Radiat Oncol Biol Phys.* 2000;47:1–12.

78. Trotti A, Bellm LA, Epstein JB, et al. Mucositis incidence, severity and associated outcomes in patients with head and neck cancer receiving radiotherapy with or without chemotherapy: a systematic literature review. *Radiother Oncol.* 2003;66(3):253–262.

79. Munter MW, Hoffner S, Hof H, et al. Changes in salivary gland function after radiotherapy of head and neck tumors measured by quantitative pertechnetate scintigraphy: comparison of intensity-modulated radiotherapy and conventional radiation therapy with and without Amifostine. *Int J Radiat Oncol Biol Phys.* 2007;67(3):651–659.

80. Braam PM, Terhaard CH, Roesink JM, Raaijmakers CP. Intensity-modulated radiotherapy significantly reduces xerostomia compared with conventional radiotherapy. *Int J Radiat Oncol Biol Phys.* 2006; 66(4):975–980.

81. Sinard RJ, Tobin EJ, Mazzaferri EL, et al. Hypothyroidism after treatment for nonthyroid head and neck cancer. *Arch Otolaryngol Head Neck Surg.* 2000;126(5):652–657.

82. Mercado G, Adelstein DJ, Saxton JP, Secic M, Larto MA, Lavertu P. Hypothyroidism: a frequent event after radiotherapy and after radiotherapy with chemotherapy for patients with head and neck carcinoma. *Cancer.* 2001;92(11):2892–2897.

19

Management of Cervical Lymph Node Metastases

Vivek V. Gurudutt
Steven J. Wang
David W. Eisele

The treatment of lymph node metastasis in head and neck cancer has evolved over the past century. Improvements in radiation and chemotherapy have made multimodal therapies common. A uniform primary surgical treatment philosophy has been supplanted by a more balanced and variable approach to treatment. Radiologic advances have allowed better tumor assessment for recurrent or persistent disease. An understanding that the approach to neck treatment is driven by the modality being used to treat the primary site has replaced the idea that radical neck dissection is required in all cases. The trend toward combining treatment modalities requires careful consideration of how to balance treatment efficacy with toxicity. Many of these issues have been explored in the recent literature. In this chapter, an analysis of the current therapeutic strategies is discussed for cervical lymph node metastases arising from squamous cell carcinoma of the upper aerodigestive tract. In addition, a review of the treatment for regional metastasis from salivary malignancies is presented. Finally, diagnostic imaging techniques involved with the assessment of neck metastases are examined.

PRIMARY SURGICAL MANAGEMENT OF CERVICAL LYMPH NODE METASTASES

Historically, surgery was the primary modality of therapy for patients with head and neck malignancies with cervical lymph node metastases. A radical neck dissection was the mainstay of treatment for the N-positive neck for many years. However, around the 1960s, therapeutic modified radical neck dissection combined with radiation therapy first began to gain favor as effective treatment. The preservation of nonlymphatic structures not involved with tumor was noted to result in no significant difference in regional control compared to standard radical neck dissection.[1,2] A review of 43 necks with N2 or N3 disease revealed a 2-year regional control rate of 91% after neck dissection with postoperative radiation—regardless of a radical or a modified radical procedure.[3] The current approach to surgical decision making in performing neck dissection is to determine need for resection of the spinal accessory nerve and internal jugular vein based on tumor involvement. The use of radiation therapy for regional control is a useful adjunct following modified radical neck dissection. Clark et al evaluated 233 modified radical neck dissections for N2 or N3 disease.[4] Extracapsular spread significantly increased regional recurrence ($p = 0.001$). Control in the neck was significantly improved with postoperative radiation ($p = 0.004$).[4] In addition, some centers advocate the use of chemotherapy with radiation post neck dissection in cases of extracapsular spread of disease.[2]

The current indications for an initial surgical management of cervical lymph node metastases include cases where the primary tumor will be treated surgically, or in select cases of bulky cervical adenopathy when a neck dissection is done prior to definitive radiation or chemoradiation therapy for a small or unknown primary. In cases of small oropharyngeal tumors to be treated with radiation therapy, the use of pretreatment neck dissection for bulky nodal disease has been suggested in the literature in order to avoid complications associated with surgical intervention in a radiated field.[5]

We described the trend from radical neck dissection to modified radical neck dissection over the past century. Recently, the use of selective neck dissection for the management of the N-positive neck has been advocated. The use of selective neck dissection for the management of the N0 neck is well accepted. For laryngeal and hypopharyngeal primary tumors, a selective neck dissection encompassing levels II to IV (lateral neck dissection) is performed. For oral cavity and oropharyngeal primary tumors, levels I to III (supraomohyoid neck dissection) are removed. The popularity of this approach has led some to advocate more limited dissections in select patients with cervical metastases. In N-positive patients without massive adenopathy, fixed nodal disease, macroscopic extracapsular spread, previous neck dissection, or disruption of fascial compartments, the use of selective neck dissection is gaining prominence.[6] Supporting the use of selective neck dissection, Pellitteri noted similar recurrence rates between N0, N1, and multiple positive nodes in patients undergoing selective neck dissection in 67 patients.[7] Traynar noted a 4% regional failure rate in 36 N1 and N2 necks after 4 years postselective neck dissection with a survival of 47% over the same

time period.[6] A retrospective review of 106 patients with N1 and N2 disease who underwent selective neck dissection demonstrated a 5-year actuarial regional control rate was 92.2%.[8] Seventy-one percent of the patients received postoperative radiation. Extracapsular spread significantly increased 5-year regional failure and disease specific mortality ($p = 0.05, 0.02$, respectively).[8] The authors of this study recommend selective neck dissection for early stage metastatic disease and encourage the use of radiation if multiple neck levels are involved or extracapsular extension is present. The concept of dissecting the next lowest level below disease down to level IV is also suggested when contemplating the use of selective neck dissection in the N-positive neck.[8]

Several studies have compared selective neck dissection and modified radical neck dissection for the treatment of lymph node metastases.[8-11] Muzaffar reported a 25-year single-institution review of therapeutic radical, modified radical, and selective neck dissections.[11] The recurrence rate was 4.9, 5.6, and 3.3% for radical, modified radical, and selective neck dissections, respectively. Overall, survival was 80% at 2 years for the selective and 64% for both radical and modified radical dissection groups. A selection bias was acknowledged as selective neck dissection only was performed in patients with N1 or N2 disease and more extensive spread mandated larger dissections. However, Muzaffar concluded that selective neck dissection with postoperative radiation is permissible in some patients.[11]

The use of radiation after surgery is an important adjuvant therapy if selective neck dissection is used for the N-positive neck. Kolli out of Roswell Park found patients with postoperative radiation had significantly improved regional control in those with N2 disease[9] and Chepeha noted a 94% neck control rate 2 years after selective neck dissection followed by radiation therapy.[10] In a review of 284 supraomohyoid neck dissections, patients with N1 disease had a regional recurrence of 5.6% in necks with radiation compared to 35.7% without. Similarly, 8.3% of N2B patients with postoperative radiation had recurrence compared to 14% without.[12]

The use of selective neck dissection for N-positive neck disease remains controversial. In contrast to the above studies, Santos and colleagues noted an 11.8% recurrence rate out of 34 necks with a median follow-up of 36 months after selective neck dissection and postoperative radiation.[13] Although small primaries and N1 disease may be amenable to limited dissection, caution is recommended when applying these principles to more advanced neck disease.[13] An algorithm for primary surgical management of neck disease is presented in Figure 19–1.

PRIMARY RADIATION-BASED MANAGEMENT OF CERVICAL LYMPH NODE METASTASES

When the primary tumor is treated with initial radiation or chemoradiation therapy, the same modality is used to treat any cervical lymph node metastases. Surgery for the primary tumor is reserved for sal-

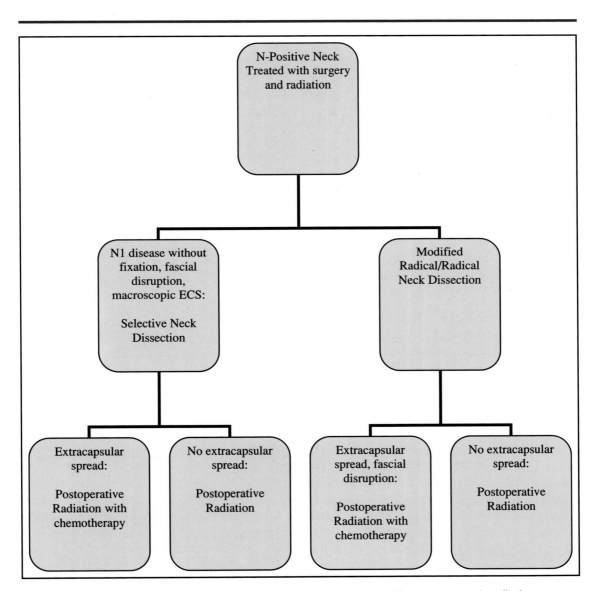

Fig 19–1. Algorithm for management of cervical metastases with surgery and radiation.

vage. However, there remains continued controversy regarding the optimal management of the neck following radiation-based initial treatment, especially for N2 or greater disease. One may perform a planned neck dissection for all patients who had pretreatment advanced nodal disease or, alternatively, neck dissections may be limited to those patients with clinically residual neck disease. Among the advocates of limiting neck dissections to partial neck responders, controversy exists regarding the optimal strategy for determining who exactly has residual disease, as physical examination alone is felt by most to be unreliable in this setting. Review of the various available imaging modalities has yet to identify the ideal noninvasive method for identifying viable residual neck disease. Finally, the type of neck dissection performed in the postradiation setting is open to discussion. An algorithm for management of the neck after a radiation based treatment regimen is presented in Figure 19–2.

RADIATION THERAPY FOR CERVICAL LYMPH NODE METASTASES

There is extensive experience described in the literature regarding the use of radiation therapy for the treatment of cervical lymph node metastases. Early reports demonstrated a clear relationship between initial neck stage and neck control with radiation therapy. Mendenhall reported the 5-year neck control rate after radiotherapy alone is 86%, 79%, 70%, and 33% for N1, N2a, N2b, and N3 disease, respectively.[14] Mendenhall also reported a neck control rate of 91% and 69%, respectively (p <0.01), for N2 and N3 necks treated with neck dissection after radiation therapy.[14] Thus, neck dissection after radiation treatment was advocated for improved regional control in N2 and N3 necks. In contrast, control of N1 disease did not significantly differ between radiation therapy alone versus radiation with planned neck dissection. Mendenhall recommended observation postradiation therapy in N1 patients with a complete clinical response (cCR).[14]

Similarly, Boyd advocated planned neck dissection in cases of initial stage N2 or greater neck disease.[15] Boyd's review of 28 neck dissections performed after radiation revealed 9 (32%) necks with residual pathologic disease after radiation therapy. Two-year regional control and disease specific survival were 93% and 60%, respectively. The relationship between cCR and pathologic complete response (pCR) in patients after radiation was addressed by Wang, who analyzed 71 neck dissections in patients with N2a or greater disease.[16] Clinical response was assessed with physical exam and CT or MRI. Of the 42 necks with cCR, 31% had malignancy noted on pathology. Seventeen of 29 patients with a partial clinical response (cPR) (59%) were positive for

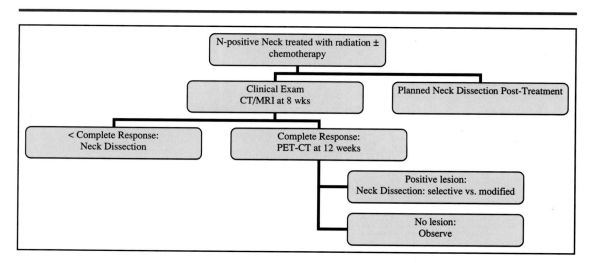

Fig 19–2. Algorithm for management of cervical metastases after radiation ± chemotherapy.

residual disease. Wang advocated planned neck dissection after radiation alone for N2a or greater neck disease because of the high rate of residual disease despite cCR.[16]

In contrast, Peters et al disputed the need for planned neck dissection for all patients treated with radiation therapy for bulky nodal disease. In their study, 75 patients underwent definitive radiotherapy with concomitant boost for node positive oropharyngeal cancer. Of the 62 patients with complete clinical and radiologic response who were observed, only 3 patients recurred in the neck.[17] The 13 partial responders undergoing neck dissection revealed disease in 6 patients, emphasizing the need for neck dissection if there is not a complete response.[17] Similarly, Narayan also concluded that neck dissection after radiation therapy should be limited to patients with residual neck disease, citing a high surgical complication rate for neck dissection after radiation of 17.3%.[18]

The feasibility of salvage treatment is important when considering observation of the neck after radiation therapy. Mabanta et al reviewed 51 patients after primary irradiation that developed regional recurrence.[19] Eighteen of the 51 patients underwent attempted salvage treatment: 4 with chemotherapy, 1 with chemotherapy and neck dissection, 11 with neck dissection, and 2 with radiation and neck dissection. The 5-year regional control rate was 9% and the 5-year absolute and cause-specific survival was only 10%. Bernier reviewed 1646 patients treated with radiation therapy.[20] Of the 116 patients with regional failure, only 32 were considered for salvage treatment. Eighteen patients underwent further radiation and 14 underwent neck dissection. Only one patient was successfully salvaged after treatment. The dismal prognosis for salvage treatment underscores the importance of adequate treatment of neck disease initially.[19]

CHEMORADIATION FOR CERVICAL LYMPH NODE METASTASES

The addition of chemotherapy to treatment of head and neck squamous cell carcinoma has increased the complexity of disease management. To address the role of chemotherapy for bulky nodal metastases, Moore and Bhattacharyya used a matched case controlled analysis to assess the sterilization capacity of concomitant chemotherapy and radiation versus radiation alone in a pathologic analysis of neck dissection specimens.[21] Ninety-seven patients treated with chemoradiation and neck dissection were matched with patients who underwent neck dissection before adjuvant therapy. Forty-one patients treated with radiation and neck dissection were matched with a control group undergoing surgery first. The postchemoradiation neck dissection group had 24.7% positive nodes versus 51.2% positive nodes among the postradiation-alone neck dissection group. Both chemoradiation and radiation significantly reduced the amount of extracapsular spread compared to the control group of patients undergoing neck dissection first. Moore concluded that there was better sterilization with chemoradiation compared to radiation alone.[21]

Chemoradiation appears to have increased therapeutic efficacy for cervical lymph node metastases compared to radiation therapy alone, indicating that neck dissection likely is not beneficial to many patients even with advanced nodal disease who are treated with primary chemoradiation. However, to limit neck dissections only to those with a cPR to chemoradiation, one must be confident of the predictive value of a cCR. Several studies have examined the accuracy of a cCR after chemoradiation by analyzing the histology of neck nodes. Using physical exam alone, Puc found 41% of patients with cCR assessed by neck palpation had positive nodes on histology.[22] Frank reported 39 patients who underwent 51 neck dissections after concomitant platinum based chemotherapy with radiation.[23] Of the 25 necks noted to be cCR, 16% had histologic evidence of malignancy. Roy assessed accuracy of palpation and CT scanning postchemoradiation. Of the 9 patients with negative disease on palpation and imaging, 33% were noted to have residual disease histologically.[24] Brizel's analysis of patients undergoing treatment with hyperfractionated radiation therapy and concurrent cisplatinum with 5-fluorouracil found significant differences in pathologic outcome between N1 disease and N2/N3 disease.[25] In this series, patients underwent a modified radical neck dissection 6 to 8 weeks post-therapy if the primary site was negative for tumor. Twelve of 13 patients with N1 disease were cCR with 11 of these patients being pathologic negative (pCR). In patients with N2 or N3 disease, 26% of cCR patients had residual tumor. Of the 16 patients with N2/N3 disease not undergoing neck dissection, 44% had recurrence. Four-year overall survival in patients with N2/N3 disease was 77% in the neck dissection group and 50% in those not undergoing surgery ($p = 0.04$). Brizel advocated neck dissection for N2/N3 disease after chemoradiation because of the poor accuracy of physical exam with imaging to predict pathologic result and the better survival seen at 4 years among patients undergoing neck dissection.[25]

In contrast, other studies support performing neck dissection for N2 or N3 disease only in patients with less than a cCR after chemoradiation.[26-29] Stenson found only 8.1% of 37 cCR patients (assessed radiographically) had positive nodes on dissection compared to 36.7 of the 30 patients that were cPR.[27] Argiris studied patients with N2/N3 disease and found that patients who underwent neck dissection after chemoradiation had a lower neck failure rate (1/92) than those without neck dissection (6/39; $p = 0.0007$).[28] However, in patients with cCR, there was no significant difference in overall survival, progression-free survival and neck control between patients with or without neck dissection. Thus, Argiris recommended that neck dissection be restricted only to those patients with cPR. Similarly, Ahmed reviewed patients undergoing chemoradiation for advanced nodal disease and also advocated neck dissection for cPR patients only.[29]

For patients who undergo surgery following chemoradiation, the type of neck dissection necessary must be determined. Historically, radical neck dissection, and more recently, modified radical neck dissections were the most often utilized. However, the oncologic justification for these procedures, considering the associated morbidity, has been called into question. In neck levels in which there were no previous pathologic nodes, the likelihood of new disease forming after radiation is rare. In addition, if isolated persistent disease is present, it is unlikely that neck recurrence will occur in levels separated by space. Thus, the use of selective neck dissections after chemoradiation has been suggested as a potential option. Using a selective dissection for disease confined to one neck level following chemoradia-

tion may reduce morbidity and spare function.[30] Robbins found that regional control rates and overall survival in patients treated with chemoradiation with planned neck dissection were better with selective and superselective neck dissections compared to those with modified radical neck dissections ($p = 0.002$, $p = 0.04$, respectively).[30] A selection bias cannot be eliminated in this study as more progressive disease required a more extensive neck dissection possibly resulting in decreased regional control and survival.[30,31]

Complications of neck dissection reported following chemoradiation have varied considerably in the literature. Robbins reported a rate of 17% after 35 neck dissections with complications including chyle leak, flap necrosis, wound dehiscence, and hematoma.[31] Brizel noted an 8% complication rate with modified radical neck dissection postchemoradiation.[25] Georgetown University reported a 22% wound complication rate postradiation with or without chemotherapy out of 41 neck dissections.[32] The use of chemotherapy did not significantly alter the complication rate among patients in this study.

CERVICAL LYMPH NODE METASTASES FROM SALIVARY MALIGNANCY

The presence of neck metastasis from salivary tumors has been shown to decrease survival as well as locoregional control.[33] Rates of neck disease vary throughout the literature with high-grade malignancies having an occult nodal rate as high as 50%.[34] For high-grade salivary malignancies, regional metastases of 29% in T1 and 54% of T2 tumors have been described with total neck spread in all tumors as high as 53%.[35] Treatment of the N positive neck from salivary malignancy is optimally treated with initial therapeutic neck dissection, typically followed by radiation therapy. Levels II and III are most often involved in the ipsilateral neck, whereas contralateral neck involvement is rare.[33] Involvement of lower levels of the neck are not common; however, skip lesions to levels III and IV can occur in up to 25% of parotid primaries.[36] The use of postoperative radiation should be considered for adjuvant therapy in patient with cervical metastases from salivary malignancy. Armstrong et al have shown an increased 5-year survival from 18.7% without to 48.9% with postoperative radiation.[37] In addition, the locoregional control increased from 40.2% to 69.1%.

IMAGING FOR CERVICAL LYMPH NODE METASTASES

Magnetic resonance imaging (MRI) or computed tomography (CT) are invaluable tools used in pretreatment planning for patients with head and neck malignancies. More recently, positron emission tomography (PET) scanning and PET-CT have been used in an attempt to better evaluate and stage the neck.[38] As use of these noninvasive imaging technologies has become more refined, their potential roles have increased. In particularly, various imaging strategies in the postradiation setting have been proposed to assess residual neck disease and need for further therapy.

Clinical assessment with physical exam even with imaging can be unreliable after radiation therapy. CT and MRI scanning alone have had variable success in assessing pathologic residual neck disease after radiation therapy. A study from the University of Texas, San Antonio noted a specificity of only 24% in 53 neck specimens with CT scanning before neck dissections performed following radiation therapy.[39] Ojiri noted that necks likely to be free of disease had lymph nodes less than 15 mm in size, lacked focal internal low attenuation or calcification, and had no evidence of extracapsular spread.[40]

With recent advances in PET scanning, the potential for detecting tumor viability in the neck has increased. Comparison of PET with CT/MRI by Kubuta revealed a significantly higher accuracy, specificity, and positive predictive value with PET scanning (p <0.05) in their study with 43 necks.[41] However, a drawback of PET to assess the neck following radiation therapy is the need to wait up to 8 to 12 weeks after completing radiation treatment before a PET scan can be obtained.[42] The delay is necessary to allow for decrease in residual inflammation from radiation, as well as to allow for some repopulation of cancer cells to enable detection by PET imaging.

When evaluating strategies for assessment of residual neck disease, the clinical utility of a high negative predictive value has been stressed. Porceddu studied 39 patients with pretreatment N-positive disease. Each of the patients in this series had a complete response at the primary site but had a residual neck lesion on physical exam or CT. PET scanning was done after a median of 12 weeks from the end of treatment. Of the 32 patients with no PET activity, 5 underwent neck dissection and were pathologic node negative, and the other 27 were observed an average of 34 months. Only 1 or the 32 PET negative patients had locoregional failure, giving a negative predictive value of 97% in patients with residual anatomical abnormality.[43] This study suggests that neck dissection can be avoided in patients with a negative PET scan.

Other studies have found PET scanning not reliable for the detection of viable residual neck disease, but have found PET to maintain a high negative predictive value.[44] Yao reviewed patients with greater than N2a disease using CT and PET to determine need for neck dissection or observation. Only 3 of 7 patients that were PET positive had pathologic nodes on subsequent neck dissection. Twenty-one necks were CT positive for cancer, but PET negative. Four were pathologically negative on neck dissection whereas the other 17 were observed for a median of 26 months and had no recurrence.[45] Forty-two were CT and PET negative and were observed without recurrence. The negative predictive value was 100% and the positive predictive value was 43%.[45] The lack of biologically active disease in the neck as measured by PET scanning may support a more observational approach for patients who have anatomic residual enlarged nodes on physical exam or imaging. On the other hand, Gourin et al found half of the 6 necks noted to be negative on PET-CT in her study were pathologically positive suggesting limitations for assessing tumor viability post-treatment.[46] Although PET and PET-CT have tremendous potential in the clinical management of the postradiated neck, further study assessing the consistency of results is needed for reliable tumor assessment.

The poor prognosis associated with cervical metastases from head and neck cancer requires careful evaluation of various therapies by the head and neck surgeon. A current knowledge of the literature is essential to assess treatment options in this continually evolving field. The use of radiation, chemotherapy, and surgery as well as combining modalities requires continued evaluation when treating neck disease. In addition, analyzing neck disease according to primary source must be included in any discussion concerning the N-positive neck. With the application of new imaging techniques, the scope of surveillance and treatment for head and neck cancer will continue to advance.

REFERENCES

1. Andersen PE, Shah JP, Cambronero E, Spiro RH. The role of comprehensive neck dissection with preservation of the spinal accessory nerve in the clinically positive neck. *Am J Surg*. 1994;168: 499–502.
2. Myers EN, Gastman BR. Neck dissection: an operation in evolution. *Arch Otolaryngol Head Neck Surg*. 2003;129:14–25.
3. Richards BL, Spiro JD. Controlling advanced neck disease: efficacy of neck dissection and radiotherapy. *Laryngoscope*. 2000;110:1124–1127.
4. Clark J, Li W, Smith G, et al. Outcome of treatment for advanced cervical metastatic squamous cell carcinoma. *Head Neck*. 2005;27:87–94.
5. Reddy AN, Eisele DW, Forastiere AA, Lee DJ, Westra WH, Califano JA. Neck dissection followed by radiotherapy or chemoradiotherapy for small primary oropharynx carcinoma with cervical metastasis. *Laryngoscope*. 2005;115:1196–1200.
6. Traynor SJ, Cohen JI, Gray J, Andersen PE, Everts EC. Selective neck dissection and the management of the node-positive neck. *Am J Surg*. 1996;172: 654–657.
7. Pellitteri PK, Robbins T, Neuman T. Expanded application of selective neck dissection with regard to nodal status. *Head Neck*. 1997;19:260–265.
8. Andersen PE, Warren F, Spiro J, et al. Results of selective neck dissection in management of the node-positive neck. *Arch Otolaryngol Head Neck Surg*. 2002;128:1180–1184.
9. Kolli VR, Datta RV, Orner JB, Hicks WL, Loree TR. The role of supraomohyoid neck dissection in patients with positive nodes. *Arch Otolaryngol Head Neck Surg*. 2000;126:413–416.
10. Chepeha DB, Hoff PT, Taylor RJ, Bradford CR, Teknos TN, Esclamado RM. Selective neck dissec-

tion for the treatment of neck metastasis from squamous cell carcinoma of the head and neck. *Laryngoscope*. 2002;112:434–438.
11. Muzaffar K. Therapeutic selective neck dissection: a 25-year review. *Laryngoscope*. 2003;113:1460–1465.
12. Byers RM, Clayman GL, McGill D, et al. Selective neck dissections for squamous carcinoma of the upper aerodigestive tract: patterns of regional failure. *Head Neck*. 1999;21:499–505.
13. de Oliveira Santos AB, Cernea CR, Inoue M, Ferraz AR. Selective neck dissection for node-positive necks in patients with head and neck squamous cell carcinoma. *Arch Otolaryngol Head Neck Surg*. 2006;132:79–81.
14. Mendenhall WM, Parsons JT, Mancuso AA, Stringer SP, Cassisi NJ, Million RR. Head and neck: management of the neck. In: Perez CA, Brady LW, eds. *Principles and Practice of Radiation Oncology*. 2nd ed. Philadelphia, Pa: JB Lippincott; 1992:790–805.
15. Boyd TS, Harari PM, Tannehill SP, et al. Planned postradiotherapy neck dissection in patients with advanced head and neck cancer. *Head Neck*. 1998;20:132–137.
16. Wang S, Wang MB, Yip H, Calcaterra TC. Combined radiotherapy with planned neck dissection for small head and neck cancers with advanced cervical metastases. *Laryngoscope*. 2000;110:1794–1797.
17. Peters LJ, Weber RS, Morrison WH, Byers RM, Garden AS, Goepfert H. Neck surgery in patients with primary oropharyngeal cancer treated by radiotherapy. *Head Neck*. 1996;18(6):552–559.
18. Narayan K, Crane CH, Kleid S, Hughes PG, Peters LJ. Planned neck dissection as an adjunct to the management of patients with advanced neck disease treated with definitive radiotherapy: for some or for all. *Head Neck*. 1999;21;606–613.
19. Mabanta SR, Mendenhall WM, Stringer SP, Cassisi NJ. Salvage treatment for neck recurrence after irradiation alone for head and neck squamous cell carcinoma with clinically positive neck nodes. *Head Neck*. 1999;21:591–594.
20. Bernier J, Bataini JP. Regional outcome in oropharyngeal and pharyngolaryngeal cancer treated with high dose per fraction radiotherapy. analysis of neck disease response in 1646 cases. *Radiother Oncol*. 1986;6(2):87–103.
21. Moore MG, Bhattacharyya N. Effectiveness of chemotherapy and radiotherapy in sterilizing cervical nodal disease in squamous cell carcinoma of the head and neck. *Laryngoscope*. 2005;115:570–573.
22. Puc MM, Chrzanowski FA, Tran HS, et al. Preoperative chemotherapy-sensitized radiation therapy for

cervical metastases in head and neck cancer. *Arch Otolaryngol Head Neck Surg.* 2000;126:337–342.

23. Frank DK, Hu KS, Culliney BE, et al. Planned neck dissection after concomitant radiochemotherapy for advanced head and neck cancer. *Laryngoscope.* 2005;115:1015–1020.

24. Roy S, Tibesar RJ, Daly K, et al. Role of planned neck dissection for advanced metastatic disease in tongue base or tonsil squamous cell carcinoma treated with radiotherapy. *Head Neck.* 2002;24:474–481.

25. Brizel DM, Prosnitz RG, Hunter S, et al. Necessity for adjuvant neck dissection in setting of concurrent chemoradiation for advanced head and neck cancer. *Int J Radiation Oncology Biol Phys.* 2004;58(5):1418–1423.

26. Lavertu P, Adelstein DJ, Saxton JP, et al. Management of the neck in a randomized trial comparing concurrent chemotherapy and radiotherapy with radiotherapy alone in resectable stage III and IV squamous cell head and neck cancer. *Head Neck.* 1997;19:559–566.

27. Stenson KM, Huo D, Blair E, et al. Planned post-chemoradiation neck dissection: significance of radiation dose. *Laryngoscope.* 2006;116:33–36.

28. Argiris A, Stenson KM, Brockstein BE, et al. Neck dissection in the combined-modality therapy of patients with locoregionally advanced head and neck cancer. *Head Neck.* 2004;26:447–455.

29. Ahmed KA, Robbins KT, Wong F, Salazar JE. Efficacy of concomitant chemoradiation and surgical for N3 nodal disease associated with upper aerodigestive tract carcinoma. *Laryngoscope.* 2000;110:1789–1793.

30. Robbins KT, Doweck I, Samant S, Vieira F. Effectiveness of superselective and selective neck dissection for advanced nodal metastases after chemoradiation. *Arch Otolaryngol Head Neck Surg.* 2005;131:965–969.

31. Robbins KT, Wong FSH, Kumar P, et al. Efficacy of targeted chemoradiation and planned selective neck dissection to control bulky nodal disease in advanced head and neck cancer. *Arch Otolaryngol Head Neck Surg.* 1999;125:670–675.

32. Davidson BJ, Newkirk KA, Harter KW, Picken CA, Cullen KJ, Sessions RB. Complications from planned, posttreatment neck dissections. *Arch Otolaryngol Head Neck Surg.* 1999;125:401–405.

33. Harrison LB, Armstrong JG, Spiro RH, Fass DE, Strong EW. Postoperative radiation therapy for major salivary gland malignancies. *J Surg Oncol.* 1990;45(1):52–55.

34. Rodriguez-Cuevas S, Labastida S, Baena L, Gallegos F. Risk of nodal metastases from malignant salivary gland tumors related to tumor size and grade of malignancy. *Eur Arch Otorhinolaryngol.* 1995;252(3):139–142.

35. Stennert E, Kisner D, Jungehuelsing M, et al. High incidence of lymph node metastasis in major salivary gland cancer. *Arch Otolaryngol Head Neck Surg.* 2003;129(7):720–723.

36. Armstrong JG, Harrison LB, Thaler HT, et al. The indications for elective treatment of the neck in cancer of the major salivary glands. *Cancer.* 1992;69(3):615–619.

37. Armstrong JG, Harrison LB, Spiro RH, Fass DE, Strong EW, Fuks ZY. Malignant tumors of major salivary gland origin. A matched-pair analysis of the role of combined surgery and postoperative radiotherapy. *Arch Otolaryngol Head Neck Surg.* 1990;116(3):290–293.

38. Jeong HS, Baek CH, Son YI, et al. Use of integrated (18) F-FDG PET/CT to improve the accuracy of initial cervical nodal evaluation in patients with head and neck squamous cell carcinoma. *Head Neck.* 2007;29:203–210.

39. Velazquez RA, McGuff HS, Sycamore D, Miller FR. The role of computed tomographic scans in the management of the N-positive neck in head and neck squamous cell carcinoma after chemoradiotherapy. *Arch Otolaryngol Head Neck Surg.* 2004;130:74–77.

40. Ojiri H, Mendenhall WM, Stringer SP, Johnson PL, Mancuso AA. Post-RT CT results as a predictive model for the necessity of planned post-RT neck dissection in patients with cervical metastatic disease from squamous cell carcinoma. *Int J Radiation Oncology Biol Phys.* 2002;52(2):420–428.

41. Kubota K, Yokoyama J, Yamaguchi K, et al. FDG-PET delayed imaging for the detection of head and neck cancer recurrence after radio-chemotherapy: comparison with MRI/CT. *Eur J Nucl Med Mol Imaging.* 2004;31:590–595.

42. Rogers JW, Greven KM, McGuirt WF, et al. Can post-RT neck dissection be omitted for patients with head and neck cancer who have a negative PET scan after definitive radiation therapy? *Int J Radiat Oncol Biol Phys.* 2004;58(3):694–697.

43. Porceddu SV, Jarmolowski E, Hicks RJ, et al. Utility of positron emission tomography for the detection of disease in residual neck nodes after (chemo) radiotherapy in head and neck cancer. *Head Neck.* 2005;27:175–181.

44. Brkovich VS, Miller FR, Karnad AB, Hussey DH, McGuff HS, Otto RA. The role of positron emission tomography scans in the management of the N-positive neck in head and neck squamous cell carcinoma after chemoradiotherapy. *Laryngoscope.* 2006;116:855–858.

45. Yao M, Smith RB, Graham MM, et al. The role of FDG PET in management of neck metastasis from head and neck cancer after definitive radiation treatment. *Int J Radiat Oncol Biol Phys.* 2005; 63(4):991–999.

46. Gourin CG, Williams HT, Seabolt WN, Herdman AV, Howington JW, Terris DJ. Utility of positron emission tomography-computed tomography in identification of residual nodal disease after chemoradiation for advanced head and neck cancer. *Laryngoscope.* 2006;116:705–710.

20

Cancer of the Unknown Primary Site

Guy J. Petruzzelli

INTRODUCTION

The evaluation and management of patients with malignant cervical adenopathy lacking an obvious primary site represents one of the most challenging yet potentially rewarding clinical presentations in head and neck oncology. These patients are best served by the multidisciplinary assessment and expertise of the head and neck cancer team. The participation of an experienced head and neck surgeon in the evaluation of these patients is important for the systematic examination of the upper aerodigestive tract which is necessary for the identification of the primary site. Close cooperation with a medical oncologist is necessary to facilitate the general physical examination, coordinate the systemic evaluation of the patient in cases of a nonsquamous cell carcinoma and to deliver and monitor chemotherapy. The detection of the site of the primary allows the radiation oncologist to carefully target postoperative radiation therapy thereby reducing the required treatment volumes and resulting treatment-related toxicities.

DEFINITION OF UNIQUE TERMS

Key Points

Occult Primary Head and Neck Cancer — metastatic cervical adenopathy without clinical obvious primary cancer, with subsequent histologic identification of the primary in directed biopsy/tonsillectomy specimens.

Cancer of the Unknown Primary Site — metastatic cervical adenopathy without clinical obvious primary cancer, without subsequent identification of primary cancer on directed biopsies or systematic physical, radiologic, and biochemical evaluation.

Patients with metastatic cervical adenopathy can be divided into three broad categories (Fig 20-1). The first group includes patients presenting with cervical metastasis in the mid to upper neck and identifiable primary tumors, most commonly of the mucosal surfaces of the upper aerodigestive tract,

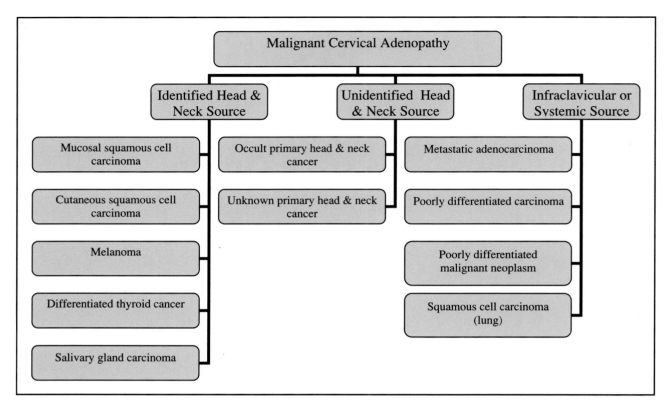

Fig 20–1. Malignant cervical adenopathy.

thyroid, parathyroid, or salivary glands. The diagnosis, evaluation, and management of these patients are reviewed in the appropriate sections of this text.

The second group is composed of patients presenting with cervical metastases without obvious primary tumors. This group of patient can be further divided into those with either an occult primary tumor or a carcinoma of an unknown primary site.

Those with histologically confirmed squamous cell carcinoma presenting in a lymph node without a clearly identified primary tumor are classified as having an occult primary head and neck carcinoma, which constitute approximately 0.5% of all cancer diagnoses and 3% to 4% of all head and neck malignancies. These tumors are not readily apparent on physical examination but are subsequently identified by histopathologic assessment of directed biopsies of the tongue base, nasopharynx (Waldeyer's ring), oro- and hypopharyngeal mucosa, and/or tonsillec-

tomy specimens. Like other upper aerodigestive tract tumors, survival in these patients correlates with the presence of extracapsular extension in nodal metastases and depends on aggressive treatment of the primary and the neck. As we describe, these patient must undergo a systematic clinical and radiographic examination for a primary source. Patients are classified as having a head and neck carcinoma of an unknown primary site when directed biopsy and tonsillectomy specimens do not reveal squamous cell carcinoma.

The final group is composed of patients presenting with cervical lymph node metastasis in the mid to lower neck or supraclavicular fossa from primary infraclavicular tumors. This category is composed primarily of adenocarcinoma, neuroendocrine carcinoma, or poorly differentiated carcinomas and this category is referred to as metastatic carcinoma of an unknown primary (CUP) site. Overall survival in this last group of patients is limited, despite intensive treatment with multidrug regimens. Primary hematologic malignancies presenting with cervical adenopathy are not included in this discussion.

This chapter reviews the evaluation and treatment of patients with either occult upper aerodigestive tract malignancies or tumors of an unknown primary site. We focus on the diagnosis, evaluation, and treatment of patients presenting with metastatic squamous cell or poorly differentiated carcinoma identified in the upper or midjugular lymph nodes. It reviews our current understanding of the clinical entity of the unknown primary tumor presenting as malignant cervical adenopathy, examines current hypotheses for the etiology and pathogenesis of these tumors, discusses the clinical and radiographic evaluation of these patients, reviews treatment alternatives, and finally discusses factors impacting survival. Patients with hematologic or lymphoreticular malignancies are not considered.

EPIDEMIOLOGY, PREVALENCE, AND ETIOLOGY

Key Points

Cancer of the unknown primary site is most often adenocarcinoma.

Unknown primary head and neck squamous cell carcinoma are rare malignancies.

Unknown primary malignancies are rare tumors accounting for approximately 2% of human cancer. Initial light microscopic examination of biopsy tissues reveals readily recognizable adenocarcinoma in approximately 60% and squamous cell carcinomas in 5% of cases. The remaining 35% of cases are defined as classified as poorly differentiated (adeno) carcinomas or poorly differentiated malignant neoplasms. Special stains may be applied to cytologic specimens or cell blocs to further differentiate these tumors into lymphomas, melanoma, sarcoma, germ

cell, and neuroendocrine tumors. This classification is based on the work of Hainsworth and Greco which has led to a classification scheme based on a comprehensive clinical evaluation of the patient and the pathologic examination of the metastatic lesion[1-3] (Table 20–1).

The development of invasive metastatic squamous cell carcinoma from the normal epithelium of the upper aerodigestive tract represents a complex

Table 20–1. Classification of Patients with Carcinoma of an Unknown Primary Site Based on Clinical Presentation, Light Microscopy, and Immunohistochemical Analysis

Adenocarcinoma
  Specific subgroup
    Women with axillary lymph node metastases
    Women with peritoneal carcinomatosis
    Men with elevated serum prostate-specific antigen (PSA) of tumors staining for PSA
    Single peripheral metastatic lesion
  No specific subgroup

Poorly Differentiated Malignant Neoplasm
  Lymphoma (anaplastic or non-Hodgkin's)
  Sarcoma
  Melanoma

Poorly Differentiated Carcinoma
  Extragonadal germ cell tumor
  Neuroendocrine carcinoma
  Lymphoma
  Melanoma
  Sarcoma

Squamous Cell Carcinoma
  Specific subgroup
    Squamous cell carcinoma involving cervical lymph nodes
    Squamous cell carcinoma involving supraclavicular lymph nodes Squamous cell carcinoma involving inguinal lymph nodes
  No specific subgroup

Schema for classifying patients with metastatic adenopathy without a clinically obvious primary site based on histologic analysis.
Source: Modified from Hainsworth and Greco, 1994.[3]

multigene series of events requiring both oncogene activation and downregulation of tumor suppressor genes. These molecular events have been linked to specific environmental factors such as the frequency of tobacco and alcohol use, history of human papilloma[4] or Epstein-Barr virus infection, immune dysregulation, dietary deficiencies, poor oral hygiene, and exposure to heavy metals or other environmental carcinogens (nickel, wood dust, petroleum distillates). A history of childhood exposure to low-dose ionizing radiation and a prior or current diagnosis of a malignancy should also be determined. Actinic particularly ultraviolet exposure should be documented to assess the risk of cutaneous malignancy. Patients should be questioned regarding their ethnicity to determine cultural risks for habitual exposure to oral carcinogens such as betel nut or pan or nasopharyngeal cancer risks such as dietary nitrosamines, EBV exposure, and southern Chinese ancestry.[5,6]

ANATOMIC BOUNDARIES AND SUBDIVISIONS OF THE REGION

Key Points

Location of metastatic cervical adenopathy is based on site of primary cancer.

Classification of cervical adenopathy is based on anatomic relationships in the neck.

The location of the malignant metastatic node(s) provides important information regarding the potential site of an initially unidentified upper aerodigestive tract tumor. The classical works by Lindberg and subsequent studies by Johnson illustrate consistent patterns of lymph node metastasis observed in head and neck squamous cell carcinoma.[7,8]

The clinical-pathologic anatomy of the neck is a based on the Memorial-Sloan Kettering Cancer Center classification modified by Robbins, Medina, Suen, and others (Fig 20-2). Zone I contains lymph nodes in the submandibular (Ia) and submental (Ib) nodal groups. Anatomic regions draining into these regions include the floor of mouth, anterior oral tongue, anterior mandibular alveolus, lower lip (Ia), and the oral cavity, cutaneous midface, upper lip, anterior nasal cavity, submandibular gland, and maxillary sinus (Ib). These anatomic regions are easy to examine and therefore are extremely rare locations for occult primary tumors. These nodes extend from the mandible to the hyoid inferiorly bounded by the digastric muscle. Zone II constitutes the upper jugular region of nodes extending from the skull base to the hyoid bone both anterior (IIa) and posterior to the spinal accessory nerves (IIb). Head and neck sites draining to these areas include the oral cavity, nasal cavity, supraglottic larynx oropharynx, parotid (IIa), and the nasopharynx, thyroid, parotid, and cutaneous metastases (IIb). Metastatic adenOopathy encountered in Zone IIb should direct attention to the nasopharynx and cause the examiner to perform carefully directed biopsies of this region. Zone III includes the middle jugular nodes, or those extending from the hyoid bone to the omohyoid tendon. This region receives lymphatics from the tonsillar fossa, tongue base, oral cavity, hypopharynx, and supraglottic larynx and represents the most common location of metastatic nodes from an unknown primary tumor. Lower jugular or Zone IV nodes extend along the jugular vein from the omohyoid muscle to the clavicle. Metastatic adenopathy in this region should direct the examiner to lesions of the hypopharynx, transglottic larynx, and cervical esophagus. Zone V encompasses the posterior neck from the posterior border of the sternocleidomastoid to the anterior border of the trapezius muscles. It is further subdivided into Zone V(a), the area above the thyroid cartilage draining the nasopharynx, oropharynx, and thyroid and Zone V(b) the region below the cricoid or the supraclavicular fossa. Metastatic adenopathy in Zone V(b) indicates an infraclavicular source for the primary tumor and most often is not a squamous cell carcinoma. Paratracheal or Zone VI adenopathy receives drainage from the thyroid gland, transglottic larynx, piriform apex, and cervical esophagus and is rarely the site of a metastatic occult node[9,10] (Table 20-2).

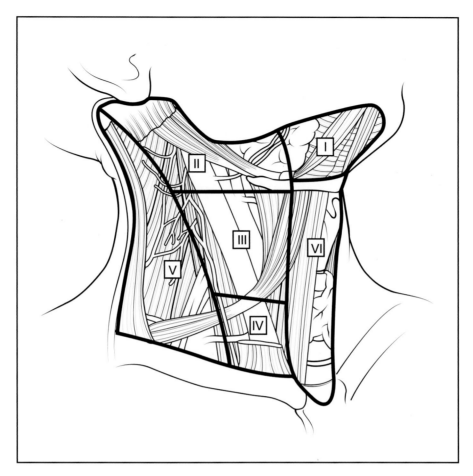

Fig 20–2. Classification of cervical nodes.

CRITICAL ELEMENTS OF THE HISTORY AND PHYSICAL EXAMINATION

Key Points

Careful history with attention to risk factors, head and neck "danger signs" (otalgia, dysphagia, dysphonia, unilateral nasal obstruction/epiphora), and comorbidities.

Systematic head and neck examination by experienced head and neck surgeon.

In cases of metastatic squamous cell cancer, primary site most often will be identified.

The evaluation of the patient with malignant metastatic cervical adenopathy must begin with a systematic and thorough history and physical examination, and in the majority of cases a primary site will be identified. Jones et al[11] identified a primary tumor site by history and physical examination in 148 of 267 (55 %) patients presenting to the University of Liverpool with squamous cell carcinoma metastatic to a cervical node.

Table 20–2. Cervical Node Classification, Anatomic Boundaries, and Site of Primary Mucosal Drainage

Level	Name	Anatomic Boundaries	Location of Primary Tumor
Level I	Submental (Ia) and Submandibular (Ib) nodes	(Ia) anterior bellies of the digastric m. laterally and the hyoid inferiorly (Ib) nodes between the anterior and posterior bellies of the digastric m. and the mandible (including facial nodes)	(Ia) floor of mouth, anterior oral tongue, anterior mandibular alveolus, lower lip (Ib) oral cavity, cutaneous midface, upper lip, anterior nasal cavity, submandibular gland, maxillary sinus
Level II	Upper jugular nodes (IIa) anterior accessory (IIb) posterior accessory	Nodes anterior and posterior to the great vessels from the skull base to the hyoid bone (or carotid bifurcation), from the sternohyoid m. anteriorly to the posterior border of the sternocleidomastoid m.	(IIa) Oral cavity, nasal cavity, supraglottic larynx oropharynx, parotid (IIb) nasopharynx, thyroid, parotid, cutaneous metastases
Level III	Middle jugular nodes	Nodes along the jugular vein from the hyoid bone (carotid bifurcation) to the omohyoid m., from the sternohyoid m. anteriorly to the posterior border of the sternocleidomastoid m.	Oropharynx, oral cavity, hypopharynx, supraglottic larynx
Level IV	Inferior jugular nodes	Nodes along the jugular vein from the omohyoid m. to the clavicle, from the sternohyoid m. anteriorly to the posterior border of the sternocleidomastoid m.	Hypopharynx, transglottic larynx, cervical esophagus
Level V	Posterior triangle nodes V (a) superior cricoid V (b) inferior cricoid	Nodes bordered anteriorly by the posterior border of sternocleidomastoid m, posteriorly by anterior border of trapezius m. and inferiorly by clavicle	(Va) nasopharynx, oropharynx, thyroid (Vb) infraclavicular sources
Level VI	Central compartment nodes	Nodes bordered superiorly by the hyoid, inferiorly by the sternal notch, and laterally by the carotid arteries	Thyroid gland, transglottic larynx, piriform apex, cervical esophagus

Summary of common predicable patterns of cervical lymph node metastases from major head and neck subsites.

When presented with a patient with a metastatic carcinoma, the minimum clinical investigations should include a careful history and complete physical examination. Individuals with squamous cell carcinoma metastatic to a cervical node should have a comprehensive head and neck examination by an experienced otolaryngologist and AP and lateral chest radiographs. Initial laboratory evaluation should include complete blood count, comprehensive metabolic profile, urinalysis, and fecal occult blood examination.[3] The initial confirmation of malignancy should be made by fine-needle aspiration biopsy

thereby minimizing distortion and oncologic "contamination" of normal tissues should definitive resection be necessary (see below).[12-14] A more detailed physical examination including pelvic, rectal, and breast examinations are indicated in cases of poorly differentiated or adenocarcinomas.

Patients or their primary care providers may have identified an otherwise asymptomatic neck mass. Failure of the neck mass to respond to a 14-day course of oral antibiotics should prompt an evaluation by an otolaryngologist-head and neck surgeon. Patients with metastatic cervical adenopathy from upper aerodigestive tract squamous cell carcinoma are by definition in stage III or IV[12] and the best chance for positive outcomes is achieved by avoiding any further delay in diagnosis and initiating multimodality treatment.

Careful inquiry regarding specific signs or symptoms may give some indication as to the site of the primary tumor. Otalgia in a normal-appearing ear, aural fullness, or decreased hearing may indicate pathology in the nasopharynx, ear, and/or the oropharynx. Dysphagia, odynophagia, persistent sore throat, or a painful foreign body sensation may indicate an occult oropharyngeal or hypopharyngeal malignancy. Hoarseness or hemoptysis are indicative of lesions of the larynx. Trismus, dysarthria, and dental pain suggest the oral cavity or tongue base as a site of the lesion. Nasal obstruction, hyponasal speech, epistaxis, and epiphora point to the nasopharynx or sinonasal tract as possible sources for the primary lesion. Finally, a history of ulcerating moles, previously excised skin lesions, or nonhealing sores may indicate cutaneous malignancies.[15]

A thorough review of systems is an integral component of any comprehensive medical history. Patients should be asked about constitutional symptoms which may be associated with hematologic malignancy, bowel and bladder habits, and when the most recent age-appropriate cancer screening examination (digital rectal, breast examination, mammography, pelvic examination with cervical Pap smear) were performed.

Concurrent diseases should be evaluated. Feinstein[16] reported the importance of symptoms as an indicator of disease progression using a simple classification of primary, systemic, and constitutional. The severity of concurrent disease may have a significant impact on the patients overall survival in addition to potential choices for cancer treatment. Several instruments are available for measuring general comorbidities and when collected in a systematic fashion comorbidity data have been shown to provide important prognostic information, independent of TNM staging, in cancers of the larynx, pharynx, and oral cavity.[17-20]

Patients with malignant cervical adenopathy should undergo a detailed examination of the head and neck prior to obtaining costly imaging studies. Mucosal surfaces of the upper aerodigestive tract should be inspected and palpated. The posterior superior lateral aspects of the nasopharynx (fossa of Rosenmüller), tonsillar fossa, walls of the oropharynx, piriform sinuses, and the base of the tongue should be carefully examined. The nasopharynx is best viewed with a rigid-Hopkins telescope which provides both excellent illumination and magnification (Fig 20-3). The tongue base, vallecula, and hypopharyngeal mucosa should be examined with a magnified angled Hopkins telescope and/or a flexible nasopharyngolaryngoscope. Areas of ulceration, induration, firmness, or erythema should be noted for biopsy. In selected patients, transoral biopsy of oropharyngeal, laryngeal, and hypopharyngeal lesions can be performed obviating the need for routine "staging triple endoscopy.[21,22]

The neck should be palpated with careful attention to the character, size, fixation, and particularly the location of the metastatic adenopathy. Mobility can give information regarding the relationship of the mass to the structures within the carotid sheath. Fixation to the skin or subcutaneous tissue indicates extracapsular extension and invasion of the subdermal lymphatics. Pulsatile masses or masses with a bruit should not be instrumented or biopsied until imaging studies have been performed.

APPROPRIATE DIAGNOSTIC OFFICE-BASED PROCEDURES

Key Points

Fine-needle aspiration biopsy should be performed prior to open biopsy.

Suspicious mucosal lesions of virtually any site in the head and neck can be safely biopsied in the office under topical anesthesia.

In the absence of an identifiable primary lesion on head and neck examination information regarding the metastatic adenopathy should be collected systematically.

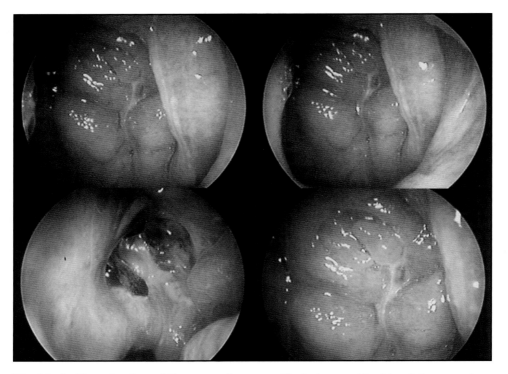

Fig 20–3. Examination of the nasopharynx with 0-degree Hopkins telescope in a patient presenting with a neck mass positive for squamous cell carcinoma on fine-needle aspiration biopsy. Nasopharyngeal biopsy showed keratinizing squamous cell carcinoma.

Fine needle aspiration (FNA) is a standard technique and should be included in the initial evaluation of all patients with suspected metastatic adenopathy. Fine-needle aspiration biopsy is the least invasive pathologic test to evaluate a suspected metastatic cervical lymph node and should be attempted prior to excisional biopsy. It can be 98% to 99% accurate in the hands of an experienced cytopathologist. The procedure, performed with a 25-gauge needle, can be carried out in the office and the aspirate can be examined immediately for rapid diagnosis using alcohol-fixed and stained tissues. Conventional cytologic examination on fixed slides, hematoxylin and eosin examination of centrifuge aspirates ("cell blocs"), and immunohistochemistry can all be used. Material obtained by FNA can be placed into appropriate in vitro transport medium (RPMI or related media) for further processing by flow cytometry or other molecular studies (gene rearrangement, in situ hybridization, PCR, etc).[23]

Adult patients with a solid neck mass should be considered to have a malignancy until proven otherwise and the majority (80%) of these will be squamous cell carcinoma. The standard examination of these patients should include careful examination under anesthesia with palpation of the oropharynx (tonsils, tongue base, lateral oropharyngeal wall). Direct laryngoscopy is performed with directed biopsies of the midline and bilateral tongue base and ipsilateral piriform sinus. Cervical esophagoscopy is performed to rule out malignancies of the pharyngoesophgeal segment. The nasopharynx can be examined and directly biopsied with the 0- and 30-degree rigid-Hopkins telescopes. Traditionally, bronchoscopy has been considered a component of the standard "panendoscopy"; however, it is no longer recommended if the preoperative chest x-ray is normal. The routine use of these modalities has been questioned on both a cost-effectiveness and therapeutic-efficacy basis.[20-23]

The majority of primary tumors are detected in the tonsillar fossa or tongue base. Bimanual palpation of the tonsils and the tongue base should be carried out under anesthesia noting areas of nodularity or induration. Despite endoscopic evaluation, some primaries may not be detected as they may be submucosal, hidden in lymphatic crypts, or have submucosally regressed.[24] This had led to bilateral tonsillectomy over tonsil biopsy in the evaluation of patients with CUP citing increased yield over conventional biopsy, an approximately 10% incidence of bilateral carcinomas, ease in follow-up examination, and no increased complications.[25,26]

Excisional Biopsy

Diagnostic excisional biopsy of a cervical lymph node should not be performed as a primary investigation of a neck mass but only after a complete head and neck examination, CT or MRI scanning of the neck, and data have been obtained from fine needle biopsy. In the case of an equivocal or nondiagnostic initial fine-needle aspiration biopsy, the FNA should be repeated using ultrasound control to identify a solid portion of the index node. Our indications for excisional biopsy and intraoperative frozen section are:

1. to obtain a definitive diagnosis of a lymphoma or other hematologic malignancy,
2. to confirm the diagnosis of head and neck squamous cell carcinoma prior to initiation of nonsurgical therapy concurrently with staging panendoscopy/tonsillectomy, airway, enteral, and vascular access,
3. to confirm the diagnosis of primary head and neck squamous carcinoma prior to concurrently initiating primary surgical therapy with staging panendoscopy/tonsillectomy and therapeutic neck dissection,
4. to confirm the diagnosis of metastatic operative head and neck salivary or endocrine carcinoma concurrently with definitive resection of the primary, and

5. to facilitate the diagnosis of an infraclavicular primary tumor.

One important consideration in this management approach is confidence in the abilities of the surgical pathologist. The pathologist must be able to distinguish squamous cell carcinoma from other malignancies and communicate clearly to the surgeon before proceeding to neck dissection. The surgeon performing the open biopsy should be prepared to proceed with definitive therapy of the neck. This includes placing the biopsy incision favorably to be included in the neck dissection and having the requisite skill to proceed safely with the type of neck dissection indicated by the pathology, including comprehensive neck dissection.

The results of treatment of squamous cell carcinoma of the head and neck following open biopsy are contradictory.[27,28] Recommendations against open biopsy are based on the initial experience reported from the University of Iowa. In this matched-pair analysis, McGuirt and McCabe[29] reported increased incidences of local recurrence and distant metastases in patients presenting for definitive treatment following open biopsy of a metastatic cervical node. The overall and disease-free survival were not reported in this study. This report led generations of head and neck surgeons to offer comprehensive neck dissection to patients following open cervical node biopsy in an effort to prevent these dire consequences.

Radical neck dissection following open biopsy has been re-examined with particular attention to the time interval between biopsy and initiation of definitive therapy. Data from both the MD Anderson Cancer Center and the University of Florida support alternative management options. Robbins et al[28] reported 192 patients treated with open biopsy prior to definitive treatment, which consisted of radiotherapy alone in 109 patients. They demonstrated no differences in wound complications, neck recurrence, distant metastasis, and 5-year survival between patients treated with open biopsy compared to age, sex, site of the primary, stage, and treatment matched controls. Data from the University of Florida also suggest that definitive radiotherapy following open biopsy can be performed without compromising outcomes. Sixty-six patients who underwent open biopsy followed by definitive radiotherapy were compared to 442 patients who did not have an open biopsy. No differences in neck control, overall risk of distant metastasis, and cause-specific survival were observed between these groups. Both these studies conclude that patients initially treated with open biopsy revealing a squamous cell carcinoma should be carefully examined for small head and neck primaries and treated aggressively in a timely fashion with neck irradiation. Open biopsy does not appear to have once dreaded consequences as previously thought.[30,31]

If lymphoma is suspected sampling of unfixed, frozen lymph node is required as an adjunct to advances in immunohistochemical techniques. The dissected specimen can be divided and a portion fixed in formalin and paraffin embedded. The formalin-fixed biopsy is used to classify the lymphoma morphologically and unfixed tissue can be banked for additional studies such as flow cytometry, determining the presence of gene rearrangements, polymerase chain reaction, and in situ hybridization which can characterize the cell lineage of lymphoma. In cases of operable solid tumors (squamous cell, thyroid/parathyroid, or salivary gland carcinomas) the surgeon must be prepared to perform a formal neck dissection and oncologically appropriate resection of the primary tumor as indicated by the frozen section.

RECOMMENDED IMAGING STUDIES

Key Points

CT scan should be performed as initial imaging on all patients with positive histology on fine needle biopsy.

PET and PET/CT scanning are not substitutes for detailed physical examination and directed biopsies.

When a metastatic neck mass is confirmed by FNA, radiographic evaluation of the head and neck is performed to identify the primary site. Imaging is performed from the skull base to the clavicles. The location of the lymph node low in the neck may dictate additional imaging of the chest, gastrointestinal tract, and prostate. Imaging may identify the primary site by showing areas of asymmetry in the nasopharynx, base of tongue, tonsil, or piriform sinus.

CT Scan

CT scan is regarded as the primary imaging modality for evaluating unknown primary tumor. Tumors and metastatic nodes appear brighter on contrast-enhanced studies than normal tissues with the exception of inflamed mucosa and blood vessels. Although MRI provides superior soft tissue detail in multiple planes with its high-contrast capabilities, CT scan is more cost effective and widely available. Certain features, such as central lymph node necrosis and size greater than 15 mm. may be more clearly visible on CT scan. CT scan is also less affected by motion artifacts. The spiral CT offers a very short examination time. Cuts ranging from 1 to 3 mm may be taken in areas of high probability. CT scans will provide additional information on the size and extension of the primary tumor including extension into paraspinal muscles, involvement of periglottic or pre-epiglottic spaces and subglottic extension in cases of laryngeal or hypopharyngeal carcinomas, and relationships to the carotid artery.[32,33] In cases of oral cavity carcinomas bone infiltration may be assessed. This may be limited by artifacts from dental and metallic implants (Figs 20–4 and 20–5).

MRI

MRI is excellent for providing soft tissue detail and contrast; however, it is susceptible to motion artifacts and cannot be used in patients with claustrophobia. CT is considered superior to MRI in detecting and evaluating neck disease. MRI is viewed primarily as a complementary imaging modality when soft tissue detail and the multiplanar image acquisition qualities of the MRI are thought to be particularly useful. MRI is particularly effective in identifying enhancement of the cranial nerve and the dura. We recommend use of MRI as an adjunctive imaging modality in the evaluation of paranasal sinus malignancies, nasopharyngeal carcinoma, and other malignancies where the skull base is at risk.[34]

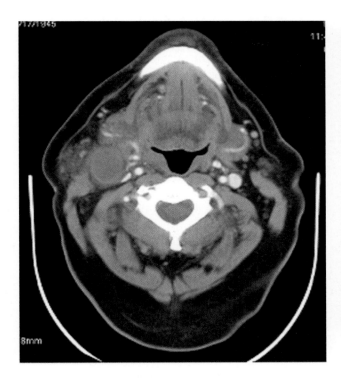

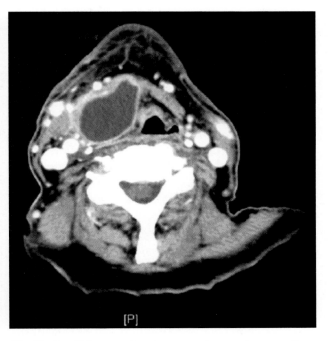

Fig 20–5. CT scan of unknown primary; large unilocular cystic neck mass with associated solid metastatic adenopathy. Bilateral tonsillectomies, nasopharyngeal and hypopharyngeal biopsies, and superficial laser excision of the tongue base did not reveal a primary source. This patient received a radical neck dissection and postoperative radiation therapy to the ipsilateral neck and oropharynx with concurrent single-agent cisplatin.

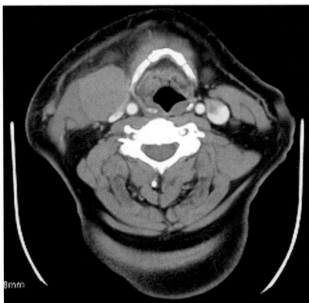

Fig 20–4. CT scan of unknown primary; 63-year-old man presenting with unilateral, unilocular cystic mass. Panendoscopy, bilateral tonsillectomy, and directed biopsies did not reveal a primary source. The patient underwent a modified radical neck dissection and postoperative radiation therapy to the ipsilateral neck and oropharynx.

No studies have advocated the routine use of MRI scans in the evaluation of patients with unknown primary tumors. Benefits of MRI include the lack of exposure to ionizing radiation, low risk of contrast hypersensity reactions, and the continued development of new technologies using metabolic and functional MR imaging. Disadvantages of the MRI include long image acquisition times, inability to image with indwelling metal objects, claustrophobia, and increased cost.

Positron Emission Tomography (PET) Scan

In 2000, the United States Food and Drug Administration (FDA) approved PET for use in the staging of head and neck cancer. PET scanning is based on the observation that there is increased uptake of glucose analogues by neoplastic cells with higher metabolism in comparison with normal tissue. The principle theoretical advantage of the PET scan is in the identification of metabolically active, small or superficial lesions not seen on conventional imaging or physical examination. The labeled glucose analogue is taken up by rapidly metabolizing tumor cells and converted to 18-F-deoxyglucose-phosphate (18F-dG6P) by hexokinase. 18F-dG6P cannot be metabolized by either glycolysis via the Krebs cycle or by phosphatase and is slowly converted to gluconate or glucuronate leading to an accumulation in metabolically active malignant cells. Qualitative evaluation of FDG-PET images is sufficient for most clinical purposes, but quantitative measurement of FDG concentration is also possible. Standardized uptake values (SUV) are used for the measurement of radioactivity concentrations at a single time point. The activity concentration is normalized to the body weight or body surface area. SUV may allow differentiation of malignant tissue from benign causes of increased uptake and can be used to measure the response to treatment.[35]

The sensitivity and specificity for identifying primary tumors were 85% and 100% for PET and 88% and 75% for CT/MRI, respectively. Accuracy was 86% for PET and 87% for CT/MRI. Sensitivity and specificity for detecting primary lymph node involvement were 71%/86 % for PET and 74%/57% for CT/MRI, resulting in an accuracy of 77% with PET and 68% with morphologic imaging. In 23 patients, histopathology revealed pT1 stages with tumor diameters <12 mm. In 8 patients CT/MRI and in 10 patients PET failed to identify small primary lesions.[35]

Miller et al[36] carried out a prospective study on 26 patients with confirmed metastatic cervical neck disease with no visible primary on comprehensive physical examination including fiberoptic laryngoscopy and nasopharyngoscopy, and imaging by CT or MRI. All patients underwent PET before panendoscopy. The overall detection rate of primary tumor was 30.8%: 3 in palatine tonsil, 2 at base of tongue, 2 in lung, and 1 in the hypopharynx. One patient had a false positive PET finding with a negative finding on pathologic analysis of the tonsil specimen.

The overall sensitivity of PET was 66% and the specificity was 92.9%. The positive predictive value of PET was 88.8% and the negative predictive value was 76.5%. The value of PET is in guiding the surgeon to a primary site and ruling out synchronous primaries.

Rustoven[37,38] completed a meta-analysis of FDG-PET in the detection of primary tumors in patients with cervical metastases from unknown primary tumors. Sixteen studies (involving a total of 302 patients) published between 1994 and 2003 were reviewed. These studies evaluated the role of FDG-PET in the detection of unknown primary tumors after conventional workup. In all studies, conventional workup included either panendoscopy or computed tomographic/magnetic resonance imaging, and in 10 of 16 studies, both of these diagnostic techniques were performed before diagnosis. The overall sensitivity, specificity, and accuracy rates of FDG-PET in detecting unknown primary tumors were 88.3%, 74.9%, and 78.8%, respectively. Furthermore, FDG-PET detected 24.5% of tumors that were not apparent after conventional workup. FDG-PET imaging also led to the detection of previously unrecognized metastases in 27.1% of patients (regional, 15.9%; distant, 11.2%). FDG-PET had notably low specificity and a high false-positive rate (39.3%) in the tonsils. In contrast, the false-positive rates for FDG-PET of the base of tongue and hypopharynx were only 21.4% and 8.3%, respectively. FDG-PET exhibited decreased sensitivity to tumors in the base of tongue (81.5%). The sensitivity of this technique at other sites was 90.5%. They concluded that FDG-PET detected primary tumors that went undetected by other modalities in approximately 25% of cases and was sensitive in the detection of previously unrecognized regional or distant metastases in 27% of cases. FDG-PET had low specificity for tonsillar tumors and low sensitivity for base-of-tongue malignancies.[37,38]

CT-PET

A major disadvantage of PET is lack of anatomic information, resulting in poor lesion localization. A number of software applications are used to "fuse" PET images with CT or MR images, which are obtained at different time points (Fig 20–6). Fusion

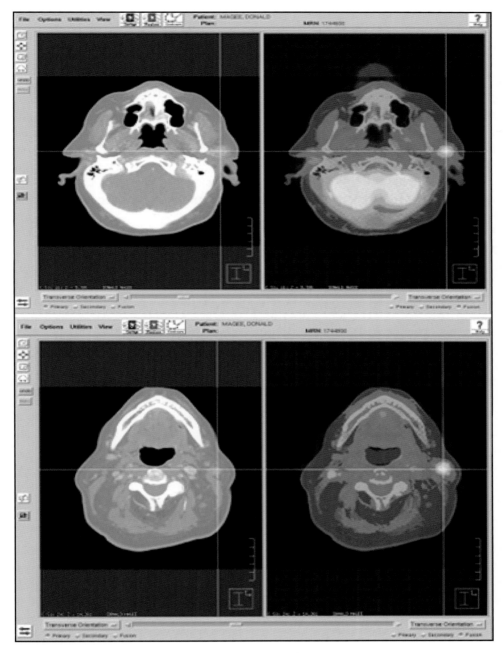

Fig 20–6. PET-CT fusion. 18-FDG-PET fused with axial CT scan in a patient following excision of neck mass revealing neuroendocrine carcinoma. Images reveal occult tumor in the ipsilateral parotid gland. Additional images in the same patient identify residual malignant in the neck. The contralateral node proved to be benign.

of anatomic and functional images significantly improves lesion localization, but is still subject to many technical difficulties and errors. Combined PET/CT units permit acquisition of both CT and PET images using a single instrument in a single session. Experience with these combined units is very promising. Errors in lesion localization are minimized, although they do occur in certain locations.[35]

Gutzeit et al[39] conducted a retrospective study to evaluate fused positron emission tomography (PET)/computed tomography (CT) in depicting the primary lesion in cancer of an unknown primary tumor, compared with PET, CT, and PET and CT side-by-side evaluation. Forty-five with metastatic cervical adenopathy ($n = 18$) or extracervical metastases ($n = 27$) of unknown primary tumor were included. PET/CT imaging was performed in all. PET/CT data sets were evaluated for the primary tumor, and imaging results were compared with those of CT, PET, and PET and CT side-by-side evaluation. PET/CT depicted the primary tumor in 15 (33%) of 45 patients. In 30 (67%) patients, the primary tumor site remained occult ($p > .05$). PET and CT side-by-side evaluation depicted 13 (29%) of 45 tumors ($p > .05$). PET alone revealed the primary tumor in 11 (24%) of 45 patients ($p > .05$), whereas CT alone helped in the correct diagnosis in eight (18%) of 45 patients ($p > .05$). There were no significant differences between the diagnostic accuracies of PET/CT and the other imaging modalities. They concluded that PET/CT was able to depict more primary tumors, though not significantly, than either of the other imaging modalities, but larger patient cohorts may be required to finally judge its value for revealing the primary tumor site.[39]

Another major limitation of PET is poor spatial resolution. Currently, the maximum spatial resolution of dedicated PET scanners is about 5 to 6 mm. It is inferior for more commonly used hybrid scanners. PET is an evolving technology with improvements in spatial resolution in the future. Because the maximum achievable spatial resolution is 1 to 2 mm, PET is poor in detection of microscopic disease.

In a series of 140 patients with cervical metastasis with unknown primaries, Mendenhall et al[33] found 58 (43%) primary head and neck cancers. Of these 58, 48 (82%) were detected in the tonsillar fossa and base of tongue. Miller recommends directed biopsies of the base of tongue, nasopharynx, and bilateral tonsillectomy routinely, adding hypopharyngeal biopsies if enhancements are seen on PET or if suspicious findings are noted on endoscopy. Miller et al[36] carried out a prospective study on 26 patients with confirmed metastatic cervical neck

disease with no visible primary on comprehensive physical examination including fiberoptic laryngoscopy and nasopharyngoscopy, and imaging by CT or MRI. All patients underwent PET before panendoscopy. 4 patients had negative PET findings, but the primary tumor was detected on panendoscopy and directed biopsies. The value of PET was in guiding the surgeon to a primary site and ruling out synchronous primaries. However, a negative PET does not preclude the need for a careful panendoscopy with directed biopsies.

Careful physical examination, CT scanning, and endoscopy with directed biopsied and bilateral tonsillectomy will identify the primary site of the tumor in between 40% and 50% of patients presenting with metastatic cervical squamous cell with an unknown primary site. The majority of these tumors will be located in the oropharynx with lower incidences identified in the nasopharynx and hypopharynx. Patients with no suggestive findings on physical examination or imaging will have a low (17%) yield on pathologic examination. Patients with suggestive finding on physical examination and CT scan will have an almost 70% chance of pathologically identifying a primary tumor. A slight improvement may result from the addition of PET scan to the evaluation of these patients; however, the marginal increase in health care costs may prove prohibitive.[33,35,36,38]

PET and PET-CT provide important information in the evaluation of the patient with a carcinoma of an unknown primary. PET and CT-PET provide overall high sensitivity (close to 90%) in the detection of occult primary tumors with the exception of the tongue base. The widespread use of this application may be limited by the overall low (75%) specificity rate and high cost. At present the greatest utility of PET scanning is as an aid in directing biopsies particular in the case of recurrent cancer.

AJCC STAGING OF MALIGNANCY

The clinical examination of the neck is incorporated into the AJCC an UICC staging systems in the following fashion. Patients in whom the status of the cervical nodes cannot be assessed are classified as NX;

this category includes patients who have undergone open excisional biopsy of a positive node with no residual palpable or radiographic apparent disease. Patients with no clinical lymph node metastasis are classified as N0. A single node less than 3 cm in diameter in the ipsilateral neck is classified as N1. N2 disease is subdivided into N2a which includes metastasis in a single ipsilateral node between 3 and 6 cm in greatest dimension, N2b which includes multiple ipsilateral nodal metastases all less than 6 cm in greatest dimension, and N2c which includes bilateral or contralateral nodal metastases all of which are less than 6 cm in greatest dimension. Patients with N3 disease are those with any node greater than 6 cm. in greatest dimension. Patients with N1 disease are at minimum stage III (T1 or T2 or T3 and N1). Cervical metastases from primary tumors located in the nasopharynx, thyroid, and cervical esophagus represent exceptions to this regional nodal staging system.[40]

EXAMPLES OF REPRESENTATIVE HISTOPATHOLOGY

Features of metastatic carcinoma including atypical squamous cells with hyperchromatic nuclei, coarser chromatin, and irregular nuclear contour may be seen. Other features include dyskeratotic cells with dense eosinophilic cytoplasm and small hyperchromatic and deformed cell nuclei. Prominent nucleoli against in a background of cellular debris are also seen[41] (Fig 20-7). Histologic features such as psamomma bodies may point to a thyroid or ovarian primary; signet ring cells may be present in gastric cancers. Diagnostic problems may arise in the case of poorly differentiated carcinomas, or when the aspirate is lymphoid.[23,41] Further evaluation by immunohistochemistry, flow cytometry, or excisional biopsy may be required. Immunohistochemical staining has confirmed the diagnosis of metastatic adenocarcinoma of the prostate,[42] seminoma,[43] and breast carcinoma[44,45] in an unknown primary cervical node.

Immunohistochemical techniques involve identifying the tissue specific marker(s) with monoclonal antibodies and localizing the antigen-antibody complex

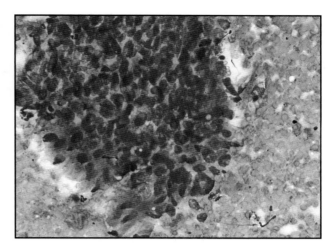

Fig 20–7. Fine-needle aspiration biopsy of squamous cell carcinoma. Appearance included atypical squamous cells with hyperchromatic nuclei, coarser chromatin, and irregular nuclear contour. Other features include dyskeratotic cells with dense eosinophilic cytoplasm and small hyperchromatic and deformed cell nuclei. Prominent nucleoli against a background of cellular debris are also seen.

with antibody-conjugated chromogen(s). Commonly employed tissue antigens include thyroglobulin for thyroid carcinomas, calcitonin for medullary thyroid carcinomas, S-100 and HMB-45 for melanoma, vimentin for sarcoma, chromogranin and synpatophysin for neuroendocrine carcinoma, and leukocyte common antigen for lymphomas. Prostate specific antigen or prostate acid phosphatase may be tested for ruling out prostate metastasis. Other special stains include estrogen/progesterone receptor for breast neoplasm and alpha-fetoprotein for liver, germ cell, and stomach neoplasm. The presence of cytokeratin and epithelial membrane antigen confirm a squamous cell carcinoma but do not provide information regarding the primary site[2,23] (Table 20-3).

IDENTIFICATION OF CRITICAL DECISION POINTS

The management of patients with occult or unknown primary head and neck is a careful endoscopic examination under anesthesia with bilateral tonsil-

Table 20–3. Specific Tissue Antibodies Used in the Diagnosis of Metastatic Carcinoma of an Unknown Primary Seen in Metastatic Cervical and Supraclavicular Adenopathy

Tissue Antigen	Tumor Type/Primary Site
Prostate specific antigen, Prostatic acid phosphatase	Prostate
Thyroid transcription factor (TTF-1)	Thyroid, Lung
Surfactant apoA1	Lung
Thyroglobulin	Papillary thyroid carcinoma
Calcitonin	Medullary thyroid carcinoma
Uroplakin	Urothelial carcinoma
Gross cystic disease fluid protein (GCDFP-15), estrogen, progesterone (ER, PR), and HER-2-neu receptors	Breast
S-100 protein, HMB-45, MelanA, tyrosinase	Melanoma
Chromogranin, synpatophysin, neuron-specific enolase (NSE), glial fibrillary acidic protein (GFAP)	Neuroendocrine carcinoma
Leukocyte common antigen (LCA), and specific cell lineage directed markers (T-cell CD3, CD 4, CD 5, CD 24; B-cell CD 20, immunoglobulin light or heavy chains)	Hematologic malignancies
Cytokeratins (CK7, 20), epithelial membrane antigen (EMA)	Squamous cell carcinoma
Vimentin, desmin, smooth muscle actin (SMA)	Sarcoma
Carcinoembryonic antigen (CEA)	Gastrointestinal adenocarcinoms
Alpha-fetoprotein (AFP), human chorionic gonadatropin (HCG), placental alkaline phosphatase	Germ cell tumor

Immunohistochemical staining of profiles and commonly recognized tumor antigens identified in metastatic cervical lymph nodes from head and neck and infraclavicular primary malignancies.

lectomies, directed biopsies of the nasopharynx and ipsilateral piriform sinus, and, in our clinic, a transoral microscopic laser excision of the tongue base.

Several management options are available to patients with confirmed metastatic squamous cell carcinoma in the neck without an identifiable mucosal primary source. Patients with N1 disease and a small primary tumor can be considered for single modality treatment with either surgery or radiation therapy. Patients with N2 disease or greater can be treated with primary nonsurgical therapy either with radiotherapy alone or concurrent chemoradiation therapy based on the size of the metastatic node. Resectable N2 and selected N3 patients can also be treated surgically with primary neck dissection and adjuvant combined modality therapy. The role of combined modality therapy in patients with advanced neck disease regardless of the site of the primary is well established. In randomized prospective trials in both Europe and the Unites States, the use of postoperative radiation therapy concurrently with platinum-based chemotherapy has been shown to reduce the rate of local recurrence and distant metastases in patients with multiple positive nodes or the extracapsular extension of cancer from the node. Although in the EORTC trial this translated into increased survival the same effect was not demonstrated in RTOG 91–05.[46,47] The use of definitive concurrent radiochemotherapy without neck dissection has also been shown to be effective for this high-risk population (see below).

ANALYSIS OF VARIOUS TREATMENT OPTIONS

Surgery Alone

Patients with isolated N1 disease from on occult primary account for between 17% and 29% of patients seen in clinical practice. The surgical treatment consists of a selective neck dissection, and adjuvant therapy is offered based on the careful histopathologic examination of a neck dissection specimen. The pathology report on a neck dissection specimen should include the number of positive lymph node(s), their size, level in the neck, presence or absence of extracapsular spread, and comment on angioinvasion and perineural invasion. Several authors have demonstrated not only that presence of extracapsular extension in cervical lymphatics portends a poor prognosis, but that extracapsular extension can be identified in up to 18% of necks clinically staged as N0. In our own experience, 27% of patients with extracapsular extension developed pulmonary metastases within 24 months of neck dissection.[48] Extracapsular extension was identified in 17% of patients clinically staged N0.

Neck dissection alone has been advocated for isolated N1 neck with no extracapsular (ECS) spread. In a retrospective study by the Mayo Clinic, 24 patients with N1 and N2 neck disease who underwent surgery but refused subsequent radiation were followed. There were no recurrences in the subset of N1 patients without extracapsular spread. The indications for radiation after neck dissection included multiple positive lymph nodes, N2 and more advanced neck disease, and the presence of extracapsular disease.[49] Grau[50] reported on 277 patients with CUP treated in 5 centers across Denmark 9% of whom received radical neck dissection as the single modality treatment. Although the overall survival was not reduced in these patients they did have a significantly 25% higher rate of the emergence of a mucosal primary than patients whose

treatment included radiotherapy.[49,50] Composite data on single modality surgical treatment of CUP are difficult to locate. We pooled data from the most often cited studies which indicated a 5-year overall survival rate of approximately 66%, a median nodal recurrence rate of 34%, and a mucosal emergence rate of 25%. These data seem to indicate that in selected cases of pN1 disease without extracapsular extension the neck can be controlled with surgery alone. These patients need continued close clinical follow-up to manage nodal recurrences and the mucosal tumors when they develop.[49-53]

Radiation Therapy Alone

Several issues exist pertaining to the application of external beam radiation therapy in the setting of CUP. The first is whether all at-risk mucosal sites should be included in the treatment fields, the second is whether or not to irradiate the nasopharynx in the face of a negative biopsy, and the third is bilateral versus unilateral neck irradiation.

Historically, radiation was delivered to bilateral cervical lymphatics and putative at-risk mucosal sites (Waldyer's ring and hypopharynx).[54] Patients are treated to a total dose of 60 Gy over 5 to 6 weeks with curative intent in patients with metastatic squamous cell carcinoma, adenocarcinoma, and undifferentiated carcinoma. The morbidity associated with this treatment is significant and has been described as "overkill". Results of treatment in this fashion have shown mucosal emergence rates between 12 to 16%, nodal failure of 20 to 50%, and overall survival at 5 years of 37 to 48%.[11,54,55]

The mean survival of patients who have radiation only to the possible primary tumor regions based on location of cervical metastasis generally is similar to survival of patients who undergo radiation to all known primary locations. Prospective studies have shown that most occult primaries lie in the base of tongue or tonsils. This has led to radiation therapy sparing the nasopharynx.[54-56]

Debate continues regarding the extent of radiation therapy to the bilateral or ipsilateral neck. Retrospective single institutional reviews seem to indicate no difference in overall and disease-free survival in patients treated with radiation therapy to the bilateral versus the ipsilateral neck. Differences in these groups have been shown in the relative rates of ipsilateral nodal failure, contralateral nodal failures, and the degree of xerostomia.[56,57]

In our practice the principal indication for single modality radiotherapy is adjuvant treatment to the neck following open biopsy and panendoscopy with directed biopsies, tongue base excision, and tonsillectomy. A "shrinking field" technique is used in current clinical practice. The whole cervical lymphatic drainage area receives a dose of 45 to 50 Gy. The oropharynx and hypopharynx are given at least 50 Gy. The ipsilateral cervical lymphatic drainage area receives 50 to 60 Gy. The affected lymph nodes are irradiated with a boost of rapid electrons to a total dose of 70 Gy, sparing the spinal cord and pharynx. When nasopharyngeal carcinoma is suspected, the nasopharynx should receive 70 Gy.

Surgery and Radiation Therapy

Patients with an N2 or N3 neck who have undergone a biopsy of a cervical node or neck dissection in the evaluation of a CUP should receive postoperative radiation therapy. Patients with metastatic lymph nodes greater than 2 cm should undergo a comprehensive neck dissection (levels I to V) with preservation of the internal jugular vein, sternoclei-

domastoid muscle, and the spinal accessory nerve as dictated by disease generally advocated, and this is followed by radiation.[58]

In a series of 136 patients reviewed from the MD Anderson, Colleteir et al[59] reported survival and patterns of failure in those receiving postoperative radiation therapy following either neck node biopsy or neck dissection. Postoperative radiation was delivered via opposed lateral fields to the bilateral necks and the naso-, oro-, and hypopharynx with a median dose to the involved neck of 63 Gy. The overall survival in this series was 60% at 5 years with 9% nodal failure, 18% distant failure, and 10% mucosal emergence rates. The overall complication rate was not reported. Similar data were reported by Strojan and Anicin[60] in a review of 125 patients treated in a similar fashion. Their results indicated an overall survival rate of 52% at 5 years with 18% nodal failure, 11% distant failure, and 9% mucosal emergence rates. Similarly, these authors did not report details of complications and reported toxicity as "acceptable.[60] We have summarized the data from these and 6 other retrospective studies examining surgery and postoperative comprehensive radiotherapy (Table 20–4). In a total of 650 patients treated the overall 5-year survival rate varied from 35 to 63%. Mean nodal failure, distant failure, and mucosal emergence rates were 18%, 19%, and 9%, respectively.[59-66]

Table 20–4. Results of Surgery (node excision or neck dissection) Followed by Comprehensive Irradiation to Bilateral Necks and At-Risk Mucosal Sites

Study (yr)	Reference	No. of Patients	Mucosal Carcinoma Emergence Rate (%)	Nodal Failure Rate (%)	Distant Metastasis Rate (%)	5-Year Survival Rate (%)
Colletier (1998)	59	136	10.0	9	18	60
Strojan (1998)	60	56	9	18	11	52
Medini (1998)	61	24	8.3	8.3	33	54
Nguyen (1994)	62	54	5.6	13	20	63
Davidson (1994)	63	73	12	26		45
Maulard (1992)	64	113	9.7	13.7	16	38
Lefebvre (1990)	66	98	16	16	30	35
Bataini (1987)	65	48	12	17	25	55

Summary of referenced publications with unknown primary squamoous cell carcinomas of the head and neck.

Neck dissection also has been performed following definitive radiation treatment. Boysen et al[67] performed neck dissection 6 weeks after radiation of 70 Gy. In 23 of 88 patients, no lymph nodes were clinically palpable, but in 5 of these 23, viable tumor was detected in neck dissection specimens. In 65 of 88 patients, cervical lymph nodes were still palpable, and 39 of these 65 had residual cancer. They found that the higher the pretherapeutic N stage, the more likely the residual cancer to be observed.[67]

A modified radical neck dissection is usually performed. Lefebvre et al[66] observed 25% higher local recurrence in modified radical neck dissections (MRND) in comparison with radical neck dissection (RND), and advocated RND in every patient. Busaba et al[58] noted that the number of surgically removed neck nodes was higher in RND in comparison with MRND. The more radical the neck dissection, the greater the yield of positive lymph nodes. However, at present, due to significant functional morbidity associated with RND, most authors advocate MRND with preservation of the internal jugular vein, sternocleidomastoid muscle, and the spinal accessory nerve as possible.

In an effort to answer particular issues regarding the delivery of postoperative radiation therapy a randomized prospective cooperative trial has been organized. The Intergroup Study (EROTC 24001–22005) is a randomized phase III trial on the selection of the target volume in postoperative radiotherapy for cervical node metastases of squamous cell carcinoma from an unknown primary. Patients with suspected CUP undergo staging endoscopy with tonsillectomy and systematic examination for a primary along with a comprehensive neck dissection. Operative procedures are performed with curative intent and include extended, radical, or modified radical neck dissections; patients with gross residual disease following resection are not eligible. Following surgery, patients are randomized to comprehensive bilateral neck and mucosal surface irradiation to 50 Gy with a 10-Gy boost to the ipsilateral neck (standard treatment arm) or selective irradiation to the ipsilateral neck to 60 Gy. Chemotherapy (cisplatin 100 mg/m^2) can only be administered concurrently with radiation and used in both treatment arms. The primary endpoint in the study is disease-free survival; secondary endpoints include control of the neck, emergence of mucosal primary tumors, overall survival, incidence of acute and late side effects, and quality of life.

Until these data are reported, we recommend that patients treated with neck dissection and postoperative comprehensive radiation therapy have improved control and survival rates. There is also agreement that local and regional failures appear to be more common in the eventual emergence of mucosal primary tumors. Although overall survival rates are not improved with bilateral neck and pharyngeal irradiation the incidence of local and contralateral neck failures are reduced. Finally, the N stage, presence of extracapsular extension of tumor, and the patient's performance status remain significant prognostic determinants.

Chemotherapy

There are few data specifically addressing the applications of systemic treatment in patients with an unknown primary squamous cell carcinoma presenting in the cervical lymphatics. What is reported represents extensions of treatment paradigms that have proven useful in patients with known primary tumors and advanced nodal disease. It is now widely accepted that in patients with advanced nodal disease significant responses can be achieved with the concurrent use of platinum-based chemotherapy with concurrent standard fractionation external beam radiation therapy.[47,48,68] Collectively, these studies show the superiority of concurrent systemic and local therapy as well as significant reductions in local failures. In two large adjuvant trials the use of concurrent cisplatin with standard fractionation radiation therapy has been shown to increase disease-free survival and reduce the incidence of local recurrence.[69-71]

In one of the few studies in this population deBraud[72,73] identified 16 (of 41) patients treated with various cisplatin-based chemotherapeutic regimens before, during, or after radiation therapy with or without neck dissection. The overall response rate and median survival times in chemotherapy-treated patients was superior to patients treated with surgery and RT or RT alone (81% vs 60%) and (37 vs 24 months), respectively.[72,73] Colletier et al[59] performed excisional biopsy only followed by chemoradiation on 39 patients. There were no locoregional relapses in any of these patients. Single lymph nodes less than 3 cm with no extracapsular spread have excellent prognosis with long-term locoregional control. Multiple lymph nodes and extracapsular spread indicated worse survival.

More recently, Argiris et al[74,75] reported 25 patients with N2 or N3 disease treated with concurrent split-course chemoradiotherapy with 5-fluorouracil/hydroxyurea (FHX) or with either paclitaxel (T-FHX) or cisplatin (C-FHX). Twenty-two of the patients underwent neck dissection, 14 of which were performed before initiating therapy. Overall actuarial survival approached 75% at 5 years and no patients have developed a metachronous cancer.

Patients with Cervical Metastases in Special Circumstances

Head and neck oncologists are frequently asked to participate in the care of patients with extremely rare malignancies metastatic to the cervical nodes. We review several of these clinical entities including carcinoma arising in a branchial cleft cyst, metastatic melanoma, and metastatic adenocarcinoma.

Carcinoma Arising in a Branchial Cleft Cyst

Controversy exists regarding whether malignant cystic neck masses represent carcinomatous degeneration of branchial cleft cyst epithelium or metastatic adenopathy from an occult primary squamous cell carcinoma.[76-79] More than 50 years ago, Martin et al[80] reviewed 225 of 250 cases of "branchiogenic carcinoma" reported in the literature and upon review was able to identify a primary tumor in 222 of the 225 cases. Martin was able to add 15 cases of his own to the 3 he had culled from this review. He thereby established the criteria for the diagnosis of this tumor, which remain in use today: (1) the tumor must originate along the anterior border of the sternocleidomastoid muscle in a line from anterior to the tragus to the sternoclavicular joint, (2) histologically the tumor must be consistent with tissue originating from a branchial cleft cyst, (3) the patient must have survived and been followed for 5 years

without the development of a carcinoma in a site that could have led to the development of the metastasis, and (4) the tumor must show squamous cell carcinoma arising in the wall of the branchial cleft cyst—this criterion has been modified by Singh et al[81] to stipulate that the normal epithelium of the cyst must demonstrate a transition to squamous cell carcinoma (Fig 20–8).

Cystic neck masses in adults should be evaluated in a careful and systematic fashion. History and careful head and neck examination remain the basis for generating the differential diagnosis. Despite earlier reports to the contrary, fine-needle aspiration biopsy appears to be helpful in differentiating benign from malignant cystic neck masses, with up to 73% sensitivity.[83,83] Unfortunately, a recent report by Ferris et al[84] indicated that combined PET-CT scans do not provide more helpful diagnostic information than CT alone, and may indeed be misleading. These authors recommend that clinical judgment, and endoscopic and CT findings are the most useful in distinguishing benign from malignant cystic neck masses and identifying a source of the primary tumor.[81] As we have discussed, primary squamous cell carcinomas of the tongue base, tonsil and nasopharynx present as cystic degeneration of a cervical lymph node in 33% to 50% of cases. Failure to perform a comprehensive physical examination, and directed biopsied and bilateral tonsillectomies on patients

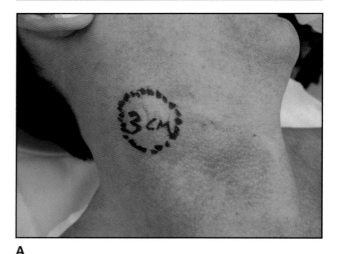

A

Fig 20–8. A. A 51-year-old man with an asymptomatic 3-cm. right neck mass. *continues*

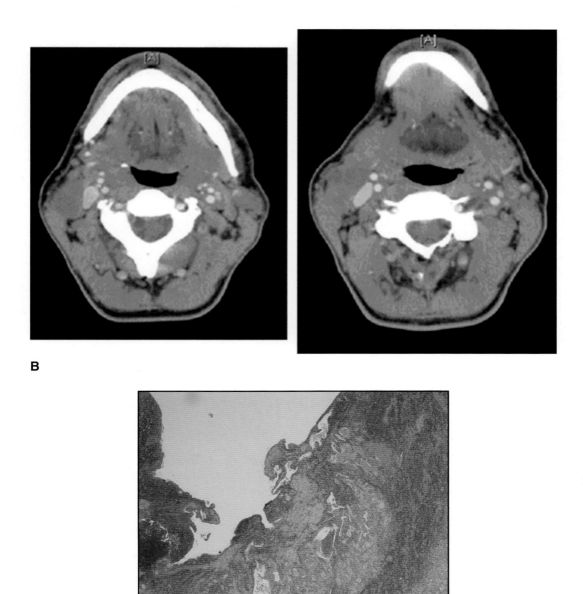

B

C

Fig 20–8. *continued* **B.** Contrast-enhanced CT scan of this patient demonstrating cystic mass anterior to the sternocleidomastoid muscle. Fine needle aspiration was performed which demonstrated "benign cystic epithelial cells and occasionally lymphocytes consistent with a branchial cleft cyst." **C.** Excisional biopsy of the cystic neck mass revealed squamous cell carcinoma arising in the cyst wall. The patient was returned to the operating room for a modified neck dissection, bilateral tonsillectomies, nasopharyngeal and piriform sinus biopsies, and a superficial laser excision (extended biopsy) of the tongue base. All biopsies were negative and the patient received external beam radiation therapy to the ipsilateral neck.

with cystic nodal metastases may delay or impair the ultimate identification of a primary site and lead to incorrect or misdirected primary therapy.[85,86]

Metastatic Melanoma

Unknown primary head and neck metastatic melanoma most often presents in the parotid bed or upper neck leading most authors to believe the initial lesion must have originated in the scalp or upper facial skin (Fig 20-9). Patients must be carefully questioned regarding sun exposure and history of repeated sunburns. Additionally, they should be questioned regarding any "moles" or other scalp or facial lesions that may have been removed in the past and not examined histologically. In addition to a comprehensive head and neck examination including fiberoptic endoscopy, the evaluation of these patients should include a total body surface area examination and combed hair scalp examination by a skilled dermatologist.

Metastatic melanoma of an unknown primary site constituted 2.2% of 84,836 cases of cutaneous and noncutaneous malignant melanoma from all sites reported to the National Cancer Data Base from 1985 to 1994. The majority (57%) of these 1,893 patients presented with distant metastases. Unknown primary metastatic melanoma of the head and neck represents approximately 5% of all head and neck melanomas. Overall 5-year survival is poor despite aggressive regimens of surgery, radiation therapy, immunotherapy, and biochemotherapy.[87] Nasri et al[88] reviewed 46 patients with unknown primary metastatic melanoma treated with primary surgery consisting of parotidectomy and neck dissection. Postoperatively, patients received 40 to 60 Gy of external beam radiation therapy and a variety of chemotherapy and immunotherapy regimens including an autologous tumor cell vaccine. The overall 5-year survival rate was 56% and 10 of 46 patients developed distant metastasis. There was no correlation between the extent of the resection and the use or type of adjuvant therapy on survival. There was a statistically significant correlation between the number of positive nodes and the likelihood of developing metastases but not on survival.[88]

Patients presenting with regionally metastatic melanoma (N1) are by definition at least stage III. In

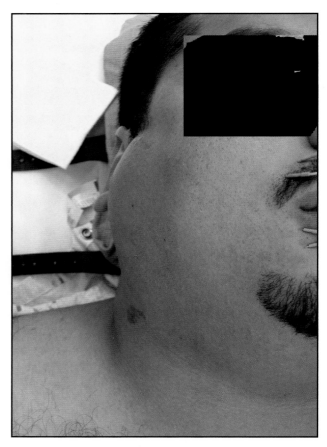

Fig 20–9. A 29-year-old man with a 3-month history of enlarging parotid tumor. On careful questioning he related that he had a "mole" excised from the right forehead 12 months prior to presentation. Parotidectomy and neck dissection revealed metastatic melanoma.

the absence of evidence of metastatic disease these patients should be treated aggressively with an oncologically appropriate regional lymphadenectomy (modified radical neck dissection is possible). Postoperative radiation therapy should be delivered to the involved lymph node basins and patients should be offered systemic therapy with interferon.

The overall survival of patients with metastatic head and neck melanoma of an unknown primary seems to be more favorable than that of similarly staged melanoma in other sites. This more favorable prognosis may be due to the ability to effectively control the cervical lymphatics or an enhanced host immune response resulting in spontaneous regression of the primary tumor and augmented tumor autoimmunity.[89,90]

Metastatic Adenocarcinoma

Although metastatic adenocarcinoma is the most commonly encountered histopathology in patients with cancer of the unknown primary, it is rarely encountered in head and neck surgical oncology practice.[91,92] A review of the Head and Neck Oncology Registry of Netherlands Cancer Center was only able to identify 15 patients treated for metastatic adenocarcinoma or undifferentiated large cell carcinoma over 24 years.[93] The majority of patients with metastatic adenocarcinoma will present with lower neck or supraclavicular fossa masses and often will have metastatic disease on initial evaluation[94] (Fig 20–10).

The initial diagnostic evaluation of patients with adenocarcinoma metastatic to a cervical node should include a complete history, comprehensive head and neck examination including fiberoptic endoscopic endoscopy, and a complete general physician examination including breast and pelvic examinations in women and rectal and testicular examinations in men. Initial biochemical investigations should include a complete metabolic panel, complete blood count, prostate-specific and carcinoembryonic antigens, and fecal occult blood examination. Initial imaging studies should include a chest radiograph and mammography in women. CT imaging of the chest, abdomen, and pelvis should be directed either by symptoms or on the basis of biochemical data. There is no demonstrated or well-studied role for PET scanning in this population.

Examination of cytologic and biopsy specimens is critically important in the identification of potentially treatable malignancies in these patients. The initial light microscopic cytologic examination should be able to classify the malignancy as either: (1) well to moderately differentiated adenocarcinoma, (2) poorly differentiated (undifferentiated) adenocarcinoma, (3) squamous cell carcinoma, or (4) undifferentiated neoplasm. Immunohistochemical stains are then applied to further characterize the malignancy in an effort to identify a potential treatable tumor (ie, lymphoma) in a cost-effective fashion. The type of immunohistochemical panel depends

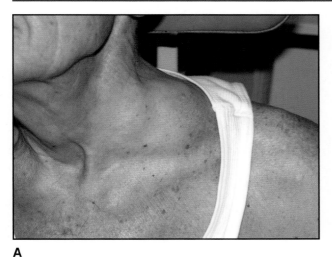
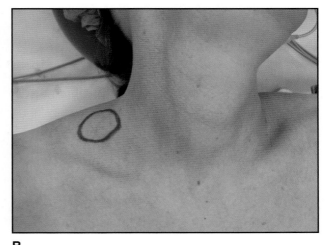

A   **B**

Fig 20–10. Clinical examples of primary infraclavicular carcinomas presenting as a supraclavicular fossa mass. **A.** An 83-year-old man with a 6-month history of an enlarging left supraclavicular fossa mass. Fine-needle aspiration biopsy demonstrated an adenocarcinoma positive for prostate specific antigen. Further examination revealed an enlarged nodular prostate, elevated serum prostate specific antigen, and lytic bone lesions consistent with metastatic prostate carcinoma. **B.** A 47-year-old woman 18 months following mastectomy and axillary node dissection for breast carcinoma. This 2-cm supraclavicular fossa mass was identified on routine follow-up examination. Excision biopsy revealed infiltrating ductal carcinoma of the breast.

on the lineage of the tumor: carcinoma, sarcoma, germ cell tumor, hematologic malignancy, and melanoma. The application of a standard series of 9 antibodies has been shown to improve the identification of primary sites from 26% to 70% in men and 54% in women (see Table 20-4).

The only role for surgery in this setting is to obtain satisfactory tissue for diagnosis. The overall prognosis for patients with metastatic adenocarcinoma is poor with mean survival less than 6 months and only 20% of patients surviving 1 year. Therefore, patients with this diagnosis are best treated by a multidisciplinary cancer team led by a medical oncologist.

SUMMARY

Patients with squamous cell carcinoma from an unknown primary site metastatic to a cervical node represent a rare malignancy. Evaluation of these patients begins with a careful history and physical examination with attention to social habits and ethic origin. Initial imaging should include a contrast-enhanced CT scan from the skull base to the upper mediastium. At this point PET-CT should be considered investigational but it is an interesting and exciting new modality. Comprehensive examination of the head and neck by an otolaryngologist should include bilateral tonsillectomies, endoscopic examination and biopsy of the nasopharynx and piriform sinus, cervical esophagoscopy, and in our clinic a generous biopsy of the tongue base with the microscope and laser.

Following examination under anesthesia, resectable patients can be treated with surgery and adjuvant treatment based on the pathologic examination of the neck nodes or definitive radiation or chemoradiation therapy. In patients with cN2 disease or greater chemoradiation should be offered. The prognosis of a patient with a metastatic cervical lymph node with unknown primary depends on the N stage and the presence of extracapsular extension. Five-year survival for pN1 disease is 68% to 80%; for pN2 disease, 40% to 60%, and for pN3, 18 to 35% when comprehensive neck dissection (levels I–V) is followed by adjuvant radiation. Many centers continue to recommend comprehensive postoperative radiation therapy to the bilateral necks and the at-risk mucosal surfaces of the head and neck. This issue may be resolved by an ongoing randomized prospective trial. The addition of adjuvant chemotherapy reduces the incidence of local recurrence and distant metastases, and increases disease-free survival but as yet has not translated into prolonged overall survival.

Patients with this unusual malignancy should be considered for clinical trials when appropriate and treated by an experienced multidisciplinary head and neck cancer team. Systematic follow-up with serial physical examinations, including fiberoptic endoscopy, should be performed to monitor for neck recurrence and the emergence of a mucosal primary tumor. Periodic chest x-rays should be obtained to survey for the development of pulmonary metastases. The failure to identify a primary site of the malignancy is a source of frequent anxiety and consternation to patients and their families. The treatment team should provide access to psychological and social support groups for patients to share these feelings. Finally, we should work to manage emotional and not just physical treatment sequelae in an effort to enhance the overall quality of life of these patients.

REFERENCES

1. Muir C. Cancer of unknown primary site. *Cancer.* 1995;75(1 suppl):353–356.
2. Ghosh L, Dahut W, Kakar S, et al. Management of patients with metastatic cancer of unknown primary. *Curr Prob Surg.* 2005;42:12–66.
3. Hainsworth JD, Greco FA. Treatment of patients with cancer of an unknown primary site. *N Engl J Med.* 1993;329:257–263.
4. Hanson BG, Rosenquisy K, Antonsson A, et al. Strong association between infection with human papillomavirus and oral and oropharyngeal squamous cell carcinoma. *Acta Oto-Laryngol.* 2005; 125:1337–1344.
5. Davidson BJ, Harter W, O'Malley BB. Cervical lymph node metastasis from squamous cell carcinoma with an unknown primary site. In: Harrison LB, Sessions RB, Hong WK, eds. *Head and Neck Can-*

cer: *A Multidisciplinary Approach.* Philadelphia, Pa: Lippincott-Raven; 1999:391–410.

6. Million RR, Cassisi NJ, Mancuso AA. The unknown primary. In: Million RR, Cassisi NJ, eds. *Management of Head and Neck Cancer: A Multidisciplinary Approach.* Philadelphia, Pa: J.P. Lippincott Company; 1994:311–320.

7. Lindberg R. Distribution of cervical lymph node metastases from squamous cell carcinoma of the upper respiratory and digestive tracts. *Cancer.* 1972;1446–1449.

8. Johnson JT, Newman RK. The anatomic location of neck metastasis from occult squamous cell carcinoma. *Otolaryngol Head Neck Surg.* 1981;89:54–58.

9. Robbins KT. Classification of neck dissection: current concepts and future considerations. *Otolaryngol Clin North Am.* 1998;31:639–655.

10. Robbins KT, Clayman G, Levine PA, et al. Neck dissection classification update: revision proposed by the American Head and Neck Society and the American Academy of Otolaryngology-Head and Neck Surgery. *Arch Otolaryngol Head Neck Surg.* 2002;128:747–748.

11. Jones AS, Cook JA, Phillips DE, Poland NR. Squamous carcinoma presenting as an enlarged cervical lymph node. *Cancer.* 1993;72:1756–1761.

12. Peters BR, Schnadig VJ, Quinn FB, et al. Interobserver variability in the interpretation of fine-needle aspiration biopsy of head and neck masses. *Arch Otolalryngol Head Neck Surg.* 1989;115:1438–1442.

13. Greene FL, Page DL, Fleming ID, et al, eds. *AJCC Cancer Staging Manual.* 6th ed. New York, NY: Springer; 2002.

14. Sheahan P, O'Leary G, Lee G, Fitzgibbon J. Cystic cervical metastases: incidence and diagnosis using fine needle aspiration biopsy. *Otolaryngol Head Neck Surg.* 2002;127:294–298

15. Mahoney EJ, Spiegel JH. Evaluation and management of malignant cervical lymphadenoapthy with an unknown primary tumor. *Otolaryngol Clin North Am.* 2005;38:87–97.

16. Feinstein AR. Symptoms as an index of biological behaviour and prognosis in human cancer. *Nature.* 1966;209:214–245.

17. Hall SF, Rochon PA, Streiner DL, et al. Measuring comorbidity in patients with head and neck cancer. *Laryngoscope.* 2002;112:1988–1996.

18. Piccirillo JF. Inclusion of comorbidity is a staging system for head and neck cancer. *Oncology.* 1995;9:831–836.

19. Piccirillo JF. Importance of comorbidity in head and neck cancer. *Laryngoscope.* 2000;110:593–602.

20. Piccirillo JF, Spitznagel EL, Vermani N, et al. Comparison of comorbidity indicies for patients with head and neck cancer. *Med Care.* 2004;42:482–486.

21. Benninger MS, Shariff A, Blazoff K. Symptom directed endoscopy: long-term efficacy. *Arch Otolaryngol Head Neck Surg.* 2001;127:770–773.

22. Shaha A, Hoover E, Marti J, Krespi Y. Is routine triple endoscopy cost-effective in head and neck cancer? *Am J Surg.* 1988;155:750–753.

23. Wenig BM. General principles of head and neck pathology. In: Harrison LB, Sessions RB, Hong WK, eds. *Head and Neck Cancer: A Multidisciplinary Approach.* Philadelphia, Pa: Lippincott-Raven; 1999:253–349.

24. McQuone SJ, Esile DW, Lee DJ, Westra WH. Occult tonsillar carcinoma in the unknown primary. *Laryngoscope.* 1998;108:1605–1610.

25. Koch WM, Bhatti N, Williams MF, Eisele DW. Oncologic rationale for bilateral tonsillectomy in head and neck squamous cell carcinoma of unknown primary source. *Otolaryngol Head Neck Surg.* 2001;124:331–333.

26. Randall DA, Johnstone PAS, Ross RD, Martin PJ. Tonsillectomy in diagnosis of the unknown primary tumor of the head and neck. *Otolaryngol Head Neck Surg.* 2000;122:52–55.

27. Mendenhall WM, Mancuso AA, Amdur RJ, Stringer SP, Villaret DB, Cassisi NJ. Squamous cell carcinoma metastatic to the neck from an unknown head and neck primary site. *Am J Otolaryngol.* 2001;22:261–267.

28. Robbins KT, Cole R, Marvel J, Fields R, Wolf P. The violated neck: cervical node biopsy prior to definitive treatment. *Otolaryngol Head Neck Surg.* 1986;94:605–610.

29. McGuirt WF, McCabe BF. Significance of node biopsy before definitive treatment of cervical metastatic carcinoma. *Laryngoscope.* 1978;88:594–597.

30. Ellis ER, Mendenhall WM, Rao PV, et al. Incisional or excisional neck node biopsy before definitive radiotherapy, alone or followed by neck dissection. *Head Neck.* 1991;13:177–183.

31. Robbins, KT. Integrating radiological criteria into the classification of cervical lymph node disease. *Arch Otolaryngol Head Neck Surg.* 1999;125:385–387.

32. Johnson J. A surgeon looks at cervical lymph nodes. *Radiology.* 1990;175:607–610.

33. Mendenhall WM, Mancuso AA, Parsons JT, et al. Diagnostic evaluation of squamous cell carcinoma

metaststic to cervical lymph nodes from an unknown head and neck primary site. *Head Neck.* 1998;20:739-744.

34. Zimmer LA, Branstetter BF, Nayak JV, Johnson JT. Current use of 18F-fluorodeoxyglucose positron emission tomography and combined positron emission tomography and computed tomography in squamous cell carcinoma of the head and neck. *Laryngoscope.* 2005;115:2029-2034.

35. Fogarty GB, Peters LJ, Stewart J, Scott C, Rischin D, Hicks RJ. The usefulness of fluorine 18-labelled deoxyglucose positron emission tomography in the investigation of patients with cervical lymphadenopathy from an unknown primary tumor. *Head Neck.* 2003;25:138-145.

36. Miller FR, Hussey D, Beeram M, et al. Positron emission tomography in the management of unknown primary head and neck cancer. *Arch Otolaryngol Head Neck Surg.* 2005;131:626-629.

37. Rusthoven KE, Koshy M, Paulino AC. The role of fluorodeoxyglucose positron emission tomography in cervical lymph node metastases from an unknown primary tumor. *Cancer.* 2004;101: 2641-2649.

38. Rusthoven KE, Koshy M, Paulino AC. The role of PET-CT fusion in head and neck cancer. *Oncology.* 2005;19:241-246.

39. Gutzeit A, Antoch G, Kuhl H, et al. Unknown primary tumors: detection with dual-modality PET/CT-initial experience. *Cancer.* 2004;101(11): 2641-2649.

40. Greene FI, Page DI, Flemming ID, et al. *AJCC Cancer Staging Manual.* 6th ed. New York, NY: Springer Science and Business Media Inc; 2002.

41. Batsakis JG. The pathology of head and neck tumors: the occult primary and metastases to the head and neck, part 10. *Head Neck Surg.* 1981; 409-423.

42. Hunt JL, Tomaszewiski JE, Montone KT. Prostatic adenocarcinoma metastatic to the head and neck and the workup of an unknown epithelioid neoplasm. *Head Neck.* 2004;26:171-178.

43. Akst LM, Discolo C, Dipasquale B, Greene D, Roberts J. Metastatic seminoma with cervical adenopathy as initial presentation. *Ear Nose Throat J.* 2004;83:356-359.

44. Chen SC, Chen MF, Hwang TL, et al. Prediction of supraclavicular lymph node metastasis in breast cancer. *Int J Radiat Oncol Biol Phys.* 2002;52: 614-619.

45. Pergolizzi S, Settineri N, Santacaterina A, et al. Ipsilateral supraclavicular lymph node metastases from breast cancer as only site of disseminated disease. *Ann Oncol.* 2001;12:1091-1095.

46. Bernier J, Domenge C, Ozahin M, et al. Postoperative irradiation with or without concomitant chemotherapy for locally advanced head and neck cancer. *N Engl J Med.* 2004;350:1945-1952.

47. Cooper JS, Pajak TF, Forastiere AA, et al. Postoperative concurrent radiotherapy and chemotherapy for high-risk squamous cell carcinoma of the head and neck. *New Engl J Med.* 2004;350: 1937-1944.

48. Viadya AM, Petruzzelli GJ, Clark J, Emami B. Patterns of spread in recurrent head and neck squamous cell carcinoma. *Otolaryngol Head Neck Surg.* 2001;125:393-396.

49. Coster JR, Foote RL, Olsen KD, et al. Cervical lymph node meastasis of unknown origin: indications for withholding radiation therapy. *Int J Radiat Oncology Biol Phys.* 1992;23:743-749.

50. Grau C, Johansen LV, Jakobsen J, et al. Cervical lymph node metastasies from unknownj primary tumours. Results from a national survey of the Danish Society for Head and Neck Surgery. *Radiother Oncol.* 2000;55:121-129.

51. Glynne-Jone RGT, Anand A, Young TE, Berry RJ. Cervical metastatic squamous cell carcinoma of unknown or occult primary source. *Head Neck.* 1990;12:440-443.

52. Inganej S, Kagan R, Anderson P, et al. Metastatic squamous cell carcinoma of the neck from an unknown primary: management options and patterns of relapse. *Head Neck.* 2002;236-246.

53. Harper CS, Mendenhall WM, Parsons JT, et al. Cancer in neck nodes with unknown primary site: role of mucosal radiotherapy. *Head Neck.* 1990;12: 436-439.

54. Mega-Marcial VA, Cardenes H, Perez CA, et al. Cervical metastases from unknown primaries: radiotherapeutic management and appearance of subsequent primaries. *Int J Radiat Oncol Biol Phys.* 1990;19:919-928.

55. Nieder C, Gregoire V, Ang KK. Cervical lymph node metastases from occult squamous cell carcinoma: cut down a tree to get an apple? *Int J Radiat Oncol Biol Phys.* 2001;50:727-733.

56. Weir L, Keanne T, Cummings B, et al. Radiation treatment of cervical node metastases from an unknown primary: an analysis of outcomes by treatment volume and other prognostic factors. *Radiother Oncol.* 1995;35:206-211.

57. Reddyt SP, Marks JE. Metastatic carcinoma in the cervical nodes from an unknown primary site:

results of bilateral neck plus mucosal irradiation vs. ipsilateral neck irradiation. *Int J Radiat Oncol Biol Phys*. 1997;37:797–802.

58. Busaba NY, Fabian LR. Extent of lymphadenectomy achieved by various modifications of neck dissection: a pathologic analysis. *Laryngoscope*. 1999;109:212–215.

59. Colletier PJ, Garden AS, Morrison WH, et al. Postoperative radiation for squamous celll carcinoma metastatic to cervical lymph nodes from an unknown primary site: outcomes and patterns of failure. *Head Neck*. 1998;20:674–681.

60. Strojan P, Anicin A. Combined surgery and postoperative radiotherapy for cervical lymph node metastases from an unknown primary tumor. *Radiother Oncol*. 1998;49:33–40.

61. Medini E, Medini AM, Lee CKK, et al. The management of metastatic squamous cell carcinoma in cervical lymph nodes from an unknown primary. *Am J Clin Oncol*. 1998; 21:121–125.

62. Nguyen C, Shenouda G, Black MJ, et al. Metastatic squamous cell carcinoma to cervical lymph nodes from unknown primary mucosal sites. *Head Neck*. 1994;16:58–63.

63. Davidson BJ, Spiro RH, Patel S, et al. Cervical metastases of occult origin: the impact of combined modality therapy. *Am J Surg*. 1994;168: 395–399.

64. Maulard C, Housset M, Brunel P, et al. Postoperative radiation therapy for cervical lymph node metastases from an occult squamous cell carcinoma. *Laryngoscope*. 1992;102:884–890.

65. Rodriguez J, Bataini JP, Jaulerry C, et al. Treatment of metastatic neck nodes secondary to an occult epidermoid carcinoma of the head and neck. *Laryngoscope*. 1987;97:1080–1084.

66. Lefebvre JL, Coche-Dequeant B, Ton Van J, Buisset E, Adenis A. Cervical lymph nodes from an unknown primary tumor in 190 patients. *Am J Surg*. 1990;160:443–446.

67. Boysen M, Lovdal O, Natvig K, Tausjo J, Jacobsen AB, Evensen JF. Combined radiotherapy and surgery in the treatment of neck node metastases from squamous cell carcinoma of the head and neck. *Acta Oncologica*. 1992;31:455–460.

68. Berneir J, Cooper JS. Chemo-radiation after surgery for high-risk head and neck cancer patients: how strong is the evidence? *Oncologist*. 2005;10: 215–224.

69. Ang KK, Harris J, Garden A, et al. Concomitant boost radiation plus concurrent cisplatin for advanced head and neck carcinoma: Radiation Therapy Oncology Group phase II trial 99-14. *J Clin Oncol*. 2005;23:3008–3013.

70. Moore MG, Bhattacharyya N. Effectiveness of chemotherapy and radiotherapy in sterilizing cervical nodal disease in squamous cell carcinoma of the head and neck. *Laryngoscope*. 2005;115: 570–573.

71. Pignon JP, Bourhis J, Domenge C, et al. Chemotherapy added to locoregional treatment for head and neck squamous-cell carcinoma: three meta-analyses of updated individual data. *Lancet*. 2000;355:949–955.

72. deBraud F, al-Sarraf M. Diagnosis and management of squamous cell carcinoma of unknown primary tumor site of the neck. *Semin Oncol*. 1993;20: 273–278.

73. de Braud F, Heilbrun LK, Ahmed K. Metastatic squamous cell carcinoma of unknown primary localized to the neck. Advantages of an aggressive treatment. *Cancer*. 1989 64: 510–515.

74. Argiris A, Haraf DJ, Kies MS, Vokes EE. Intensive concurrent chemoradiotherapy for head and neck cancer with 5-fluorouracil- and hydroxyurea-based regimens: reversing patterns of failure. *Oncologist*. 2003;8:350–360.

75. Argiris A, Smith SM, Stenson K, et al. Concurrent chemoradiotherpay for N2 or N3 squamous cell carcinoma of the head and neck from an occult primary. *Ann Oncol*. 2003;14:1306–1311.

76. Devaney KO, Rinaldo A, Ferlito A, et al. Squamous carcinoma arising in a branchial cleft cyst: Have you ever treated one? Will you? *J Laryngol Otol*. 2008;122:547–550.

77. Barrie JR, Knapper WH, Strong EW. Cervical nodal metastases of unknown origin. *Am J Surg*. 1970;120:466–470.

78. Briggs, RD, Pou AM, Schnadig J. Cystic metastasis versus branchial cleft carcinoma: a diagnostic challenge. *Laryngoscope*. 2002;112:1010–1014.

79. Mallet Y, Lallemant B, Robin YM, Lefebvre JL. Cystic lymph node metastases of head and neck squamous cell carcinoma: pitfalls and controversies. *Oral Oncol*. 2005;41:429–434.

80. Martin H, Morfit HM, Ehrlich H. The case of malignant branchiogenic carcinoma (malignant branchioma). *Ann Surg*. 1950;132:867–887.

81. Singh B, Bawally, Sundaran K, Har-El G, Krgin Bl. Branchial cleft cyst carcinoma: myth or reality? *Ann Otol Rhinol Laryngol*. 1998;107:519–524.

82. Sheahan P, O'Lery G, Lee G, Fitzgibbon J. Cystic cervical metastases: incidence and diagnosis using fine needle aspiration biopsy. *Otolaryngol Head Neck Surg*. 2002;127:294–298.

83. Thompson LD, Heffner DK. The clinical importance of cystic squamous cell carcinomas in the neck. *Cancer.* 1998;82:944-956.

84. Ferris RL, Branstetter BF, Nayak JV. Diagnostic utility of positron emission tomography-computed tomography for predicting malignancy in cystic neck masses in adults. *Laryngoscope.* 2005;115: 1979-1982.

85. Winegar LK, Griffin W. The occult primary tumor. *Arch Otolaryngol Head Neck Surg.* 1973;98: 159-163.

86. Wang RC, Goepfert H, Barber AE, Wolf P. Unknown primary squamous cell carcinoma metastatic to the neck. *Arch Otolaryngol Head Neck Surg.* 1990;116:1388-1393.

87. Chang AE, Karnell LH, Menck HR. The National Cancer Data Base report on cutaneous and noncutaneous melanoma. *Cancer.* 1998;83:1664-1678.

88. Nasri S, Namazie A, Dulguerov P, Mickel R. Malignant melanoma of cervical and parotid lymph nodes with an unknown primary site. *Laryngoscope.* 1994;104:1194-1198.

89. Balm AJ, Kroon BB, Hilgers FJ, et al. Lymph node metastases in the neck and parotid gland from an unknown primary melanoma. *Clin Otolaryngol Allied Sci.* 1994;19:161-165.

90. http://www.nccn.org/professionals/physician_gls/PDF/melanoma.pdf

91. Moertel CG, Reitemeier RJ, Schutt AJ, Hahn RG. Treatment of the patient with adenocarcinoma of unknown origin. *Cancer.* 1972;30:1469-1472.

92. Templer J, Perry MC, Davis WE. Metastatic cervical adenocarcinoma from unknown primary tumor. *Arch Otolaryngol.* 1981;107:45-47.

93. Zuur CL, van Velthuysen ML, Schornagel JH, et al. Diagnosis and treatment of isolated neck metastases of adenocarcinomas. *Eur J Surg Oncol.* 2002; 28:147-152.

94. Giridharan W, Hughes J, Fenton JE, Jones AS. Lymph node metastases in the lower neck. *Clin Otolaryngol Allied Sci.* 2003;28:221-226.

21

Salivary Gland

Kevin S. Emerick
Daniel G. Deschler

INTRODUCTION

Salivary gland malignancies are a heterogeneous group of tumors. They are varied in their histological composition, clinical presentation, and natural history. Because of this variability it is important for clinicians to be aware of the different histologic subtypes of salivary gland malignancies and the impact of histology on treatment. Treatment varies from wide local excision to aggressive surgical resection including neck dissection and adjuvant (chemo) radiation therapy. As diagnostic tools such as imaging techniques and fine needle aspiration evolve in the workup of salivary gland malignancies, the clinician must determine the appropriate role for each of these modalities in their assessment of patients with salivary gland neoplasm. This chapter outlines the appropriate workup of a salivary gland malignancy and reviews the different histologic subtypes and their appropriate treatments based on the evidence to date.

DEFINITIONS OF UNIQUE TERMS

The discussion of salivary gland malignancy often involves the terms major salivary gland and minor salivary gland. These distinctions become important when considering the specific histologic diagnosis and prognosis for an individual patient. Major salivary glands refer to the parotid, submandibular, and sublingual glands, whereas minor refers to nests of salivary tissue which can be found throughout the upper aerodigestive tract from the lip to the larynx. They also have a different histologic composition, varying from predominantly serous acini in the parotid gland to predominantly mucinous in the sublingual and minor salivary glands.

Parotid gland tumors and surgery often refer to either the deep or superficial lobe of the parotid gland. It is important to recognize that "lobe" in this case does not refer to an anatomically independent region, but rather to whether one is discussing the parotid tissue deep or superficial to the plane of the facial nerve.

The embryology and ultrastructure of the salivary gland provide a framework for understanding how and where these tumors develop. Major salivary glands are ectodermal in origin. They begin as solid ingrowths and develop into tubules that become the ductal system. Into these ducts drain serous and mucinous cells that are arranged into clusters called acini. The ducts are arranged in a series beginning with the acini which drain into an intercalated duct which drains into a striated duct and ultimately into the excretory duct.[1] This is outlined in Figure 21–1.

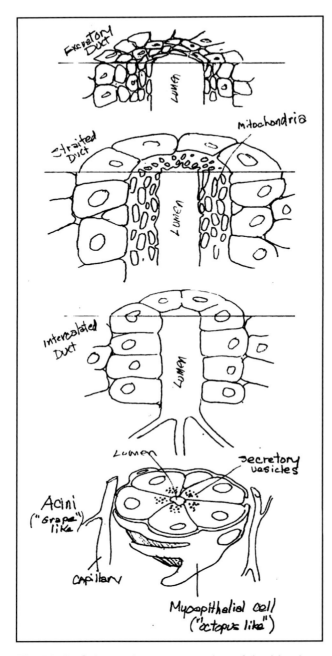

Fig 21–1. Schematic representation of the histology of the normal salivary gland.

EPIDEMIOLOGY, PREVALENCE

Salivary gland malignancies are not common. They account for only 1 to 6% of head and neck cancer and 0.3% of all cancer. The relatively small number of patients with salivary gland malignancy has made it difficult to thoroughly describe the epidemiology and prevalence of these malignancies. Data from SEER show a mean incidence of 0.89 per 100,000 per year,[2] and several smaller series have found similar incidence.[3,4] Salivary glands malignancies typically present in the sixth decade of life. One large population based study demonstrated that more aggressive tumors tend to present at an older age, usually in the seventh decade.[3] According to the SEER data there is a male predominance for malignant tumors. However, a recent analysis of over 2000 patients in Europe found an equal incidence among males and females. SEER data also show a greater incidence in whites, 1.4 times that of black patients.[2,3]

Among salivary gland malignancies most, 50% to 60%, occur in the parotid gland. Thirty percent arise in the submandibular gland and the remaining 10% to 15% arise in the sublingual and minor salivary glands. These overall numbers are important to consider when assessing a neoplasm in each of these different sites. The parotid gland is the most common site for salivary gland malignancy as well as benign tumors. Benign neoplasm predominate in the parotid gland with only 15% of parotid tumors classified as malignant. Submandibular malignancies are present in approximately 50% of submandibular neoplasm. Neoplasm of the sublingual gland and minor salivary glands are infrequent, but when they occur, 70% to 80% are malignant.[5-7]

ANATOMIC BOUNDARIES AND SUBDIVISIONS

The parotid glands are paired structures found in the preauricular region. They are primarily composed of serous acini. The parotid gland is surrounded by a fascial layer which is contiguous with the superficial layer of the deep cervical fascia. This fascia invests the sternocleidomastoid and trapezius muscles and then splits to surround the parotid gland forming a tough connective tissue capsule. The posterior aspect of the gland lies posterior to the ramus of the mandible and abuts the tragal cartilage of the auricle. Posteroinferiorly, it overlies the anterior aspect of the sternocleidomastoid muscle. Anteriorly, the gland overlies the posterior aspect of the masseter muscle. Superiorly, it approaches the zygomatic arch. The medial, deep border of the gland is defined by the lateral pharyngeal space, styloid muscles, stylomandibular ligament, and the carotid sheath.[8]

The parotid gland is unilobular with three to five processes, but without a true superficial or deep lobe. However, for surgical purposes, the gland is frequently considered as having a superficial compartment, which involves the parotid tissue lateral to the facial nerve and a deep compartment, which extends medial to the facial nerve. In addition to parotid tissue, the superficial compartment contains the great auricular nerve and auriculotemporal nerve. Several veins run within the gland between the superficial and deep compartments including the superficial temporal vein, internal maxillary vein, posterior facial vein (or retromandibular vein), and external jugular vein. These veins can be helpful to identify the general plane of the facial nerve radiographically and intraoperatively. Within the deep compartment, the external carotid artery, internal carotid artery, and superficial temporal artery can be found.[8]

Lymph nodes are intimately associated with the region of the parotid gland. Because of its embryologic development, the parotid gland is unique in that lymph nodes are located intraparenchymally, as well as in the periparotid region. The majority of these intraparenchymal lymph nodes rest in the superficial lobe and become an important consideration as they may harbor metastases from not only salivary gland tumors, but also other locations such as the skin, scalp, auricle, and orbit which have lymphatic drainage to the parotid region.

Stenson's duct can be found in the superficial compartment at the anterior border of the gland. It is 4 to 7 cm long and traverses superficial to the masseter muscle about halfway between the zygomatic arch and the corner of the mouth. At the anterior border of the masseter it turns medially and pierces the buccinator muscle to enter the oral cavity.[8]

The critical anatomic structure to consider during parotid surgery is the facial nerve. The safest approach to the facial nerve is to identify the main trunk. Three landmarks are routinely identified to direct safe surgical dissection to the main trunk. The first is the posterior belly of the digastric muscle, which helps provide the depth of the nerve. Its insertion into the digastric groove of the temporal bone is at the level where the nerve exits the stylomastoid foramen. The tragal pointer refers to the medial end of the tragal cartilage in the tympanomastoid notch. The nerve is located one centimeter medial and slightly anteroinferior to the pointer. The most consistent landmark is the tympanomastoid suture. It can be readily palpated, but it is not routinely visualized because of overlying soft tissue. The nerve is located 1 to 4 mm medial to the inferior end of the suture line. A study comparing the proximity and consistency of the tympanomastoid suture line and the posterior belly of the digastric, found the former to be the closest and most consistent landmark. On average, the nerve could be found within 2 mm of the tympanomastoid suture line in live patients, whereas the mean distance from the posterior belly of the digastric to the facial nerve trunk was 10.7 mm.[9]

If tumor or previous surgery obscures these landmarks or makes it unsafe to approach the main trunk in this fashion, a distal branch can be identified and dissected proximally. This can be most safely done with the marginal mandibular nerve which can be identified posterior and superficial to the facial vein within approximately 1 cm of the angle of the mandible. The buccal branch also can be identified coursing parallel to Stenson's duct.[8] Similarly the main trunk of the facial nerve can be identified it its course through the temporal bone and traced toward the stylomastoid foramen.

The submandibular gland is invested by the same superficial layer of the deep cervical fascia which encompasses the parotid gland. The anterior aspect of the gland is at the anterior belly of the digastric muscle. Inferiorly and posteriorly, the stylohyoid and posterior belly of digastric muscle border the gland. The inferior portion of the gland is covered on its lateral surface by investing fascia, platysma, and skin. Within this tissue, the anterior facial vein, the marginal mandibular, and cervical branches of the facial nerve course. The nerves lie superficial to the vein. Superiorly, the gland is covered laterally by the mandible. The gland is bordered medially by the floor of mouth mucosa and mylohyoid muscle.

Several important structures course along the medial aspect of the gland, including the hypoglossal nerve, lingual nerve, submandibular ganglion, and submandibular duct.

To prevent injury to these nerves they should be routinely identified during dissection of the gland. The hypoglossal nerve enters from a course inferior to the posterior belly of the digastric muscle and courses along the medial aspect of the gland and then medial to the mylohyoid muscle. The nerve can be identified with anterior and superior retraction of the mylohyoid muscle. The lingual nerve has a course along the superior medial aspect of the gland. In distinction to the parotid anatomy, lymph nodes do not have an intraparenchymal position in the submandibular gland. They are closely associated with the submandibular gland but not within the gland itself.[10] The sublingual glands are paired structures located in the anterior floor of the mouth. Each gland is bordered laterally by the mandible and medially by the styloglossus and hyoglossus muscles. The genioglossus near its attachment to the mandible defines the anterior extent. The deep or inferior surface of the gland abuts the mylohyoid muscle. Superficially the gland is covered by mucosa. The gland has 12 or more sublingual (Rivinius) ducts which open individually into the oral cavity or sometimes join to a common duct of Bartholin.

The minor salivary glands are distributed throughout the oral cavity, oropharynx, hypopharynx, and larynx. Typically they are organized in small clusters in a submucosal location.

CRITICAL ELEMENTS OF THE HISTORY AND PHYSICAL

Because of the varied locations for salivary glands, the history and physical examination appropriate for each site also can be quite varied. The major salivary glands are relatively superficial in their location and therefore masses often are recognized on self-palpation by the patient. As with any neck mass it is important to ascertain the key elements of the mass: size, nature of the progression, firmness, associated pain, overlying skin changes, and previous presence

of masses. Because of the critical location of the cranial nerves with respect to the major salivary glands it is important to ask patients about symptoms associated with the cranial nerves. The examiner should inquire and assess for facial twitching or facial asymmetry, dysarthria, limited tongue mobility, dysphagia, facial dysesthesia or hypoesthesia, and changes in the sensation of the tongue and floor of mouth. Cranial nerves II through XII should be fully assessed on examination in all patients with a suspected salivary gland neoplasm. The history should also ascertain information about potential systemic manifestations such as unintentional weight loss, fatigue, pulmonary symptoms, bone pain, and focal neurologic deficits.

Although the most common presentation is an asymptomatic mass, other signs and symptoms will help suggest a malignancy. Up to one-third of malignancies have pain associated with the mass. Twenty percent have some cranial nerve symptoms and 10% have overlying skin involvement.[5] See Table 21–1.

APPROPRIATE DIAGNOSTIC OFFICE-BASED PROCEDURES

Certain elements of the history and physical can be helpful in identifying which masses are benign or malignant, but ultimately a tissue diagnosis is needed. Second, even when the history and physical exam suggest a malignancy, the specific histology can impact a treatment plan. Lesions suspicious for minor salivary gland tumors in the oral cavity or oropharynx often can be biopsied in a traditional fashion in the office using injectable anesthetic and biopsy for-

Table 21–1. Symptoms Associated with Malignancy

Symptom	Percent of Patients with Malignancy
Asymptomatic mass	65%
Painful mass	30%
Cranial nerve deficit	21%
Overlying skin involvement	11%

ceps or dermal punches. With regard to parotid and submandibular lesions, fine needle aspiration has been widely reported in the recent literature. This appears to be a safe and cost-effective diagnostic tool. It also appears to be quite feasible as a nondiagnostic or nonsatisfactory result occurs in only 2% to 12% of specimens.[12-14] Figure 21–2 demonstrates a representative example of benign and malignant cytology from FNA.

When the specimen is diagnostic, several studies have shown a consistent sensitivity, specificity and accuracy. In a large study from the Netherlands, Postema summarized the results from several large series.[12] All of the series had at least 151 patients. The mean sensitivity was 81%, specificity 95%, accuracy 91%, and positive predictive value 86%. In addition Postema's series demonstrated their ability to further identify malignant histologic subtypes. They correctly identified 99% of the adenomas (pleomorphic and monoadenomas) in the study as well as 90% of Warthin's tumors. For malignant tumors, they were also very successful with a positive predictive value of 95%. Exact type-specific concordance with the histology was 81%. Importantly, FNA also correctly diagnosed 6 cases of lymphoma and 15 cases of metastasis in their series.

It is apparent from several studies that the presence of a cytopathologist can decrease the number of nondiagnostic specimens, by providing immediate feedback while the patient is still present. In addition, cystic lesions appear to be more difficult to accurately assess. Benign cysts on FNA can turn out to be Warthin's tumor, acinic cell carcinoma, or mucoepidermoid carcinoma on surgical pathology. Several other pitfalls should be mentioned. In a report from the College of American Pathologists, they identified the most common false positive result for pleomorphic adenoma was adenoid cystic carcinoma and the most common false positive result for Warthin's tumors was lymphoma.[15] They reported the overall false positive rates were highest for monomorphic adenoma (53%), intraparotid lymph node (31%), oncocytoma (18%), and granulomatous lesion (10%). Accurate FNA results will depend on quality achieved at three levels: acquisition of appropriate specimen material, proper fixation of that material, and skilled cytopathologic interpretation.

Concerns about tumor seeding with FNA have largely been alleviated by the growing experience of FNA using higher gauge needles than those used in core needle biopsies. There are reported complications with FNA which include hemorrhage, facial

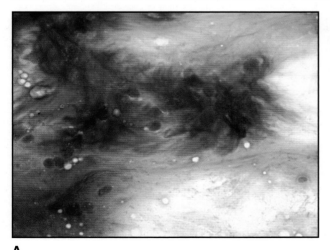

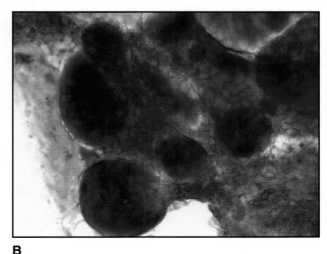

A   B

Fig 21–2. **A.** FNA of pleomorphic adenoma. Cytologically bland myoepithelial cells are embedded within a metachromatic fibrillar matrix. (Diff-Quik, 600×) **B.** FNA of adenoid cystic carcinoma. Cellular aspirate of basaloid cells surrounding acellular spheres of metachromatic matrix material. (Diff-Quik, 600×)

nerve injury, cellulites, and parotitis, but all are considered rare.[16] Ultimately, the decision to proceed with a fine needle aspiration of a parotid mass depends on two factors: Is the result dependable? Will the information obtained from the FNA affect management decisions? The answer to the first point will depend on the practitioner's experience with FNA in their specific clinical setting. In certain academic centers, literature and experience prove FNA to be highly accurate and dependable, whereas in other practice settings such dependability cannot be achieved and the information from the test can be misleading and have the potential to adversely affect care. Accurate results from FNA of parotid tumors can allow for appropriate preparation and operative intervention. This could range from a limited biopsy in the setting of a lymphoma to limited parotidectomy in the setting of a small pleomorphic adenoma to potential radical parotidectomy with neck dissection and appropriate facial nerve reconstruction. Such knowledge allows for appropriate preoperative consultation of the patient and possible coordination with other services such as reconstructive or otologic surgery.

Another office-based technique that has received attention is ultrasound. It has two potential roles. The first is to provide guidance for the FNA. Salivary gland masses can sometimes be difficult to fully define by palpation because of neighboring normal gland and structures and ultrasound can help ensure the FNA is from the desired tissue. Ultrasound also has a potential diagnostic radiographic role. However, as discussed in the next section, ultrasound is not the desired radiographic study of choice.

RECOMMENDED IMAGING STUDIES

Imaging studies can be very useful for salivary gland malignancies in all sites. Computed tomography is most familiar to head and neck surgeons because it is the first-line imaging study for malignancies of the upper aerodigestive tract. For minor salivary gland tumors or sublingual gland lesions this is still an excellent first mode of imaging. However, in recent years MRI has become the modality of choice. CT is typically able to accurately define the presence and extent of tumors; however, MRI may offer more diagnostic information.[17] Figure 21–3 shows a typical well circumscribed benign parotid tumor on CT whereas Figures 21–4 and 21–5 demonstrate MRI images of benign and malignant tumors.

Several recent publications have outlined potentially diagnostic features on MR imaging which could be used in the preoperative assessment of these patients. Malignant lesions are hypointense on T2 imaging which is helpful in distinguishing between benign tumors (see Fig 21–4). High-grade malignant tumors usually have an irregular border and infiltrate Stenson's duct or surrounding structures. Low-grade malignancies are usually well circumscribed but they are not encapsulated.[18,19] Additional findings can be indicative of specific histologic subtypes. Mucoepidermoid tumors may demonstrate a significant cystic component which has high intensity on both T1 and T2 imaging due to the mucin content.[19] Adenoid cystic tumors that are predominantly solid

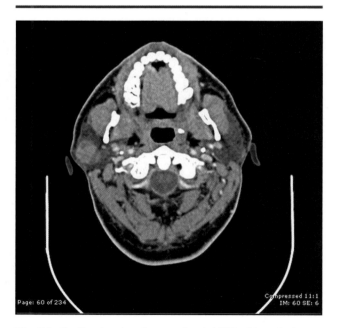

Fig 21–3. Contrast-enhanced axial CT with soft tissue windows revealing well-circumscribed pleomorphic adenoma of the right parotid gland.

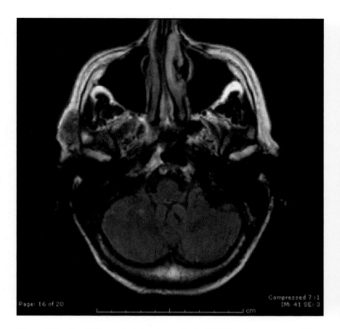

Fig 21–4. T2-weighted axial MRI demonstrating hypointense malignant mass with irregular borders in superior right parotid gland.

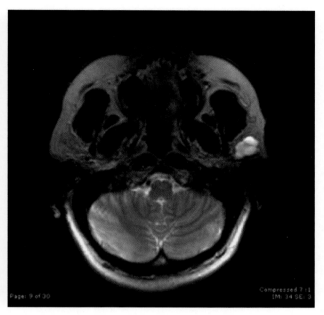

Fig 21–5. T2-weighted axial MRI demonstrating hyperintense, well-circumscribed, and bosselated pleomorphic adenoma of the left parotid gland.

type histology have low signal intensity on T2 imaging whereas cribriform and tubular types have a higher intensity on T2 because of their lack of cellularity.[19] Primary salivary lymphoma can be distinguished when it arises in a periparotid lymph node. There is typically a distinct plane separating the mass from the gland. This is more difficult to assess when the node is intraparotid; however, it is usually low signal intensity on both T1 and T2 imaging with limited enhancement with contrast.[18,19]

As benign tumors represent the majority of salivary gland tumors there are several important features to point out in benign lesions. Pleomorphic adenomas characteristically have a bright intensity on T2-weighted images with inhomogeneity and a well-defined capsule and margin. They also have a typical lobulated or bosselated contour which occurs from the variable growth rate within the tumor (see Fig 21–5). The only other tumors which could also have high signal intensity on T2 are vascular lesions such as hemangiopericytoma and hemangioma. See Table 21–2.

Table 21–2. MRI Characteristics of Malignant and Benign Salivary Gland Neoplasms

Malignant Characteristics	Benign Characteristics
Hypointense on T2	Hyperintense on T2
Indistinct borders	Lobulated or bosselated (pleomorphic adenoma)
Infiltrate surrounding tissue or Stenson's duct	
Not encapsulated	

STAGING

Table 21–3 summarizes the American Joint Committee on Cancer sixth edition staging for salivary gland malignancies.[20] Although much of the literature and discussion about treatment and prognosis of salivary gland malignancies focuses on histologic grading, TNM staging remains an important and useful tool.

Table 21–3. Salivary Gland Staging

Primary Tumor (T)

T1	Tumor 2 cm or less in greatest dimension, without extraparenchymal extension*
T2	Tumor more than 2 cm but less than 4 cm in greatest dimension, without extraparenchymal extension*
T3	Tumor more than 4 cm and/or extraparenchymal extension*
T4a	Tumor invades skin, mandible, ear canal, and/or facial nerve
T4b	Tumor invades skull base and/or pterygoid plates and/or encases carotid artery

Note: Extraparenchymal extension is clinical or macroscopic evidence of invasion of soft tissues. Microscopic evidence alone does not constitute extraparenchymal extension for classification purposes.

Regional Lymph Nodes (N)

N0	No regional lymph node metastasis
N1	Metastasis in a single ipsilateral lymph node, 3 cm or less in greatest dimension
N2a	Metastasis in a single ipsilateral lymph node, more than 3 cm but not more than 6 cm in greatest dimension
N2b	Metastasis in multiple ipsilateral lymph nodes, none more than 6 cm in greatest dimension
N2c	Metastasis in bilateral or contralateral lymph nodes, none more than 6 cm in greatest dimension
N3	Metastasis in a lymph node greater than 6 cm in greatest dimension

Distant Metastasis (M)

Mx	Distant metastasis cannot be assessed
M0	No distant metastasis
M1	Distant metastasis

Source: Used with permission of the American Joint Committee on Cancer (AJCC), Chicago, Illinois. The original source for this material is the AJCC Cancer Staging Manual, Sixth Edition (2002) published by Springer Science and Business Media LLC, www.springerlink.com

HISTOPATHOLOGY

The histologic composition of the salivary unit is outlined in Fig 21-1. Malignant salivary gland tumors arise from these cells in a predictable fashion. There are currently two theories on how salivary gland malignancies arise.[21] The multicellular theory suggests each type of neoplasm originates from a different cell type within the glandular unit, whereas the bicellular reserve cell theory suggests that all salivary neoplasm originate from either an excretory or intercalated duct cell which functions as a reserve cell with the ability to differentiate into different epithelial or epidermoid cells.[22-24]

Regardless of the exact mechanism of histogenesis, there are several histologic subtypes which are important to be aware of and understand. This understanding will help facilitate appropriate workup and treatment of these tumors.

Mucoepidermoid Carcinoma

Mucoepidermoid carcinoma (MEC) is the most common salivary gland malignancy overall. It comprises up to 15% of all salivary gland neoplasm and 29% of all salivary gland malignancies. Mucoepidermoid carcinoma is notably the most common malignant salivary gland tumor to arise in patients younger than 20 years of age. Greater than 80% of MEC occur in the parotid gland, 10% in the submandibular gland, and less than 5% in minor salivary glands.[25] It is clearly the most common parotid gland malignancy; however, there are series which support both MEC and adenoid cystic carcinoma as the most common submandibular and minor salivary gland malignancies. Among the minor salivary gland sites of MEC, the palate is the most common with rare occurrences on the retromolar trigone, floor of mouth, buccal mucosa, lip, and tongue.

Mucoepidermoid carcinomas are composed of three different cell types: mucin-secreting, epidermoid, and intermediate. Figure 21-6 shows an example of mucoepidermoid histology. Intermediate cells likely arise from pluripotent reserve cells in the salivary duct unit and then give rise to the mucous and epidermoid cells. It is important to distinguish that epidermoid cells are not squamous cells, but their similar appearance in high-grade tumors can make them difficult to distinguish. It is the variable composition of these cell types which creates the variable histologic appearance of these tumors.[26]

Stewart et al[27] were the first to coin the term "mucoepidermoid tumor" in 1945 and shortly thereafter Foote and Frazell established a two-tier grading system, one grade thought to be benign and the other malignant.[25] However, it became clear to the authors that, in fact, all of these tumors were malignant, but in varying degrees of low, intermediate, and high grades. Future data then demonstrated that grading was a key prognostic factor for these tumors. However, as several grading systems have been proposed it remains unclear exactly which grading system should be applied.

The two main grading systems were developed by Healey and modified by Batsakis[28] (Table 21-4) and the system developed by Goode et al at the AFIP[25] (Table 21-5). Each system grades tumors based on tumor architecture, pattern of invasion, cell type composition, histocytologic pleomorphism, and frequency of mitotic figures. Based on several studies using these grading systems it has become clear there is a significant difference in the clinical behavior of these tumors depending on their grade. Figure 21-6 demonstrates examples of both a low-grade and high-grade MEC.

However, stage is also important. Survival for stage I/II tumors is above 90%, whereas stage III/IV tumors have a 5-year survival in the 25% range.[29] Tumor site has been described as prognostic by some authors. Spiro found that the only low-grade

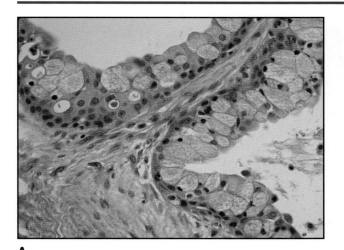

A

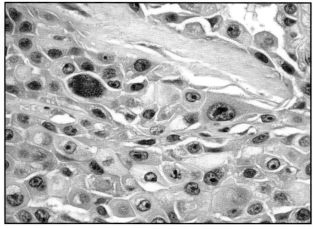

B

Fig 21–6. **A.** Low-grade mucoepidermoid carcinoma. Cystic neoplasm containing a proliferation of epidermoid, intermediate, and mucinous epithelial cells. (H&E, 400×) **B.** High-grade mucoepidermoid carcinoma. Markedly atypical malignant neoplasm composed of sheets of squamoid cells with rare mucin-containing epithelial cells. (H&E, 600×)

Table 21–4. Histocytologic Criteria for Grading Mucoepidermoid Carcinoma Based on Batsakis and Luna Modification of Healey System

---

Grade 1 (low-grade) Mucoepidermoid Carcinoma

- Macrocysts and microcysts with areas of transition from adjacent excretory ducts
- Proliferation of daughter cysts from larger cysts
- Equal proportion of differentiated mucous and epidermoid (squamoid) cells with minimal to moderate numbers of intermediate cells.
- Minimal to absent pleomorphism and rare mitoses
- Often circumscribed, broad-front infiltration of tissue
- Extravasated mucin pools with fibrosis and chronic inflammation with or without foreign body giant cells and cholesterol clefts

Grade 2 (intermediate-grade) Mucoepidermoid Carcinoma

- Solid nests of cells with few microcysts and no macrocysts
- Predominantly intermediate cells with or without epidermoid differentiation; sparse mucous cells
- Mild to moderate pleomorphism with identifiable mucleoli and occasional mitoses
- Well-defined, noncircumscript infiltration of tissue
- Fibrosis separating cell nests and groups
- Chronic inflammation at periphery (advancing front) of neoplasm

Grade 3 (high-grade) Mucoepidermoid Carcinoma

- Predominantly solid nests and/or microcystic glandular with no macrocysts
- Range of cellular composition from poorly differentiated to epidermoid and intermediate cells to ductal-type adenocarcinoma admixed with epidermoid and intermediate cells
- Rare mucin-positive cells
- Marked pleomorphism with prominent, easily identified nucleoli and frequent mitoses (may be atypical, bizarre mitotic figures)
- Definite invasion of soft tissue with or without perineural and vascular invasion
- Desmoplasia accompanying invasive cell clusters and groups
- Less prominent chronic inflammation

MEC which metastasized, recurred, or caused the death of the patient occurred in the submandibular gland; however, other studies have not found the same correlation.[29]

Low-grade MEC has the best prognosis ranging from a reported 92% to 100% 5-year survival. These patients are usually younger in their fifth decade and there appears to be strong female predominance, 6:1 as reported by Hicks.[28] These tumors uniformly present as stage I.[29] Surgical excision of these tumors with negative margins yields an excellent local control rate, nearing 100%.[25,28,29] These tumors rarely metastasize to regional lymph nodes or to distant sites.

High-grade MEC behave very differently then their low-grade counterparts. Survival is very poor in this group with most groups reporting on the order of 22 to 43% 5-year survival.[25-30] These tumors usually present in patients in the sixth decade of life and tend to have a male predominance. They present at a higher stage than low-grade tumors, usually stage III or IV. Up to 85% of these tumors have

Table 21–5. Histocytologic Criteria for Grading Mucoepidermoid Carcinoma Based on Armed Forces Institute of Pathology Grading System

Parameter	Point Value
Intracystic component	+2
Neural invasion present	+2
Necrosis present	+3
Mitosis (4 or more per high-power field)	+3
Anaplasia present	+4

Grade	Point Score
Low	0–4
Intermediate	5–6
High	7–14

regional metastasis. Not surprisingly, they have higher local and regional recurrences despite aggressive treatment. Failure rates have been reported from 33% locally and 55% distantly. Of patients with MEC who present or develop distant metastasis, they are nearly all high-grade. Because these tumors frequently have poorly differentiated epidermoid cells and rare mucin-positive cells they can be confused with other high-grade carcinomas such as squamous cell carcinoma, salivary ductal carcinoma, adenocarcinoma, and malignant mixed tumors.

They require a more aggressive treatment than low-grade MEC. In addition to wide local excision, selective neck dissection is also recommended for the N0 neck given the high incidence of occult metastasis. Postoperative radiation therapy to both the primary site and ipsilateral neck usually is administered even for early T-stage disease.

Intermediate-grade tumors are the least well described of the three grades. Their clinical features also appear intermediate. Patients present with smaller tumors than high-grade MEC, usually less than 3 cm. Neck metastasis is not uncommon, occurring in almost 20% of patients.[29] The local and regional/distant recurrence rates are 22% to 30% and 39%, respectively, which fall in between the incidence reported for high-grade and low-grade tumors. Similarly, survival is intermediate, generally reported in

the 70% range for these tumors.[28,29] There appears to be a population of intermediate grade MEC which does well, much like low-grade MEC, and a population which does quite poorly, behaving more like a high-grade MEC. Further studies into biochemical markers may help distinguish these tumors in the future. Presently, treatment is variable among institutions. However, many favor an approach based on stage. Small tumors with a benign clinical picture can be treated with wide local excision; however, increasing size, neck metastasis, and aggressive pathologic features should direct a more aggressive treatment course similar to a high-grade tumor.

Adenoid Cystic Carcinoma

Adenoid cystic carcinoma (ACC) was first recognized in 1854, but the term adenoid cystic carcinoma was not coined until 1953 by Foote and Frazell.[6] It is the second most common salivary gland malignancy, accounting for 10% of nonsquamous cell head and neck carcinomas.[6] It occurs most commonly in the minor salivary glands, particularly intraoral sites and specifically the hard palate, followed by the parotid gland, submandibular gland, extraoral minor salivary glands, and the sublingual glands. Although rare, it can present in sites such as the lacrimal gland, esophagus, and tracheobronchial tree. There does not seem to be a sex predilection and patients usually present in their fifth and sixth decades of life. Overall these tumors are characterized by slow local growth with rare spread to regional lymphatics. However, they are well known for their propensity for perineural invasion and distant metastasis.[31-33]

The grading of ACC is much less controversial than other salivary gland malignancies. It is characterized by three histologic subtypes: solid, tubular, and cribriform. The solid type demonstrates solid sheets and nests of atypical basaloid cells with an undifferentiated appearance and many mitoses.[34] Several large series have demonstrated that the solid-type histology imparts a worse prognosis with 5-year survival as low as 17% in some studies.[31-33] Tubular histology has the best survival. Its appearance is characterized by small tubules and well-defined ductal architecture and no mitoses. The cribriform pattern, seen in Figure 21–7, is considered the classic

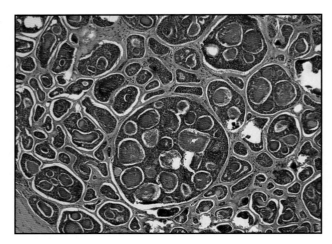

Fig 21–7. Adenoid cystic carcinoma. Classic cribriform pattern of basaloid cells surrounding myxoid matrix material. (H&E, 100×)

ACC and occurs in up to 64% of reported cases of ACC.[34] It has a "Swiss-cheese" appearance. It is considered an intermediate grade when comparing survival among all three of these subtypes. Appearance of a pure subtype is less common than a mixed pattern of two or more of the subtypes.

Overall survival varies widely from different series and subsites. Several studies have identified poor prognostic features for ACC. Clinical stage, solid histologic subtype, and increased p53 expression are independent significant prognostic factors in one large series.[31] Others have shown T stage, age >45, paresthesias, pain, perineural invasion and margin status to correlate with survival.[32] Unlike most head and neck malignancies the survival for ACC does not plateau at 5 years. This is attributable to late local recurrences, late development of distant metastasis, and the slow growth of distant metastasis when they do occur.

Adenoid cystic carcinoma is usually treated with surgical resection followed by radiation therapy. Because of the propensity for perineural spread, negative margins can be a challenge to obtain. Despite the overall high-grade nature of this tumor, elective neck dissection for the N0 patient is not recommended for these tumors because of the low incidence of lymphatic spread. Postoperative radiation is important for improving both local control and

overall survival.[31] Because of the slow growing nature of this tumor neutron beam therapy has been investigated.[35] However, its overall benefit has yet to be determined in the postoperative setting and it is only available in a few sites worldwide.

Adenocarcinoma

An adenocarcinoma is a tumor arising from a glandular unit. Previously, the term adenocarcinoma incorporated a very heterogeneous group of tumors. Today, there are several well-described classifications of adenocarcinomas which arise from different salivary subglandular units such as the different cells within the acini or different salivary ducts. These include tumors such as salivary duct carcinoma, polymorphous low-grade adenocarcinoma, and epithelial-myoepithelial carcinoma. Those tumors which do not fall into recently described classifications are still collectively referred to as adenocarcinoma, not otherwise specified.

As more tumors are classified the number of adenocarcinomas becomes much fewer and they now represent the least common salivary gland tumor. However, they are still a heterogeneous group with variable cytoarchitecture ranging from low grade to high grade in differentiation, solid or cystic, and papillary and nonpapillary features. They occur in older patients in their seventh decade of life, with a 4:1 male predominance, and predominantly in major salivary glands.[36] Poor prognostic features have previously been described and include: advanced stage, high histologic grade, infiltrative growth factor, and tumor DNA content.[37]

Unfortunately, most of these tumors are high grade with a propensity for cervical metastasis, 23%, and distant metastasis, 37%. They have an overall poor prognosis with survival 10 to 60%.[36,38] Treatment is correspondingly aggressive with wide local excision, elective neck dissection, and postoperative radiation therapy.

Acinic Cell

Acinic cell carcinomas (AC) account for 1 to 17% of all salivary malignancies. Because of this wide disparity, it is considered the third, fourth, or fifth most common salivary gland tumor. However, in children, it is second only to mucoepidermoid carcinoma in incidence. It is thought to arise from progenitor reserve cells of the terminal tubules and intercalated ducts of salivary tissue.[39] Batsakis went on to further describe the histomorphology of these tumors and create a grading scale. Low-grade tumors closely resemble normal salivary tissue whereas high-grade tumors are poorly differentiated and resemble the early stages of embryonic development of the acini. The prognostic importance of this grading remains unclear. As 90% of tumors are low grade it is difficult to accumulate enough data for a statistically significant comparison to high-grade tumors.[39]

A recent National Cancer Data Base review of 1,353 cases has helped characterized this tumor.[40] It arises at a younger age than most other salivary gland malignancies with a median age of 52 and has a female predilection. One study has also shown a large Caucasian predominance. It has been reported to occur in all salivary glands but is predominantly a tumor of the parotid gland, 86% of cases. This is likely attributable to the predominance of serous-type acini in the parotid compared to other salivary glands. It is notable for an incidence of bilateral tumors in up to 3% of cases, making it the second most common salivary neoplasm to occur bilaterally. Regional metastasis is not common. Studies report varying incidence from 0% to 17%, with most series reporting less than 10% and the National Cancer Data Base review identifying a 9.9% incidence.[40-42]

Acinic cell carcinoma is considered the least aggressive of all salivary gland malignancies. Five-year disease-free survival for AC is greater than 90%.[40] However, several factors do portend a poorer outcome including high-grade histology, regional or distant metastasis at presentation, primary tumor in the submandibular gland, and age greater than 30 years.[40] Those patients considered high-grade did have a significantly lower survival ranging from 30% to 40%. The overall recurrence rate from the Armed Forces Institute of Pathology series was 35%, yet within this group of recurrent disease only 16% died of this disease.[42] Other reports have also highlighted that prolonged survival is possible despite persistent disease. This has led many surgeons to consider palliative surgery for patients with incurable disease.

First-line treatment is surgical excision. Because the incidence of regional metastasis is less than 10%, routine elective neck dissection is not recommended. Adjunctive radiation therapy is reserved for high-grade tumors, recurrent tumors, positive margins, and stage III or IV tumors.[40-42]

Salivary Duct Carcinoma

Although salivary duct carcinoma was first described in the 1960s, it was not until the 1990s that pathologists began more frequently recognizing and reporting this distinct salivary gland malignancy. The tumor is best known histologically for its resemblance to ductal carcinoma of the breast, from which it is indistinct.[43] It has varying forms of cribriform, papillary, and solid growth patterns embedded in a sclerotic stroma. Comedonecrosis, perineural invasion, and periglandular infiltration are common.

It is an aggressive tumor characterized by rapid onset and progression frequently associated with pain and cranial nerve involvement. Patients typically present at an advanced stage with approximately half presenting with stage IV disease.[44,45] Some series report a male predominance. It occurs most commonly, 80% to 90%, in the parotid gland, but has been reported in all major salivary glands and in minor salivary glands. Neck metastasis is not uncommon occurring in 43% to 58% of patients at the time of diagnosis.[43,44] Increasing T stage correlates with increased risk of neck metastasis, but even T1 tumors have a 30% incidence of cervical metastasis. Cervical metastasis is also prognostic for distant metastasis, as 50% of patients with neck disease also had distant disease. Current treatment strategies provide good local regional control; unfortunately, distant metastasis are not uncommon and make overall survival poor for these patients, 40% by 2 years and 20% by 5 years.[44,45]

All salivary duct tumors are treated as aggressive high-grade tumors. Aggressive surgical excision with facial nerve sacrifice, if clinically involved, and routine neck dissection are the standard first modality of treatment even for early T-stage tumors. Radiation to the primary and ipsilateral neck is also considered standard. Because of the poor survival and high incidence of distant metastasis, chemotherapy also should be considered. However, there is limited data on its efficacy, but a trial using cisplatin and 5-fluorouracil is underway to investigate its use.[45]

Mixed Malignant Tumor and Carcinoma ex Pleomorphic Adenoma

The term mixed malignant tumor encompasses two types of tumors. The first is a true mixed malignant carcinoma in which the primary tumor consists of malignant epithelial component and a malignant mesenchymal component. The second type is best referred to as carcinoma ex pleomorphic adenoma, which is an epithelial malignancy that arises from a benign pleomorphic adenoma. The former is considered extremely rare and therefore the discussion focuses on the latter. However, one should be aware of the histologic distinction between these tumors, and not use the terms mixed malignant tumor and carcinoma ex pleomorphic interchangeably.

Carcinoma ex pleomorphic adenoma is an aggressive tumor with variable histology. Figure 21–8 shows an example of this histology. Typically, pleomorphic adenoma can still be identified within the

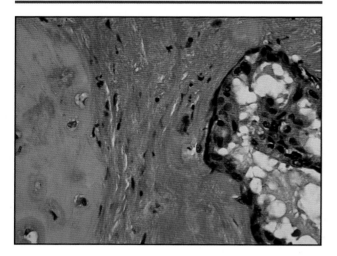

Fig 21–8. Carcinoma ex pleomorphic adenoma. High-grade malignant glandular cells (*right*) are present adjacent to an area of conventional pleomorphic adenoma (*left*) with chondromyxoid matrix and myoepithelial cells. (H&E, 400×)

mass, but typically the malignant component will compose greater than 50% of the mass. This malignant component is most commonly adenocarcinoma (40-44%), salivary duct carcinoma (25-33%), adenoid cystic (14%), or adenosquamous cell carcinoma (7%).[46,47]

The exact pathogenesis of these tumors remains unknown. However, Eneroth and Zetterberg studied the DNA content of mixed tumors and found that over time the cells increasing anaploidy suggests that as mixed tumors grow the may undergo transformation that could induce a carcinomatous component of the neoplasm.[48] This is supported by the clinical data which reports these tumors frequently arise in a long-standing mass and that up to 10% of recurrent pleomorphic adenomas have carcinoma ex pleomorphic.

Like other aggressive malignancies, rapid growth, pain, and cranial nerve involvement are not uncommon, although asymptomatic neck mass remains the most common presentation. Several of these clinical features have been shown to have a significant effect on survival including pain, skin ulceration, and cranial nerve deficit. There appears to be a subset which is particularly aggressive and progresses rapidly in the first year. These patients have approximately a 25% survival at one year.[46] Neck metastasis occurs in 20 to 30% of patients and distant spread eventually occurring in over 40% of patients.[46,47] As a group, survival is poor with 39% alive at 3 years and 30% at 5 years. Several pathologic features predict worse outcome including T stage, N stage, extent of carcinoma (>50% vs <50%) and extent of invasion.[46] Metastasis is a very poor prognostic factor. Spiro et al reported only 1 of 31 patients with neck metastasis alive at 10 years.[49]

Treatment of carcinoma ex pleomorphic begins with surgical resection of the primary tumor and all at-risk lymph nodes given the high rate of metastasis. For parotid malignancies this would entail a total parotidectomy in order to address all intraparotid lymph nodes as well as a neck dissection. Sacrifice of cranial nerves is reserved only for cases with clinical involvement. Radiation therapy is employed when the final histology is a high-grade subtype, positive margins or perineural invasion, invasion of surrounding extraparenchymal tissue, or lymph node metastasis. For histologic subtypes such salivary ductal carcinoma chemotherapy may have a role. The best treatment of these tumors is prevention. Appropriate, timely surgical excision of benign pleomorphic adenomas should eliminate a significant number of these tumors.

Polymorphous Low-Grade Adenocarcinoma

Unlike most of the other salivary gland malignancies, polymorphous low-grade adenocarcinoma is notable for its propensity to arise in minor salivary glands, specifically those in the oral cavity.[51] Within the oral cavity, the palate is the most common site, followed by the lip and buccal mucosa. Its name is both clinically and histologically descriptive. Histologically they are well circumscribed but not encapsulated. A mixture of growth patterns can be displayed within a single tumor including solid islands, glandular profiles, tubules, trabeculae, cribriform nests, and single file lines of infiltration. They have an infiltrative periphery and a characteristic perineural targetoid pattern of growth. Generally the histologic diagnosis is not difficult to make, but these tumors can overlap with pleomorphic adenoma and adenoid cystic carcinoma. Immunohistochemistry can be helpful with the histologic diagnosis. Glial fibrillary acidic protein, S-100, and SMA are nonspecific but can assist in the diagnosis.[51] Of note, there is discussion in the literature about the significance of the papillary component of these tumors and its prognostic importance.[52] Some studies suggest a significant component of papillary invasion may correlate with increased neck metastasis.

Clinically, these tumors have a slow growth and indolent biology. Typical presentation is that of an asymptomatic mass in the oral cavity that has often been present for years. Infrequently, patients will have pain, bleeding, or ulceration, but this does not portend a more aggressive tumor or worse outcome. These tumors do not commonly metastasize. In a series of 164 patients from the AFIP, there was no cervical or distant metastasis.[51] Other series have reported up to a 12% neck metastasis incidence and 6% distant metastasis.

The overall prognosis for these tumors is quite good, greater than 90%. Initial treatment is usually wide local excision. Because of their predilection for oral cavity sites, this may entail partial maxillectomy or mandibulectomy (Fig 21–9). With a low rate of neck metastasis, elective neck treatment is not indicated. Evans and Luna demonstrated these tumors can have a propensity for recurrence, most of which can be controlled with re-excision.[52] However, a small portion of these recurrent tumors lead to uncontrollable disease and death. Therefore, more aggressive treatment at the primary site and postoperative radiation should be considered for recurrences.

Primary Lymphoma

Primary lymphoma of the salivary glands is uncommon, comprising only 1.7 to 3.1% of salivary neoplasm. Nearly all of them occur in the parotid gland, but there are reports of their occurrence in all of the various salivary glands. Salivary gland sites represent only 10% of all head and neck lymphomas.[53] Greater than 85% are non-Hodgkin B-cell lymphomas, either nodular or diffuse. The remainder is nearly all Hodgkin disease. Parotid lymphomas can arise from intraglandular lymph nodes or can arise from the parenchyma itself. The latter is referred to as mucosa-associated lymphoid tissue and makes up the majority of cases. Salivary gland lymphoma is rare in patients under 50. Their presentation is quite similar to other salivary gland malignancies. Most have a progressively enlarging painless mass. Reports of cervical lymphadenopathy vary widely from 9% to 69%. There are clinical features, which may suggest a lymphoma diagnosis preoperatively. A previous history of underlying coexistent autoimmune disorder such as Sjögren's syndrome or rheumatoid arthritis has been reported in up to 44% of patients. A mass occurring in a patient with a previous diagnosis of benign lymphoepithelial lesion, multiple masses in a unilateral parotid gland or bilateral parotid masses, or a mass associated with multiple, enlarged unilateral or bilateral cervical lymph nodes should all raise the suspicion of lymphoma.[54] Figure 21–10 shows a representative example of a lymphoma of the parotid gland on MRI. The mass is isointense to the adenoidal tissue on T1-weighted imaging which may also help preoperative planning.

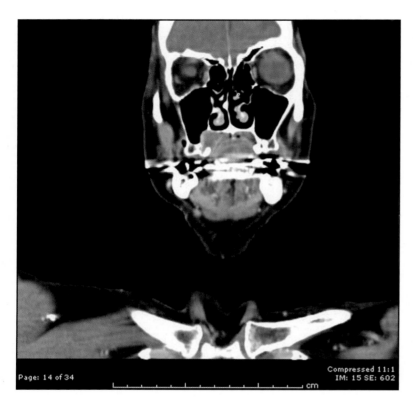

Fig 21–9. Contrast-enhanced coronal CT demonstrating asymptomatic low-grade polymorphous adenocarcinoma of the right hard palate.

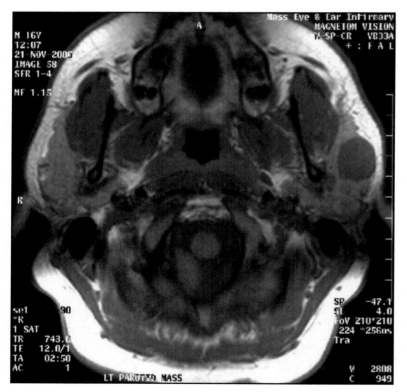

Fig 21–10. T1-weighted MRI in axial plane demonstrating a well-circumscribed mass of the left parotid gland which is isointense with the adenoidal lymphoid tissue and found to be a lymphoma upon removal.

Salivary gland lymphomas are staged according to traditional lymphoma staging systems and not the TNM staging applied to other salivary gland malignancies. Survival ranges from 52 to 83% at 5 years.[53,54] These masses should be approached with surgical excision. This will allow adequate tissue for flow cytometry and other diagnostic tests. Even in the setting of a known diagnosis of lymphoma elsewhere in the body, one should consider surgical excision, as not all parotid masses in this setting will be lymphoma. Depending on the stage of the tumor, radiotherapy and/or chemotherapy constitute the primary treatment.

IDENTIFICATION OF CRITICAL DECISION POINTS

The first key in management of salivary gland malignancies is recognizing when they are present. Although this is straightforward for a patient with a large mass in the preauricular region which is rapidly expanding and the facial nerve is weak, it is not always quite as clear. Asymptomatic parotid masses are typically benign; however, certain clinical features, radiographic findings, and FNA results can increase suspicion for a malignancy and impact a treatment plan. Tumors arising in the submandibular triangle, floor of the mouth, and sites of minor salivary glands have a relatively broad neoplastic differential diagnosis. For example, it is important to separate salivary gland malignancies from oral cavity and oropharynx squamous cell carcinomas. As discussed in previous sections the role of FNA and imaging is evolving; however, they each offer additional information to aid in the diagnosis of malignancy.

With the recognition of a malignancy, the next critical step is treatment planning, specifically, determining extent of local resection and need for neck dissection. In terms of local resection, particular focus is on resection of cranial nerves. Resection of the nerve is indicated when the nerve is involved clinically, as demonstrated by paresis, hypoesthesia, or dysesthesia, radiographically, or grossly at the time of resection when verified unequivocally on frozen section analysis. However, even high-grade tumors do not mandate nerve resection if there is not clinical, radiographic, or intraoperative pathologic evidence of malignant involvement. Nerve resection was standard many years ago for any malignancy; however, this is no longer the case.

Neck dissection is indicated for any cervical metastasis. The treatment of potential occult cervical metastasis with neck dissection, however, varies based on the tumor grade and histology. The details of this are discussed within each histology section. Table 21–6 gives general guidelines for when to consider a neck dissection. Table 21–7 provides additional data on incidence for cervical metastasis.

A consideration of surgery-related deficits and potential reconstructive options that may be re-

Table 21–6. Indications for Neck Dissection

Clinicopathologic Indications
Palpable nodal disease
Radiographic evidence of nodal disease
Any high-grade tumor (except adenoid cystic carcinoma)
Consideration for any T3 or T4
Consideration for tumors with aggressive features such as nerve invasion and extraparenchymal invasion

Table 21–7. Incidence of Neck Metastasis by Histology

Histologic Type	Lymph Node Involvement (%)
High-Grade Mucoepidermoid	70–80
Intermediate-Grade Mucoepidermoid	20
Low-Grade Mucoepidermoid	0
Adenoid Cystic	4
Adenocarcinoma	18–23
Acinic Cell Carcinoma	<10
Salivary Duct Carcinoma	48–53
Carcinoma Ex Pleomorphic Adenoma	20–30
Polymorphous Low-Grade Adenocarcinoma	<10

quired at the time of surgery is another important preoperative consideration. Such issues require introduction at the time of preoperative counseling. Although many attempt to preserve the great auricular nerve during standard parotidectomy, this often is not achievable or advisable in the setting of malignancy. The resultant sensory deficit should be discussed as should issues of trismus. Trismus is more common with more extensive resections requiring resection into the parapharyngeal space or involving the muscles of mastication. Contour deficits in these cases may also be more noticeable and require soft tissue reconstruction with a pedicled flap or free tissue transfer. Finally, for cases involving the facial nerve directly and necessitating resection, planning for potential otologic surgery, discussion of its potential sequelae and appropriate specialist availability is essential. Similarly, a discussion of facial nerve reconstructive options should be engaged preoperatively and appropriate reconstructive services aligned. Cervical nerve graft sites such as great auricular nerve or ansa cervicalis and noncervical nerve graft donor sites such as sural nerve and cutaneous nerve of the upper arm should be discussed.

ANALYSIS OF TREATMENT OPTIONS

For resectable tumors, surgery remains the primary treatment modality. The extent of surgery and need for neck dissection is determined by the stage, grade, and histology of the tumor. Details of surgical management are included in each histologic discussion.

Although salivary gland tumors are considered to be relatively radioresistant, radiation therapy still plays an important role in the treatment of salivary gland malignancies as an adjunctive treatment. There are no randomized studies to determine the exact benefit of postoperative radiation. However, several series have shown improved 5-year local control and survival.[55-58] Several prognostic factors have now been well established for poor outcome with salivary gland malignancy: high-grade histology, locally or regionally advanced disease (T3, T4, N1, or greater), positive surgical margins, perineural/angiolymphatic invasion, cranial nerve involvement, and extraglandular extension. It is recommended that all

patients with any of these features undergo postoperative radiation therapy to least 66 Gy. Because of risk of occult metastasis, this would include treatment of the ipsilateral neck as well, if neck dissection has not been performed. Radiation therapy alone has been shown to be less effective than surgery and radiation. Therefore, it is reserved for patients with advanced, potentially unresectable tumors. It is estimated that 20% of stage IV disease is curable by radiation alone.[55]

There has been recent interest in neutron beam therapy for salivary gland malignancies. Neutron beam therapy works by directly disrupting DNA thereby limiting the sublethal damage and recovery from potentially lethal damage. This is an appealing mechanism given the slow growth rate and apparent lack of radiosensitivity for many salivary malignancies. The results of a combined Radiation Therapy Oncology Group and Medical Research Council trial found 10-year locoregional control rates were superior to conventional radiation for patients with inoperable or recurrent tumors.[59] However, survival was not improved and the incidence of severe complications was much higher. In addition to the increase in toxicity, there is an additional drawback to this modality. There are currently only a few centers in the world with the ability to administer neutron therapy. At this point, the role for those centers with neutron capability is for treating adenoid cystic carcinoma and unresectable tumors.[60] Experience with proton beam irradiation continues to grow at a limited number of centers throughout the United States and specific benefit has been noted in the treatment of salivary gland malignancies of the sinonasal cavity such as adenoid cystic carcinoma.[61]

The role of chemotherapy in the treatment of salivary gland carcinomas is very poorly established. Given that many patients with advanced stage disease and aggressive high-grade histology die of distant metastasis, further investigation is needed in this area. Many salivary gland tumors have overexpression of EGFR, c-kit, or her-2; unfortunately, chemotherapeutic agents directed at these targets have had a limited impact.[62] Most show no response or at best a slowing of the progression of the disease. Cisplatin-based regimens have shown some antitumor activity and ability to limit disease progression and palliate symptoms for adenoid cystic carcinoma.[62] Paclitaxel has been shown to have moderate activity against recurrent or metastatic mucoepidermoid and adenocarcinomas.[63] Unfortunately, this is a rare group of heterogeneous tumors which makes prospective studies of chemotherapeutic agents very difficult. At this point, patients with recurrent tumors or distant disease should be considered for treatment with chemotherapy in a clinical trial setting.

CONCLUSION

Salivary gland malignancies are uncommon tumors, which affect both the major and minor salivary glands. They are a heterogeneous group ranging from benign clinical features with nearly 100% survival to aggressive tumors with difficult to control local disease, frequent distant metastasis, and overall poor survival. Treatment varies from simple wide local excision to aggressive surgery requiring sacrifice of cranial nerves, neck dissection, and postoperative radiation therapy. It is important to be aware of the impact of specific histologic subtypes, grades, stages, and clinical features which are prognostic for poor outcome. This will help direct appropriate diagnosis and treatment of these challenging malignancies.

REFERENCES

1. Carlson GW. The salivary glands. Embryology, anatomy, and surgical applications. *Surg Clin North Am.* 2000;80:261-273.
2. Wahlber P, Anderson H, Biorklund A, Moller T, Perfekt R. Carcinoma of the parotid and submandibular glands—a study of survival in 2465 patients. *Oral Oncol.* 2002;38:706-713.
3. Pinkston JA, Cole P. Incidence rates of salivary gland tumors: results from a population-based study. *Otolaryngol Head Neck Surg.* 1999;120:834-840.
4. Ries LAG, Hankey BF, Miller BA, et al. *Cancer statistics review. 1973-88.* Bethesda Md: National Cancer Institute; 1991. NIH Publication No. 91-2789
5. Rinaldo A, Shaha AR, Pellitteri PK, Bradley PJ, Ferlito A. Management of malignant sublingual salivary gland tumors. *Oral Oncol.* 2004;40:2-5.
6. Foote FS, Frazell EL. Tumors of the major salivary glands. *Cancer.* 1953;6:1065.
7. Batsakis JG. Carcinomas of the submandibular and sublingual glands. *Ann Otol Rhinol Laryngol.* 1986;95:211-212.
8. Janfaza P, Nadol JB, Fabian RL, Montgomery WW. *Surgical Anatomy of the Head and Neck.* Philadelphia, Pa: Lippincott Williams & Wilkins; 2000.
9. Witt RL, Weinstein GS, Reyto LK. Tympanomastoid suture and digastric muscle in cadaver and live parotidectomy. *Laryngoscope.* 2005;115:574-577.
10. Spiegel JH, Brys AK, Bhatki A, Singer MI. Metastasis to the submandibular gland in head and neck carcinoma. *Head Neck.* 2004;26:1064-1068.
11. Terhaard CHJ, Lubsen H, Van der Tweel I, et al. Dutch Head and Neck Oncology Cooperative Group. Salivary gland carcinoma: independent prognostic factors for locoregional control, distant metastases, and overall survival: results of the Dutch Head and Neck Oncology Cooperative Group. *Head Neck.* 2004;26:681-693.
12. Seethala RR, LiVolsi VA, Baloch ZW. Relative accuracy in fine needle aspiration and frozen section in the diagnosis of lesions in the parotid gland. *Head Neck.* 2005;27:217-223.
13. Cohen EG, Patel SG, Lin O, et al. Fine-needle aspiration of the salivary gland lesions in a selected patient population. *Arch Otolaryngol Head Neck Surg.* 2004;130:773-778.
14. Postema RJ, van Velthuysen MF, van den Brakel MWM, Balm AJM, Peterse JL. Accuracy of fine-needle aspiration cytology of salivary gland lesions in the netherlands cancer institute. *Head Neck.* 2004;26: 418-424.
15. Hughes JH, Volk EE, Wilbur DC. Pitfalls in salivary gland fine-needle aspiration cytology. *Arch Pathol Lab Med.* 2005;129:26-31.
16. Bahar G, Dudkiewicz M, Feinmesser R, et al. Acute parotitis as a complication of fine-needle aspiration in warthin's tumor. A unique finding of a 3-year experience with parotid tumor aspiration. *Otolaryngol Head Neck Surg.* 2006;134:646-649.
17. Koyuncu M, Sesen T, Akan H, et al. Comparison of computed tomography and magnetic resonance imaging in the diagnosis of parotid tumors. *Otolaryngol Head Neck Surg.* 2003;129:726-732.
18. Kinoshita T, Ishii K, Naganuma H, Okitsu T. MR image findings on parotid tumors with pathologic diagnostic clues. A pictoral essay. *J Clin Imaging.* 2004;28:93-101.
19. Okohara M, Kiyosue H, Hori Y, et al. Parotid tumors: MR imaging with pathologic correlation. *Eur Radiol.* 2003;13:25-33.

20. *Major Salivary Glands (Parotid, Submandibular, and Sublingual): AJCC Cancer Staging Manual.* 6th ed. New York, NY: Springer-Verlag; 2002.

21. Levin, RJ, Bradley MK. Neuroectodermal antigens persist in benign and malignant salivary gland tumor cultures. *Arch Otolaryngol Head Neck Surg.* 1996;122:551-557.

22. Dardick I. Mounting evidence against current histogenetic concepts for salivary gland tumorigenesis. *Eur J Morphol.* 1998;36:257-261.

23. Batsakis JG, Regezi JA, Luna MA, et al. Histogenesis of salivary gland neoplasms: a postulate with prognostic implications. *J Laryngol Otol.* 1989;103: 939-944.

24. el-Naggar AK, Klijanienko J. Advances in clinical investigations of salivary gland tumorigenesis. *Ann Pathol.* 1999;19:19-22.

25. Goode RK, Auclair PL, Ellis GL. Mucoepidermoid carcinoma of the major salivary glands. Clinical and histopathologic analysis of 234 cases with evaluation of grading criteria. *Cancer.* 1998;82: 1217-1224.

26. Batsakis JG, Luna MA. Histopathologic grading of salivary gland neoplasms: I. Mucoepidermoid carcinomas. *Ann Otol Rhinol Laryngol.* 1990;99: 835-838.

27. Stewart FW, Foote FW, Becker WF. Mucoepidermoid tumors of salivary glands. *Ann Surg.* 1945;122:820-844.

28. Hicks MJ, El-Naggar AK, Flaitz CM, et al. Histologic grading of mucoepidermoid carcinoma of major salivary glands in prognosis and survival: a clinicopathologic and flow cytometric investigation. *Head Neck.* 1995;17:89-95.

29. Brandwein MS, Ivanov K, Wallace DI, et al. Mucoepidermoid carcinoma. A clinicopathologic study of 80 patients with special reference to histological grading. *Am J Surg Pathol.* 2001;25:835-845.

30. Spiro RH, Huvos AG, Berk R, et al. Mucoepidermoid carcinoma of salivary origin: a clinicopathologic study of 367 cases. *Am J Surg.* 1978;136:461-468.

31. da Cruz Perez DE, de Abreu Alves F, Nishimoto IN, Paes de Almeida O, Kowalski LP. Prognostic factors in head and neck adenoid cystic carcinoma. *Oral Oncol.* 2006;42:139-146.

32. Khafif A, Anavi Y, Haviv J, Fienmesser R, Calderon S, Marshak G. Adenoid cystic carcinoma of the salivary glands: a 20-year review with long term follow-up. *ENT.* 2005;84:662-667.

33. Gurney TA, Eisele DW, Weinberg V, Shin E, Lee N. Adenoid cystic carcinoma of the major salivary glands treated with surgery and radiation. *Laryngoscope.* 2005;115:1278-1282.

34. Batsakis JG, Luna MA, El-Naggar A. Histopathologic grading of salivary gland neoplasms: III. Adenoic cystic carcinoma. *Ann Otol Rhinol Laryngol.* 1990;99:1007-1009.

35. Brackrock S, Krull A, Roser K, Schwarz R, Riethdorf L, Alberti W. Neutron therapy, prognostic factors and dedifferentiation of adenoid cystic carcinomas of salivary glands. *Anticancer Res.* 2005;25: 1321-1326.

36. Li J, Wang BY, Nelson M, Hu Y, Urken ML, Brandwin-Gensler M. Salivary adenocarcinoma, not otherwise specified. A collection of orphans. *Arch Pathol Lab Med.* 2004;128:1385-1394.

37. Batsakis JG, wl-Naggar AK, Luna MA. "Adenocarcinoma not otherwise specified": A diminishing group of salivary carcinomas. *Ann Otol Rhinol Laryngol.* 1992;101:102-104.

38. Wahlber P, Anderson H, Bjorklund A, et al. Carcinoma of the parotid and submandibular glands: a study of survival in 2465 patients. *Oral Oncol.* 2002;38:706-713.

39. Batsakis JG, Luna MA, El-Naggar A. Histopathologic grding of salivary gland neoplasms: II. acinic cell carcinomas. *Ann Otol Rhinol Laryngol.* 1990;99: 929-933.

40. Hoffman HT, Karnell LH, Robinson RA, Pinkston JA, Menck HR. National Cancer Center Data Base report on cancer of the head and neck: acinic cell carcinoma. *Head Neck.* 1999;21:297-309.

41. Kim SA, Mathog RH. Acinic cell carcinoma of the parotid gland: a 15-year review limited to a single surgeon at a single institution. *ENT.* 2005;84: 597-602.

42. Mehta RP, Faquin WC, Deschler DG. Acinic cell of the parotid gland with ductal extension. *Arch Otolaryngol Head Neck Surg.* 2004;130:790, 792-793.

43. Ellis GL, Auclair PL. Malignant epithelial tumors. In: Armed Forces Institute of Pathology, eds. *Atlas of Tumor Pathology: Tumors of the Salivary Glands, 3rd Series*, fascicle 17. Bethesda, Md: Universities Associated for Research and Education in Pathology, Inc; 1996:183.

44. Hosal AS, Fan C, Barnes L, Myers EN. Salivary duct carcinoma. *Otolaryngol Head Neck Surg.* 2003; 129:720-725.

45. Guzzo M, Di Palma S, Grandi C, Molinari M. Salivary duct carcinoma: clinical characteristics and treatment strategies. *Head Neck.* 1997;19:126-133.

46. Olsen KD, Lewis JE. Carcinoma ex pleomorphic adenoma: a clinicopathologic review. *Head Neck.* 2001;23;705-712.

47. Chen AM, Garcia J, Bucci MK, Quivey JM, Eisele DW. The role of postoperative radiation therapy in carcinoma ex pleomorphic adenoma of the parotid gland. *Int J Radiat Oncol Biol Phys.* 2006;13.

48. Eneroth CM, Zetterberg A. Malignancy in pleomorphic adenoma. A clinical and microspectrophotometric study. *Acta Otolaryngol.* 1974;77:426-432.

49. Spiro RH, Huvos AG, Strong EW. Malignant mixed tumor of salivary origin: a clinicopathologic study of 146 cases. *Cancer.* 1977;39:388-396.

50. Thackray AC, Lucas RB. Tumors of the major salivary glands. *Atlas of Tumor Pathology.* Washington DC: Armed Forces Institute of Pathology; 1983:107-117.

51. Castle JT, Thompson LDR, Frommelt RA, Wenig BM, Kessler HP. Polymorphous low grade adenocarcinoma. A clinicopathologic study of 164 cases. *Cancer.* 1999;86:207-219.

52. Evans HL, Luna MA. Polymorphous low-grade adenocarcinoma. A study of 40 cases with long-term follow up and an evaluation of the importance of papillary areas. *Am J Surg Pathol.* 2000;24:1319-1328.

53. Jaehne M, Ubmuller J, Jakel KT, Zschaber R. The clinical presentation of non-Hodgkin lymphomas of the major salivary glands. *Acta Otolaryngol.* 2001;121:647-651.

54. Barnes L, Myers EN, Prokopakis EP. Primary malignant lymphoma of the parotid gland. *Arch Otolaryngol Head Neck Surg.* 1998;124:573-577.

55. Mendenhall WM, Morris CG, Amdur RJ, Werning JW, Villaret DB. Radiotherapy alone or combined with surgery for salivary gland carcinoma. *Cancer.* 2005;103:2544-2550.

56. Armstrong JG, Harrison LB, Spiro RH, Fass DE, Strong WE, Fuks Z. Malingngt tumors of major salivary gland origin: a matched-pair analysis of the role of combined surgery and postoperative radiotherapy. *Arch Otolaryngol Head Neck Surg.* 1990;116:290-293.

57. North CA, Lee DJ, Piantadosi S, Zahurak M, Johns ME. Carcinoma of the major salivary glnads treated by surgery or surgery plus postoperative radiotherapy. *Int J Radiat Oncol Biol Phys.* 1990;18:1319-1326.

58. Garden AS, El-Naggar AK, Morrison WH, Callender DL, Ang KK, Peters LJ. Postoperative radiotherapy for malignant tumors of the parotid gland. *Int J Radiat Oncol Biol Phys.* 1997;37:79-85.

59. Griffin TW, Pajak TF, Laramore GE, et al. Neutron vs. photon irradiation of inoperable salivary gland tumors: results of an RTOG-MRC cooperative randomized study. *Int J Radiat Oncol Biol Phys.* 1988;15:1085-1090.

60. Brackrock S, Krull A, Roser K, Schwarz R, Riethdorf L, Alberti W. Neutron therapy, prognostic factors and dedifferentiation of adenoid cystic carcinomas (ACC) of salivary glands. *Anticancer Res.* 2005;25:1321-1326.

61. Pommier P, Liebsch NJ, Deschler DG, et al. Proton beam radiation therapy for skull base adenoid cystic carcinoma. *Arch Otolaryngol Head Neck Surg.* 2006;132:1242-1249.

62. Laurie SA, Licitra L. Systemic therapy in the palliative management of advanced salivary gland cancers. *J Clin Oncol.* 2006;24:2673-2678.

63. Gilbert J, Li Y, Pinto HA, et al. Phase II trial of taxol in salivary gland malignancies (E1394): a trial of the Eastern Cooperative Oncology Group. *Head Neck.* 2006;28:197-204.

22

Diagnosis and Management of Head and Neck Endocrine Malignancies

Jeffrey S. Moyer
Theodoros N. Teknos

EPIDEMIOLOGY OF THYROID MALIGNANCIES

Thyroid cancer is the most common endocrine malignancy in the United States accounting for 1.9% of all new malignant tumors (excluding in situ cancers and skin malignancies).[1] In 2006, there will be approximately 30,180 new cases of thyroid carcinoma in the United States (prevalence of 292,555) with 1,500 expected deaths among persons diagnosed with the disease.[2] The incidence of thyroid cancer has more than doubled over the last 30 years from 3.6 cases per 100,000 people in 1973 to 8.7 per 100,000 in 2002[3] (Fig 22–1). Although the incidence of thyroid carcinoma appears to be on the rise, mortality has been constant during the same period (Fig 22–2). Thyroid cancer-specific mortality was approximately 0.5 deaths per 100,000 in both 1973 and 2002.[3] As mortality has remained relatively stable, the increasing incidence most likely partially reflects the earlier detection of subclinical disease

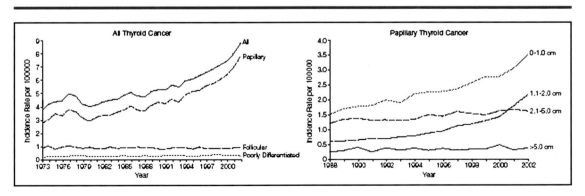

Fig 22–1. Increasing incidence of thyroid cancer in the United States, 1973–2002. Used with permission. Davies, L. and Welch H.G., Increasing incidence of thyroid cancer in the United States, 1973-2002. *JAMA*, 2006;295(18):2164–2167.

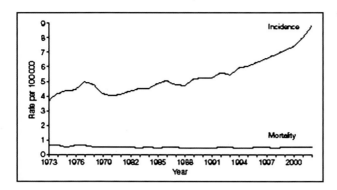

Fig 22–2. Thyroid cancer incidence and mortality, 1973–2002. Used with permission. Davies, L. and Welch H.G., Increasing incidence of thyroid cancer in the United States, 1973-2002. *JAMA*, 2006;295(18): 2164–2167.

with increased diagnostic scrutiny and the use of more sophisticated imaging modalities. It has long been known that the true incidence of thyroid cancer is probably much higher given autopsy data suggesting rates of papillary microcarcinomas (tumors = 1-cm diameter) as high as 36%.[4-8]

Thyroid cancer is two to three times more common in women than men and has a peak incidence at 50 to 54 years of age in women and 65 to 69 years in men.[3] Although thyroid carcinoma is more common in females, mortality rates are higher for men due, in part, to the later age of presentation.[9] In addition, male patients have a relatively higher proportion of malignant nodules when compared with female patients.[10]

The risk factor most strongly associated with thyroid malignancy is radiation exposure.[11] Thyroid glands exposed to external beam or systemically administered ^{131}I radiation develop multinodularity, fibrosis, oncocytic change, and chronic inflammation.[12-14] After radiation, new nodules develop at a rate of 2% annually with a peak incidence at 30 years after radiation.[15] In a large study of childhood thyroid cancer that began in 1948,[11] the authors noted a significant increase in the incidence of thyroid cancer between 1946 and 1959 and that 76% of the children included in this study had a history of neck irradiation. Between 1920 and 1960, gamma radiation was commonly used for a variety of head and neck conditions, including enlarged tonsils and adenoids. The incidence of radiation-induced thyroid carcinomas has decreased since 1970 with the discontinuation of this practice.[16] However, after the Chernobyl nuclear accident in 1986, it became apparent that ^{131}I and other radioiodines are also potent thyroid carcinogens in children in addition to external beam radiation.[17] The risk of radiation-induced thyroid carcinoma appears to be greater in children, women, certain Jewish populations, and patients with a family history of thyroid malignancies.[18]

Genetic factors also appear to be strongly associated with the development of certain thyroid malignancies. Familial, nonmedullary thyroid carcinoma accounts for approximately 5% of papillary carcinomas.[19] The familial form of this disease appears to behave more aggressively with high rates of local recurrence as well as regional and distant metastases.[20] Other familial syndromes such as familial adenomatous polyposis (Gardner's syndrome), familial hamartomas (Cowden's disease), and Carney complex (multiple neoplasia and lentiginosis syndrome) are also associated with papillary carcinoma. Medullary carcinoma is also present in a familial form in 20% of medullary cancers (MEN2A, MEN2B, and familial non-MEN medullary carcinoma) and involves a mutation in the RET oncogene. MEN2A-related medullary carcinomas present in the first and second decades whereas MEN2B-associated medullary carcinomas present primarily during the first decade of life. In contrast, familial non-MEN medullary carcinoma presents during the sixth decade and later and occurs equally in males and females.[21]

The relative proportion of differentiated thyroid cancers (papillary and follicular) in a given population is dependent on dietary iodine intake.[22] Papillary carcinoma predominates in populations with sufficient iodine intake[23] whereas iodine-deficient regions typically have a higher proportion of follicular carcinomas.[22] Surveillance, Epidemiology, and End Results (SEER) data from the National Cancer Institute for the period 1973 to 2002[3] found the most common histologic category in the United States to be papillary carcinoma (88%), followed by follicular carcinoma (9%), and poorly differentiated tumors-medullary/anaplastic carcinoma (3%).

EVALUATION OF THYROID NODULE (FIG 22–3)

A thyroid nodule is a distinct lesion within the thyroid parenchyma that can be detected on physical examination by palpation or is visualized on a radi-ographic imaging study such as ultrasonography, computerized tomography, or magnetic resonance imaging. Solitary nodules of the thyroid gland are present in 6.4% of women and 1.5% of men in the United States[24-26] and high-resolution ultrasound has found rates as high as 27% in some populations.[27] Of palpable nodules (typically >1 cm), cancer is

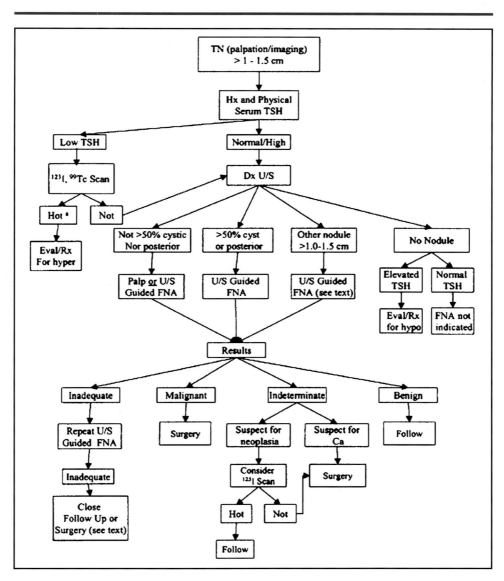

Fig 22–3. Management guidelines for patients with thyroid nodules and differentiated thyroid cancer. Reprinted with permission. Cooper, D.S., et al., Management guidelines for patients with thyroid nodules and differentiated thyroid cancer. *Thyroid*, 2006;16(2):109–142.

present 10 to 14% of the time whereas the overwhelming majority are follicular adenomas, colloid adenomas, or cysts.[24-26] Nonpalpable nodules found incidentally on imaging studies ("incidentalomas") have the same risk of malignancy as similarly sized nodules that are easily palpated and should be fully evaluated.[28] However, a nodule less than 1 cm in an otherwise low-risk, asymptomatic patient has a very low risk of malignancy and usually does not require biopsy.[29,30] In patients with suspicious radiographic findings, a family history of thyroid cancer, or prior neck radiation, a more thorough evaluation is warranted. Patients with multiple thyroid nodules also have the same risk of malignancy as patients with solitary nodules.[31,32]

History and Physical Examination

A complete history and head and neck physical examination is mandatory for patients presenting with a thyroid nodule, but as few as 5% to 10% of patients with a malignancy present with symptoms. Numerous retrospective and prospective studies have found the sensitivity and specificity of history and physical examination in predicting thyroid malignancy to be approximately 60% and 80%, respectively.[33-37]

Relevant historical factors that might suggest thyroid malignancy are previous neck irradiation or environmental radiation exposure, family history of thyroid cancer in a first-degree relative, and rapid growth of the nodule/mass (Table 22-1). The inci-

dence of thyroid cancer increases with age, but a higher percentage of nodules in patients less than 20 years of age will also demonstrate malignancy.[38] A family history of pheochromocytoma, hypercalcemia, mucosal abnormalities, or medullary carcinoma may suggest the possibility of multiple endocrine neoplasia (MEN) syndrome or hereditary medullary carcinoma. Patient's with benign goiter in Pendred's syndrome also have a higher cancer risk than the general population.[24]

Pertinent review of symptoms findings that are more worrisome for malignancy include hoarseness or voice change, dysphagia, shortness of breath, and pain, but are typically more common in locally advanced disease. Thyroid lymphoma also should be considered in patients with a history of Hashimoto's thyroiditis who have rapid thyroid enlargement, particularly in women over 50.

The physical exam of a patient with a thyroid nodule should involve visualization of the endolarynx as well as a careful inspection of the thyroid gland and regional lymphatics. The presence of cervical lymphadenopathy, fixation of the nodule, and vocal fold paralysis are all highly suggestive of a malignancy. Investigation of substernal extension is best evaluated on radiographic imaging, but the presence of thoracic inlet obstruction can be elicited by Pemberton's maneuver. This technique has patients raise their hands over their head; subsequent respiratory discomfort or venous engorgement suggests significant substernal involvement and compression.

Thyroid Function and Other Laboratory Studies

The discovery of a thyroid nodule should elicit a thyrotropin (TSH) level evaluation to determine whether or not the patient is euthyroid. A low TSH level suggesting clinical hyperthyroidism should be followed by a radionucleotide thyroid scan to document whether the nodule is functioning ("hot"), nonfunctioning ("cold"), or isofunctioning ("warm"). Patients with a functioning nodule and hyperthyroidism rarely harbor malignancy and frequently can be spared surgery given the high incidence of follicular adenoma.[39] Thyroid function studies should be reserved for patients with abnormal screening TSH levels.

Table 22-1. High-Risk Features in a Thyroid Nodule

History	Physical Exam
Neck irradiation	Neck lymphadenopathy
Family history of MEN2	Rapid growth
Dysphagia	Vocal fold paralysis
Odynophagia	Firm and fixed
Hoarseness	Stridor
Dyspnea	
Growth with thyroxine	

The routine use of serum thyroglobulin for the intial evaluation of a thyroid nodule is not helpful in determining the relative risk of malignancy given the fact that it is routinely elevated in many thyroid diseases.[40] Thyroglobulin levels, however, may be useful in the post-total thyroidectomy patient where elevated levels are associated with residual or recurrent disease.[41]

Unless there is a history of medullary carcinoma or MEN 2 syndrome, the evidence for routine calcitonin testing is currently limited in the initial evaluation of a thyroid nodule. Several recent large prospective studies, however, have shown that routine testing may result in the early diagnosis of medullary carcinoma and improved survival.[42-44] Based on issues of sensitivity, specificity, and cost effectiveness, the American Thyroid Association (ATA) Guidelines Taskforce could not recommend either for or against its routine use in screening routine thyroid nodules.[45]

FINE-NEEDLE ASPIRATION BIOPSY

Fine-needle aspiration biopsy (FNAB) should be performed in the initial evaluation of thyroid nodules and is the best nonsurgical method for diagnostic evaluation. For the best results, FNAB should be performed by an experienced clinician and interpreted by a seasoned pathologist who evaluates a large, continuous patient volume. In the best of hands, the negative predicative value of FNAB for thyroid nodules approaches 100%, but the positive predictive value ranges from 33% to 85%.[46] Many studies have demonstrated that ultrasound (US)-guided FNAB is more precise and offers better sampling of thyroid nodules compared to palpation-guided FNAB.[47-56] This is particularly true for cystic and solid lesions in multinodular goiter as well as Hashimoto's thyroiditis or Graves' disease.[57,58]

Results of FNAB are typically divided into four categories: benign, nondiagnostic, suspicious/indeterminate, and malignant. Nodules characterized as benign on cytopathology are typically nodular goiter, hyperplastic nodules, or thyroiditis but false negatives do occur and a benign FNAB should not take precedence over a clinical scenario that suggests malignancy. In addition, benign nodules require follow-up with serial ultrasounds to detect changes in the nodule due to the possibility of false-negative FNAB ranging from 1% to 11%.[59,60] Nodules that change in size should have a repeat FNAB performed. Nondiagnostic FNABs are frequently the result of aspirates with an inadequate number of cells to make a diagnosis.[59,61] Nondiagnostic aspirates should be repeated until a diagnostic sample is obtained and should not be construed as a negative result. Nodules with repeated nondiagnostic specimens have malignancy rates in some studies as high as 5% in women and 30% in men.[62] The ATA Guidelines Task Force recommends surgical excision of solid nodules with repeatedly nondiagnostic FNAB and close observation or excision for cystic nodules with repeatedly nondiagnostic FNAB.[45] FNAB interpreted as "suspicious for papillary carcinoma or Hurthle cell neoplasm" should have surgical excision.[45] Cytopathology revealing "follicular lesion" or "follicular neoplasm" is seen in 15% to 30% of FNAB specimens and patients without an autonomously functioning nodule ("cold nodule") should also undergo surgical excision.[45] A number of studies have looked at cytometric DNA analysis[63] and biomarkers[64-68] as a way to confirm a malignancy in suspicious/indeterminate specimens, but the diagnostic accuracy has not yet been fully established. If cytology reveals a malignancy, surgical excision is indicated.[69]

Imaging Techniques

Ultrasonography

Ultrasonography is a relatively low-cost, widely available technique that should be performed in all patients to better characterize a thyroid nodule as well as assess for other nodules. Sonographic characteristics such as microcalcifications, hypoechogenicity of a solid nodule, and intranodular hypervascularity are associated with malignancy.[32,56] Ultrasound also can be used to evaluate regional lymph nodes and certain US-features (narrowing of fatty hilum/widening of cortex, increased vascularity, rounded node configuration, and pinhead size calcifications) are associated with nodal metastasis.[70,71] US-guided

FNAB is also helpful when palpation FNAB is difficult due to a patient's body habitus, small size of the nodule, or to reduce the likelihood of obtaining nondiagnostic specimens.

Thyroid Scanning

Thyroid scanning utilizes radionucleotide isotopes (most commonly ^{131}I, ^{99m}TcO$_4$, and ^{123}I) to determine the functional state of a thyroid nodule. Based on the uptake of the nucleotide, the nodule is designated hyperfunctioning ("hot"), hypofunctioning ("cold"), or isofunctioning ("warm"). On radionucleotide scanning, 5% of nodules are "hot," 10% are "warm," and 85% are "cold." Most thyroid carcinomas and adenomas have defects in iodine accumulation and/or organification are found to be "cold" nodules. However, cold nodules are still benign in over 80% of cases. In contrast, "hot" nodules rarely represent malignancy. Thus, the sensitivity and specificity of this test is relatively poor when compared with FNAB for the diagnosis of malignancy.

The utility of thyroid scanning in the routine workup of a thyroid nodule is limited and is most useful in particular clinical situations such as a hyperfunctioning nodule in patients with hyperthyroidism, suppressed TSH levels, or FNAB suggestive of a follicular neoplasm.

CT/MRI

CT or MRI is not routinely used in the initial evaluation of thyroid nodules. Larger thyroid cancers with aggressive characteristics on physical exam (fixation, dyspnea, dysphagia) may require CT or MRI to assess thyroid cartilage invasion, tracheal invasion, or esophageal involvement. This information helps with extirpative and reconstructive planning for lesions found to be surgically resectable. In addition, CT or MRI allows for better visualization of the substernal component of the tumor. The main disadvantage of CT scanning is the need for iodinated contrast. Iodine uptake may be blunted in patients given contrast for up to 8 weeks after the scan, making diagnostic and therapeutic ^{123}I or ^{131}I ineffective. MRI with gadolinium does not suffer from this limitation and a number of studies have found it to be up to 95% sensitive and specific for detecting invasion of surrounding structures.[72-74] The main disadvantages of MRI relative to CT are increased cost, length of time required to perform the scan, and inability to image patients with certain implanted metal devices.

TUMOR CLASSIFICATION AND STAGING

TNM System

The TNM system was developed by the American Joint Committee on Cancer (AJCC) in conjunction with the International Union Against Cancer (UICC) and uses local tumor growth (T), spread to regional lymph nodes (N), and/or distant metastasis (M) to classify and stage tumor extent[75] (Tables 22-2 through 22-5). Although anatomic extent is a key feature in many head and neck sites for TNM staging, thyroid cancer is unique in that the histologic diagnosis and the age of the patient are taken into consideration when determining the stage of the tumor. For well-differentiated thyroid carcinoma (papillary and follicular carcinoma), patients less than 45 years of age have either stage I or stage II disease regardless of TNM extent. Anaplastic carcinoma is also staged differently in that all patients are considered stage IV due to the aggressiveness of the disease and are stratified by resectability into stage IVa (surgically resectable), stage IVb (surgically unresectable), or stage IVc (distant disease).

Many prognostic scoring systems have been developed and none are universally accepted; however, the TNM staging method is the most widely used system. Brierley et al[76] evaluated six different staging systems and found poor predictive value among the groups studied and found no single one that offered an advantage over the TNM system. The authors advocated its universal use to improve standardization between medical centers. However, no staging system adequately addresses variants of papillary and follicular carcinoma whose clinical behavior can be markedly different. In addition, staging systems demonstrate inconsistent findings when applied to populations different than the original study populations.[77]

Table 22–2. AJCC Staging for Thyroid Cancer

Primary Tumor (T)	
T1	Tumor 2 cm or less in greatest dimension limited to the thyroid
T2	Tumor more than 2 cm but not more than 4 cm in greatest dimension limited to the thyroid
T3	Tumor more than 4 cm in greatest dimension limited to the thyroid or any tumor minimal extrathyroidal extension (eg, extension to the sternothyroid muscle or perithyroid soft tissue
T4a	Tumor of any size extending beyond the thyroid capsule to invade subcutaneous soft tissues, larynx, trachea, esophagus, or recurrent laryngeal nerve
T4b	Tumor invades prevertebral fascia or encases carotid artery or mediastinal vessels
All anaplastic carcinomas are considered T4 tumors regardless of size	
T4a	Intrathyroidal anaplastic carcinoma—surgically respectable
T4b	Extrathyroidal anaplastic carcinoma—surgically unresectable
Regional Lymph Nodes (N)	
Regional lymph nodes are the central compartment, lateral cervical, and upper mediastinal lymph nodes	
N0	No regional lymph node metastasis
N1	Regional lymph node metastasis
N1a	Metastasis to Level VI (pretracheal, paratracheal, and prelaryngeal/Delphian lymph nodes
N1b	Metastasis to unilateral, bilateral, or contralateral cervical or superior mediastinal lymph nodes
Distant Metastasis	
M0	No distant metastasis
M1	Distant metastasis

Source: AJCC Staging Handbook (2002).

AMES System

The AMES system stratifies patients into high risk and low risk based on a patient's age (A), metastases (M), extent of tumor (E), and tumor size (S).[78] Low-risk patients are men less than 40 years old and women less than 50 years old without evidence of metastasis, papillary carcinoma without extrathyroidal invasion or follicular carcinoma without major vascular or capsular invasion, and tumor size less than 5 cm. Sanders and Cady[79] examined 1,019 patients with well-differentiated thyroid cancer treated between 1940 and 1990 and found during the period from 1980 to 1990, survival rates (mean follow-up of 8 years) in the high-risk and low-risk group of 47% and 98%, respectively. Recurrences occurred in 5% of low-risk patients and were typically curable while recurrences in the high-risk group were associated with a 75% mortality rate.

AGES/MACIS System

The Mayo clinic initially published a staging system for papillary carcinoma based on age (A), histologic grade (G), extent (E), and tumor size (S).[80] This

Table 22–3. AJCC Staging for Well-Differentiated Thyroid Carcinoma

	Papillary or Follicular Under 45 Years		
Stage I	Any T	Any N	Any M0
Stage II	Any T	Any N	M1
	Papillary or Follicular 45 Years and Older		
Stage I	T1	N0	M0
Stage II	T2	N0	M0
Stage III	T3	N0	M0
	T1	N1a	M0
	T2	N1a	M0
	T3	N1a	M0
Stage IVa	T4a	N0	M0
	T4a	N1a	M0
	T1	N1b	M0
	T2	N1b	M0
	T3	N1b	M0
	T4a	N1b	M0
Stage IVb	T4b	Any N	M0
Stage IVc	Any T	Any N	M1

Table 22–4. AJCC Staging for Medullary Thyroid Carcinoma

Stage I	T1	N0	M0
Stage II	T2	N0	M0
Stage III	T3	N0	M0
	T1	N1a	M0
	T2	N1a	M0
	T3	N1a	M0
Stage IVa	T4a	N0	M0
	T4a	N1a	M0
	T1	N1b	M0
	T2	N1b	M0
	T3	N1b	M0
	T4a	N1b	M0
Stage IVb	T4b	Any N	M0
Stage IVc	Any T	Any N	M1

system was modified due to the infrequency of tumor grading by pathologists and a new system termed MACIS was advocated based on metastases (M), age (A), completeness of resection (C), invasion (I), and tumor size (S)[81] (Table 22-6). The Mayo group identified three factors that were considered to be most important in predicting prognosis: presence of postoperative local metastatic nodes, postoperative distant metastases, and local recurrence in the thyroid bed or adjacent tissue other than lymph nodes (Table 22-7).

Table 22–5. AJCC Staging for Anaplastic Thyroid Carcinoma

Stage IVa	T4a	Any N	M0
Stage IVb	T4b	Any N	M0
Stage IVc	Any T	Any N	M1

Table 22–6. MACIS Scoring System

Metastases	Absent	0
	Present	3
Patient age	<40	3.1
	>40	0.08 × age
Resection	Complete	0
	Incomplete	1
Invasion	Absent	0
	Present	1
Tumor size		0.3 × size in cm

Table 22–7. MACIS and Mortality Rates[81]

Score	AMES (High Risk) [%]	20-yr Mortality Rates (%)
<6	1.7	0.9
6–6.99	39.2	11.3
7–7.99	86.4	44.4
>8	100	76.5

MANAGEMENT OF DIFFERENTIATED THYROID MALIGNANCIES

Much of the controversy in the management of differentiated thyroid carcinoma exists because of the lack of large phase III studies to support a definitive treatment approach. However, there are considerable data from retrospective studies from large patient cohorts where treatment was not randomly assigned. To interpret these sometimes conflicting data, a number of groups have developed treatment guidelines to guide therapy including: the American Thyroid Association (ATA),[45] American Association of Clinical Endocrinologists and the American Association of Endocrine Surgeons,[82] the British Thyroid Association and the Royal College of Physicians,[83] and the National Comprehensive Cancer Network (NCCN).[84]

The goals of the initial management of well-differentiated thyroid carcinoma were well delineated by the most recent ATA Guidelines Task Force[45] and consist of: (1) Removal of the primary tumor, disease that extends beyond the thyroid capsule, and involved lymph nodes; (2) Minimize treatment- and disease-related morbidity; (3) Permit accurate staging of the disease; (4) Facilitate postoperative treatment with radioactive iodine, where appropriate; (5) Permit accurate long-term surveillance for disease recurrence; and (6) Minimize the risk of disease recurrence and metastatic spread.

Papillary Carcinoma

Clinical Presentation

Papillary carcinoma is the most common type of thyroid malignancy in the United States and comprises over 80% of all thyroid cancers, depending on the study cited.[3,85,86] One of the largest cohorts of patients with papillary carcinoma was studied at the Mayo Clinic and the ratio of women to men was 2:1 and most patients presented between the ages of 30 and 60 (range 5 to 93).[87] Papillary carcinoma is the also the most common thyroid malignancy in children, comprising 70 to 90% of cases.[88,89]

The most common presentation is that of a thyroid nodule found on physical examination or by an imaging study performed for another purpose in a patient who is otherwise asymptomatic and euthyroid. The management of a thyroid nodule was described previously, but all thyroid nodules should have a FNAB in an attempt to pathologically characterize the abnormality. Cervical lymphadenopathy is also a relatively common presentation for papillary carcinoma and an FNAB of the lymph node frequently leads to the discovery of the primary thyroid malignancy.[90] Nodal metastases are present clinically in close to 40% of patients with papillary carcinoma and are routinely present ipsilateral to the tumor and inferiorly into the superior mediastinum.[24] The frequency of micrometastases may be closer to 90% if more sensitive testing methods are employed.[91,92] Contralateral metastases tend to occur with more aggressive tumors or more advanced disease. Ultrasonography of the contralateral lobe and bilateral necks should be performed to identify occult cervical metastases in patients with an FNAB positive or suspicious for papillary carcinoma prior to thyroidectomy in order to properly prepare for the extent of surgery. In the Mayo series,[87,93] distant metastases were present in approximately 2% of the patients studied.

Although most patients are asymptomatic, symptoms are usually suggestive of either an aggressive form of papillary carcinoma or a large tumor. Symptoms are typically related to increasing size or invasion and consist of dysphagia, cough, dysphonia/hoarseness, or a dull ache. Frank pain is rare from papillary carcinoma and suggests subacute thyroiditis, hemorrhage within a nodule or cyst, or a less differentiated malignancy such as medullary or anaplastic carcinoma.

Papillary carcinoma can be classified based on size and local aggressive behavior into three groups. The first group consists of tumors less than 1.0 cm and are frequently found incidentally and are termed "microcarcinomas" or "incidentalomas." Their recurrence and cancer-specific mortality rates are near zero.[94] Intrathyroidal tumors are greater than 1.0 cm and are confined to the thyroid gland whereas extrathyroidal tumors can be of any size but demonstrate extension to the soft tissues or lymph nodes of the neck. There is a linear relationship between tumor size and recurrence and cancer-specific mortality.[9] Extrathyroidal tumors have recurrence rates two times higher than intrathyroidal tumors and as many as 33% of patients die within 10 years.[9,95]

Histologic Variants

Although overall survival rates for papillary carcinoma are good compared to other head and neck malignancies, certain histologic subsets have a much poorer prognosis.

Tall cell variant (TCV) of papillary carcinoma was originally described by Hazard in 1964 and at least 30% of the tumor must be involved to be classified in this manner.[96] However, these pathologic assessments are subjective accounting for variability across institutions with regard to TCV's true natural history. Most studies report the incidence of TCV to be roughly 5% to 10% of papillary carcinomas. Whereas most studies of clinical behavior are small, Sywak et al reviewed the literature on 209 cases of TCV and found the rate of distant metastasis and tumor-related mortality to be 22% and 16%, respectively.[97] This study found TCV to be a poor prognostic sign that was independent of patient age or tumor size.

Columnar-cell variant of papillary carcinoma is uncommon and has a similar appearance to tall cell variants but the nucleus is stratified and the cytoplasm is clear. The mortality rate for this variant is 32% and poorly encapsulated tumors had extrathyroidal spread in 67% and distant metastases in 87% of patients.[97] Well-encapsulated tumors had a prognosis similar to other papillary carcinomas.

Diffuse sclerosing variant of papillary carcinoma is relatively rare, tends to occur in younger patients, and is characterized by pronounced fibrosis and extensive lymphocytic infiltration.[98] Patients tend to have greater regional and distant metastases, but mortality rates are similar to pure papillary carcinoma.[97,98]

Follicular cell variant of papillary carcinoma is present when more than 70% of the histologic pattern is composed of neoplastic follicles. The prognosis for this variant is similar to pure papillary lesions and is thought not to behave differently.[24,99,100]

Surgical Management

Most surgeons agree that the appropriate surgery for papillary carcinoma of the thyroid is either near-total or total thyroidectomy, but controversy still exists due to the lack of definitive phase III data. Near-total thyroidectomy should only leave 1gram or less of tissue near the insertion of the recurrent laryngeal nerve into the cricothyroid muscle whereas total thyroidectomy is the complete removal of all visible thyroid tissue. Completion thyroidectomy should be performed after a lobectomy for an indeterminate or nondiagnostic FNA whenever the resulting pathology, if it had been known prior to the lobectomy, would have warranted a near-total or total thyroidectomy. Lobectomy may be appropriate definitive treatment for intrathyroidal tumors in low-risk patients that are smaller than 1 cm in the absence of cervical metastases. Lobectomy, however, frequently confounds postoperative thyroglobulin and ^{131}I scan interpretation due to the large remnant of thyroid tissue. In addition, evidence exists that rates of recurrence are lower with near-total or total thyroidectomy even in patients considered low-risk.[79,101,102] In contrast to these findings, Haigh et al[103] studied more than 5,000 patients who underwent partial thyroidectomy and found that there were no survival differences between low- and high-risk patients.

Depending on the study and the techniques used, lymph node metastases are present in up to 90% of patients.[24,104,105] Central compartment dissection (level VI) should be performed in all patients regardless of nodal status and has been shown in some studies to decrease nodal recurrence and improve survival.[106,107] Preoperative ultrasound should be performed to evaluate the lateral neck compartments and patients with either clinical or radiographic evidence of cervical metastases should undergo an ipsilateral selective neck dissection (II–V). Level I is rarely involved and should be dissected only when there is clinical evidence of disease. Selective neck dissection in this patient population has been shown to decrease nodal recurrence and mortality.[104,108,109]

Complication rates after near-total or total thyroidectomy have been used as justification by some clinicians for more limited surgery in low-risk, well-differentiated thyroid carcinoma. Injury to the recurrent laryngeal nerve or permanent hypoparathyroidism are the most common complications after total thyroidectomy and occur with rates of 3% and 2.6%, respectively.[110] Surgical experience has a significant impact on these complication rates and surgeons performing fewer than 10 thyroidectomies a year had four times the complication rate as those surgeons performing more than 100 a year.[111]

Radioactive Iodine

Radioactive iodine is used postoperatively in a whole-body scan to look for remnant thyroid tissue in the surgical bed as well as look for metastatic disease in the neck or at distant sites. These findings might alter management by suggesting the need for additional surgery or altering the dose of radioiodine used in thyroid ablation. Radioactive iodine is also used in the postoperative setting for the ablation of remaining thyroid tissue to facilitate future detection of recurrence through subsequent scans and thyroglobulin assays as well as to possibly decrease disease recurrence and mortality. In a review of 1,543 articles on the efficacy of radioactive iodine ablation, Sawka et al[112] concluded that "the effectiveness of radioiodine ablation decreasing recurrence and possibly mortality in low-risk patients with well-differentiated thyroid carcinoma, although suspected, cannot be definitely verified by summarizing the current body of observational patient data." The greatest benefit of ablation appears to be in patients with larger tumors (>1.5 cm) or with residual disease after surgery.[101,113,114]

In centers that perform preablation whole-body iodine scans, ^{123}I is frequently used rather than ^{131}I due to the risk of "thyroid stunning." Thyroid stunning occurs when diagnostic doses of radioiodine are used resulting in a short-term reduction of radioiodine uptake leading to impaired thyroid ablation. Patients undergoing whole-body iodine scans or ablation require elevated TSH levels. This can be achieved by the withdrawal of levothyroxine (LT_4) for 3 weeks prior to radioiodine or the use of levotriiodothyronine (LT_3) for 4 weeks and then removal of the LT_3 for 2 weeks prior to the radioiodine. Alternatively, some studies suggest the usefulness of recombinant TSH (Thyrogen) instead of thyroid hormone withdrawal to achieve an elevated TSH level.[115,116] Many centers currently recommend a postablation whole-body iodine scan after approximately 1 week to look for additional metastatic foci that is seen in up to 26% of patients.[117,118]

External Beam Radiation and Chemotherapy

The role for fractionated radiotherapy and/or chemotherapy in papillary carcinoma typically is reserved for patients with extensive locoregional or metastatic disease that is refractory to surgery and radioiodine therapy as well as in patients receiving palliative treatment. The true benefit of radiotherapy and chemotherapy is unclear, however, due to the retrospective nature of the studies and the highly selected patient populations.

Some centers recommend external-beam radiation for patients 45 years and older who have extrathyroidal extension and gross or microscopic disease after resection, particularly in patients where further surgery or radioactive iodine would not be beneficial. Several studies have demonstrated that external-beam radiation improves both local control and survival in patients at high risk of recurrence in the thyroid bed.[119-123]

Chemotherapy generally is reserved for palliation in patients who are symptomatic from disease progression. There are no current data that clearly demonstrate a survival advantage for patients receiving chemotherapy, but tumor response and palliation of symptoms has been observed in several studies. The most commonly used chemotherapeutic agents in this setting are doxorubicin, bleomycin, and cisplatin with response rates from 17% to 37%, but treatment is limited by performance status and chemotherapy-induced toxicities.[124-126]

Surveillance

The decision on how to follow patients after treatment for papillary thyroid carcinoma centers on the likelihood of recurrence based on individual patient and tumor characteristics. The NCCN currently recommends the following for surveillance after treatment for papillary carcinoma: (1) long-term surveillance and maintenance with a physical examination, TSH, and Tg measurements with anti-Tg antibodies every 6 to 12 months for 2 years, then annually if patients remain disease free. Serum-Tg has a high sensitivity and specificity for detecting thyroid cancer, particularly when performed after thyroid hormone withdrawal or recombinant TSH.[41]

In addition, anti-Tg antibodies are important to assess because they are present in up to 25% of thyroid cancer patients[127] and will falsely lower serum-Tg levels in laboratory assays[128]; (2) periodic neck ultrasound. Ultrasound is very sensitive for detecting cervical metastases and may even uncover neck disease in a patient who otherwise has a negative stimulated TSH level[129]; (3) recombinant-TSH-stimulated Tg in low-risk patients with recent negative neck ultrasound and with negative TSH-suppressed Tg without distant metastases or soft tissue invasion on initial staging; (4) regular diagnostic whole-body ^{131}I scans every 12 months until absence of treatable disease for patients with detectable Tg, distant metastases, or soft tissue invasion on initial staging; and (5) consider additional nonradioiodine imaging for patients whose ^{131}I scans are negative and stimulated Tg is increased more than 2 to 5 ng/mL. FDG-PET has sensitivities ranging from 60% to 94% and specificities from 25% to 90% for detecting residual/recurrent papillary cancer in Tg-positive patients who have a negative diagnostic iodine scan.[130] False-negative scans are more common in well-differentiated tumors and lesions smaller than 5 to 6 mm.

TSH Suppression Therapy

There are data to support the suppression of TSH with levothyroxine in patients with persistent disease or high risk features. A prospective study by the National Thyroid Cancer Treatment Cooperative Study Group found improved progression-free survival in high-risk stage III and stage IV patients but no significant improvement in the low-risk patients (stage I and II).[131] A number of other studies have found similar results with decreased recurrence and mortality in patients with well-differentiated thyroid carcinoma.[9,114,132,133]

Follicular Carcinoma

Clinical Presentation

Follicular thyroid carcinoma typically presents as a solitary, well-circumscribed soft lesion in a patient 50 years of age or older. Women are affected three times as often as men, but men tend to have a worse

prognosis.[134] Follicular carcinomas are also more common during pregnancy and, taken together, suggest a possible role of higher endogenous estrogen levels in its pathogenesis. In contrast to papillary carcinoma, the incidence of follicular carcinoma of the thyroid appears to be decreasing.[135]

Follicular thyroid carcinoma in the United States is less common than papillary carcinoma and accounts for approximately 10% of thyroid cancer cases. However, in countries where iodine deficiency is endemic, follicular carcinomas are more common than papillary carcinomas.[22] Unlike papillary carcinoma, cervical metastases are relatively uncommon but distant metastases to the lung or bone are present at the time of initial presentation in 10 to 20% of patients.[123,136-139] Follicular thyroid carcinoma metastasizes more frequently through local extension and hematogenous spread rather than via the lymphatics.

Of the FNABs that are interpreted as follicular neoplasm, roughly 80% will prove to be a benign follicular adenoma on definitive pathology. The diagnosis of follicular carcinoma cannot be made on FNAB and the demonstration of tumor invasion into or through the capsule is a key aspect of the histopathologic diagnosis. This finding requires a thorough analysis of the entire tumor capsule for evidence of invasion and frozen section analysis is insufficient for definitive diagnosis. D'Avanzo et al[140] risk-stratified three groups based on findings at the time of pathologic analysis: minimally invasive (only capsular invasion), moderately invasive (blood vessel invasion with or without capsular invasion), and widely invasive. The authors reported 5-year survival rates of 98%, 80%, and 38%, respectively.

Hürthle Cell Variant

Hürthle cell tumors are considered a subtype of follicular carcinomas by the World Health Organization classification scheme and most studies demonstrate a worse prognosis than for other follicular tumors.[141,142] These tumors are often multifocal and bilateral at initial presentation. Lymph node metastases are more common in Hürthle cell tumors than with other follicular carcinomas and occur in approximately 30% of cases.[143-146] Histologically, the cells of this tumor exhibit abundant granular eosinophilic cytoplasm, hyperchromatic nuclei, and numerous mitochondria. Capsular invasion must also be present as is the case with other follicular carcinomas.[147]

Hürthle cell tumors account for roughly 3% of all thyroid tumors and tend to have less radioactive iodine avidity, making treatment of residual and metastatic disease more difficult.[148] In a recent series from the Memorial Sloan-Kettering Cancer Center, tumors with only capsular invasion or minimal vascular invasion had a low incidence of recurrence and disease-related death whereas tumors with extensive capsular and vascular invasion had recurrence and mortality rates of 80% and 60%, respectively.[149]

Surgical Management

Patients with an FNAB that is interpreted as follicular neoplasm should have a thyroid lobectomy with isthmusectomy. The one possible exception to this is in patients with a low TSH and a "hot" nodule on radioiodine scan when the lesion is less than 3 cm. The likelihood of a nodule being malignant in this clinical situation is approximately 1% and careful observation may be warranted. In older patients (>50 years) with a nodule greater than 4 cm, a total thyroidectomy can be considered given that the likelihood of malignancy is approximately 50%.[150] In the 20% of cases when the diagnosis of follicular carcinoma is made on permanent pathology after a FNAB demonstrated follicular neoplasm and a thyroid lobectomy has been performed, a completion total thyroidectomy should be undertaken.

There is generally less disagreement among physicians in this clinical situation given the more aggressive behavior of follicular carcinoma. Although patients with minimally invasive follicular carcinoma generally have a very good prognosis, the level of invasiveness is directly correlated with decreased survival. Total thyroidectomy, unlike subtotal or near-total thyroidectomy, typically allows the detection of residual thyroid malignancy on radionucleotide scan given the absence of remnant normal thyroid tissue. Elective neck dissection in patients with follicular carcinoma without cervical adenopathy is unwarranted given the low risk of cervical metastases.

In patients with known Hürthle cell carcinoma, a total thyroidectomy should be performed along with an ipsilateral central compartment neck dissection given the higher rate of cervical metastases. For patients with known positive lymphadenopathy, an ipsilateral modified neck dissection should be performed.

Radioactive Iodine

The use of radioiodine is similar for follicular carcinoma as it is for papillary carcinoma. One of the major differences between follicular carcinoma and papillary carcinoma is the much higher risk of distant metastases given the angioinvasive nature of follicular carcinoma and its proclivity to metastasize hematogenously to the lung, bone, liver, brain, and kidney. The use of radioiodine in these situations can be both diagnostic as well as therapeutic. As previously mentioned, Hürthle cell carcinoma tends to be less sensitive to radioiodine and only 36% of patients have radioiodine avid tumors as compared to 60% and 64% of papillary and non-Hürthle cell follicular carcinomas, respectively.[142]

As in patients with papillary carcinoma, the decision for radioactive iodine scanning and therapeutic ablation is based on risk stratification. Patients at higher risk of recurrence or distant disease based on tumor behavior or patient characteristics should be considered for radioactive iodine treatment.

External Beam Radiation and Chemotherapy

The role for adjuvant radiotherapy in advanced follicular carcinoma (T4a) is not as well established as it is for papillary carcinoma. In the two studies that demonstrated a benefit of adjuvant external-beam radiation in papillary carcinoma, neither showed efficacy in follicular carcinoma.[119,122] In patients with unresectable tumors, however, radiation may offer some benefit. Patients with large, invasive Hürthle cell tumors may benefit from external-beam radiation. In a small study of 18 patients with Hürthle cell carcinoma, there was a 50% local regional control rate at 5 years in patients who received radiation after treatment for a recurrence.[151]

Surveillance

The level of surveillance after the treatment of follicular carcinoma is determined by the prognostic risk of tumor recurrence and death based on tumor and patient characteristics and is similar to the surveillance for patients with papillary carcinoma. Many of the same determinants of prognosis in papillary carcinoma also apply to follicular carcinoma.

Patients can be grouped by tumor histology into two groups: minimally invasive and widely invasive. Widely invasive tumors behave much more aggressively and have a higher incidence of cancer-related death than patients with papillary carcinoma.[152,153] Patients at high risk of recurrence with poor prognostic variables should undergo regular whole-body scanning and serum-Tg measurements looking for evidence of recurrence or metastatic disease as would be performed for papillary carcinoma. Fifty to 80% of the adverse events after follicular carcinoma treatment occurred during the first 2 years after diagnosis whereas patients with papillary carcinoma experience adverse events up to 40 years after treatment.[143,153]

FDG-PET scanning is also helpful in the surveillance of patients with follicular carcinoma, particularly when tumors are not radioiodine sensitive. In patients with Hürthle cell tumors, FDG-PET can be extremely helpful as many tumors are not radioiodine avid. In one study, 20 patients with Hürthle cell tumors were evaluated by PET and the test was found to have a sensitivity of 87% and positive predictive value of 100%.[154]

MANAGEMENT OF MEDULLARY THYROID CARCINOMA

Medullary thyroid carcinoma (MTC) accounts for approximately 5% of all thyroid cancers and arises from the neuroendocrine parafollicular C cells that secrete calcitonin. As medullary thyroid carcinoma typically secretes calcitonin, calcitonin levels are almost always elevated in patients with clinically evident MTC and generally increase with the degree of tumor burden.[155] With occult or early disease, basal levels of calcitonin tend to be in the upper lim-

its of normal. MTC also secretes proteins other than calcitonin including corticotrophin, carcinoembryonic antigen (CEA), histamines, and vasoactive peptides.[156] The ability to secrete these hormonally active peptides can contribute to the development of paraneoplastic syndromes such as diarrhea, Cushing's syndrome, or facial flushing in patients with advanced disease.

Sporadic MTC accounts for roughly 80% of cases, but nearly 1 in 5 cases will be hereditary. Hereditary forms of MTC consist of multiple endocrine neoplasia type 2A (MEN2A), MEN2B, and familial medullary thyroid carcinoma (FMTC). Somatic mutations of the RET proto-oncogene in tumor DNA account for roughly 50% of the cases of sporadic MTC.[157] In contrast, germline mutations of the RET proto-oncogene are found in at least 98% of patients with MEN 2A and FMTC.[158]

Lymph node metastases are identified in approximately 50% of patients at presentation and distant metastases to the lungs or bone occur in 5% to 10% of patients.[159] Survival rates are closely linked to early diagnosis and tumor stage. Patients younger than 40 years of age have a 5-year disease-specific survival rate of 95% as compared to patients older than 40 where the survival drops to 65%.[159] The overall 10-year survival rate of patients with MTC ranges from 50% to 80% and vary significantly among patients with sporadic and familial MTC.[156] The presence of cervical metastases decreases survival to approximately 45%.[159,160] In addition, studies have correlated the exon of the RET proto-oncogene mutation with disease aggressiveness in hereditary MTC.[161]

The workup for patients with MTC centers around the determination of whether or not the disease is sporadic or hereditary and whether or not the patient is at risk for existing pheochromocytoma or hyperparathyroidism. Determining the risk of family members is also crucial (Table 22–8). Patients should be screened for germline RET proto-oncogene mutations even if there is no family history of FTC, because 3% to 6% of patients will be found to harbor the mutation.[162] In addition to RET proto-oncogene screening of patients and first-degree relatives, testing for calcitonin, CEA, serum calcium, and 24-hour urine metanephrines (or plasma-fractionated metanephrines) is helpful for risk strat-

Table 22–8. Indications for RET Proto-oncogene Testing

Presumed sporadic MTC
First-degree relatives of patients with known MTC
All patients who have pheochromocytoma
Children with Hirschsprung's disease

ification. As is true with other thyroid cancers, ultrasound of the thyroid and surrounding lymphatics is also helpful for surgical planning.

Sporadic Medullary Thyroid Carcinoma

Sporadic medullary thyroid carcinoma accounts for roughly 80% of MTC and tends to be unifocal without C-cell hyperplasia.[156] Patients tend to be older with presentation in the mid-50s with more advanced disease than hereditary MTC.[163] There is an equal prevalence between men and women. The most common presentation is with an asymptomatic thyroid nodule alone or in the context of a multinodular goiter. However, some studies have found lymph node metastases in up 80% of cervical nodes with 20% progressing to distant sites.[164] Occasionally, patients with a significant tumor burden will present with hoarseness, dysphagia, or a paraneoplastic syndrome such as flushing, secretory diarrhea, or hypercortisolism. Of the patients with systemic symptoms at presentation, 33% will die within 5 years.[165]

The diagnosis of MTC can be made by FNAB and the sensitivity appears to be equivalent to that in papillary carcinoma, but the cytopathologist needs a degree of suspicion to use calcitonin immunostaining. RET somatic mutations at codon 918 found in tumor cells after FNAB can also be diagnostic.[166] Plasma calcitonin measurements also can be confirmatory because virtually all patients with clinically evident MTC have elevated levels. As previously mentioned, a thorough workup needs to be completed to eliminate the possibility of a hereditary form of MTC that may impact the treatment of the patient and family members. Ultrasound is helpful in defining the size of the thyroid tumor as well as looking for adenopathy in the central and lateral portions of the neck.

Total thyroidectomy with a central compartment nodal dissection is the minimal treatment for patients with sporadic MTC. Patients with evidence of enlarged central or lateral lymph nodes on exam should have an ipsilateral function neck dissection. In addition, patients with tumors greater than 1 to 1.5 cm in diameter should have an ipsilateral neck dissection. Modified radical neck dissection with preservation of uninvolved structures provides the best outcome in patients with regional metastases.[165,167,168]

The role for postoperative external beam radiotherapy is somewhat controversial but several studies have demonstrated improved locoregional recurrence when surgical excision is incomplete or in patients with ipsilateral lymph node metastases.[167,169,170] Radioactive iodine does not appear to offer any benefit in MTC.

Patients should be monitored postoperatively for serum calcitonin and CEA levels on a regular basis. Patients with elevated levels should undergo a high-quality neck ultrasound to look for adenopathy in the neck. Neck CT and MRI also can be helpful in the localization of pathologically enlarged lymph nodes. The chest and abdomen should be included to look for distant metastases. FDG-PET is also helpful in identifying areas of increased calcitonin production.

Hereditary Medullary Thyroid Carcinoma

Approximately 20% to 40% of MTC cases are inherited in an autosomal dominant pattern and can occur as familial MTC (FMTC), MEN2A, or MEN2B.[158] A RET proto-oncogene germ-line mutation is responsible for these syndromes but the exact mutation and clinical features of these syndrome differs between families. MTC is highly penetrant with 90% of carriers eventually developing thyroid carcinoma.[158]

MEN2A accounts for more than 75% of MEN2 syndromes and consists of MTC, pheochromocytoma, and hyperparathyroidism.[158] Either unilateral or bilateral pheochromocytoma develops in 50% of carriers[158] whereas multiglandular parathyroid tumors develop in approximately 30% of carriers.[171,172] Both pheochromocytoma and hyperparathyroidism, however, occur later than MTC. MEN2A carriers typically develop bilateral MTC prior to 10 years of age.

Mutations in the RET proto-oncogene at exon 11 in codon 634 account for 70% of MEN2A cases.[173]

MEN2B is the most aggressive from of MEN2 and has the worse prognosis of all MTC with many patients developing thyroid carcinoma during the first year of life.[174] MEN2B is characterized by MTC, pheochromocytoma in half of carriers, and a connective tissue abnormality that results in a marfanoid habitus. Mucosal neuromas and ganglioneuromas also are quite common. More than 95% of MEN2B cases are due to a single germ-line point mutation in the RET proto-oncogene at exon 16 in codon 918.[175]

FMTC is not associated with other syndromic findings such as pheochromocytoma or hyperparathyroidism and thyroid carcinoma typically manifests later than the MEN2 syndromes, occurring in the third or fourth decade of life.[176] Most criteria for diagnosing FMTC are quite conservative due to the fact that clinicians do not want to miss an occult pheochromocytoma that could affect patient outcome. A concensus meeting in Gubbio, Italy in 1999 of the Seventh International Workshop of Multiple Endocrine Neoplasia categorized MEN kindred as FMTC if it met the following criteria: (1) more than 10 carriers in the kindred, (2) multiple carriers or affected members over age 50 years, and (3) an adequate medical history, particularly in older kindred members.[158]

There is a direct correlation between early diagnosis of MTC and clinical outcome. Thus, the goal of management should be to prevent or cure MTC in all patients with MEN by performing genetic testing and prophylactic thyroidectomy based on the timing of MTC development. As most carriers of the MEN2A mutation develop MTC by 10 years of age, the Gubbio consensus panel recommended total thyroidectomy be done before 5 years of age.[158] Mortality rates appear to have decreased from 20% to less than 5% with this treatment strategy in patients with MEN2A.[156] In contrast, MEN2B patients can develop MTC with metastases during the first year of life. Based on this observation, total thyroidectomy is recommended within the first 6 months of life and ideally within the first month of life.[158] The need to perform surgery at such an early age reinforces the importance of RET proto-oncogene screening in family members to determine the level of risk. Known FMTC carriers develop MTC later in life and the decision of when to perform total thyroidectomy is based on pentagastrin testing starting around 10 years of age. Surgery should be performed when the pentagastrin test becomes positive (calcitonin >10 pg/mL) or the patient reaches the third decade of life when the likelihood of disease is more prevalent.[158] The management of the neck in prophylactic total thyroidectomy remains controversial. Most surgeons, however, favor a central node dissection during the initial surgery because of the difficulty and morbidity associated with reoperation.

MANAGEMENT OF ANAPLASTIC CARCINOMA

Anaplastic carcinoma fortunately is rare in comparison to other differentiated carcinomas with a mean survival of 3 to 7 months and 5-year survival rates ranging between 1% and 7.1%.[177] Although anaplastic carcinoma accounts for only 1% of thyroid cancers, deaths from this disease account for roughly half of the 1200 deaths per year from thyroid cancer.[178] Cervical lymph node involvement is present in up to 75% of patients at presentation and distant metastases are present in over 50% of cases with the most common site being the lungs (80%) followed by bone and brain.[178]

Anaplastic carcinoma typically presents during the sixth to seventh decade of life with a rapidly enlarging thyroid mass in 97% of patients.[179] Many patients have an existing goiter and/or thyroid nodule. Involvement of the surrounding anatomic structures is quite common with recurrent laryngeal nerve involvement in 30% of cases and esophageal and tracheal involvement in approximately 45% of cases.[180] Symptoms associated with compression and/or invasion are also common including dyspnea, stridor, dysphagia, hoarseness, and pain. Diagnosis is typically confirmed with an FNAB which has been shown to be accurate in 90% of patients.[178] Failure to obtain a diagnosis on FNAB may necessitate an open biopsy for definitive diagnosis.

Controversy exists with regard to the timing and extent of surgery in patients with anaplastic carcinoma. Most agree that multimodality treatment is the best treatment approach given the universally poor outcomes with single modality therapy. If the tumor is surgically resectable, surgery should be followed by radiation. In a Dutch review of 67 cases of anaplastic carcinoma,[181] complete resection followed by radiation was associated with 1 and 3-year survival rates of 92% and 83%, respectively. However, 3-year survival rates after debulking and radiation or radiation alone fell to 0%. However, complete resections are uncommon in anaplastic carcinoma and some studies suggest no benefit between radical and marginal resections.[179] The recent concensus panel on the treatment of anaplastic thyroid carcinoma recommends complete surgical resection whenever possible in selected patients where all gross cervical and mediastinal disease can be resected without excessive morbidity.[82] A neck dissection should be performed only when macroscopic disease has been resected.

As many anaplastic tumors are not resectable at presentation, radiation and combined chemotherapy and radiation are the mainstay for local control and palliation. Perhaps the most successful regimen was reported by investigators in Sweden. Tennvall et al[182] reported on their experience with 55 patients treated between 1984 and 1999 with neoadjuvant doxorubicin with daily hyperfractionated radiation followed by debulking surgery. In the group that only received preoperative chemoradiation followed by debulking surgery, 17 of 17 patients had no evidence of local recurrence. Even if debulking surgery was not performed after chemoradiation, 17 of 22 patients had no signs of local recurrence. Despite improvements in local recurrence, median survival in this population was only 3.5 months with 2-year survival rates approximately 9%. These findings were confirmed in a nonrandomized retrospective study in which chemoradiation followed by surgery tended to offer better outcomes, but overall prognosis was still extremely poor.[183] Based on the still universal poor prognosis with combined chemotherapy and radiation, some clinicians still prefer radiation alone to avoid the possible dose-limiting toxicities associated with combined regimens.

MANAGEMENT OF THYROID LYMPHOMA

Primary thyroid non-Hodgkin's lymphoma is quite rare and tends to be from the B-cell lineage. T-cell lymphomas of the thyroid have been reported, but tend to occur in areas endemic for human T-cell lymphotropic virus-I (HTLV-1)-associated T-cell leukemia/lymphoma.[184] The median age of presentation is 75 years with a 4:1 female predominance.[185] Hashimoto's thyroiditis is the most common predisposing condition in patients developing thyroid lymphoma and these patients have a 60-fold relative risk compared to patients without Hashimoto's disease.[185]

The most common presenting symptom is a rapidly enlarging thyroid with symptoms of compression and/or invasion that are also commonly seen in patients with anaplastic thyroid carcinoma. Approximately 50% of patients will have associated cervical adenopathy and approximately 10% of patients will have "B" symptoms consisting of fever, sweats, and weight loss. Half of patients will have disease limited to the thyroid gland and approximately 45% will have disease limited to the thyroid and locoregional nodes. Only about 5% of patients will have disease above and below the diaphragm or diffuse organ involvement.[185]

Diagnosis can often be made with FNAB and flow cytometry, but occasionally more tissue is needed and a large-bore needle biopsy or surgical excision is required for definitive diagnosis. The initial staging workup should include a complete blood count, serum chemistries (including TSH, LDH, and uric acid), and CT of the neck, chest, and abdomen. Some centers also advocate bone marrow examination in the intial workup. Staging is most commonly performed using the Ann Arbor stage classification.

Treatment is typically either radiation or combined chemotherapy and radiation. The role for surgery at most centers is for diagnostic purposes only. External beam radiation that includes the neck and mediastinal nodes is advocated for stage I disease whereas the addition of chemotherapy to stage II to IV disease is associated with improved outcomes in some studies.[186] The disease-specific 5-year survival of all patients with primary thyroid lymphoma is

45 to 65%.[185,187-191] However, patients with stage IIIE or stage IV disease have a 5-year survival of only 15 to 35%.[185,187]

MANAGEMENT OF PARATHYROID CARCINOMA

Parathyroid carcinoma accounts for between 0.1% and 5% of all patients with primary hyperparathyroidism and occurs equally in both men and women.[192-194] Patients typically present in the fifth and sixth decades of life.[195] The main distinguishing features of parathyroid carcinoma from parathyroid adenoma is the magnitude of symptomatic hypercalcemia and a frequently palpable neck mass. This is in contrast to benign primary hyperparathyroidism in which hypercalcemia is typically found incidentally and the adenoma is rarely palpable on clinical exam. Patients with parathyroid carcinoma often have severe nephrolithiasis and nephrocalcinosis as well as severe ostopenia due to the high levels of parathyroid hormone and calcium. Lymph node metastases are present in 17% to 32% of patients at diagnosis.[196,197]

If a diagnosis of parathyroid carcinoma is suspected, FNAB is contraindicated due to the risk of seeding. As intraoperative frozen sections are unreliable, clinical evaluation of the suspected parathyroid gland is extremely important. Typically, parathyroid carcinoma is adherent, firm, and whitish-gray, in contrast to normal parathyroid glands which have the color of peanut butter and have a soft consistency.[198] Identification at the time of surgery is extremely important because en bloc resection at the time of initial surgery provides the best chance for a durable cure. En bloc resection includes the preservation of the parathyroid capsule along with the removal of the ipsilateral thyroid lobe and any contiguous lymph nodes and fibrofatty tissue.[198] Of patients who have parathyroid carcinoma and have only routine parathyroidectomy, 50% will suffer local recurrence within a mean time of 41 months with a mean survival of only 62 months. In contrast, en bloc resection improves the local recurrence rate to 10% to 33% with an improvement in long-term

survival.[199,200] Attempts to remove recurrent disease are nearly universally unsuccessful.[201]

Adjuvant radiotherapy appears to offer some benefit. Studies at Princess Margaret Hospital, Mayo Clinic, and the M.D. Anderson Cancer Center have demonstrated decreased local recurrence and improved long-term survival with the use of external beam radiotherapy.[202-205]

SUMMARY

The diagnosis and management of thyroid malignancies continues to be a challenge to clinicians given the relatively high prevalence of thyroid nodules in the population. Epidemiologic studies have found palpable thyroid nodules in up to 5% of women and 1% of men in iodine-sufficient regions and with current imaging techniques, thyroid nodules can be found in over 60% of randomly selected patients. The challenge has been to identify the 5% to 10% of nodules that harbor a malignancy while minimizing the morbidity to the roughly 90% of patients whose nodules ultimately turn out to be benign. In addition, the lack of phase III clinical trial data on the relative efficacy of the various thyroid cancer management strategies has added to the controversy.

Currently, fine-needle aspiration (FNA) biopsy remains one of the key diagnostic tools for the evaluation of thyroid nodules. In the future, the use of molecular markers will almost assuredly increase our ability to correctly identify those patients at greatest risk of malignancy and ultimately decrease the need for unnecessary thyroidectomy. However, until these markers have achieved the required diagnostic accuracy, the key diagnostic step will be fine needle aspiration by routine cytologic analysis and thyroidectomy for those lesions that are repeatedly nondiagnostic, suspicious, or malignant. Most centers now recommend a total thyroidectomy for a known thyroid cancer at the time of FNA as well as completion thyroidectomy for nodules that are found to be malignant at the time of hemithyroidectomy. The use of neck dissection for regional metastases has been shown to be of high value in the treatment of most thyroid malignancies. In addition, postoperative radionucleotide scanning and ablation continue to play an important role in the management of many well-differentiated thyroid malignancies. Close surveillance of the postoperative patient is important to address recurrences that can be managed at an early, treatable stage.

REFERENCES

1. Jemal A, Murray T, Ward E, et al. Cancer statistics, 2005 [erratum appears in *CA: Cancer J Clin.* 2005;55(4):259]. *CA: Cancer J Clin.* 2005;55:10-30.

2. Jemal A, Siegel R, Ward E, et al. Cancer statistics, 2006. *CA: Cancer J Clin.* 2006;56:106-130.

3. Davies L, Welch HG. Increasing incidence of thyroid cancer in the United States, 1973-2002 [see Comment]. *JAMA.* 2006;295:2164-2167.

4. Harach HR, Franssila KO, Wasenius VM. Occult papillary carcinoma of the thyroid. A "normal" finding in Finland. A systematic autopsy study. *Cancer.* 1985;56:531-538.

5. Bondeson L, Ljungberg O. Occult thyroid carcinoma at autopsy in Malmo, Sweden. *Cancer.* 1981;47: 319-323.

6. Heitz P, Moser H, Staub JJ. Thyroid cancer: a study of 573 thyroid tumors and 161 autopsy cases observed over a thirty-year period. *Cancer.* 1976; 37:2329-2337.

7. Sobrinho-Simoes MA, Sambade MC, Goncalves V. Latent thyroid carcinoma at autopsy: a study from Oporto, Portugal. *Cancer.* 1979;43:1702-1706.

8. Solares CA, Penalonzo MA, Xu M, Orellana E. Occult papillary thyroid carcinoma in postmortem species: prevalence at autopsy. *Am J Otolaryngol.* 2005;26:87-90.

9. Mazzaferri EL, Jhiang SM. Long-term impact of initial surgical and medical therapy on papillary and follicular thyroid cancer [see Comment] [erratum appears in *Am J Med.* 1995;98(2):215]. *Am J Med.* 1994;97:418-428.

10. Belfiore A, La Rosa GL, La Porta GA, et al. Cancer risk in patients with cold thyroid nodules: relevance of iodine intake, sex, age, and multinodularity [see Comment]. *Am J Med.* 1992;93:363-369.

11. Winship T, Rosvoll RV. Cancer of the thyroid in children. *Proc Natl Canc Conf.* 1970;6:677-681.

12. Hanson GA, Komorowski RA, Cerletty JM, Wilson SD. Thyroid gland morphology in young adults: normal subjects versus those with prior low-dose neck irradiation in childhood. *Surgery.* 1983;94: 984-988.

13. Spitalnik PF, Straus FH 2nd. Patterns of human thyroid parenchymal reaction following low-dose childhood irradiation. *Cancer.* 1978;41:1098-1105.

14. Freedberg AS, Kurland GS, Blumgart HL. The pathologic effects of I131 on the normal thyroid gland of man. *J Clin Endoc Metab.* 1952;12: 1315-1348.

15. Ron E, Lubin JH, Shore RE, et al. Thyroid cancer after exposure to external radiation: a pooled analysis of seven studies. *Radiat Res.* 1995;141: 259-277.

16. Mehta MP, Goetowski PG, Kinsella TJ. Radiation induced thyroid neoplasms 1920 to 1987: a vanishing problem? *Int J Radiat Oncol Biol Phys.* 1989;16:1471-1475.

17. Jacob P, Goulko G, Heidenreich WF, et al. Thyroid cancer risk to children calculated. *Nature.* 1998; 392:31-32.

18. Wong FL, Ron E, Gierlowski T, Schneider AB. Benign thyroid tumors: general risk factors and their effects on radiation risk estimation. *Am J Epidemiol.* 1996;144:728-733.

19. Frankenthaler RA, Sellin RV, Cangir A, Goepfert H. Lymph node metastasis from papillary-follicular thyroid carcinoma in young patients. *Am J Surg.* 1990;160:341-343.

20. Agostini L, Mazzi P, Cavaliere A. Multiple primary malignant tumours: gemistocytic astrocytoma with leptomeningeal spreading and papillary thyroid carcinoma. A case report. *Acta Neurologica.* 1990;12:305-310.

21. Ledger GA, Khosla S, Lindor NM, Thibodeau SN, Gharib H. Genetic testing in the diagnosis and management of multiple endocrine neoplasia type II. *Ann Int Med.* 1995;122:118-124.

22. Lohrs U, Permanetter W, Spelsberg F, Beitinger M. Investigation of frequency and spreading of the different histological types of thyroid cancer in an endemic goiter region [in German]. *Verhandlungen der Deutschen Gesellschaft fur Pathologie.* 1977;61:268-274.

23. Hrafnkelsson J, Jonasson JG, Sigurdsson G, Sigvaldason H, Tulinius H. Thyroid cancer in Iceland 1955-1984. *Acta Endocrinologica.* 1988;118: 566-572.

24. Mazzaferri EL. Management of a solitary thyroid nodule [see Comment]. *New Engl J Med.* 1993; 328:553-559.

25. Burch HB. Evaluation and management of the solid thyroid nodule. *Endocrinol Metab Clin North Am*. 1995;24:663-710.

26. Ridgway EC. Clinical review 30: Clinician's evaluation of a solitary thyroid nodule. *J Clin Endocrinol Metab*. 1992;74:231-235.

27. Brander A, Viikinkoski P, Nickels J, Kivisaari L. Thyroid gland: US screening in a random adult population. *Radiology*. 1991;181:683-687.

28. Hagag P, Strauss S, Weiss M. Role of ultrasound-guided fine-needle aspiration biopsy in evaluation of nonpalpable thyroid nodules. *Thyroid*. 1998;8:989-995.

29. Tan GH, Gharib H. Thyroid incidentalomas: management approaches to nonpalpable nodules discovered incidentally on thyroid imaging. *Ann Int Med*. 1997;126:226-231.

30. Ezzat S, Sarti DA, Cain DR, Braunstein GD. Thyroid incidentalomas. Prevalence by palpation and ultrasonography [see Comment]. *Arch Int Med*. 1994;154:1838-1840.

31. Marqusee E, Benson CB, Frates MC, et al. Usefulness of ultrasonography in the management of nodular thyroid disease [see Comment]. *Ann Int Med*. 2000;133:696-700.

32. Papini E, Guglielmi R, Bianchini A, et al. Risk of malignancy in nonpalpable thyroid nodules: predictive value of ultrasound and color-Doppler features. *J Clin Endocrinol Metab*. 2002;87:1941-1946.

33. Blum M, Rothschild M. Improved nonoperative diagnosis of the solitary 'cold' thyroid nodule. Surgical selection based on risk factors and three months of suppression. *JAMA*. 1980;243:242-245.

34. Belanger R, Guillet F, Matte R, Havrankova J, d'Amour P. The thyroid nodule: evaluation of fine-needle biopsy. *J Otolaryngol*. 1983;12:109-111.

35. Hugues FC, Baudet M, Laccourreye H. [The thyroid nodule. A retrospective study of 200 cases] [in French]. *Ann Oto-Laryngol Chirurg Cervico-Facial*. 1989;106:77-81.

36. Okamoto T, Yamashita T, Harasawa A, et al. Test performances of three diagnostic procedures in evaluating thyroid nodules: physical examination, ultrasonography and fine needle aspiration cytology [erratum appears in *Endocr J*. 1995; 42(4):following 586]. *Endoc J*. 1994;41:243-247.

37. Piromalli D, Martelli G, Del Prato I, Collini P, Pilotti S. The role of fine needle aspiration in the diagnosis of thyroid nodules: analysis of 795 consecutive cases. *J Surg Oncol*. 1992;50:247-250.

38. McHenry C, Smith M, Lawrence AM, Jarosz H, Paloyan E. Nodular thyroid disease in children and adolescents: a high incidence of carcinoma. *Am Surgeon*. 1988;54:444-447.

39. Cersosimo E, Gharib H, Suman VJ, Goellner JR. "Suspicious" thyroid cytologic findings: outcome in patients without immediate surgical treatment. *Mayo Clinic Proc*. 1993;68:343-348.

40. Pacini F, Pinchera A, Giani C, et al. Serum thyroglobulin in thyroid carcinoma and other thyroid disorders. *J Endocrinol Investig*. 1980;3:283-292.

41. Eustatia-Rutten CFA, Smit JWA, Romijn JA, et al. Diagnostic value of serum thyroglobulin measurements in the follow-up of differentiated thyroid carcinoma, a structured meta-analysis. *Clin Endocrinol*. 2004;61:61-74.

42. Elisei R, Bottici V, Luchetti F, et al. Impact of routine measurement of serum calcitonin on the diagnosis and outcome of medullary thyroid cancer: experience in 10,864 patients with nodular thyroid disorders [see Comment]. *J Clin Endocrin Metab*. 2004;89:163-168.

43. Hahm JR, Lee MS, Min YK, et al. Routine measurement of serum calcitonin is useful for early detection of medullary thyroid carcinoma in patients with nodular thyroid diseases. *Thyroid*. 2001; 11:73-80.

44. Niccoli P, Wion-Barbot N, Caron P, et al. Interest of routine measurement of serum calcitonin: study in a large series of thyroidectomized patients. The French Medullary Study Group [see Comment]. *J Clin Endocrinol Metab*. 1997;82:338-341.

45. Cooper DS, Doherty GM, Haugen BR, et al. Management guidelines for patients with thyroid nodules and differentiated thyroid cancer. *Thyroid*. 2006;16:109-142.

46. Yang GC, Liebeskind D, Messina AV. Ultrasound-guided fine-needle aspiration of the thyroid assessed by Ultrafast Papanicolaou stain: data from 1135 biopsies with a two- to six-year follow-up. *Thyroid*. 2001;11:581-589.

47. Cochand-Priollet B, Guillausseau PJ, Chagnon S, et al. The diagnostic value of fine-needle aspiration biopsy under ultrasonography in nonfunctional thyroid nodules: a prospective study comparing cytologic and histologic findings [see Comment] [erratum appears in *Am J Med*. 1994;97(3):311]. *Am J Med*. 1994;97:152-157.

48. Takashima S, Fukuda H, Kobayashi T. Thyroid nodules: clinical effect of ultrasound-guided fine-needle aspiration biopsy. *J Clin Ultrasound*. 1994; 22:535-542.

49. Yokozawa T, Miyauchi A, Kuma K, Sugawara M. Accurate and simple method of diagnosing thy-

roid nodules the modified technique of ultrasound-guided fine needle aspiration biopsy. *Thyroid*. 1995;5:141–145.

50. Khurana KK, Richards VI, Chopra PS, et al. The role of ultrasonography-guided fine-needle aspiration biopsy in the management of nonpalpable and palpable thyroid nodules. *Thyroid*. 1998;8:511–515.

51. Carmeci C, Jeffrey RB, McDougall IR, Nowels KW, Weigel RJ. Ultrasound-guided fine-needle aspiration biopsy of thyroid masses. *Thyroid*. 1998;8:283–289.

52. Danese D, Sciacchitano S, Farsetti A, Andreoli M, Pontecorvi A. Diagnostic accuracy of conventional versus sonography-guided fine-needle aspiration biopsy of thyroid nodules. *Thyroid*. 1998;8:15–21.

53. Mikosch P, Gallowitsch HJ, Kresnik E, et al. Value of ultrasound-guided fine-needle aspiration biopsy of thyroid nodules in an endemic goitre area. *Eur J Nucl Med*. 2000;27:62–69.

54. Newkirk KA, Ringel MD, Jelinek J, et al. Ultrasound-guided fine-needle aspiration and thyroid disease. *Otolaryngol Head Neck Surg*. 2000;123:700–705.

55. Deandrea M, Mormile A, Veglio M, et al. Fine-needle aspiration biopsy of the thyroid: comparison between thyroid palpation and ultrasonography. *Endocr Pract*. 2002;8:282–286.

56. Leenhardt L, Hejblum G, Franc B, et al. Indications and limits of ultrasound-guided cytology in the management of nonpalpable thyroid nodules. *J Clin Endocrinol Metab*. 1999;84:24–28.

57. Sidawy MK, Del Vecchio DM, Knoll SM. Fine-needle aspiration of thyroid nodules: correlation between cytology and histology and evaluation of discrepant cases. *Cancer*. 1997;81:253–259.

58. Hall TL, Layfield LJ, Philippe A, Rosenthal DL. Sources of diagnostic error in fine needle aspiration of the thyroid. *Cancer*. 1989;63:718–725.

59. Baloch ZW, Sack MJ, Yu GH, Livolsi VA, Gupta PK. Fine-needle aspiration of thyroid: an institutional experience. *Thyroid*. 1998;8:565–569.

60. Gharib H, Goellner JR. Fine-needle aspiration biopsy of the thyroid: an appraisal [see Comment]. *Ann Int Med*. 1993;118:282–289.

61. Lachman MF, Cellura K, Schofield K, Mitra A. On-site adequacy assessments for image-directed fine needle aspirations: a study of 341 cases. *Connecticut Med*. 1995;59:657–660.

62. McHenry CR, Walfish PG, Rosen IB. Non-diagnostic fine needle aspiration biopsy: a dilemma in management of nodular thyroid disease. *Am Surgeon*. 1993;59:415–419.

63. Backdahl M, Wallin G, Lowhagen T, Auer G, Granberg PO. Fine-needle biopsy cytology and DNA analysis. Their place in the evaluation and treatment of patients with thyroid neoplasms. *Surg Clin North Am*. 1987;67:197–211.

64. Finley DJ, Zhu B, Fahey TJ 3rd. Molecular analysis of Hürthle cell neoplasms by gene profiling. *Surgery*. 2004;136:1160–1168.

65. Finley DJ, Zhu B, Barden CB, Fahey TJ 3rd. Discrimination of benign and malignant thyroid nodules by molecular profiling. *Ann Surg*. 2004;240:425–436; discussion 36–37.

66. Finley DJ, Arora N, Zhu B, Gallagher L, Fahey TJ 3rd. Molecular profiling distinguishes papillary carcinoma from benign thyroid nodules. *J Clin Endocrinol Metab*. 2004;89:3214–3223.

67. Finley DJ, Lubitz CC, Wei C, Zhu B, Fahey TJ, 3rd. Advancing the molecular diagnosis of thyroid nodules: defining benign lesions by molecular profiling. *Thyroid*. 2005;15:562–568.

68. Lubitz CC, Gallagher LA, Finley DJ, Zhu B, Fahey TJ 3rd. Molecular analysis of minimally invasive follicular carcinomas by gene profiling. *Surgery*. 2005;138:1042–1048; discussion 48–49.

69. Gharib H, Goellner JR, Johnson DA. Fine-needle aspiration cytology of the thyroid. A 12-year experience with 11,000 biopsies. *Clin Lab Med*. 1993;13:699–709.

70. Vassallo P, Wernecke K, Roos N, Peters PE. Differentiation of benign from malignant superficial lymphadenopathy: the role of high-resolution US. *Radiology*. 1992;183:215–220.

71. Bruneton JN, Roux P, Caramella E, et al. Ear, nose, and throat cancer: ultrasound diagnosis of metastasis to cervical lymph nodes. *Radiology*. 1984;152:771–773.

72. Wang J, Takashima S, Matsushita T, et al. Esophageal invasion by thyroid carcinomas: prediction using magnetic resonance imaging. *J Comp Assis Tomog*. 2003;27:18–25.

73. Takashima S, Matsushita T, Takayama F, et al. Prognostic significance of magnetic resonance findings in advanced papillary thyroid cancer. *Thyroid*. 2001;11:1153–1159.

74. Wang JC, Takashima S, Takayama F, et al. Tracheal invasion by thyroid carcinoma: prediction using MR imaging. *AJR American Journal of Roentgenology*. 2001;177:929–936.

75. Cancer AJCo. *AJCC Cancer Staging Manual*. 6th ed. New York, NY: Springer-Verlag; 2002.

76. Brierley JD, Panzarella T, Tsang RW, Gospodarowicz MK, O'Sullivan B. A comparison of different

staging systems predictability of patient outcome. Thyroid carcinoma as an example. *Cancer*. 1997; 79:2414-2423.

77. Hannequin P, Liehn JC, Delisle MJ. Multifactorial analysis of survival in thyroid cancer. Pitfalls of applying the results of published studies to another population. *Cancer*. 1986;58:1749-1755.

78. Cady B, Rossi R. An expanded view of risk-group definition in differentiated thyroid carcinoma. *Surgery*. 1988;104;947-953.

79. Sanders LE, Cady B. Differentiated thyroid cancer: reexamination of risk groups and outcome of treatment. *Arch Surg*. 1998;133:419-425.

80. Hay ID, Grant CS, Taylor WF, McConahey WM. Ipsilateral lobectomy versus bilateral lobar resection in papillary thyroid carcinoma: a retrospective analysis of surgical outcome using a novel prognostic scoring system. *Surgery*. 1987;102: 1088-1095.

81. Hay ID, Bergstralh EJ, Goellner JR, Ebersold JR, Grant CS. Predicting outcome in papillary thyroid carcinoma: development of a reliable prognostic scoring system in a cohort of 1779 patients surgically treated at one institution during 1940 through 1989. *Surgery*. 1993;114:1050-1057; discussion 1057-1059.

82. Thyroid Carcinoma Task F. AACE/AAES medical/ surgical guidelines for clinical practice: management of thyroid carcinoma. American Association of Clinical Endocrinologists. *Am Coll Endocrinol Endocr Prac*. 2001;7:202-220.

83. British Thyroid Association and Royal College of Physicians 2002 Guidelines for the management of thyroid cancer in adults. Available from http:// www.british_thyroid_association.org/guidelines .htm2002

84. National Comprehensive Cancer Network. Thyroid carcinoma. Available from http://www .nccn.org/professionals/physician_gls/PDF/ thyroid.pdf

85. Schlumberger MJ. Papillary and follicular thyroid carcinoma. *New Engl J Med*. 1998;338: 297-306.

86. Ain KB. Papillary thyroid carcinoma. Etiology, assessment, and therapy. *Endocrinol Metab Clin North Am*. 1995;24:711-760.

87. Hay ID. Papillary thyroid carcinoma. *Endocrinol Metab Clin North Am*. 1990;19:545-576.

88. Samuel AM, Sharma SM. Differentiated thyroid carcinomas in children and adolescents. *Cancer*. 1991;67:2186-2190.

89. Ceccarelli C, Pacini F, Lippi F, et al. Thyroid cancer in children and adolescents. *Surgery*. 1988;104: 1143-1148.

90. De Jong SA, Demeter JG, Jarosz H, Lawrence AM, Paloyan E. Primary papillary thyroid carcinoma presenting as cervical lymphadenopathy: the operative approach to the "lateral aberrant thyroid." *Am Surgeon*. 1993;59:172-176; discussion 176-177.

91. Arturi F, Russo D, Giuffrida D, et al. Early diagnosis by genetic analysis of differentiated thyroid cancer metastases in small lymph nodes. *J Clin Endocrinol Metab*. 1997;82:1638-1641.

92. Qubain SW, Nakano S, Baba M, Takao S, Aikou T. Distribution of lymph node micrometastasis in pN0 well-differentiated thyroid carcinoma. *Surgery*. 2002;131:249-256.

93. Hay ID, McConahey WM, Goellner JR. Managing patients with papillary thyroid carcinoma: insights gained from the Mayo Clinic's experience of treating 2,512 consecutive patients during 1940 through 2000. *Trans Am Clin Climatol Assoc*. 2002;113: 241-260.

94. Baudin E, Travagli JP, Ropers J, et al. Microcarcinoma of the thyroid gland: the Gustave-Roussy Institute experience [see Comment]. *Cancer*. 1998;83:553-559.

95. Salvesen H, Njolstad PR, Akslen LA, et al. Papillary thyroid carcinoma: a multivariate analysis of prognostic factors including an evaluation of the p-TNM staging system. *Eur J Surg*. 1992;158:583-589.

96. Hazard JB. Classification and staging of thyroid cancer. *J Surg Oncol*. 1981;16:255-257.

97. Sywak M, Pasieka JL, Ogilvie T. A review of thyroid cancer with intermediate differentiation. *J Surg Oncol*. 2004;86:44-54.

98. Soares J, Limbert E, Sobrinho-Simoes M. Diffuse sclerosing variant of papillary thyroid carcinoma. A clinicopathologic study of 10 cases. *Pathol Res Prac*. 1989;185:200-206.

99. Tielens ET, Sherman SI, Hruban RH, Ladenson PW. Follicular variant of papillary thyroid carcinoma. A clinicopathologic study. *Cancer*. 1994; 73:424-431.

100. van Heerden JA, Hay ID, Goellner JR, et al. Follicular thyroid carcinoma with capsular invasion alone: a nonthreatening malignancy. *Surgery*. 1992;112:1130-1136; discussion 1136-1138.

101. Hay ID, Thompson GB, Grant CS, et al. Papillary thyroid carcinoma managed at the Mayo Clinic during six decades (1940-1999): temporal trends in initial therapy and long-term outcome in 2444

consecutively treated patients. *World J Surg.* 2002;26:879-885.

102. Shaha AR, Shah JP, Loree TR. Differentiated thyroid cancer presenting initially with distant metastasis. *Am J Surg.* 1997;174:474-476.

103. Haigh PI, Urbach DR, Rotstein LE. Extent of thyroidectomy is not a major determinant of survival in low- or high-risk papillary thyroid cancer. *Ann Surg Oncol.* 2005;12:81-89.

104. Kouvaraki MA, Shapiro SE, Fornage BD, et al. Role of preoperative ultrasonography in the surgical management of patients with thyroid cancer. *Surgery.* 2003;134:946-954; discussion 954-955.

105. Grebe SK, Hay ID. Thyroid cancer nodal metastases: biologic significance and therapeutic considerations. *Surg Oncol Clin North Am.* 1996;5:43-63.

106. Tisell LE, Nilsson B, Molne J, et al. Improved survival of patients with papillary thyroid cancer after surgical microdissection. *World J Surg.* 1996;20:854-859.

107. Scheumann GF, Gimm O, Wegener G, Hundeshagen H, Dralle H. Prognostic significance and surgical management of locoregional lymph node metastases in papillary thyroid cancer. *World J Surg.* 1994;18:559-567; discussion 567-568.

108. Ito Y, Tomoda C, Uruno T, et al. Preoperative ultrasonographic examination for lymph node metastasis: usefulness when designing lymph node dissection for papillary microcarcinoma of the thyroid. *World J Surg.* 2004;28:498-501.

109. Gemsenjager E, Perren A, Seifert B, et al. Lymph node surgery in papillary thyroid carcinoma. *J Am Coll Surg.* 2003;197:182-190.

110. Udelsman R, Lakatos E, Ladenson P. Optimal surgery for papillary thyroid carcinoma. *World J Surg.* 1996;20:88-93.

111. Sosa JA, Bowman HM, Tielsch JM, et al. The importance of surgeon experience for clinical and economic outcomes from thyroidectomy. *Ann Surgery.* 1998;228:320-330.

112. Sawka AM, Thephamongkhol K, Brouwers M, et al. Clinical review 170: a systematic review and metaanalysis of the effectiveness of radioactive iodine remnant ablation for well-differentiated thyroid cancer [see Comment]. *J Clin Endocrinol Metab.* 2004;89:3668-3676.

113. DeGroot LJ, Kaplan EL, McCormick M, Straus FH. Natural history, treatment, and course of papillary thyroid carcinoma. *J Clin Endocrinol Metabol.* 1990;71:414-424.

114. Mazzaferri EL. Thyroid remnant 131I ablation for papillary and follicular thyroid carcinoma. *Thyroid.* 1997;7:265-271.

115. Robbins RJ, Larson SM, Sinha N, et al. A retrospective review of the effectiveness of recombinant human TSH as a preparation for radioiodine thyroid remnant ablation. *J Nucl Med.* 2002;43:1482-1488.

116. Pacini F, Molinaro E, Castagna MG, et al. Ablation of thyroid residues with 30 mCi (131)I: a comparison in thyroid cancer patients prepared with recombinant human TSH or thyroid hormone withdrawal [see Comment]. *J Clin Endocrinol Metab.* 2002;87:4063-4068.

117. Fatourechi V, Hay ID, Mullan BP, et al. Are posttherapy radioiodine scans informative and do they influence subsequent therapy of patients with differentiated thyroid cancer? *Thyroid.* 2000;10:573-577.

118. Sherman SI, Tielens ET, Sostre S, Wharam MD Jr., Ladenson PW. Clinical utility of posttreatment radioiodine scans in the management of patients with thyroid carcinoma. *J Clin Endocrinol Metab.* 1994;78:629-634.

119. Tsang RW, Brierley JD, Simpson WJ, et al. The effects of surgery, radioiodine, and external radiation therapy on the clinical outcome of patients with differentiated thyroid carcinoma. *Cancer.* 1998;82:375-388.

120. Phlips P, Hanzen C, Andry G, Van Houtte P, Fruuling J. Postoperative irradiation for thyroid cancer. *Eur J Surg Oncol.* 1993;19:399-404.

121. Benker G, Olbricht T, Reinwein D, et al. Survival rates in patients with differentiated thyroid carcinoma. Influence of postoperative external radiotherapy. *Cancer.* 1990;65:1517-1520.

122. Farahati J, Reiners C, Stuschke M, et al. Differentiated thyroid cancer. Impact of adjuvant external radiotherapy in patients with perithyroidal tumor infiltration (stage pT4). *Cancer.* 1996;77:172-180.

123. Simpson WJ, Panzarella T, Carruthers JS, Gospodarowicz MK, Sutcliffe SB. Papillary and follicular thyroid cancer: impact of treatment in 1578 patients. *Int J Radiat Oncol Biol Phys.* 1988;14:1063-1075.

124. Hoskin PJ, Harmer C. Chemotherapy for thyroid cancer. *Radiother Oncol.* 1987;10:187-194.

125. Gottlieb JA, Hill CS, Jr. Chemotherapy of thyroid cancer with adriamycin. Experience with 30 patients. *New Engl J Med.* 1974;290:193-197.

126. Shimaoka K, Schoenfeld DA, DeWys WD, Creech RH, DeConti R. A randomized trial of doxorubicin versus doxorubicin plus cisplatin in patients with advanced thyroid carcinoma. *Cancer.* 1985;56: 2155-2160.

127. Spencer CA, LoPresti JS, Fatemi S, Nicoloff JT. Detection of residual and recurrent differentiated thyroid carcinoma by serum thyroglobulin measurement. *Thyroid.* 1999;9:435-441.

128. Spencer CA. Challenges of serum thyroglobulin (Tg) measurement in the presence of Tg autoantibodies [Comment]. *J Clin Endocrinol Metab.* 2004;89:3702-3704.

129. David A, Blotta A, Rossi R, et al. Clinical value of different responses of serum thyroglobulin to recombinant human thyrotropin in the follow-up of patients with differentiated thyroid carcinoma. *Thyroid.* 2005;15:267-273.

130. Khan N, Oriuchi N, Higuchi T, Zhang H, Endo K. PET in the follow-up of differentiated thyroid cancer. *Br J Radiol.* 2003;76:690-695.

131. Cooper DS, Specker B, Ho M, et al. Thyrotropin suppression and disease progression in patients with differentiated thyroid cancer: results from the National Thyroid Cancer Treatment Cooperative Registry. *Thyroid.* 1998;8:737-744.

132. McGriff NJ, Csako G, Gourgiotis L, et al. Effects of thyroid hormone suppression therapy on adverse clinical outcomes in thyroid cancer. *Ann Med.* 2002;34:554-564.

133. Pujol P, Daures JP, Nsakala N, et al. Degree of thyrotropin suppression as a prognostic determinant in differentiated thyroid cancer. *J Clin Endocrinol Metab.* 1996;81:4318-4323.

134. Brennan MD, Bergstralh EJ, van Heerden JA, McConahey WM. Follicular thyroid cancer treated at the Mayo Clinic, 1946 through 1970: initial manifestations, pathologic findings, therapy, and outcome [see Comment]. *Mayo Clinic Proc.* 1991;66:11-22.

135. LiVolsi VA, Asa SL. The demise of follicular carcinoma of the thyroid gland. *Thyroid.* 1994;4: 233-236.

136. Jensen MH, Davis RK, Derrick L. Thyroid cancer: a computer-assisted review of 5287 cases. *Otolaryngol Head Neck Surg.* 1990;102:51-65.

137. Ruegemer JJ, Hay ID, Bergstralh EJ, et al. Distant metastases in differentiated thyroid carcinoma: a multivariate analysis of prognostic variables. *J Clin Endocrinol Metab.* 1988;67:501-508.

138. Schlumberger M, Tubiana M, De Vathaire F, et al. Long-term results of treatment of 283 patients with lung and bone metastases from differentiated thyroid carcinoma. *J Clin Endocrinol Metab.* 1986;63:960-967.

139. Young RL, Mazzaferri EL, Rahe AJ, Dorfman SG. Pure follicular thyroid carcinoma: impact of therapy in 214 patients. *J Nucl Med.* 1980;21: 733-737.

140. D'Avanzo A, Treseler P, Ituarte PHG, et al. Follicular thyroid carcinoma: histology and prognosis. *Cancer.* 2004;100:1123-1129.

141. Samaan NA, Schultz PN, Hickey RC, et al. The results of various modalities of treatment of well differentiated thyroid carcinomas: a retrospective review of 1599 patients. *J Clin Endocrinol Metab.* 1992;75:714-720.

142. Samaan NA, Schultz PN, Haynie TP, Ordonez NG. Pulmonary metastasis of differentiated thyroid carcinoma: treatment results in 101 patients. *J Clin Endocrinol Metabol.* 1985;60:376-380.

143. DeGroot LJ, Kaplan EL, Shukla MS, Salti G, Straus FH. Morbidity and mortality in follicular thyroid cancer. *J Clin Endocrinol Metabol.* 1995;80: 2946-2953.

144. Kushchayeva Y, Duh Q-Y, Kebebew E, Clark OH. Prognostic indications for Hürthle cell cancer. *World J Surg.* 2004;28:1266-1270.

145. Cooper DS, Schneyer CR. Follicular and Hürthle cell carcinoma of the thyroid. *Endocrinol Metab Clin North Am.* 1990;19:577-591.

146. Azadian A, Rosen IB, Walfish PG, Asa SL. Management considerations in Hürthle cell carcinoma. *Surgery.* 1995;118:711-714; discussion 714-715.

147. Kinder BK. Well differentiated thyroid cancer. *Curr Opin Oncol.* 2003;15:71-77.

148. Bhattacharyya N. Survival and prognosis in Hürthle cell carcinoma of the thyroid gland. *Arch Otolaryngol Head Neck Surg.* 2003;129: 207-210.

149. Stojadinovic A, Ghossein RA, Hoos A, et al. Hürthle cell carcinoma: a critical histopathologic appraisal. *J Clin Oncol.* 2001;19:2616-2625.

150. Lang W, Choritz H, Hundeshagen H. Risk factors in follicular thyroid carcinomas. A retrospective follow-up study covering a 14-year period with emphasis on morphological findings. *Am J Surg Pathol.* 1986;10:246-55.

151. Foote RL, Brown PD, Garces YI, McIver B, Kasperbauer JL. Is there a role for radiation therapy in the management of Hürthle cell carcinoma? *Int J Radiat Oncol Biol Phys.* 2003;56:1067-1072.

152. Chow S-M, Law SCK, Au S-K, et al. Differentiated thyroid carcinoma: comparison between papil-

lary and follicular carcinoma in a single institute. *Head Neck*. 2002;24:670–677.

153. Grebe SK, Hay ID. Follicular thyroid cancer. *Endocrinol Metab Clin North Am*. 1995;24:761–801.

154. Grunwald F, Kalicke T, Feine U, et al. Fluorine-18 fluorodeoxyglucose positron emission tomography in thyroid cancer: results of a multicentre study. *Eur J Nucl Med*. 1999;26:1547–1552.

155. Cohen R, Campos JM, Salaun C, et al. Preoperative calcitonin levels are predictive of tumor size and postoperative calcitonin normalization in medullary thyroid carcinoma. Groupe d'Etudes des Tumeurs a Calcitonine (GETC). *J Clin Endocrinol Metab*. 2000;85:919–922.

156. Massoll N, Mazzaferri EL. Diagnosis and management of medullary thyroid carcinoma. *Clin Lab Med*. 2004;24:49–83.

157. Blaugrund JE, Johns MM, Jr., Eby YJ, et al. RET proto-oncogene mutations in inherited and sporadic medullary thyroid cancer. *Hum Molec Gen*. 1994;3:1895–1897.

158. Brandi ML, Gagel RF, Angeli A, et al. Guidelines for diagnosis and therapy of MEN type 1 and type 2 [see Comment]. *J Clin Endocrinol Metab*. 2001; 86:5658–5671.

159. Saad MF, Ordonez NG, Rashid RK, et al. Medullary carcinoma of the thyroid. A study of the clinical features and prognostic factors in 161 patients. *Medicine*. 1984;63:319–342.

160. Kakudo K, Carney JA, Sizemore GW. Medullary carcinoma of thyroid. Biologic behavior of the sporadic and familial neoplasm. *Cancer*. 1985;55: 2818–2821.

161. Machens A, Niccoli-Sire P, Hoegel J, et al. Early malignant progression of hereditary medullary thyroid cancer [see Comment]. *N Engl J Med*. 2003;349:1517–1525.

162. Wohllk N, Cote GJ, Bugalho MM, et al. Relevance of RET proto-oncogene mutations in sporadic medullary thyroid carcinoma. *J Clin Endocrinol Metab*. 1996;81:3740–3745.

163. Beressi N, Campos JM, Beressi JP, et al. Sporadic medullary microcarcinoma of the thyroid: a retrospective analysis of eighty cases. *Thyroid*. 1998; 8:1039–1044.

164. Moley JF, DeBenedetti MK. Patterns of nodal metastases in palpable medullary thyroid carcinoma: recommendations for extent of node dissection. *Ann Surg*. 1999;229:880–887; discussion 887–888.

165. Kebebew E, Ituarte PH, Siperstein AE, Duh QY, Clark OH. Medullary thyroid carcinoma: clinical

166. Russo D, Arturi F, Chiefari E, et al. A case of metastatic medullary thyroid carcinoma: early identification before surgery of an RET proto-oncogene somatic mutation in fine-needle aspirate specimens. *J Clin Endocrinol Metab*. 1997; 82:3378–3382.

167. Hyer SL, Vini L, A'Hern R, Harmer C. Medullary thyroid cancer: multivariate analysis of prognostic factors influencing survival. *Eur J Surg Oncol*. 2000;26:686–690.

168. Weber T, Schilling T, Frank-Raue K, et al. Impact of modified radical neck dissection on biochemical cure in medullary thyroid carcinomas. *Surgery*. 2001;130:1044–1049.

169. Rougier P, Parmentier C, Laplanche A, et al. Medullary thyroid carcinoma: prognostic factors and treatment. *Int J Radiat Oncol Biol Phys*. 1983;9:161–169.

170. Sarrazin D, Fontaine F, Rougier P, et al. Role of radiotherapy in the treatment of medullary cancer of the thyroid. *Bull Cancer*. 1984;71:200–208.

171. Schuffenecker I, Virally-Monod M, Brohet R, et al. Risk and penetrance of primary hyperparathyroidism in multiple endocrine neoplasia type 2A families with mutations at codon 634 of the RET proto-oncogene. Groupe D'etude des Tumeurs a Calcitonine. *J Clin Endocrinol Metab*. 1998;83: 487–491.

172. Gagel RF, Tashjian AH, Jr., Cummings T, et al. The clinical outcome of prospective screening for multiple endocrine neoplasia type 2a. An 18-year experience. *New Engl J Med*. 1988;318:478–484.

173. Eng C. Seminars in medicine of the Beth Israel Hospital, Boston. The RET proto-oncogene in multiple endocrine neoplasia type 2 and Hirschsprung's disease. *New Engl J Med*. 1996;335: 943–951.

174. Skinner MA, DeBenedetti MK, Moley JF, Norton JA, Wells SA Jr. Medullary thyroid carcinoma in children with multiple endocrine neoplasia types 2A and 2B. *J Pediat Surg*. 1996;31:177–181; discussion 181–182.

175. Rossel M, Schuffenecker I, Schlumberger M, et al. Detection of a germline mutation at codon 918 of the RET proto-oncogene in French MEN 2B families. *Hum Genet*. 1995;95:403–406.

176. Fugazzola L, Cerutti N, Mannavola D, et al. Multi-generational familial medullary thyroid cancer (FMTC): evidence for FMTC phenocopies and

association with papillary thyroid cancer [erratum appears in *Clin Endocrinol (Oxf)*. 2002 Apr;56(4):563]. *Clin Endocrinol*. 2002;56:53-63.

177. O'Neill JP, O'Neill B, Condron C, Walsh M, Bouchier-Hayes D. Anaplastic (undifferentiated) thyroid cancer: improved insight and therapeutic strategy into a highly aggressive disease. *J Laryngol Otol*. 2005;119:585-591.

178. Are C, Shaha AR. Anaplastic thyroid carcinoma: biology, pathogenesis, prognostic factors, and treatment approaches. *Ann Surg Oncol*. 2006;13: 453-464.

179. McIver B, Hay ID, Giuffrida DF, et al. Anaplastic thyroid carcinoma: a 50-year experience at a single institution. *Surgery*. 2001;130:1028-1034.

180. Giuffrida D, Gharib H. Anaplastic thyroid carcinoma: current diagnosis and treatment. *Ann Oncol*. 2000;11:1083-1089.

181. Pierie J-PEN, Muzikansky A, Gaz RD, Faquin WC, Ott MJ. The effect of surgery and radiotherapy on outcome of anaplastic thyroid carcinoma. *Ann Surg Oncol*. 2002;9:57-64.

182. Tennvall J, Lundell G, Wahlberg P, et al. Anaplastic thyroid carcinoma: three protocols combining doxorubicin, hyperfractionated radiotherapy and surgery. *Br J Canc*. 2002;86:1848-1853.

183. Besic N, Auersperg M, Us-Krasovec M, et al. Effect of primary treatment on survival in anaplastic thyroid carcinoma. *Eur J Surg Oncol*. 2001;27:260-264.

184. Coltrera MD. Primary T-cell lymphoma of the thyroid. *Head Neck*. 1999;21:160-163.

185. Pedersen RK, Pedersen NT. Primary non-Hodgkin's lymphoma of the thyroid gland: a population based study. *Histopathol*. 1996;28:25-32.

186. Harrington KJ, Michalaki VJ, Vini L, et al. Management of non-Hodgkin's lymphoma of the thyroid: the Royal Marsden Hospital experience. *Br J Radiol*. 2005;78:405-410.

187. Pyke CM, Grant CS, Habermann TM, et al. Non-Hodgkin's lymphoma of the thyroid: is more than biopsy necessary? *World J Surg*. 1992;16:604-609; discussion 609-610.

188. Logue JP, Hale RJ, Stewart AL, Duthie MB, Banerjee SS. Primary malignant lymphoma of the thyroid: a clinicopathological analysis. *Int J Radiat Oncol Biol Phys*. 1992;22:929-933.

189. Tsang RW, Gospodarowicz MK, Sutcliffe SB, et al. Non-Hodgkin's lymphoma of the thyroid gland: prognostic factors and treatment outcome. The Princess Margaret Hospital Lymphoma Group. *Int J Radiat Oncol Biol Phys*. 1993;27: 599-604.

190. Derringer GA, Thompson LD, Frommelt RA, et al. Malignant lymphoma of the thyroid gland: a clinicopathologic study of 108 cases. *Am J Surg Pathol*. 2000;24:623-639.

191. DiBiase SJ, Grigsby PW, Guo C, Lin HS, Wasserman TH. Outcome analysis for stage IE and IIE thyroid lymphoma. *Am J Clin Oncol*. 2004;27: 178-184.

192. Kebebew E. Parathyroid carcinoma. *Curr Treat Options Oncol*. 2001;2:347-354.

193. Obara T, Fujimoto Y, Ito Y. Primary hyperparathyroidism in patients with multiple endocrine neoplasia type 1: experience by a single surgical team in Japan. *Henry Ford Hospital Med J*. 1992;40:191-194.

194. Favia G, Lumachi F, Polistina F, D'Amico DF. Parathyroid carcinoma: sixteen new cases and suggestions for correct management. *World J Surg*. 1998;22:1225-1230.

195. Babar-Craig H, Quaglia A, Stearns M. Parathyroid carcinoma: a report of two cases and a concise review and update of the literature. *J Laryngol Otol*. 2005;119:577-580.

196. Shaha AR, Shah JP. Parathyroid carcinoma: a diagnostic and therapeutic challenge [Comment]. *Cancer*. 1999;86:378-380.

197. Hundahl SA, Fleming ID, Fremgen AM, Menck HR. Two hundred eighty-six cases of parathyroid carcinoma treated in the U.S. between 1985-1995: a National Cancer Data Base Report. The American College of Surgeons Commission on Cancer and the American Cancer Society [see Comment]. *Cancer*. 1999;86:538-544.

198. Rodgers SE, Perrier ND. Parathyroid carcinoma. *Curr Opin Oncol*. 2006;18:16-22.

199. Wang CA, Gaz RD. Natural history of parathyroid carcinoma. Diagnosis, treatment, and results. *Am J Surg*. 1985;149:522-527.

200. Koea JB, Shaw JH. Parathyroid cancer: biology and management. *Surg Oncol*. 1999;8:155-165.

201. Iacobone M, Ruffolo C, Lumachi F, Favia G. Results of iterative surgery for persistent and recurrent parathyroid carcinoma. *Langenbecks Arch Surgery*. 2005;390:385-390.

202. Busaidy NL, Jimenez C, Habra MA, et al. Parathyroid carcinoma: a 22-year experience. *Head Neck*. 2004;26:716-726.

203. Clayman GL, Gonzalez HE, El-Naggar A, Vassilopoulou-Sellin R. Parathyroid carcinoma: evaluation and interdisciplinary management. *Cancer*. 2004;100:900-905.

204. Chow E, Tsang RW, Brierley JD, Filice S. Parathyroid carcinoma—the Princess Margaret Hospital experience. *Int J Radiat Oncol Biol Phys*. 1998; 41:569-572.

205. Munson ND, Foote RL, Northcutt RC, et al. Parathyroid carcinoma: is there a role for adjuvant radiation therapy? *Cancer*. 2003;98:2378-2384.

23

Malignant Neoplasms of the Temporal Bone

Sam J. Marzo
John P. Leonetti
Guy J. Petruzzelli

INTRODUCTION

The contemporary management of malignant neoplasms of the ear and temporal bone has evolved with advances in neurotology, skull base surgery, head and neck oncology, neurosurgery, plastic and reconstructive surgery, diagnostic and therapeutic radiology, and adjuvant chemoradiotherapy. En bloc oncologic resection with negative margins is now possible in the majority of lesions affecting this area. Regional rotational and free-flap reconstruction can be performed after surgical resection. Cranial nerve deficits (facial and lower cranial nerves) resulting from treatment of neoplasms in this area can now be addressed with acceptable rehabilitative outcomes. The goals of minimizing patient morbidity and maximizing quality of life remain important. This chapter discusses the modern evaluation and management of malignant lesions of the ear and lateral temporal bone.

SURGICAL ANATOMY

A correct understanding of the surgical anatomy of the temporal bone is critical to successful treatment and management of malignant lesions in this region.

The temporal bone has five divisions: mastoid (posterior), squamous (superior), petrous (medial), tympanic (lateral), and zygomatic (anterior). Each of these anatomic areas contains critical structures and is adjacent to important areas of the lateral skull base. Figure 23-1 is a sagittal section of the human temporal bone highlighting the relationships between the ossicular chain, facial nerve, cochlea, and carotid artery. The middle cranial fossa is superior to the temporal bone, the sigmoid sinus and posterior

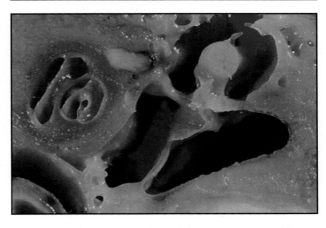

Fig 23–1. Sagittal section of human temporal bone showing relationships of facial nerve, cochlea, ossicular chain, and carotid artery.

cranial fossa are posterior and medial, the mandible, glenoid fossa, and parotid gland are anterior, and the cartilaginous pinna with overlying squamous epithelium is lateral.

Tumors of the temporal bone often can be relatively asymptomatic; therefore, patients can present with advanced disease. Also, the temporal bone has several anatomic relationship-preformed end pathways predisposing to local and regional spread of disease. Many tumors begin in the external auditory canal (EAC). The EAC is lined by a thin layer of periosteum and squamous epithelium. The medial border of the EAC is the tympanic membrane (TM), which has an outer squamous layer, a middle fibrous layer, and a medial layer of columnar epithelium. Once the TM is breached, the tumor can spread medially along the petrous apex into the carotid canal and along the petrous carotid artery. Posterior extension into the mastoid can lead to facial nerve invasion and paralysis. Inferior invasion into the jugular foramen can result in lower cranial nerve paralysis. Anterior extension through the tympanic bone can result in glenoid fossa/temporomandibular joint involvement and then invasion of the infratemporal fossa. Superior extension through the squamous portion of the temporal bone overlying the middle ear can result in invasion of the middle cranial fossa dura and brain parenchyma.

A critical understanding of the course of the infratemporal facial nerve is very important in addressing management of lesions in this area. Figure 23-2 shows an axial section of the facial nerve as it courses through the temporal bone. The facial nerve has several divisions within the temporal bone. The meatal segment is within the internal auditory canal. Next is the labyrinthine (or geniculate) segment, which gives rise to the geniculate ganglion and greater superficial petrosal nerve. The tympanic segment begins at the cochleaform process and traverses between the horizontal semicircular canal and stapes superstructure. At the pyramidal process (through which courses the stapes tendon) the nerve becomes the descending mastoid segment. Finally, the nerve leaves the temporal bone through the stylomastoid foramen and enters the substance of the parotid gland, forming the extratemporal segment.

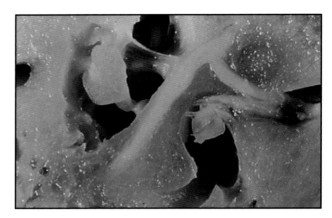

Fig 23–2. Axial section of human temporal bone showing course of infratemporal facial nerve.

REGIONAL PATHOLOGY AND DIFFERENTIAL DIAGNOSIS

The complete differential diagnosis of temporal bone neoplasms is extensive and is presented in Table 23-1.[1] As the temporal bone contains bony, cartilaginous, epithelial, respiratory, vascular, paraganglioma, and neural tissues, virtually every type of tumor can occur. Tumors can be benign or malignant, can arise from tissues within or adjacent to the temporal bone, and can also metastasize to the temporal bone.

An understanding of the regional tissue histology can help one develop an effective differential diagnosis when treating patients with temporal bone neoplasms. The EAC, tympanic membrane, and pinna are covered by squamous epithelium, which can give rise to squamous cell carcinoma. Neoplastic change within epidermal elements can also result in basal cell carcinoma and melanoma. The middle ear mucosa is lined by a nonstratified columnar respiratory epithelium. Neoplastic change of this tissue fortunately is rare, but can result in adenomatous tumors of the middle ear. Glomus tumors, which are the most common benign tumors of the temporal bone, arise from paraganglioma along Jacobson's nerve (glomus tympanicum tumors) and along the jugular bulb (glomus jugulare tumors). Hemangiomas and schwannomas

Table 23–1. Differential Diagnosis of Temporal Bone Neoplasms

EXTERNAL AUDITORY CANAL

Benign:	Pleomorphic adenoma
	Ceruminous adenoma
Malignant:	Squamous cell carcinoma
	Basal cell carcinoma
	Sarcoma
	Melanoma
	Lymphoma
	Adenocarcinoma
	Adenoid cystic carcinoma
	Ceruminous adenocarcinoma

MIDDLE EAR AND MASTOID

Epithelial neoplasms

Benign:	Mucosal adenoma
	Papillary adenoma
	Papilloma
Malignant:	Squamous cell carcinoma
	Basal cell carcinoma
	Adenocarcinoma
	Carcinoid tumor

Soft tissue neoplasms

Benign:	Paraganglioma
	Myxoma
	Lipoma
	Hemangioma
	Schwannoma
	Neurofibroma
Malignant:	Rhabdomyosarcoma
	Malignant paraganglioma
	Malignant schwannoma
	Hemangiopericytoma

Tumors of bone and cartilage

Benign:	Osteoma
	Chondroblastoma
	Giant cell tumor
Malignant:	Osteosarcoma
	Chondrosarcoma

Miscellaneous

Benign:	Meningioma
	Teratoma
Malignant:	Malignant germ cell tumor

Malignant lymphomas

Metastatic neoplasms—Breast, prostate, lung, kidney

involving the facial nerve can also rarely occur. In children, the most common malignant tumor of the temporal bone is a rhabdosarcoma. Primary tumors of the endolymphatic sac are possible but fortunately are rare. Chondrosarcomas can arise from cartilaginous elements of the lateral skull base. Meningiomas of the posterior fossa and middle fossa can involve the temporal bone. Advanced or recurrent benign and malignant tumors of the parotid gland can involve the temporal bone. Finally, metastatic tumors (breast, prostate, lung, and kidney) are possible, as well as recurrent head and neck carcinoma.

CLINICAL PRESENTATION

Symptoms and signs of malignant lesions of the temporal bone are varied and depend on the location of the tumor. Table 23–2 lists the various clinical presentations.[2] Tumors originating in the ear canal can present with a nonhealing lesion, otorrhea, otalgia, or a conductive hearing loss. The most common malignant neoplasm in this location is squamous cell carcinoma. It often arises in a patient with long-standing otorrhea or chronic otitis media. Persistent granulation tissue in the external auditory canal represents squamous cell carcinoma until proven otherwise. As the tumor breaches the tympanic membrane, or the posterior ear canal, it can then spread relatively unobstructed into the mastoid air cell system. Posterior invasion into the mastoid also may result in facial nerve paresis or paralysis. Trismus may signify anterior invasion into the glenoid fossa.

Tumors neighboring the temporal bone also can cause otologic symptoms.[3] Lesions of the nasopharynx and infratemporal fossa can cause a middle ear effusion from involvement of the eustachian tube. Tumors of the parotid gland involving the temporal bone can present with a fixed mass within the parotid gland, occasionally with facial paralysis. Tumors of the deep lobe of the parotid and infratemporal fossa involving the temporal bone can be present with referred otalgia and can mimic trigeminal neuralgia. Hoarseness and dysphagia can signify involvement of the jugular foramen and adjacent cranial nerves.

Table 23–2. Clinical Symptoms of Temporal Bone Neoplasms

SYMPTOMS:	Otorrhea
	Pain
	Facial weakness
	Facial numbness
	Hearing loss
	Vertigo, imbalance
	Trismus
	Hoarseness
	Dysphagia
SIGNS:	EAC mass
	Bloody otorrhea
	Facial paralysis
	Other cranial nerve deficits
	Parotid mass
	Cervical mass
	Middle ear mass
	Middle ear effusion
	Conductive hearing loss
	Sensorineural hearing loss

CLINICAL ASSESSMENT

Evaluating patients with malignant neoplasms of the ear and temporal bone requires a thorough assessment of the presenting symptoms, duration, and prior treatment. It is also important to assess for any prior surgery, radiotherapy, and/or chemotherapy, which can potentially impact the current treatment and necessitate additional reconstructive options after surgery. Other important aspects of the medical history include assessing comorbidities such as hypertension, cardiac disease, cerebrovascular disease, diabetes, chronic pulmonary disease, liver disease, and obstructive sleep apnea.

Once a complete history is taken, a complete otolaryngologic examination is performed including microscopic otoscopy and cranial nerve testing. Special attention is directed to the facial and lower cranial nerve[7-12] examination. Flexible examination of the larynx is sometimes necessary to accurately assess the vagus nerve. Because the proposed surgery may result in an additional partial or complete unilateral hearing deficit, binaural audiometric testing is required.

Some patients will be referred with a tissue diagnosis. Outside pathology should be reviewed for accuracy by the treating institution's pathology department. In some cases, pathology will not be known before the initial consultation. Granulation tissue in the ear canal (suggesting squamous cell carcinoma) can be biopsied in the office or under general anesthesia if inconclusive. Masses of the pinna can be biopsied in the office. Palpable parotid and/or neck masses may be amenable to fine needle aspiration. The symptom of recurrent pain in the context of prior treatment for malignant lesions of the ear and/or temporal bone necessitates evaluation for persistent or residual disease.

DIAGNOSTIC IMAGING

Several key studies are required for management of malignant lesions of the ear and temporal bone. A computed tomographic (CT) scan of the temporal bone will delineate the bony confines of the lesion. It is important to assess for extension of the tumor posteriorly into the mastoid and medially through the tympanic membrane. The carotid canal and jugular bulb should also be assessed on the CT scan. Figure 23-3 shows a SCCA of the right temporal bone with extensive bony erosion.

MRI is best at showing the soft tissue extent of the lesion. An MRI of the parotid gland with contrast will identify anterior soft tissue extension into the parotid gland and glenoid fossa, inferior extension into the infratemporal fossa, superior extension into the middle fossa, and posterior extension into the posterior fossa. Figure 23-4 shows superior extension of a SCCA of the temporal bone into the middle cranial fossa.

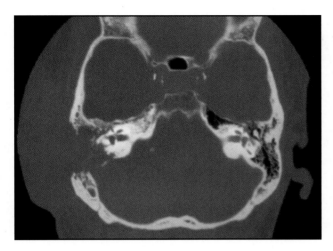

Fig 23–3. Axial CT scan showing an erosive SCCA of the right temporal bone.

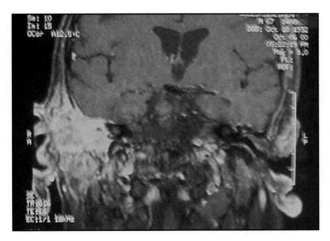

Fig 23–4. Coronal MRI of lesion of right skull base with intracranial extension.

THERAPEUTIC IMAGING

A recurrent or advanced squamous cell carcinoma involving the petrous carotid artery may necessitate preoperative sacrifice of the carotid artery within the petrous portion of the temporal bone with detachable coils, provided the patient has passed a preoperative balloon occlusion test with cerebral blood flow studies.[4,5]

OTHER IMAGING STUDIES

Further imaging is dictated by the clinical and radiographic assessment. Neck and parotid disease can be assessed by CT and/or MRI. Patients with presumed metastatic lesions should undergo a metastatic survey, which may include CT scan imaging of the chest, and abdomen, and positron emission tomography (PET) scan.

STAGING /PREOPERATIVE PREPARATION, AND ASSESSMENT

Staging and a treatment plan are next formulated, based on a review of the clinical and radiographic data. Table 23–3 lists staging of SCCA of the temporal bone. Prior to initiating treatment all patients should be presented at a multidisciplinary tumor board conference. Many patients with malignant lesions of the temporal bone will require adjuvant radiation therapy and possibly chemotherapy. The clinical and radiographic assessment of the patient will allow the surgeon to decide if the lesion is technically resectable. The more difficult question is whether surgery should be undertaken in every case. In certain circumstances, surgery may not be advisable. Relative contraindications for surgical resection include malignant lesions involving the cavernous sinus, carotid artery, infratemporal fossa, and paraspinus musculature.[6] However, some authors have reported extended survival even with intracranial extension.[7] Some of these patients may also benefit from palliative chemoradiotherapy.

Also important in the preoperative assessment of patients is to determine potential reconstructive options. It may be possible to close the defect primarily by oversewing the ear canal and obliterating the mastoid cavity with nonvascularized abdominal fat. However, if postoperative radiotherapy is required, a better option may be a local regional flap (temporalis), or rotational pedicle flap (trapezius or latissimus dorsi), or a microvascular free tissue transfer (rectus abdominus). Patients who have undergone prior radiotherapy will benefit from a vascularized

Table 23–3. SCCA Stage and Surgical Approach

Stage	Definition	Surgical Approach
T1	Limited to EAC without bony erosion or evidence of soft tissue extension	Lateral temporal bone resection
T2	Limited bony EAC erosion or limited <5 mm soft tissue involvement	Lateral temporal bone resection
T3	Full thickness EAC erosion with limited <5 mm soft tissue involvement or middle ear involvement, or facial paresis	Subtemporal temporal bone resection
T4	Erosion of cochlea, petrous apex, medial wall of middle ear, carotid canal, jugular foramen dura, >5 mm soft tissue involvement	Total temporal bone resection

tissue closure to decrease postoperative complications. Involving a reconstructive surgeon in the patient's care preoperatively is important in assessing the various reconstructive options.

For lesions involving or abutting the middle fossa or posterior fossa, a preoperative neurosurgical consultation also will be beneficial. Finally, patients with significant comorbidies can benefit from a preoperative medical, pulmonary, or cardiac consultation. Finally, as many of these surgical cases can last several hours, patients with poor pulmonary reserve should be offered a temporary tracheotomy, which can reduce postoperative pulmonary complications.

Once the treatment plan has been formulated, a detailed discussion with the patient and supporting family members is important. The goals, risks, potential complications, and expected postoperative course should be discussed. Also, if cranial nerve deficits are anticipated, a treatment plan to address these deficits is discussed preoperatively. If multiple lower cranial nerve deficits are possible, the discussion should mention the possibility of tracheotomy and feeding tube placement for airway protection and nutrition, respectively. If postoperative radiotherapy is likely to be needed, the patient should undergo a preoperative consultation with radiation oncology.

As treatment of patients with such tumors is a multidisciplinary effort, communication and coordination between disciplines is essential. This best occurs through the development of skull base teams involving head and neck surgical oncologists, neu-

rotologists, neuroanesthesiologists, interventional neuroradiologists, radiation oncologists, plastic and reconstructive surgeons, surgical assistants, and intraoperative cranial nerve monitoring personnel.

SURGICAL TECHNIQUE

General Principles

The clinical assessment, pathology review, and radiographic assessment will dictate the extent of surgery. Important considerations include the status of the ear canal, middle ear and conductive hearing apparatus, cochlea and vestibular apparatus, and potential for cerebrospinal fluid otorrhea or rhinorrhea. For example, if a SCCA of the ear canal is treated with a sleeve resection of the ear canal, skin grafting, and postoperative radiotherapy, the patient may likely develop a chronic problematic mastoid cavity that has to be debrided at regular intervals, hears poorly, periodically drains or gets infected, and is prone to serous middle ear effusions. This patient may have been better served with a lateral temporal bone resection with oversewing of the ear canal, obliteration of the mastoid cavity with abdominal fat, and hearing rehabilitation with a bone-anchored hearing aid (BAHA).[8]

The best way to address potential postoperative problems with CSF is preoperatively. CSF wound accumulations and fistulae can be problematic and eventually lead to meningitis. Therefore, incisions should be multilayered. Abdominal fat sometimes can be utilized to obliterated dead space. If the surgical field will be radiated, obliteration of the surgical defect is best accomplished with a rotational flap or free flap. Finally, the eustachian tube and middle ear may need to be obliterated with muscle to prevent postoperative CSF rhinorrhea.

The location of tumors within and adjacent to the temporal bone determines the surgical approach. In general, tumors limited to the ear canal can be treated with a temporal bone resection. The ear canal is oversewn and the cavity is packed with abdominal fat. Depending on the stage of the tumor, a parotidectomy and neck dissection may also be required. If the pinna or a significant portion of the external auditory meatus are involved and have to be resected, the surgical procedure is as above; however, a rotational flap (trapezius) or free flap reconstruction (rectus abdominus) generally is required to reconstruct the cutaneous component of the defect.

Tumors involving the jugular foramen are medial to the descending mastoid segment of the facial nerve and therefore may require that the nerve be mobilized anteriorly. The ear canal limits the potential mobilization. For tumors involving the petrous carotid artery, the ear canal is removed and the facial nerve is mobilized at the tympanic segment and/or resected if involved with disease. Craniotomies may be necessary for temporal bone tumors with posterior or superior extension.

Patient Positioning

Preoperative consultation with the anesthesiologist is critical to ensure that short-acting paralytics are used for the anesthetic induction so that cranial nerve monitoring will be possible throughout the case. If a tracheotomy is planned, it is generally done after induction of anesthesia. The operative table is then turned 180 degrees so that the scrub nurse is positioned opposite the surgeon. Most patients will be positioned supine, with the treated ear up, and the head gently turned to the opposite side. Overtorsion of the head can occlude the contralateral jugular venous system, which can cause cerebral edema if the ipsilateral venous system will be taken surgically. The head can be immobilized with tape, placed in a Mayfield head-holder, or even secured with pins (if a craniotomy is anticipated). If an abdominal free flap is anticipated for wound closure, it can be harvested with the patient supine. If the reconstructive option is a pedicled flap such as a trapezius or latissimus, the patient can be positioned on his or her side for both the surgical resection and reconstruction. All bony prominences are padded. Arterial lines are placed. A Foley catheter is placed for monitoring urine output. Cranial nerve monitoring electrodes are also placed. If a rectus abdominus free-tissue transfer or fat graft is anticipated for wound closure, the abdomen is also prepared accordingly. Figure 23–5 shows patient positioning and room set-up for a lateral temporal bone resection.

Surgical Incision

The best way to prevent postoperative wound healing issues and wound complications is by accurate planning of the surgical incisions and approach. Most tumors of the temporal bone can be approached through a C-shaped postauricular incision. The incision can be modified as needed. It is placed further behind the ear if more access is required posteriorly, along the sigmoid sinus. If superior extension is required (such as for a middle fossa craniotomy), the incision is placed more superiorly, within the temporal hairline. If access to the neck and great vessels is required, the incision gently curves into a cervical neck crease. If the ear canal is to be part of the surgical resection, an incision is made in the cartilaginous EAC encompassing the lesion (Fig 23–6).

The incision is made initially with a 10-bladed scalpel. Undermining of the skin above the temporalis fascia is then quickly performed for approximately 1 cm. Manual pressure on the wound edges will temporarily tamponade arterial bleeding. Hemostatic clips are then placed. These are preferred to electrocautery of the skin edges as the former will allow for improved vascularity of the skin incision and thus quicker wound healing. This is especially important if the middle or posterior fossa dura needs to be opened as part of the surgical procedure and CSF can enter the wound.

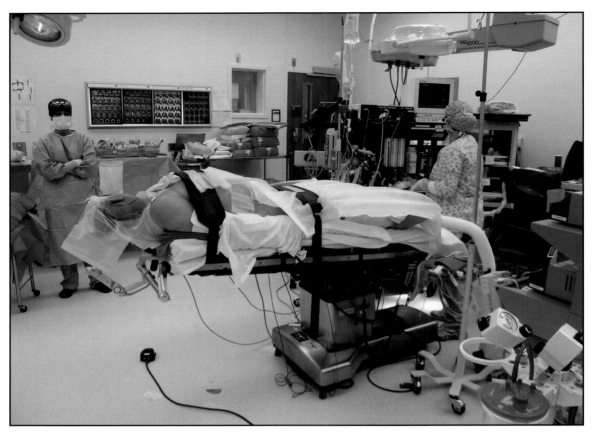

Fig 23–5. Patient positioning for temporal bone surgery.

Soft Tissue Dissection

The soft tissue dissection should be planned to incorporate stepped incisions and multiple layers to allow water-tight closure, especially if CSF can enter the wound. Next, a scalpel, dissection scissors, or electrocautery is used to develop the plane above the temporalis fascia. A stepped incision is made through the fascia, muscle, and periosteum. A C-shaped incision 1 cm inside the surgical incision is easier to close in a water-tight fashion than a T-shaped incision, which is commonly used in otologic surgery. This flap is elevated anteriorly until the root of the zygoma, soft tissue entering the ear canal, and mastoid tip are identified. Elevation of the soft tissues overlying the mastoid cortex should be done in the subperiosteal plane. The soft tissues are reflected anteriorly, out of the surgical field, moistened with gauze-soaked saline, and secured with hooks.

Access to the neck contents and great vasculature is possible through a cervical extension of the incision. If ear canal sacrifice is required, it is sectioned at the bony cartilaginous junction, and closed in multiple layers. Carrying this dissection forward above the parotid fascia will allow further anterior extension, especially if a parotidectomy is required.

Modifications of the soft tissue dissection are also possible depending on the anticipated size of the surgical defect. The temporoparietal fascia can be preserved and reflected forward as a rotational flap reconstruction. The temporalis muscle can also be utilized as a rotational flap, based on its deep vascular supply.

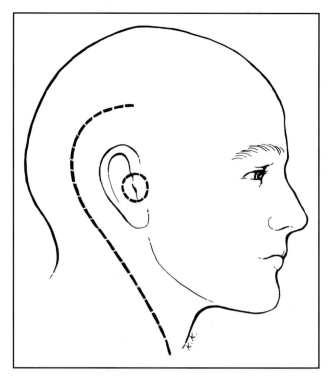

Fig 23–6. Outline of skin incisions for a lateral temporal bone resection including resection of skin of the external auditory canal.

Bony Dissection and Osteotomies

Once the soft tissues dissection is completed, the bony dissection begins with a large cutting bur and copious irrigation. Most approaches to temporal bone neoplasms will require some form of mastoidectomy. Principles of safe bony dissection include wide saucerization and the utilization of constant landmarks for finding key structures. The deepest portion of the dissection should always be anterosuperior, as the facial nerve and horizontal semicircular canal are deepest here. Superiorly, the tegmen, or bony plate overlying the middle cranial fossa dura is carefully skeletonized. This plate usually has an irregular shape (like that of a potato chip) rather than a flat plane, so care is taken to avoid dural injury. Anteriorly, the bony ear canal, which is cylindrically shaped, is also carefully skeletonized.

Posteriorly, the sigmoid sinus is identified and skeletonized. Finally, inferiorly the mastoid tip is identified. Figure 23-7 shows the relationships of the mastoid, middle ear, facial nerve, and ear canal within the temporal bone. As the dissection proceeds medially, the drill size and suction irrigator size are decreased accordingly, as the size of the surgical field narrows. Also, although the surgeon can perform a simple mastoidectomy without magnification, using an operating microscope will allow safe dissection of the infratemporal facial nerve, middle ear, and inner ear structures.

For tumors with extension near the petrous carotid artery, or into the infratemporal fossa it is necessary to perform an infratemporal fossa approach, as described by Fisch.[9] This approach involves a wide mastoidectomy as described above, resection of the tympanic bone, and soft tissue of the ear canal with oversewing of the soft tissue of the external auditory meatus. The facial nerve is skeletonized within the tympanic and mastoid segments and mobilized anteriorly. Using continuous facial nerve monitoring and preserving the periosteum of the stylomastoid foramen during this portion of the rerouting can decrease incidence of postoperative facial nerve paresis.[10] The internal jugular vein, internal carotid artery, and lower cranial nerves are identified in the neck. The internal jugular vein is divided.

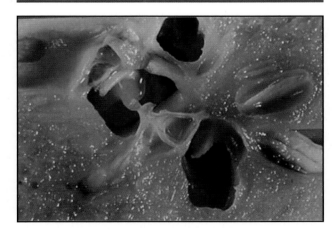

Fig 23–7. Axial section of a right temporal bone showing relationships between ear canal, facial nerve, and middle and inner ear.

The sigmoid sinus is occluded. The adventitia of the lateral portion of the jugular bulb is removed with the tumor, with attempted preservation of the lower cranial nerves and internal carotid artery. Bleeding from the inferior petrosal sinus and condylar vein can be quite brisk and is controlled with oxidized cellulose. Intracranial extension of the tumor is resected in conjunction with neurosurgery after the temporal portion of the tumor is removed.

Closure includes obliteration of the eustachian tube with muscle, waxing of open mastoid air cells, temporalis fascia grafting of any dural defect, and obliteration of the cavity with abdominal fat. A pressure dressing is also placed for several days postoperatively. Postoperative care is described in the next section.

Although benign tumors of the temporal bone can be resected in a piecemeal approach, malignant tumors, such as squamous cell carcinoma, or advanced parotid malignancies require an en bloc approach. See Table 23–3 for the clinical stage and corresponding surgical approach for SCCA of the temporal bone.[11] For T1 and T2, lesions, a lateral temporal bone resection is performed.[12] A negative surgical margin is obtained at the ear canal and the canal is oversewn. A partial or total auriculectomy may be necessary depending on tumor extension. An intact canal wall tympanomastoidectomy is performed with an extended facial recess. Dissection continues around the bony ear canal into the glenoid fossa anteriorly. The incudostapedial joint is sectioned and the incus is removed. The tensor tympani is sectioned. The stylomastoid foramen is widely exposed and decompressed. The disgastric muscle is exposed in the mastoid tip. A chisel is used to section the tympanic bone. The specimen is then reflected anteriorly. A parotidectomy and supraomohyoid neck dissection are performed for staging purposes (Fig 23–8). Closure is as described for the infratemporal fossa approach. A trapezius rotational flap or rectus flap may be required if an auriculectomy has also been performed. Most patients will also undergo postoperative radiotherapy, and the 5-year survival for tumor limited to the EAC is approximately 50 to 70%.[13,14] Figures 23–9 through 23–13 detail a lateral temporal bone resection in a patient with SCCA of the temporal bone involving the pinna and reconstruction with a pedicled trapezius myocutaneous flap.

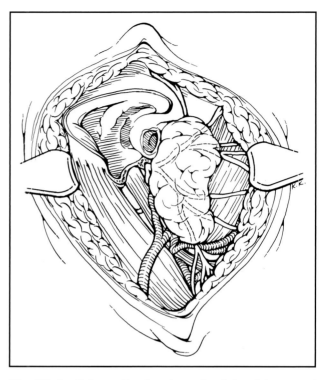

Fig 23–8. Schematic drawing of a lateral temporal bone resection. The specimen has been reflected anteriorly and includes a lateral parotidectomy.

Once SCCA breaches the ear canal and enters the mastoid and middle ear, it can spread easily within the temporal bone. For tumors limited to the middle ear and mastoid, a subtotal temporal bone resection is performed, which removes the temporal bone lateral to the petrous apex, including the otic capsule. This operation includes mobilization of the petrous carotid artery as well as an infratemporal fossa dissection (Fig 23–14). Five-year survival for patients treated with subtotal temporal bone resection ranges from 35 to 41.7%.[13,14]

Once the tumor invades the petrous apex, it can invade the dura, brain parenchyma, and internal carotid artery. The only hope of cure is a total temporal bone resection, which includes resection of the petrous apex with or without resection of the petrous carotid artery.[15] This approach involves an extensive infratemporal fossa dissection with carotid artery mobilization and/or resection, and middle and posterior fossa craniotomies, Five-year survival

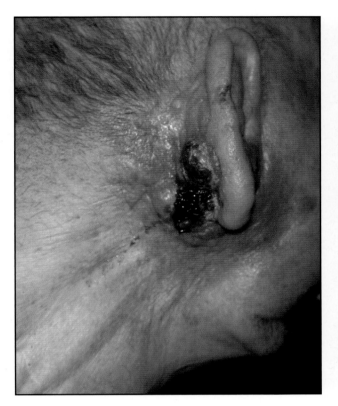

Fig 23–9. Photograph of a patient with SCCA of the pinna, fixed to mastoid bone.

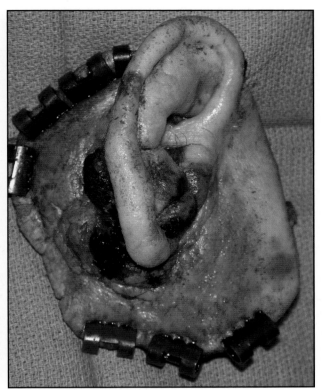

Fig 23–10. Resected surgical specimen.

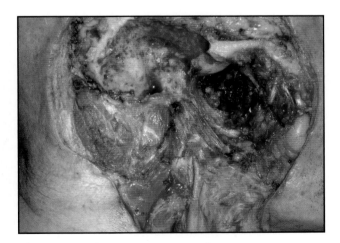

Fig 23–11. Intraoperative photograph of surgical defect.

is poor and ranges from 0 to 11%.[13] Some authors believe that invasion of the cavernous sinus, carotid artery, paraspinal musculature, and infratemporal fossa are contraindications to surgical resection.[6] Other authors have reported extended survival with dural and intracranial extension treated with surgery and postoperative radiotherapy.[7] Preoperative chemoradiotherapy combined with surgical resection may have a role in some of these patients.[16] Closure is as above.

Postoperative Care

The care varies with the extent of the surgery. Patients undergoing lateral temporal bone resection should be observed in the hospital until the wound is stable. If the patient has undergone pedicled or free-flap reconstruction, jugular venous system dissection, carotid artery dissection, or transdural surgery, the patient should be observed in the neurologic intensive care unit and watched closely hemodynamically and neurologically. Any change in the patient's mental status should be addressed

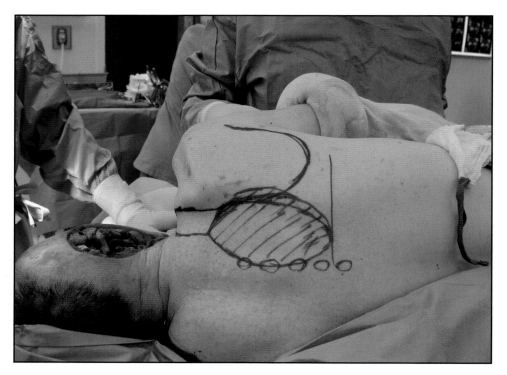

Fig 23–12. Outline of skin incisions for trapezius myocutaneous rotational flap.

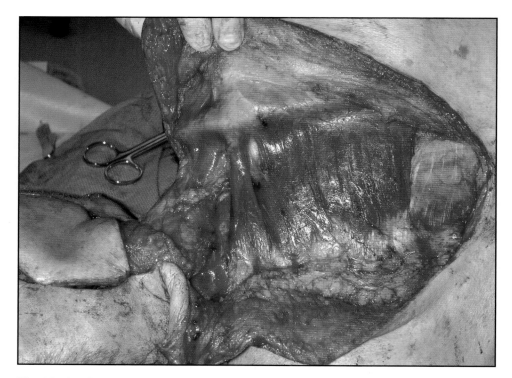

Fig 23–13. Trapezius flap delivered into surgical defect.

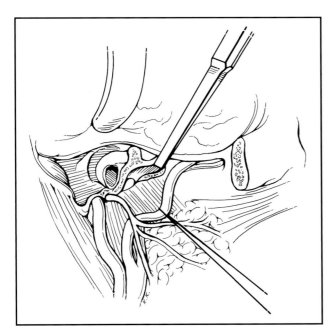

Fig 23–14. Schematic drawing of subtotal temporal bone resection. The petrous carotid artery has been preserved and mobilized inferiorly. An osteotome is placed in the petrous canal and angled toward the internal auditory canal.

immediately, as this may suggest intracranial hemorrhage and/or meningitis. Postoperative cranial nerve deficits are addressed as described below.

Discharge planning includes education of the patient and caretakers as to what to watch for regarding the wound and other issues. Redness, purulent drainage, clear drainage, fluid accumulations under the wound, changes in mental status, fever, difficulty breathing, and calf pain all merit evaluation in the office and appropriate intervention. CSF wound accumulations can be managed with repeated sterile aspiration and pressure dressings. The patient is followed closely until the wound is completely healed. Stitches and staples are removed 1 to 2 weeks after surgery.

Surgical Complications and Avoidance

Any surgical team that treats patients with temporal bone neoplasms will encounter complications. One should continually strive to decrease the complication rate. The first place to start is to spend time preoperatively making sure the patient is adequately prepared for surgery from a medical standpoint and that the patient and family members understand the goals of surgery and potential complications. The surgeon should also thoroughly review the imaging studies to make sure the proposed surgical approach will be ideal. Communication between all members of the surgical team is essential.

Intraoperatively, the patient is carefully positioned to avoid potential cervical spine and brachial plexus injury. Cranial nerve monitoring can facilitate cranial nerve preservation. The patient is kept stable hemodynamically during the procedure. Care is taken around the dural venous sinuses. Overpacking the sigmoid sinus can lead to obstruction of the vein of Labbe and venous infarction of the temporal lobe. Excessive packing of the inferior petrosal sinus can injure the 9th, 10th, and 11th cranial nerves. Judicious use of mannitol during the surgical procedure can decrease the volume of the intracranial space in patients requiring transdural procedures.

Postoperative cerebrospinal fluid wound issues may lead to meningitis. Sterile wound CSF accumulations may be treated with repeated sterile aspiration and pressure dressings. CSF wound fistulae may require reapproximation of the wound edges. Persistent fistulae or wound accumulations may require continuous lumbar drainage. As humans produce about 18 cc of CSF per hour, less than this is removed, typically 10 cc per hour. Removing CSF too rapidly can lead to tension pneumocephalus, mental status changes, and even brain herniation.[17,18] CSF rhinorrhea should be treated with reoperation and packing of the middle ear, eustachian tube, and opened mastoid air cells.

OUTCOMES OF THERAPY

There are several difficulties when analyzing results of treatment for SCCA of the temporal bone. The tumor is relatively rare, most centers have only small case series, most studies are retrospective, staging may not be completely accurate (especially in those receiving radiotherapy alone, in which imaging and physical exam are used for staging), and studies may not adequately stratify patients according to disease staging and treatment. Although radiotherapy is often used postoperatively in the treatment of malignant temporal bone neoplasms, in some centers, or in patients who refuse surgery, it has been used as primary therapy. Pemberton et al reviewed 123 patients with SCCA of the middle ear and external auditory canal treated only with fractionated radiotherapy (median dose of 55 Gy given over 16 days).[19] At 5 and 10 years, respectively, freedom from local recurrence was 56% and 56%, whereas disease-free survival was 45% and 43%, cancer-specific survival was 53% and 51%, and overall survival was 40% and 21%. Radionecrosis as a complication occurred in 6% of patients.

Hashi et al reviewed 20 patients with SCCA of the EAC treated with radiotherapy versus radiotherapy and surgery.[20] Most patients had T1 or T2 tumors. Patients treated by radiotherapy alone received 65 Gy in 26 fractions over 6.5 weeks. Those treated with surgery and radiotherapy received 30 to 75 Gy in 12 to 30 fractions. The mean follow-up was 71 months. Five of eight patients with T1 tumors treated with radiotherapy alone had 100% survival. Patients with T2 tumors treated with radiotherapy alone had much worse 5-year survival (38%). The authors believe that when the tumor invades the EAC, radiotherapy as a single treatment modality is not as good as surgery and radiotherapy combined.

Testa et al assessed prognostic factors in carcinoma of the EAC.[21] They evaluated 79 patients. There were 34 patients with stage T1 and T2 tumors, 43 patients with T3 and T4 tumors, and 2 patients with Tx tumors; 68 patients had N0 tumors and 11 patients had stage N1 tumors. Fifty-nine patients had surgery whereas 9 patients had radiotherapy. Eleven patients did not have any treatment. The 5-year survival rates were 65% for those undergoing surgery, 29% for those undergoing radiotherapy, and 63% for those undergoing surgery and radiotherapy. Bone involvement and tumor stage were significant prognostic indicators.

In a 1999 study of 27 patients with carcinoma of the ear canal and middle ear with a median follow-up of 2.7 years, treatment by surgery and radiotherapy yielded a 5-year survival of 61%.[22] For T1 and T2 tumors, the survival was 86%, for T3 tumors 50%, and for T4 tumors 41%. For tumors limited to the EAC, the 5-year survival was 100%. Once tumor invaded the temporal bone, 5-year survival was 63%; and 37% once tumor infiltrated beyond the temporal bone. Prognostic factors included unresectability by dural or cerebral invasion with all of these patients dead within 2.2 years. The authors concluded that surgery and postoperative radiotherapy is the preferred treatment.

In a multimodality study, Nakagawa et al reviewed 25 patients with SCCA of the EAC and middle ear.[16] Seven of 12 patients received preoperative chemoradiotherapy. The 3-year estimated survival for T1 and T2 lesions was 100%. The 5-year estimated survival for T3 and T4 lesions was 80% and 35%, respectively. The 5-year estimated survival improved up to 75% for those patients with T4 tumors who had surgery, whereas it was 16% for those who did not undergo surgery. Positive surgical margin, concomitant chronic otitis media, and positive lymph nodes were significantly associated with poorer survival.

The above studies suggest that primary surgery followed by postoperative radiotherapy is the treatment of choice for carcinoma of the temporal bone. For patients with invasion of the carotid canal, petrous apex, and dura, prognosis is poor regardless of treatment. These patients may be candidates for preoperative chemoradiotherapy, followed by surgery in selected cases.

FOLLOW-UP AND REHABILITATION

Patients with tumors involving the jugular foramen may have pre and/or postoperative deficits of the lower cranial nerves, with resultant speech and swallowing difficulty, with the potential for aspiration. These patients should undergo a bedside vocal and swallowing evaluation using flexible fiberoptic laryngoscosopy postoperatively before being allowed to take oral feeding.[23] Some patients will require adjunctive procedures including thyroplasty[24] and possibly palatal adhesion.[25] Feeding tube placement may be necessary in some patients. Ultimately, time and speech therapy will improve postoperative lower cranial nerve function.

Rehabilitation of the facial nerve and eye begins immediately postoperatively. A paralytic eyelid risks exposure keratitis and possible blindness. Oculoplastic consultation can be very helpful. For temporary facial paresis, the eye is lubricated and taped closed at night. Long-standing paresis is best treated with a gold weight[26] and possible canthoplasty.[27] Lower facial paresis is managed conservatively when the nerve is intact. If the nerve function fails to improve, nerve substitution procedures (7–12 grafting), or static suspension procedures may be required.

Return to work status depends on the vigor of the work activity and the patient's motivation to return to work. Patients working at heights or using heavy machinery in whom a postoperative vestibular or neurologic deficit exists may not be able to return to these jobs, but may perform some form of sedentary or office work. Temporary or short-term disability may be necessary in other patients.

Postoperative radiotherapy is often required in patients with malignant neoplasms of the temporal bone. This usually begins at about 6 weeks postoperatively, as the wound is usually healed at this point. It is important to follow the patient closely during postoperative radiotherapy as breakdown of the skin of the postauricular area and pinna can occur. This is initially managed conservatively. Exposed cartilage of the pinna may require debridement.

Postoperative imaging studies are necessary in some patients to assess for recurrent or residual disease. MRI is usually performed 6 months after the initial procedure and then biannually or annually. Postsurgical changes will generally remain stable over time, whereas lesions that enhance and enlarge represent residual or recurrent disease.

CONCLUSION

In summary, patients with malignant neoplasms of the temporal bone often require multidisciplinary management. A thorough understanding of the microsurgical anatomy and various pathologies of the temporal bone and neighboring lateral skull base is critical for proper treatment of diseases in this area. Surgical resection with negative margins followed by postoperative radiotherapy is the preferential treatment. Survival is related to stage of disease and completeness or surgical resection. Unilateral hearing deficits are common, secondary to resection of the ear canal and postoperative radiotherapy. Lower cranial nerve deficits will require time and possibly further adjunctive surgical procedures for adequate rehabilitation.

REFERENCES

1. Wackym PA, Friedman I. Unusual tumors of the middle ear and mastoid. In: Jackler RK, Driscol CLW, eds. *Tumors of the Ear and Temporal Bone.* Philadelphia, Pa; Lippincott Williams & Wilkins; 2000:128–145.
2. Leonetti JP, Marzo SJ. Malignancy of the temporal bone. *Otolaryngol Clin North Am.* 2002;35:405–410.
3. Leonetti JP, Smith PG, Kletzker R, Izquierdo R. Invasion patterns of advanced temporal bone malignancies. *Am J Otol.* 1996;17:438–442.
4. Peterman SB, Taylor A, Hoffman JC. Improved detection of cerebral hypoperfusion with internal carotid balloon test occlusion and ^{99m}Tc-HMPAO SPECT imaging. *AJNR.* 1991;12:1035–1044.
5. Monsein LH, Jeffery PJ, Van Heerden BB, et al. Assessing adequacy of collateral circulation during balloon test occlusion of the internal carotid artery with ^{99m}Tc-HMPAO SPECT. *AJNR.* 1991;12:1045–1051.
6. Pensak ML, Gleich LL, Gluckman JL, Shumrick KA. Temporal bone carcinoma:contemporary perspectives in the skull base surgical area. *Laryngoscope.* 1996;106:1234–1237.
7. Moffat DA, Grey P, Ballagh RH, et al. Extended temporal bone resection for squamous cell carcinoma. *Otolaryngol Head Neck Surg.* 1997;116:617–623.
8. Tjellstrom A. Osseointegrated systems and their application in the head and neck. *Adv Otolaryngol Head Neck Surg.* 1989;3:39–70.
9. Fisch U. Infratemporal fossa approach for glomus tumors of the temporal bone. *Ann Otol Rhinol Laryngol.* 1982;91:474–479.
10. Leonetti JP, Brackmann DE, Prass RL. Improved preservation of facial nerve function in the infratemporal approach to the skull base. *Otolaryngol Head Neck Surg.* 1989;101:74.
11. Arriaga M, Curtin H, Hirsch BE, Takahashi H, Kamerer D. Staging proposal for external auditory meatus carcinoma based on preoperative clinical examination and CT findings. *Ann Otol Rhinol Laryngol.* 1990;99:714–721.

12. Crabtree JA, Britton BH, Pierce MK. Carcinoma of the external auditory canal. *Laryngoscope.* 1976; 86:405-415.

13. Prasad S, Janecka IP. Efficacy of surgical treatments for squamous cell carcinoma of the temporal bone: a literature review. *Otolaryngol Head Neck Surg.* 1994;110:270-280.

14. Lewis JS. Temporal bone resection:review of 100 cases. *Arch Otolaryngol.* 1975;101:23-25.

15. Graham MD, Sataloff RT, Kemik JL, Wolf GT, McGillicuddy JE. Total en bloc resection of the temporal bone and carotid artery for malignant tumors of the ear and temporal bone. *Laryngoscope.* 1984; 94:528-533.

16. Nakagawa T, Kumamoto Y, Natori Y, et al. Squamous cell carcinoma of the external auditory canal and middle ear: an operation combined with preoperative chemoradiotherapy and a free surgical margin. *Otol Neurotol.* 2006;27:242-249.

17. Effron MZ, Black FO, Burns D. Tension pneumocephalus complicating the treatment of postoperative CSF otorrhea. *Arch Otolaryngol Head Neck Surg.* 1981;107:579-580.

18. Graf CJ, Gross CE, Beck DW. Complication of spinal drainage in the management of cerebrospinal fluid fistula: report of three cases. *J Neurosurg.* 1981; 54:392-395.

19. Pemberton LS, Swindell R, Sykes AJ. Primary radical radiotherapy for squamous cell carcinoma of the middle ear and external auditory canal: an historical series. *Clin Oncol.* 2006;18:390-394.

20. Hashi N, Shirato H, Omatsu T, et al. The role of radiotherapy in treating squamous cell carcinoma of the external auditory canal, especially in the early stages of disease. *Radiother Oncol.* 2000;56: 221-225.

21. Testa JR, Fukuda Y, Kowalski LP. Prognostic factors in carcinoma of the external auditory canal. *Arch Otolaryngol Head Neck Surg.* 1997;123: 720-724.

22. Pfreundner L, Schwanger K, Willner J, et al. Carcinoma of the external auditory canal and middle ear. *Int J Radiat Oncol Biol Phys.* 1999;44:77-88.

23. Bastian RW. Videoendoscopic evaluation of patients with dysphagia: an adjunct to the modified barium swallow. *Otolaryngol Head Neck Surg.* 1991;104: 339-342.

24. Netterville JL, Jackson CG, Civantos FJ. Thyroplasty in the functional rehabilitation of neurotologic skull base surgery patients. *Am J Otol.* 1993;14:460-465.

25. Netterville JL, Vrabec JT. Unilateral palatal adhesion for paralysis after high vagal injury. *Arch Otolaryngol Head Neck Surg.* 1994;120:218-224.

26. Jobe RP. A technique for lid-loading in the management of lagophthalmos in facial paralysis. *Plast Reconstr Surg.* 1974;53:29-31.

27. Tenzel RR. Treatment of lagophthalmos of the lower lid. *Arch Ophthalmol.* 1969;81:366-368.

24

Management of Malignant Head and Neck Tumors in Children

John Maddalozzo
Amy Anstead
Sheri Poznanovic

INTRODUCTION

Pediatric head and neck malignancy is a rare condition that most commonly presents with an enlarging mass, and therefore is associated with a diverse and extensive differential diagnosis. The more common of these entities are explored in this chapter. Thyroid malignancy and nasopharyngeal carcinoma are important elements in the differential diagnosis of pediatric head and neck malignancy and are discussed in their respective chapters in this text.

It is important to highlight the fact that the majority of the pediatric head and neck masses encountered will be benign inflammatory processes and that the following malignant diagnoses, although important to consider and rule out, will make up the minority of cases. An in-depth discussion of each disease process is beyond the scope of this text and each condition is the subject of active investigation by multiple research groups; therefore, it is important to review the current available literature before initiating a treatment program.

NON-HODGKIN'S LYMPHOMA

After the age of 6, lymphoma becomes the most common pediatric head and neck malignancy. Overall, it is the third most common childhood malignancy in the United States.[1] Non-Hodgkin's lymphoma (NHL) represents 60% of these lymphoma cases.[2-3] The average annual incidence of pediatric NHL rose by almost 30% in the United States between 1973 and 1991.[4] The annual incidence in children younger than 15 years of age is 7 to 8 per 1,000,000, with peak ages between 7 and 11 years. Boys are affected by a margin of 3:1.[5,6] It is half as common in blacks as in whites.[7] NHL accounts for approximately 10% of solid tumors in childhood, and almost 10% of all these arise in the head and neck.[8]

Specific populations at increased risk are children with deficient T-cell function including patients previously treated with chemotherapy or with congenital immunodeficiency syndrome (ataxia–telangiectasia, the Wiskott-Aldrich syndrome, or X-linked lymphoproliferative disease), HIV/AIDS or other acquired immunodeficiency syndrome, and those who have received immunosuppressive therapy after transplantation.[2,9]

Presenting symptoms vary with location of disease. Children typically present with extranodal disease involving the abdomen (in 31% of cases), the head and neck (in 29%), or the mediastinum (in 26%).[2,10,11] Extranodal sites in the head and neck (nasopharynx, Waldeyer's ring, oral cavity, orbit, scalp, sinuses, and larynx) manifest frequently as a submucosal mass or by a polypoid, bulky mass with a smooth mucosal surface. Clinically aggressive lymphomas are characterized by destruction of the maxilla, mandible, and bones around the paranasal sinuses.[12] Central nervous system involvement can present with malignant pleocytosis or cranial nerve palsies. Pancytopenia suggests bone marrow involvement. The tumor often grows rapidly, and the disease spreads by blood-borne dissemination. Ninety percent of children have high-grade tumors. This predominance is thought to reflect maturational changes taking place in the cellular composition and function of the maturing immune system.[2] As a result, almost two-thirds of children and adolescents with non-Hodgkin's lymphoma have locally advanced or metastatic disease at the time the diagnosis is made.

The gold standard for diagnosis remains the open surgical biopsy, obtaining enough fresh tissue for morphologic, immunophenotypic, cytogenetic, and molecular studies. The role of FNA with the application of immunocytochemistry has borne diagnostic accuracy as ancillary tests continue to become more sophisticated.[13,14]

On CT and MRI studies, the lymph nodes of HL and NHL are homogeneous and variable in size. They may enhance slightly or moderately, display necrosis before and after treatment, and display calcification post-treatment. Contrast CT is indicated for evaluation of cervical lymph nodes, paranasal sinuses, and orbits. CT is also useful for detection of bone destruction involving the base of the skull, paranasal sinuses, and the mandible or maxilla. MR imaging is preferred for the assessment of extension of lymphomas to different fascial spaces and for intracranial extension. Lymphomas are isodense to muscle on CT and circumscribed with distinct margins that occasionally display extranodal extension with less well-defined margins and areas of necrosis within the tumor matrix. Lymphomas appear low in signal intensity on T1-weighted images and low to high in signal intensity on T2-weighted images, with variable, but usually low, enhancement following introduction of gadolinium-DTPA (Gd-DTPA) contrast material.[12]

Staging studies include a CBC with a differential count, HIV testing, a blood-chemistry panel (including uric acid, calcium, phosphorus, and lactate dehydrogenase), UA, examination of cerebrospinal fluid, and bilateral bone marrow aspiration and biopsy are important not only to determine the stage of the disease but also to identify metabolic abnormalities that could complicate the administration of chemotherapy. Diagnostic imaging includes CT of the chest, abdomen, and pelvis as well as bone scanning.[15]

Bone marrow involvement has been defined as 5% malignant cells in an otherwise normal bone marrow with normal peripheral blood counts and smears. Patients with lymphoblastic lymphoma with more than 25% malignant cells in the bone marrow are considered to have leukemia. CNS disease in lymphoblastic lymphoma is defined by criteria similar to that used for acute lymphocytic leukemia, that is, white blood cell count of at least 5/μL and malignant cells in the cerebrospinal fluid (CSF). For any other NHL, the definition of CNS disease is any malignant cell present in the CSF regardless of cell count.[10]

The most widely used staging scheme for childhood NHL is that of the St. Jude Children's Research Hospital (Murphy Staging).

Stage I: a single tumor or nodal area is involved, excluding the abdomen and mediastinum.

Stage II: disease extent is limited to a single tumor with regional node involvement or 2 or more tumors or nodal areas involved on one side of the diaphragm.

Stage III: tumors or involved lymph node areas occur on both sides of the diaphragm or any primary intrathoracic (mediastinal, pleural, or thymic) disease, extensive primary intra-abdominal disease, or any paraspinal or epidural tumors.

Stage IV: tumors involve bone marrow and/or CNS disease regardless of other sites of involvement.[10]

Over the years, different classification systems have been used to differentiate lymphomas including the Rappaport Classification (used until the 1970s), the Working Formulation, the National Cancer Institute Working Formulation, and Revised European-American Lymphoma Classification (REAL). In 2001, a modern comprehensive classification system was published under the World Health Organization (WHO). The committee recognized that specific disease entities could be defined by a combination of morphology, immunology, genetic features, and clinical features. Childhood NHL's fall into four broad categories (with approximate percentage of occurrence): lymphoblastic lymphoma (30%), Burkitt's lymphoma (40%), anaplastic large cell lymphoma (10%), and large B-cell lymphoma (20%).[15]

Because hematogenous dissemination occurs early in the course of non-Hodgkin's lymphoma in children, systemic treatment is the cornerstone of therapy. Investigators in the United States have focused on multiagent chemotherapy directed to the histologic subtype, whereas French and German investigators have chosen an immunophenotype-directed approach. Irradiation of the primary sites of disease is usually restricted to emergency situations such as airway compression. The tumor burden, reflected by both the stage of the disease and the serum lactate dehydrogenase concentration, are the most important predictors of the outcome.[2,10] Autologous bone marrow transplantation has been effective in selected children who have a partial remission with induction therapy or selected patients with relapse.

Despite improvements in the treatment of non-Hodgkin's lymphoma in children over the past 25 years, approximately 30% of patients relapse or do not have a first remission.[4] A significant number of patients also suffer severe late effects after cure, including cardiomyopathy and secondary acute myeloid leukemia.[16,17]

HODGKIN'S DISEASE

In children, Hodgkin's disease (HD) almost always presents in the second decade of life. Overall, approximately 4% of cases occur in children younger than 10 years of age, and 11% are found in children between 10 and 16 years of age. Children tend to have a better survival and freedom from relapse than their adult counterparts.[18]

HD usually presents as a nodal disease and only approximately 5% arise in extranodal sites.[19] The classically described rubbery, nontender, mobile lymph node of the neck and supraclavicular region is the most common presentation. The presence or absence of systemic "B" symptoms should be elucidated as they have implications on staging and thus on treatment and prognosis. These include drenching night sweats, loss of greater than 10% body weight over a 6-month period, and unexplained fever greater than 38 degrees Celsius for 3 consecutive days.

The gold standard of diagnosis is excisional surgical biopsy of an involved node. Enough material should be obtained to provide material for fresh, frozen, and formalin-fixed samples.[3] The presence of Hodgkin's cells (mononuclear cells) and Reed-Sternberg cells (binucleated or multinucleated tumor cells) in a background of reactive cells will confirm the diagnosis.

HD is separated into classical (nodular sclerosing, mixed cellularity, lymphocyte-rich classical, and lymphocyte-depleted) and lymphocyte predominant (LPHD) by the World Health Organisation (WHO).[20] For staging purposes CXR, CT of the chest, and MRI abdomen/pelvis, as well as bone marrow biopsy must be completed. PET scan is optional. CBC, ESR, CRP, alkaline phosphatase, albumin, LDH, and complete blood chemistry also need to be completed.[20]

The accepted staging system is the Ann Arbor system:

Stage I: Single lymph node region or extralymphatic organ site.

Stage II: Involvement of two or more lymph node regions on the same side of the diaphragm or localized involvement of extralymphatic organ or site and/or one or more lymph node regions on the same side of the diaphragm.

Stage III: Involvement of lymph node regions on both sides of the diaphragm which may also be accomplished by localized involvement of extralymphatic organ or site or by involvement of the spleen or both spleen and extralymphatic organ.

Stage IV: Diffuse or disseminated involvement of one or more extralymphatic organs or tissue with or without associated lymph node enlargement.

Each stage is qualified by the presence or absence of B symptoms: A—absent, B—present. Also qualified by E for extranodal site of disease, most commonly the spleen.

Additional risk factors which require more aggressive treatment include large mediastinal mass, extranodal involvement, massive involvement of the spleen, elevated ESR, and extensive lymph node involvement.[20] Treatment of HD depends on stage and risk stratification. In some stages chemotherapy: doxorubicin, bleomycin, vincristine, and dacarbazine (ABVD)-only is an option. A combination of low-dose radiation therapy and chemotherapy commonly is used with generally more cycles for more advanced disease. As the long-term effects of radiation on growing children are well documented many researchers are searching for ways to treat these young patients with chemotherapy alone.

RHABDOMYOSARCOMA

Childhood rhabdomyosarcoma (RMS) is a soft tissue malignant tumor of mesenchymal skeletal muscle origin. It is the most common soft tissue sarcoma in children and adolescents, accounting for approximately 3.5% of cases of cancer among children below age 14, and 2% of the cases among adolescents and young adults 15 to 19 years of age.[21,22] About 35% of all RMSs arise in the head and neck region. These tumors can then be further divided into three different groups based on location: parameningeal

(40%), orbital (30%), and nonorbital/nonparameningeal (30%).[23]

Presentation is dependent on site of origin. Orbital tumors most often present with proptosis, strabismus, or visible lid lesions and thus are usually diagnosed in a relatively early stage of the disease process.[24] Conversely, parameningeal tumors of the nasopharynx/nasal cavity, paranasal sinuses, middle ear, mastoid, and the pterygopalatine and infratemporal fossae present with a wide variety of signs and symptoms depending on location and extent of tumor infiltration: isolated cranial nerve palsy, painless enlarging cervical of facial/cranial mass, meningeal symptoms, or chronic otitis media not responsive to standard treatment are among the possible presenting signs.[25] These patients can also present with ophthalmic symptoms due to extension of the tumor along the skull base or through the paranasal sinuses. Symptoms are often nonspecific: airway obstruction, persistent upper respiratory tract symptoms, sinusitis, epiphora, epistaxis, nasal obstruction, and nasal discharge can all occur with nasal and paranasal sinus involvement.[26] Nonorbital, nonparameningeal tumors including the oral cavity, larynx, parotid region, cheek, scalp and soft tissue of the neck, usually present with a painless enlarging mass in the involved region.

CT scan and MRI are complementary imaging modalities necessary to delineate the anatomic extent of the tumor and thus have accurate staging information. On CT RMS appears as a homogeneous mass with very mild contrast enhancement. With MRI there is better resolution of soft tissues which is useful when attempting to delineate recurrence from postradiation changes. RMS enhances significantly with gadolinium and has intermediate signal on both T1 and T2 scans. Also included in the standard workup are CXR and bone scan. Bone marrow biopsy is performed when skeletal lesions are identified. Lumbar puncture should be included if intracerebral extension is suspected.[25,27]

Rhabdomyosarcomas are staged with a TNM staging system developed by the Intergroup Rhabdomyosarcoma Study Group (IRS). Stage 1 includes patients with head and neck tumors (excluding parameningeal sites) either confined to their site of origin or with extension to local tissues (including regional lymph node metastasis). Stage 2 includes patients with parameningeal tumors with no lymph node involvement and stage 3 comprises those parameningeal tumors with lymph node spread. Stage 4 are those patients with distant metastases.[28,29] In addition, in an anatomic staging paradigm, the IRS has also grouped patients based on surgical pathology. Group I includes patients with localized disease, completely resected. Group II are patients with total gross resection with evidence of regional spread. Patients in group III have tumors that have been incomplete resected with gross residual disease. Patients in group IV have distant metastatic disease at presentation.[29]

Biopsy is critical to make a definitive diagnosis and initiating combined modality treatment. Core needle biopsy may be performed in select cases and pathologic diagnosis can be made using H&E staining. Microscopically, RMS is composed primarily of small, anaplastic, round and spindle-shaped cells exhibiting hyperchromic nuclei and granular acidophilic cytoplasm. However, in certain instances immunohistochemical staining is necessary to identify the presence of desmin and myoglobin in the malignant spindle cells. These reactions can sometimes occur focally which can lead to misdiagnosis; therefore, multiple areas from the specimen should be sampled and examined.[30]

Embryonal (spindle cell and botryoid are variants), alveolar, and undifferentiated are the three distinct histologic types of rhabdomyoscaroma described. Embryonal is the most common making up 70% of cases, with alveolar contributing approximately 20% and undifferentiated 4%. The IRS combines the alveolar and undifferentiated types due to their similar clinical behavior and response to treatment. Specific translocations and immunohistochemical staining patterns have been identified within each group.[29]

Treatment consists of a combination of surgery, multiagent chemotherapy (vincristine, dactinomycin, and cyclophosphamide) with or without the addition of radiation treatment. Since the formation of the IRS the cure rate has increased from 25% in 1970 to 70% in 1991. As this text is published, the IRS has now completed five large consecutive trials and is currently pursuing Study VI. Risk factors associated with reduction in overall and disease-free survival include age <1 year, adolescent age (>10 years), parameningeal site, advanced tumor stage and group, and undifferentiated or alveolar histologic type. Toxicity of chemotherapy frequently consists of myelosuppression. Fifty-five percent of patients treated in IRS IV developed severe infections with treatment-related mortality of less than 1%. The 3-year estimated cumulative incidence of a secondary malignancy was 2%. Survival after relapse is dependent on group, with 40% 3-year survival after relapse in group 1 and 2 versus 22% for group 3.[31]

NEUROBLASTOMA

Neuroblastic tumors are the third most common cause of solid tumors in early childhood. They originate from the sympathetic chains and are located on the adrenal glands in 75 to 90% of cases. Cervical primary tumors account for only 5% of cases.[32]

Presenting symptoms generally are the result of mass effect either on the nearby cranial nerves or on the upper aerodigestive tract. Horner's syndrome as well as compression of CNs IX to XII have been reported. Airway compromise in the form of sleep apnea, stridor, and stertor are all possible symptoms. Solitary neck mass can also be the presentation. Generally, neuroblastic tumors that present themselves in the head and neck are more likely metastasis from a nonhead and neck primary and thus the chest, abdomen, and pelvis must be imaged as part of the routine workup.

Essential laboratory testing includes serum LDH, ferritin, and urine catecholomines. Amplification of the N-myc oncogene is evaluated.[33]

US, CT, or MRI can be used to delineate the extent of disease. Calcifications are commonly seen. Imaging of the abdomen and pelvis are essential to rule out primary abdominal tumors and/or liver metastasis.[34] Bone marrow biopsy and myelogram are part of the staging process. Scintiscan with [131]iodine-methyliodobenzylguanidine (MIBG) is useful before and after treatment to discriminate active residual tumor from scar formation. It also serves the dual purpose as a screen for bone involvement.

There is no TNM staging for these malignancies. The International Neuroblastoma staging system is a clinical pathologic classification based on completeness of surgical resection, status of margins, and regards nodal involvement and the presence of metastasis.

Stage 1 includes patients with localized tumor with complete gross excision, with or without microscopic residual disease; ipsilateral lymph nodes negative for malignancy.

Patients in *Stage 2A* have localized tumor with incomplete gross excision; ipsilateral lymph nodes negative for tumor.

In *Stage 2B* ipsilateral lymph nodes are positive for disease. Enlarged contralateral lymph nodes are negative for disease.

Stage 3 includes patients with unresectable unilateral tumor infiltrating across midline, with or without regional lymph node involvement; localized tumor with contralateral lymph node involvement; or midline tumor with bilateral extension by infiltration or lymph node involvement.

Stage 4 includes any primary tumor with distant metastasis to lymph nodes, bone marrow, liver, skin, and/or other organ, and

Stage 4S specifies infants <1year of age: with localized primary tumor (stages 1, 2A, or 2B) with dissemination limited to skin, liver, and/or <10% bone marrow involvement. "S" indicates the higher rate of spontaneous regression among this group.

Neuroblastic tumors are derived from a nine precursor uptake and distribution of cells of neural crest origin. Neuroblastic tumors are classified into three histologic subgroups from least to most differentiated, neuroblastomas, ganglioneuroblastomas, and ganglioneuromas. The three histologic types are different developmental stages of the same disease.[35] Treatment is based on stage, age, and the presence of N-myc amplification. In the absence of N-myc amplification, surgical extirpation should be attempted in resectable tumors. In these cases, microscopic residual disease appears to have little impact on prognosis.[36] Unfavorable prognostic indicators in stage 2 disease after gross surgical resection include N-myc amplification, undifferentiated histologic types, age older than 2 years, and lymph node metastasis.[37] Survival in more advanced stages depends on combined treatment with surgery and chemotherapy.[38]

Surveillance is mandatory and studies include urine catecholamine levels (if originally an amine-secreting tumor), MIBG scintiscans, and MRI.

SARCOMA

Non-rhabdomyosarcoma soft tissue sarcomas (NRSTS) are a heterogeneous group of tumors that account for 3% to 5% of childhood malignancies.[39] NRSTS's arising in the head and neck include fibrosarcoma, synovial sarcoma, neurofibrosarcoma, or malignant schwannoma, hemangiopericytoma, chondrosarcoma, and extraosseous Ewing's sarcoma. These tumors are more common in the adolescent age group and cannot be differentiated from RMS on a clinical basis; therefore, pathologic examination of representative biopsy material is critical.

Similar to RMS these tumors typically present as firm enlarging masses in the head and neck. Their symptoms generally are related to that of mass effect on surrounding vital structures.

The diagnostic workup for non-RMS is essentially the same as that for RMS and has been outlined previously in this chapter. MRI is the preferred imaging modality to define extent of disease. Staging is similar to that of RMS. T1 tumors are confined to one anatomic site of origin. T2 demonstrates extension or infiltration into surrounding tissue. The A subtype refers to tumors less than or equal to 5 cm. B refers to tumors larger than 5 cm. Orbital and head and neck tumors are considered stage 1. Cranial parameningeal tumors are considered stage 2 if there are no involved nodes or stage 3 if there are positive lymph nodes. Tumors are considered stage 4 only when metastasis is present.[40]

Due to the great biological diversity of these tumors, histopathologic identification of the particular tumor type is critical to treatment planning. Fibrosarcoma consists of small uniform spindle or round cells arranged in fascicular-like groups. Desmoid fibromatosis appear as fascicles of spindle fibroblasts in a myxoid background. Malignant schwannoma or neurofibrosarcoma shows a plexiform, swirling pattern of fusiform cells with elongated nuclei and variable collagen content with abundant mitotic figures. Other histopathologic variants include synovial sarcoma, hemangiopericytoma, and extraosseous Ewing's sarcoma among others.

Currently, the most important factors determining the likelihood of cure are histologic grade and tumor resectability.[41] Local control with surgical resection, with or without radiation therapy, is the cornerstone of treatment for patients with localized disease. The 5-year survival in children with completely resected tumors approaches 90% in some series[42,43] and the administration of adjuvant chemotherapy does not appear to improve the outcome in this group.[44] In contrast, children with incompletely resected tumors or metastatic disease fair poorly, with fewer than one-third of patients surviving long term.[45-48]

SALIVARY GLAND MALIGNANCIES

Salivary gland malignancies are exceedingly rare in children, and fewer than 5% of all malignant parotid tumors occur in the pediatric population.[49] Vascular lesions far outnumber solid tumors in parotid and submandible regions.[50] The most common solid salivary tumors in children are pleomorphic adenomas, followed by the malignant tumors: mucoepidermoid and acinic cell carcinomas.[50,51] In children, the risk of cancer of the salivary gland increases with age.[49] According to one study, 73% of tumors occurred in children over the age of 10. A 2006 study reviewed the Surveillance, Epidemiology, and End Results (SEER) database for the time period 1988 through 2001 and found 113 primary salivary gland malignancies (103 parotid, 10 submandibular) in children under the age of 18. There was a 10:1 ratio between parotid and submandibular gland incidence. Mean age of presentation was 13.2 years. Female: male ratio of 5:4.[52] Additional risk factors included

previous radiation therapy to the head and neck and a history of multiagent chemotherapy treatment.[50]

Slowly enlarging salivary mass is the most common presenting symptom. These masses persist after empiric antibiotic treatment. They may be tender or nontender. Facial nerve paralysis and skin tethering are rarely reported.[49] However, these masses may be firm and fixed to the skin.[53] Extraglandular tumor extension may be found in approximately 20% of tumors. Shapiro and Bhattacharyya found that 8.7% of parotid malignancies presented with localregional lymphadenopathy, whereas none of the submandibular gland malignancies presented with pathologic lymphadenopathy.[52]

Fine needle aspiration may be attempted. However, definitive tissue diagnosis is made at the time of surgery by complete excision. Incisional biopsies are contraindicated due to the risk of tumor spillage and facial nerve injury.

Ultrasound, CT scan, and MRI can all be used to image the parotid and submandibular gland lesions. MRI may have some advantages in viewing soft tissue infiltration but generally one of the three imaging modalities is adequate for preoperative evaluation.[54,55]

TNM staging is the same as that used in adults and can be referenced in the chapter on salivary gland malignancies.

The most common malignant histologic types are mucoepidermoid carcinomas (MEC) followed by acinic cell carcinomas.[52] Other salivary gland cancers reported are rhabdomyosarcoma, lymphoma, adenocarcinoma, Hodgkin's disease, adenoid cystic carcinoma, and embryomas among others.[52,56] Recurrence and overall survival in MEC are linked to tumor size, histocytologic grade, clinical stage of disease, perineural and vascular involvement, as well as lymph node and distant metastasis. Low-grade histologies are more frequent in pediatric mucoepidermal carcinoma than in adults conveying a survival advantage.[50] In contrast, the survival for rhabdomyosarcoma involving the major salivary glands tends to be poorer than that of epithelial salivary gland neoplasms.[52]

For parotid disease either superficial or total parotidectomy is the mainstay of treatment. Submandibular gland excision is the gold standard for submandibular involvement. Neck dissection is of limited value and is only recommended when there are clinically positive lymph nodes.[51,57] Postoperative radiotherapy is recommended for high-grade lesions or those with adverse prognostic factors, such as soft-tissue extension and perineural invasion, microscopic residual disease, or lymph node involvement.[57,58]

Complications of treatment include those commonly encountered during parotidectomy or submandibular gland excision. Facial nerve paralysis/paresis, hypertrophied/keloid scar formation, and Frey's syndrome are among the possible complications of surgery. If radiation therapy is required, risks include long-term trismus, dentofacial deformity, osteoradialnecrosis, and development of secondary malignancies.[49]

MALIGNANT TERATOMAS

Cervicofacial teratoma is a rare condition accounting for one in 20,000 to 40,000 live births.[59] Three to 6% of all teratomas are thought to involve the head and neck.[59,60] An even smaller subset of these tumors (20%) are found to be malignant.[59]

Craniofacial teratomas may manifest prenatally on ultrasound with macrocrania or polyhydramnios. They also may present during delivery or postnatally as a life-threatening mass causing brain herniation, hydrocephalus, respiratory distress, or feeding difficulty. Due to the increased use of prenatal ultrasound, early diagnosis can help alert the medical team to prepare for ex utero intrapartum treatment procedure. This necessitates the presence of a pediatric otolaryngologist ready to obtain a surgical airway at the time of delivery while maternal fetal circulation is still intact.[59]

Metastatic malignant teratomas are rare and generally consist of neuroectodermal elements and immature neural tissue. In aproximately one-third of cases the metastatic tissue was more differentiated than the primary tumor and did not necessarily confer a poor prognosis.[59]

Prenatal ultrasound is essential to establish the diagnosis of teratoma. However, distinguishing malignant from benign teratoma is difficult because tumor size, presence of calcification, and gross appearance (cystic or solid) do not relate to the tumor's benign or malignant nature.[61] Elevated alpha fetal protein (AFP) can be seen in patients with malignancy and in patients with immature lesions. Postoperative rise in AFP level is a good indicator of malignant recurrence in those tumors that are AFP secretors.[62]

CT and MRI can be used to delineate the extent of teratoma. The masses are usually multiloculated, often large, with complex radiologic characteristics. Determining intracranial involvement through imaging is imperative in the preoperative planning.

Teratoma is the most common type of germ cell tumor, derived from pluripotent cells, and can be seen with varying degrees of differentiation. They contain a medley of heterogeneous tissues, typically reflecting more than one of the three embryonic germ layers (endoderm, mesoderm, and ectoderm). Malignancy is not equated with the degree of immaturity of the tissue elements.

After an airway is secured and the extent of the lesions has been delineated by imaging complete surgical resection followed by multiagent chemotherapy with or without radiation for malignant lesions is the mainstay of therapy. Early complete resection of all teratomas is advocated for several reasons. One being that there is a high potential for malignant transformation in cervical lesions not treated before adolescence or adulthood; this potential is greater than 90% in some reports.[59] Removal of the mass may also aid and relieve aerodigestive tract obstruction.

Complications from surgery are related to location and extent of the lesion. These include nerve injury to branches of the facial nerve and recurrent laryngeal nerve, as well as cosmetic deformity from resection. Brain ischemia at the time of delivery due to delay in obtaining an adequate airway is a possible and potentially devastating complication. Long-term surveillance should be conducted to monitor for the late effects of chemotherapy and radiation as well as for recurrence.

POST-TRANSPLANT LYMPHOPROLIFERATIVE DISORDERS

Post-transplant lymphoproliferative disorder (PTLD) is an unusual entity that has emerged as a significant complication of solid organ transplantation. PTLD is a term that collectively describes all abnormal proliferation of lymphoid tissue seen in the post-transplant population. The normal prominence of Waldeyer's ring lymphoid tissue and PTLD has high morbidity and mortality rates secondary to difficulty in diagnosis, prevention, treatment, and potential for graft loss. The increasing process of pediatric transplantation are reasons accounting for the observation that PTLD may first present in the tonsils and adenoids in the pediatric transplant population.

The incidence of PTLD has risen since the mid-1980s. Data from the North American Pediatric Renal Transplant Cooperative Study (NAPRTCS) showed a significant doubling of incidence density from 320 cases per 100,000 years of patient follow-up from 1987 to 1992 to 630 cases per 100,000 years of patient follow-up from 1992 to 1997.[63] With the introduction of prophylactic measures recently, however, some centers, have reported a reduction in prevalence of PTLD at their institutions.[64] Current prevalence rates range from 1% to 15%, depending on the organ transplanted and the immunosuppressive agents used.

The single most important risk factor is the lack of previous exposure to Epstein-Barr virus (EBV). Prevalence in EBV-seronegative recipients ranges from 23% to 50%, compared to 0.7% to 1.9% for seropositive recipients. The highest rates of PTLD are reported for intestinal transplantation followed by heart, lung, and liver.[65] Prevalence in kidney and bone marrow transplants are usually lower. Prevalence is highest in the pediatric age group, with a relative risk of 2.81 as compared to adult recipients.[65] Caucasian children also appear to have a higher relative risk.[65] The immunosuppressive agents muromonab-Cd3 (OKT3) and tacrolimus (FK506) have been reported to increase the risk of PTLD.

The pathogenesis of PTLD is intimately linked to EBV. Persistence of the EBV genome in the latent state in transformed B cells occurs following a primary EBV infection and results in a permanent carrier state in which small numbers of latently infected B cells circulate in seropositive individuals. Elimination of these cells is usually carried out by cytotoxic T lymphocytes. With immunosuppression, however, these infected cells are allowed to proliferate.

According to the above paradigm, all PTLDs should represent B-cell proliferation secondary to EBV infection; however, T cell and natural killer cell PTLDs have also been reported. Furthermore, PTLDs not associated with EBV have been noted. A higher proportion of late-developing PTLDs (>2 years post-transplant) are more likely to be non-B cell or non-EBV related.

Signs and symptoms of PTLD are usually vague and include fever, poor appetite, weight loss, irritability, diarrhea, and impaired general condition. PTLD has been noted to present with adenotonsillar hypertrophy (ATH) in several recent reports.[66] Patients can also present with sudden onset lymphoid hyperplasia either externally (cervical lymph nodes) or internally (abdominal or intracranial). Occasionally, these masses may develop within the graft. PTLD may also present as fever of unknown origin in the transplant recipient or may mimic graft rejection, particularly late rejection. Depending on location, symptoms may range from abdominal pain, respiratory difficulty, stridor, and seizures. The time to diagnosis can be highly variable, ranging from a few months to several years posttransplant. The mean time in most series is 20 to 35 months.

Serological tests (immunoglobulin G and M) should be performed to determine recent EBV infection. The serum can also be analyzed for EBV viral capsid antigen (EB-VCA). Multiple studies have demonstrated that increased EBV viral loads can be used to differentiate between latent infection and PTLD. Rooney et al[67] showed that levels of EBV DNA between 20,000 and 200,000 copies per microgram of peripheral blood DNA were associated with subsequent PTLD. In pediatric patients, however, viral load monitoring is associated with high sensitivity but poor specificity. Many pediatric patients exhibit higher viral loads than adults because of a primary EBV infection or a chronic high viral load state without ever developing PTLD.

Monoclonal proteins, particularly IgM related, have been reported to appear with greater frequency in serum and urine of patients with PTLD.

Initial studies are often focused on the manifesting symptoms, such as imaging localization of the mass and determination of its extent, invasiveness, and homogenicity. Ultrasound, CT scanning, or MRI can be used depending on the area of interest.

Histopathologic diagnosis of biopsy tissue remains the criterion standard for making the diagnosis of PTLD. By light microscopy, infiltrates of polymorphous or monomorphous mononuclear cells are observed that disrupt the architecture of the invaded tissue. Depending on the degree of proliferation and dedifferentiation, lesions may be characterized as hyperplastic, lymphomatous, or intermediate. EBV can frequently be demonstrated within the abnormal cells. PTLD may coexist with acute rejection, and the diagnoses may be difficult to separate. The features that favor the diagnosis of PTLD include nodular infiltrates, serpiginous necrosis, plasmacytoid and immunoblastic cells, and absence of ancillary cells such as neutrophils.

The World Health Organization (WHO) classifies PTLD into 4 major categories: (1) early lesions, which encompass reactive lymphoplasmacytic hyperplasia and infectious mononucleosis-like lesions; (2) polymorphous PTLD; (3) monomorphic PTLD, which should be classified according to the WHO classification of lymphoma; and (4) Hodgkin lymphoma and Hodgkin lymphoma-like PTLD.

Adenotonsillar hypertrophy may be the earliest sign of PTLD. Several studies have demonstrated that adenotonsillar tissue is a principal reservoir for EBV replication.[68] Prompt adenotonsillectomy may initiate management of PTLD in its earliest forms.

No uniform consensus exists regarding optimal treatment options for PTLD. Treatment is often based on WHO classification.[69] Type 1 disease usually requires no therapy, whereas type 2 disease requires reduction of immunosuppresion. There may also be a role for antiviral medication (acyclovir and ganciclovir). Types 3 and 4 are the most controversial groups. Some advocate the use of an escalating approach consisting of reduction of immunosuppression followed by chemotherapy or radiation therapy for nonresponders.

Anti-CD20 monoclonal antibody has recently been used, with promising results, to neutralize the CD20-expressing B cells. Interferon-alfa is also reported to be efficacious in treatment of PTLD that is unresponsive to immunosuppressive dose reduction alone. Some protocols combine this agent with intravenous immunoglobulin.

Standard cancer chemotherapy is reserved for patients with definitive features of malignancy. The usual regimen used has been the CHOP regimen for non-Hodgkin lymphoma.

Recent attention has focused on prophylactic treatment with the use of concomitant antiviral therapy (ganciclovir, acyclovir, or valacyclovir) in adult transplant recipients.[70] Using routine viral load monitoring and pre-emptive therapy, several studies have shown a reduction in PTLD prevalence based on historical controls, particularly in the pediatric liver transplant population.[71] These results have led many centers to perform routine viral load monitoring, particularly for pre-emptive interventions including reduction in immunosuppression or initiation of antiviral therapy when a significant rise in EB viral load occurs.

The prognosis of PTLD is highly variable. Most mild cases regress. The outlook for more severe cases is less favorable, particularly in frank malignancies or CNS PTLD. Non-EBV positive or late onset cases have a poorer prognosis.

Graft rejection is an obvious risk with reduction of immunosuppression. Surprisingly, however, it is not observed in every patient. Immunomodulation by the underlying disease is speculated to prevent the normal alloimmune response in these patients. Retransplantation has been performed successfully.

THYROGLOSSAL DUCT CARCINOMA

Thyroglossal duct carcinoma (TGD carcinoma) is rare, occurring in approximately 1% of all thyroglossal duct cysts. It is usually diagnosed postoperatively. Eighty-five to 90% are papillary carcinomas of thyroid origin. The thyroid gland is first identifiable as a median thickening of the endoderm in the floor of the pharynx between the first and second pharyngeal pouches. This tissue mass forms a diverticulum and descends to the level of the laryngeal primordium. The thyroglossal tract is normally obliterated but, when it persists, may increase the likelihood of the formation of a thyroglossal duct cyst. Accessory thyroid tissue may be found along the path of migration.

The etiology of the disease process is controversial. Theories include metastasis, direct extension through the thyroglossal duct, or primary development of carcinoma in the cyst wall or ectopic thyroid tissue.

The clinical presentation of TGD carcinoma is often very similar to that of its benign counterpart, with a gradually enlarging, painless midline neck mass. It may present in childhood, but the median age for development is 40 years. Uncommonly, dysphagia, voice change, or a draining cutaneous sinus can be seen. Carcinoma should be suspected in any cyst that is hard, fixed, irregular, or is associated with lymphadenopathy.

In most cases TGD carcinoma is an incidental finding after surgical excision. On the rare occasion when malignancy is suspected clinically, fine-needle aspiration (FNA) cytology or imaging may possibly help. Seventeen cases of preoperative FNA cytology of TGD papillary carcinoma have been reported in the literature, with a true-positive rate of 53% and a false-negative rate of 47%.[72] Hypocellular cystic fluid was aspirated in many of the reported false-negative cases.

In the workup of a thryoglossal duct cyst, an ultrasound is warranted to identify normal thyroid tissue anterior to the trachea. Occasionally, the only functioning thyroid tissue may be found within the tract itself.

Imaging in the form of CT is rarely justified during the preoperative assessment of a presumed TGD cyst. However, if it is performed, a TGD cyst is seen as well-circumscribed, and low-density with a smooth, thin wall. Rim contrast enhancement may also be observed. The most common CT findings in the presence of malignancy include a solid nodule within the cyst, calcification, an irregular margin, and a thick wall.[73]

Positive identification of a thyroglossal duct cyst is accomplished by demonstrating an epithelial lining of the duct and/or cyst and normal thyroid follicles in its wall. TGD carcinoma is, consequently, generally either of thyroid or squamous cell origin. Thyroid papillary carcinoma is the most common type, followed by mixed papillary/follicular carcinoma, and squamous cell carcinoma. Uncommonly, Hürthle cell, follicular, and anaplastic carcinoma can be seen.

Widstrom et al[74] described the criteria that should be fulfilled for a definitive diagnosis of primary TGD carcinoma: First, the carcinoma should be in the wall of the TGD cyst. Second, the TGD carcinoma must be differentiated from a cystic lymph node metastasis by histologic demonstration of a squamous or columnar epithelial lining and normal thyroid follicles in the wall of the cyst. And third, there should be no malignancy in the thyroid gland or any other possible primary site.

Much of the controversy in the management of this neoplasm surrounds the optimal surgical management of the thyroid gland. Advocates of total thyroidectomy point to an associated 25% to 30% incidence of papillary carcinoma in thyroid glands removed in the setting of TGD carcinoma.[75]

A Sistrunk procedure, which involves en bloc resection of the thyroglossal duct cyst, mid-portion of the hyoid bone, and tract, is the treatment of the primary lesion. In a retrospective review conducted by Patel et al, prognostic factors predictive of overall survival in patients with TGD carcinoma revealed that the only significant predictor of outcome was the extent of surgery for the TGD cyst.[75] Those who had a simple excision faired significantly worse than those who had a Sistrunk operation, with 10-year overall survival rates of 75% and 100%, respectively. Also, the addition of total thyroidectomy to the Sistrunk procedure did not have significant impact on outcome.

If the TGD carcinoma focus is well-differentiated carcinoma, microscopic, without invasion of the cyst wall, and if there are no palpable masses in the thyroid or neck, then an en bloc resection without thyroidectomy should suffice. In the setting of carcinoma in the thyroid gland or cervical lymph nodes, a total thyroidectomy, followed by postoperative radioiodine therapy and thyroid-stimulating hormone suppression, appears warranted. Modified neck dissection should be considered in the setting of palpable cervical lymphadenopathy. The reported cure rate for TGD carcinoma is 95%. All patients require close postoperative follow-up.

Complications involve those related to the surgical procedures performed. A Sistrunk procedure carries with it the risk of recurrence, hypothyroidism (if the only functioning thyroid tissue is within the TGD cyst), and less commonly, fistula, abscess, airway injury, and recurrent laryngeal nerve injury.

LANGERHANS' CELL HISTIOCYTOSIS

Langerhans' cell histiocytosis (LCH) is a rare group of diverse disorders with the common primary event of the accumulation and infiltration of Langerhans' cells in the affected tissues. The etiology and pathogenesis remain largely unknown. The incidence of LCH is 4.0 to 5.4 per million of population. The estimated incidence of neonatal LCH is 1 to 2 per million neonates. The male-to-female ratio is 2:1. The incidence peaks in children aged 1 to 3 years; however, the disease can be seen in neonates to adults.

Normally, Langerhans' cells act as antigen-presenting cells in the skin, and are found in the skin, lymph nodes, bronchial mucosa, and thymus. LCH cells are nonfunctioning, and appear to be arrested in an activated state. They have a wider tissue distribution than normal Langerhans' cells and consequently present in a variety of ways. The cells lack histologic evidence of malignancy but behave in an aggressive manner.

LCH can be local and asymptomatic, as in isolated bone lesions, or it can involve multiple organs and systems. The clinical manifestations, therefore, can vary. Bone involvement is observed in 78% of patients and often includes the skull 49%, innominate bone 23%, femur 17%, and orbit 11%. On clinical examination, the lesions can be singular or multiple. Asymptomatic or painful involvement of vertebrae can occur and result in collapse. Long bone involvement can induce fractures. Purulent otitis media may occur. Maxillary, mandibular, and gingival disease may cause loss of teeth, hemorrhagic gum, and mucosal ulceration. Patients may present with brown to purplish papules over any part of the body (Hashimoto-Pritzker disease). Pulmonary involvement is observed in 20% to 40% and may result in cough, tachypnea, dyspnea, and pneumothorax. GI bleeding may be the presenting sign of patients with GI involvement. Liver, spleen, and marrow involvement may cause hematologic changes. Lymph node enlargement is observed in 30% of patients. Infiltration of various areas of the brain gives rise to corresponding signs and symptoms. The most common site of CNS involvement is the hypothalamic-pituitary axis resulting in diabetes insipidus and delayed puberty. Patients with periorbital lesions often have proptosis because of a tumor mass behind the eye.

Despite variability in its presentation, one area that is commonly affected is the head and neck region.

The reported incidence of temporal bone involvement ranges from 15% to 61%, with an initial otologic presentation in as many as 25%. Common aural symptoms include otorrhea unresponsive to medical therapy, postauricular swelling, conductive hearing loss, and aural polyp or granulation tissue. Facial nerve paralysis, vertigo, or sensorineural loss is rare.

The cause of LCH is unknown. Factors implicated in the etiology include viral infections, cellular and immune dysfunction, neoplastic mechanisms, genetic factors, and dysfunction of cellular adhesion molecules.

All patients should receive a complete evaluation, including general pediatric examination, hematologic evaluation, ESR, liver function tests, coagulation studies, urinalysis, chest radiography, and bone marrow biopsy. A skeletal survey or radionucleotide study to detect skeletal lesions should be performed. Depending on location, other studies that may be performed include PFTs, small bowel series, hepatic ERCP, MRI of brain, CT imaging of head/neck/chest, audiogram, and endocrine investigation. Radiographic imaging of lytic lesions of the skull reveals a punched-out pattern without evidence of periosteal reaction or marginal sclerosis. Ultimately, however, biopsy is needed to establish the diagnosis of LCH.

The histologic hallmark of this disease is a proliferation of the Langerhans' dendritic cell in a background of inflammatory cells with sheets of eosinophils, as well as presence of Birbeck granules on electron microscopy. Immunohistochemical staining demonstrates positivity for CD1a and S-100. The histopathology of LCH does not appear to be prognostic of the outcome of the disease.

Physicians should be aware of the multiple ways in which LCH can present to help with expediting the diagnosis and treatment of the disease.

The entity now referred to as LCH was initially divided into eosinophilic granuloma, Hand-Schuller-Christian disease, and Letterer-Siwe disease, depending on the sites and severity. Most recently, this designation was changed to LCH to reflect the recognition of the primary cell involved and the pathophysiology of the disease. Hand-Schuller-Christian disease represents the more severe, systemic form of LCH. It classically involves the triad of diabetes insipidus, proptosis, and bone disease and is characterized by multifocal osseous lesions with limited extraskeletal involvement of skin, lymph nodes, and viscera. Letterer-Siwe disease is the disseminated form of LCH with multiorgan involvement that characteristically presents with fever, rash, lymphadenopathy, hepatosplenomegaly, dyspnea, and blood dyscrasias. Historically, the disease course was rapidly progressive with a high mortality rate.

LCH is now classified as a single-system disease (unifocal or multifocal) or a multisystem disease if more than one system is involved. The presence of organ function failure in the liver, lung, or bone marrow identifies LCH with "organ dysfunction."

Patients are stratified by The Histiocyte Society into three groups: (1) at-risk patients, or those with multisystemic involvement including 1 or more at-risk organs; (2) low-risk patients, or those with multisystem involvement not including at-risk organs; and (3) other patients, or those with single-system multifocal bone disease or localized involvement of special sites (intraspinal extension or involvement of the paranasal, parameningeal, periorbital, or mastoid region) that can lead to persistent, soft-tissue swelling.

Optimal treatment of LCH has not been established. Substantial variation of the disease and the fact that 10% to 20% of patients achieve spontaneous regression complicates the comparison of current therapies.

If a patient clearly has only one site involved (eg, skin, lymph nodes, non-CNS risk bone lesion), therapy may consist of only prednisone, Velban and prednisone, or curettage of the bone lesions. Lesions limited to the mastoid cortex may be treated by cortical mastoidectomy. These patients should be watched carefully for evidence of disease in other organs.

In patients with multiple bone lesions or multisystem (nonrisk organ) involvement, a short treatment course with only a single agent (eg, prednisone) is not sufficient, and relapses commonly occur in these patients. These patients should receive treatment with Velban and prednisone for 6 or 12 months.

Patients with multisystem disease and risk organ involvement can be difficult to treat. If they do not respond in the first 6 to 12 weeks to treatment with Velban and prednisone, a salvage protocol, including the use of cladribine, is instituted.

Special sites have been designated because of the recognition that patients with multifocal bone disease and those patients with disease at the base of the skull need to have systemic therapy, not just local therapy or single-drug administration. Patients with only skin involvement, especially difficult ulcerative lesions of the scalp or inguinal region, may respond well to topical nitrogen mustard or corticosteroids. Thalidomide has proven to be an effective therapy for patients with skin and/or bone involvement, but is not indicated for those with high-risk lesions. Some evidence exists that bone marrow transplantation can be effective if performed when patients are in remission. At this time, no standard approach exists and data are insufficient to give survival estimates.

Radiation therapy has fallen out of favor, except for patients with bone lesions of the vertebrae or femoral neck, which are at risk of collapse. If a patient has vertebra plana, the disease likely has "burned out" and therapy will enhance the possibility of vertebral restoration. When instability of the cervical vertebrae and neurologic symptoms are present, spinal fusion is indicated.

Children with low-risk disease most often complete treatment and have no long-term sequelae beyond some obesity from treatment with prednisone. Those with diabetes insipidus (DI) are at risk for panhypopituitarism and should be monitored carefully for adequacy of growth and development. Hearing loss, neurocognitive and psychological problems, and orthopedic defects may be seen. Diffuse pulmonary disease may leave a patient with poor lung function. Liver disease may lead to ascending cholangitis, which is not amenable to any treatment other than liver transplant. Patients with LCH have a higher than normal risk of developing secondary cancers. Leukemia (usually acute myeloid) occurs after treatment as does lymphoblastic lymphoma. Concurrent LCH/malignancy has been reported in a few patients, and some patients have had their malignancy first, and developed LCH at a later date. Solid tumors associated with LCH include retinoblastoma, brain tumors, hepatocellular carcinoma, Askin tumor, and Ewing's sarcoma.

REFERENCES

1. Robison LL. General principles of the epidemiology of childhood cancer. In: Pizzo PA, Poplack DG, eds. *Principles and Practice of Pediatric Oncology.* 2nd ed. Philadelphia, Pa: JB Lippincott; 1993:3-10.

2. Magrath IT. Malignant non-Hodgkin's lymphomas in children. In: Pizzo PA, Poplack DG, eds. *Principles and Practice of Pediatric Oncology.* 2nd ed. Philadelphia, Pa: JB Lippincott; 1993:537-575.

3. Young JL Jr, Ries LG, Silverberg E, Horm JW, Miller RW. Cancer incidence, survival, and mortality for children younger than age 15 years. *Cancer.* 1986;58 (suppl):598-602.

4. Ries LAG, Miller BA, Hankey BF, Kosary CL, Harras A, Edwards BK, eds. SEER cancer statistics review, 1973-1991: tables and graphs. Bethesda, Md: National Cancer Institute; 1994. (NIH publication no. 94-2789.)

5. Murphy SB. Classification, staging and end results of treatment of childhood non-Hodgkin's lymphomas: similarities and differences from lymphomas in adults. *Semin Oncol.* 1980;7:332-339.

6. Young Jr JL, Miller RE. Incidence of malignant tumors in US children. *J Pediatr.* 1975;86:254-258.

7. Sandlund JT, Downing JR, Crist WM. Non-Hodgkin's lymphoma in childhood. *N Engl J Med.* 1996;334:1238-1248.

8. LaQuaglia MP. Non-Hodgkin's lymphoma of the head and neck in childhood. *Semin Pediatr Surg.* 1994;3:207-215.

9. Ellaurie M, Wiznia A, Bernstein L, Rubinstein A. Lymphoma in pediatric HIV infection. *Pediatr Res.* 1989;25:150A.

10. Murphy SB, Fairclough DL, Hutchison RE, Berard CW. Non-Hodgkin's lymphomas of childhood: an analysis of the histology, staging, and response to treatment of 338 cases at a single institution. *J Clin Oncol.* 1989;7:186-193.

11. Sandlund JT, Hutchison RE, Crist WM. Non-Hodgkin's lymphoma. In: Fernbach DJ, Vietti TJ, eds. *Clinical Pediatric Oncology.* 4th ed. St. Louis, Mo: Mosby-Year Book; 1991:337-353.

12. Weber AL, Rahemtullah A, Ferry JA. Hodgkin and non-Hodgkin lymphoma of the head and neck: clinical, pathologic, and imaging evaluation. *Neuroimaging Clin North Am.* 2003;13(3):371-392.

13. Jeffers MD, Milton J, Herriot R, McKean M. Fine needle aspiration in the investigation of non-hodgkin's lymphoma. *J Clin Pathol.* 1998;51:189-196.

14. Safley AM, Buckley PJ, Creager AJ, et al. The value of FISH and PCR in diagnosis of B-cell NHL by FNA. *Arch Pathol Lab Med.* 2004;128:1395-1403.

15. www.lymphomainfo.net

16. Lipshultz SE, Colan SD, Gelber RD, Perez-Atayde AR, Sallan SE, Sanders SP. Late cardiac effects of doxorubicin therapy for acute lymphoblastic leukemia in childhood. *N Engl J Med.* 1991;324:808-815.

17. Pui C-H, Ribeiro RC, Hancock ML, et al. Acute myeloid leukemia in children treated with epipodophyllotoxins for acute lymphoblastic leukemia. *N Engl J Med.* 1991;325:1682-1687.

18. Cleary SF, Link MP, Donaldson SS. Hodgkin's disease in the very young. *Int J Radiat Oncol Biol Phys.* 1994;28:77-83.

19. Weber AL, Rahemtullah A, Ferry JA. Hodgkin and non-Hodgkin lymphoma of the head and neck: clinical, pathologic, and imaging evaluation. *Neuroimaging Clin North Am.* 2003;13(3):371-392.

20. Jost LM, Stahel RA; ESMO Guidelines Task Force. ESMO Minimum Clinical Recommendations for diagnosis, treatment and follow-up of Hodgkin's disease. *Ann Oncol.* 2005;16(suppl 1):54-55.

21. JG Gurney, Severson RK, Davis S, et al. Incidence of cancer in children in the United States. Sex-, race-, and 1-year age-specific rates by histological type. *Cancer.* 1995;75(8)2186-2195.

22. LA Ries, BF Hankey, CL Kosary, et al, eds, SEER Cancer Statistics Review, 1973-1996. Bethesda, Md: National Cancer Institute; 1999. (Also available online.)

23. Dickson PV, Davidoff AM. Malignant neoplasms of the head and neck 2006. *Sem Pediatr Surg.* 2006;15:92-98.

24. Oberlin O, Rey A, Anderson J, et al. Treatment of orbital rhabdomyosarcoma: survival and late effects of treatment: results of an international workshop. *J Clin Oncol.* 2001;19:197-204.

25. Sbeity S, Abella A, Arcand P, et al. Temporal bone rhabdomyosarcoma in children. *J Ped Otorhinolaryngol.* In press.

26. Mullaney PB, Nabi, NU, Thorner P, et al. Ophthalmic involvement as a presenting feature of nonorbital childhood parameningeal embryonal rhabdomyosarcoma. *Ophthalmology.*2001;108(1):179-182.

27. Klem ML, Grewal RK, Wexler LH, Schoder H, Meyers PA, Wolden SL. PET for staging in rhabdomyosarcoma: an evaluation of PET as an adjunct to

current staging tools. *J Pediatr Hematol Oncol.* 2007;29(1):9-14.

28. Maurer HM, Beltangady M, Gehan EA, et al. The Intergroup Rhabdomyosarcoma Study—1. A final report. *Cancer.* 1988;61:209-220.

29. Pappo AS, Meza JL, Donaldson, SS, et al. Treatment of localized nonorbital, nonparameningeal head and neck rhabdomyosarcoma: lessons learned from intergroup rhabdomyosarcoma Studies III and IV. *J Clin Oncol.* 2003;21(4):638-645.

30. Salwa-Zurawska W, Biczysko W, Wozniak A, Janicka-Jedynska M, Trejster E. Usefulness of immunohistochemical testing and electron microscopy in the diagnosis of embryonal rhabdomyosarcoma. *Med Sci Monit.* 2002;8(1):BR39-BR46.

31. Crist WM, Anderson JR, Meza JL et al. Intergroup Rhabdomyosarcoma Study-IV: results for patients with nonmetastatic disease. *J Clin Oncol.* 2001; 19(12):3091-3102.

32. Jaffe N. Neuroblastoma: review of the literature and an examination of factors contributing to its enagmatic character. *Cancer Treat Rev.* 1976;3:61-62.

33. Triglia JM, Bernard JL, Scheiner C. Cervical neuroblastoma and multiple endocrine neoplasia type 2a. *Int J Pediatr Otorhinolaryngol.* 1993;26(1): 71-77.

34. Smith MCF, Smith RJH, Bailey M. Primary cervical neuroblastoma in infants. *J Laryngol Otol.* 1985; 99:209-214.

35. Shimada H, Ambros I, Dehner L, Hata J-I, Joshi VV, Roald B. Terminology and morphologic criteria of neuroblastic tumors. *Cancer.* 1999;86:349-363.

36. Koneko M, Ohakawa H, Iwakawa M. Is extensive surgery required for treatment of advanced neuroblastoma? *J Pediatr Surg.* 1997;32:1616-1619.

37. Perez CA, Matthay KK, Atkinson JB, et al. Biologic variables in the outcome of stages I and II neuroblastoma treated with surgery as primary therapy: a Children's Cancer Group study. *J Clin Oncol.* 2000;18:18-26.

38. Haase GM, O'Leary MC, Ramsay NKC, et al. Aggressive surgery combined with intensive chemotherapy improves survival in poor risk neuroblastoma. *J Pediatr Surg.* 1991;26:1119-1124.

39. Smith MA, Gloeckler Ries LA. Childhood cancer: Incidence, survival, and mortality. In: Pizzo PA, Poplack DG, eds. *Principles and Practice of Pediatric Oncology.* 4th ed. Philadelphia, Pa: Lippincott Williams & Wilkins; 2002:1-12.

40. Pappo AS, Shapiro DN, Crist WM. Biology and therapy of pediatric rhabdomyosarcoma. *J Clin Oncol.* 1995;13:2123.

41. Hayani A. Soft-tissue sarcomas other than rhabdomyosarcoma in children. *Med Pediatr Oncol.* 1992;20:114-118.

42. Spunt SL, Poquette CA, Hurt YS, et al. Prognostic factors for children and adolescents with surgically resected nonrhabdomyosarcoma soft tissue sarcoma: an analysis of 121 patients treated at St Jude Children's Research Hospital. *J Clin Oncol.* 1999;17:3697-3705.

43. Ben Arush MW, Nahum MP, Meller I, et al. The role of chemotherapy in childhood soft tissue sarcomas other than rhabodmyosarcomas. *Pediatr Hematol Oncol.* 1999;16:397-406.

44. Pratt CB, Pappo AS, Gieser P, et al. Role of adjuvant chemotherapy in the treatment of surgically resected pediatric nonrhabdomyosarcomatous soft tissue sarcomas: a Pediatric Oncology Group Study. *J Clin Oncol.* 1999;17:1219.

45. Pappo AS, Rao BN, Jenkins JJ, et al. Metastatic nonrhabdomyosarcomatous soft-tissue sarcomas in children and adolescents: The St. Jude Children's Research Hospital experience. *Med Pediatr Oncol.* 1999;33:76-82.

46. Pratt CB, Maurer H, Gieser P, et al. Treatment of unresectable or metastatic pediatric soft tissue sarcomas with surgery, irradiation, and chemotherapy: A Pediatric Oncology Group study. *Med Pediatr Oncol.* 1998;30:201-209.

47. Wexler LH, Helman LJ. Pediatric soft tissue sarcomas. *Calif Cancer J Clin.* 1994;44:211.

48. Dillion PW. Nonrhabdomyosarcoma soft tissue sarcomas in children *Semin Pediatr Surg.* 1997;6(1): 24-28.

49. Ethunandan M, Ethunandan A, Macpherson D, Conroy B, Pratt C. Parotid neoplasms in children: experience of diagnosis and management in a district general hospital. *Int J Oral Maxillofac Surg.* 2003;32(4):373-377.

50. J. Hicks, Flaitz C. Mucoepidermoid carcinoma of salivary glands in children and adolescents assessment of proliferation markers. *Oral Oncol.* 2000; 36(5):454-460.

51. Bentz BG, Hughes CA, Ludemann JP, Maddalozzo J. Masses of the salivary gland region in children. *Arch Otolaryngol Head Neck Surg.* 2000;126: 1435-1439.

52. Shapiro NL, Bhattacharyya N. Clinical characteristics and survival for major salivary gland malignancies in children. *Otolaryngol Head Neck Surg.* 2006;134(4):631-634.

53. Bianchi A, Cudmore RE. Salivary gland tumors in children. *J Pediatr Surg.* 1978;13:519-521.

54. Byrne MN, Spector JG, Garvin CF, Gado MH. Preoperative assessment of parotid masses: a comparative evaluation of radiologic techniques to histopathologic diagnosis. *Laryngoscope.* 1989; 99(3):284-292.

55. Koyuncu M, Sesen T, Akan H, et al. Comparison of computed tomography and magnetic resonance imaging in the diagnosis of parotid tumors. *Otolaryngol Head Neck Surg.* 2003;129(6):726-732.

56. Baker SR, Malone B. Salivary gland malignancies in children. *Cancer.* 1985;55(8):1730-1736.

57. Callender DL, Frankenthaler RA, Luna MA, et al. Salivary gland neoplasms in children. *Arch Otolaryngol Head Neck Surg.* 1992;118:472-476.

58. Kessler A, Handler SD. Salivary gland neoplasms in children: a 10-year survey at the Children's Hospital of Philadelphia. *Int J Pediatr Otorhinolaryngol.* 1994;29(3):195-202.

59. Azizkhan RG, Haase GM, Applebaum H, et al. Diagnosis, management, and outcome of cervicofacial teratomas in neonates: a Children's Cancer Group study. *J Pediatr Surg.* 1995;30:312-316.

60. Dehner LP, Mills A, Talerman A, Billman GF, Krous HF, Platz CE. Germ cell neoplasms of head and neck soft tissues: a pathologic spectrum of teratomatous and endodermal sinus tumors. *Hum Pathol.* 1990;21(3):309-318.

61. Grosfeld JL, Ballantine TV, Lowe D, Baehner RL. Benign and malignant teratomas in children: analysis of 85 patients. *Surgery.* 1976;80(3):297-305.

62. Billmire DF, Grosfeld JL. Teratomas in childhood: analysis of 142 cases. *J Pediatr Surg.* 1986;21(6): 548-551.

63. Dharnidharka VR, Ho PL, Stablein DM, et al. Mycophenolate, tacrolimus and posttransplant lymphoproliferative disorder: a report of the North American Pediatric Renal Transplant Cooperative Study. *Pediatr Transplant.* 2002;6(5):396-399.

64. Brennan DC, Schnitzler MA, Ceriotti C, et al. The Barnes-Jewish Hospital/Washington University Renal Transplant Program: comparison of two eras 1991-1994 and 1995-2000. *Clin Transpl.* 2001; 131-141.

65. Dharnidharka VR, Tejani AH, Ho PL, Harmon WE. Posttransplant lymphoproliferative disorder in the United States: young Caucasian males are at highest risk. *Am J Transplant.* 2002;2(10):993-998.

66. Shapiro NL, Strocker AM, Bhattacharyya N. Risk factors for adenotonsillar hypertrophy in children following solid organ transplantation. *Int J Ped Otorhinol.* 2003;67:151-155.

67. Rooney CM, Loftin SK, Holladay MS, et al. Early identification of Epstein-Barr virus-associated posttransplantation lymphoproliferative disease. *Br J Haematol.* 1995;89(1):98-103.

68. Williamson RA, Huang RY, Shapiro NL. Adenotonsillar histopathology after organ transplantation. *Otolaryngol Head Neck Surg.* 2001;125:231-240.

69. Mourad WA, Tulabah A, Sayed AA, et al. The impact of the world health organization classification and clonality assessment of posttransplant lymphoproliferative disorders on disease management. *Arch Pathol Lab Med.* 2006;130:1649-1653.

70. Darenkov IA, Marcarelli MA, Basadonna GP, et al. Reduced incidence of Epstein-Barr virus-associated posttransplant lymphoproliferative disorder using preemptive antiviral therapy. *Transplantation.* 1995;59(4):524-529.

71. McDiarmid SV, Jordan S, Kim GS, et al. Prevention and preemptive therapy of posttransplant lymphoproliferative disease in pediatric liver recipients. *Transplantation.* 1998;66(12):1604-1611.

72. Yang YJ, Haghir S, Wanamaker JR, et al. Diagnosis of papillary carcinoma in a thyroglossal duct cyst by fine needle aspiration biopsy. *Arch Pathol Lab Med.* 2000;124:139-142.

73. Branstetter BF, Weismman JL, Kennedy TL, et al. The CT appearance of thyroglossal duct carcinoma. *AJNR.* 2000:1547-1550.

74. Widstrom A, Magnusson P, Hallberg O, et al. Adenocarcinoma originating in the thyroglossal duct. *Ann Otol.* 1976;85:286-290.

75. Patel SG, Escrig M, Shaha AR, et al. Mangement of well-differentiated thyroid carcinoma presenting within a thyroglossal duct cyst. *J Surg Oncol.* 2002;79:134-139.

25

Head and Neck Lymphomas and Lymphoreticular Neoplasms

Andrew C. Urquhart

INTRODUCTION/DEFINITIONS

Lymphomas are a heterogeneous group of lymphocytic neoplasms that are typically divided into two major groups, Hodgkin's disease (HD) and non-Hodgkin's lymphoma (NHL). Within each of these groups there are multiple subtypes that are determined by their histopathology and cytoarchitecture, and more recently by their molecular phenotype and genetic profile. These tumors arise from the various types of lymphocytes that compose the lymphocyte-rich lymphoid tissues of the body, that is, lymph nodes, spleen, tonsils, bone marrow, and so forth. When these tumors arise from the bone marrow and the malignant cells are found in the blood, it is then called leukemia which may be acute or chronic, that is, acute lymphocytic leukemia (ALL) or chronic lymphocytic leukemia (CLL). Because plasma cells represent activated end-stage B lymphocytes, it is reasonable to consider multiple myeloma, Waldenström's macrogammoglobulinemia (lymphoplasmacytic lymphoma), and plasmacytomas as being integral components of the lymphoid neoplasms. These maladies are discussed only briefly in this review as they are not commonly found presenting as head and neck tumors.

Over the past 3 to 4 decades the classification of these tumors has evolved and there have been numerous published reclassifications of lymphomas over that span of time. With continued progress made in the ability to differentiate and predict the behavior of the various types of lymphomas, revisions and newer classifications became necessary to provide the oncologist with important information to manage and select the appropriate therapy.[1] Much of this progress has been the direct result of new technology applied to the unique molecular and genetic features of these tumors including flow cytometry to study the immunophenotype and cytogenetics of the tumor cells. Computerized tomographic (CT) scanning and magnetic resonance imaging (MRI) have provided vital information in assessing the extent or stage of the disease.

All lymphoid neoplasms represent a proliferation of a single transformed cell and are therefore monoclonal. However, each of these malignant clones has its own unique histopathologic and molecular features that enable accurate differentiation using immunophenotyping and histochemical staining. Cytogenetics or karyotyping of the tumor cell also can provide important information in predicting prognosis and response to therapy. Thus, because of the difficulty in differentiating lymphomas, especially NHL, it is imperative that adequate tissue be obtained from the tumor and a careful examination of the tissue by an experienced pathologist be made along with histochemical staining, immunophenotyping, and cytogenetic analysis to achieve an accurate diagnosis.

The spectrum of lymphoid neoplasms is derived from the various subtypes of lymphocytes, that is, B-cells, T-cells, and natural killer (NK) cells. The vast majority of NHL in adults (80–85%) are of B-cell origin and there is now ample information that the malignant cell of HD is also a transformed B-cell. Focusing specifically on lymphomas in this review, it is important to understand some of the basic differences within the two major groups, that is, NHL and HD.

NHLs have a characteristic histologic pattern of infiltration that is either nodular or diffuse. This effacement of the normal architecture of a lymph node has important therapeutic and prognostic implications. Second, the pathologist must decide if the malignant cells are large or small lymphocytes and in some instances an admixture of both. Details and further differentiation into the various subtypes can be determined with immunophenotyping and cytogenetics. These data serve as the foundation upon which the more recent classifications have been devised to provide great assistance to the oncologist who must manage and treat the patient.

HD or Hodgkin's lymphoma arises in a single lymphoid aggregate, usually a lymph node, and spreads to the contiguous nodal chains and adjacent tissues. The disease is frequently localized to one or multiple nodes in a single anatomic site or node-bearing region that may be above or below the diaphragm. This is considered "local or early stage disease" and accounts for approximately 50% of cases. However, the disease may be more wide-spread and involve both nodal and extranodal tissue above and below the diaphragm, and is then considered advanced stage.

The classification of HD consists of four major subtypes based on the histopathologic appearance of the tumor: (1) nodular sclerosis, (2) mixed cellularity, (3) lymphocyte predominance, and (4) lymphocyte depleted. The nodular sclerosis subtype makes up approximately 70% of HD, whereas the mixed cellularity subtype is next most common. The lymphocyte predominance and lymphocyte depleted are distinctly less common, making up greater than 10% of all cases of HD.

EPIDEMIOLOGY/PREVALENCE

Lymphomas are the most common nonepithelial tumors occurring in the head and neck[2] and are the leading cause of death due to cancer in adolescents and young adults. Although the incidence of lymphomas has increased over the last 5 years,[3] the frequency of HD has declined over the last 2 decades. NHL is more common than HD with an incidence of 16 cases per 100,000 per year in the United States, whereas the incidence of HD is lower with 3 cases per 100,000 per year.[4] There is a steady rise in the incidence of NHL with increasing age[5] with peaks in the 5th, 6th, and 7th decades.[6] There is a slightly higher incidence in males than females. Interestingly, the incidence of NHL has been increasing since the 1970s.[7] This may be explained by a number of factors, including the human immunodeficiency virus (HIV) epidemic[8-10] in which it is the second most common malignancy[11] with up to 15% of AIDS patients presenting with lymphoma.[12] HIV testing should be considered in newly diagnosed NHL patients. Similarly, in transplant patients on immunosuppressive treatment, lymphoproliferative disorders, including lymphomas are more common. There has been a direct association shown with *Helicobacter pylori* infection for patients with mucosa associated lymphoid tissue (MALT) lymphomas.[13] There is an increased incidence of lymphomas of the salivary glands in patients with Sjögren's syndrome.[14]

Hodgkin's disease makes up less than 1% of all new annual cancers in the United States with approximately 7,500 new cases reported annually.[15] The etiology of HD remains an enigma and the usual candidates have been speculated on, that is, environmental toxins and infectious diseases. However, there is mounting data suggesting that the Epstein-Barr virus (EBV) may play a causative role in the etiology of HD because of its ability to transform B-cells into a malignant clone. Additionally, EBV has been implicated as a causative agent in HD because of the frequency with which genetic material from the virus is found in the malignant cells. Viral integration into the genome of the malignant cell of HD has been found in 20% to 80%, depending on the histopathologic subtype.[16-20]

HD has a bimodal incidence pattern with most cases occurring during the third and fourth decades and a second peak occurring after age 55 years. It represents one of the most common malignancies of young adults and is more common in young adult females than men. The histopathology is usually that of nodular sclerosis and involves the mediastinal and cervical lymph nodes. However, in older individuals with HD, the gender incidence is reversed, with men being affected more frequently than women and the histopathology more often that of mixed cellularity.[21]

The median age of diagnosis for multiple myeloma is 70 years.[22] It is more common in people of African descent.

ANATOMIC BOUNDARIES AND SUBDIVISIONS OF THE REGION

There is a rich network of lymph channels that drain into the lymph nodes forming an extensive lymphatic system in the head and neck. The lymph nodes can be divided into a superficial and deep group. The superficial nodes form a circle beginning on the face extending posteriorly to the occipital area. These include the buccal, facial, submandibular, anterior cervical, sublingual, parotid (within the superficial aspect of the parotid gland), retroauricular, and occipital nodes.

The deep cervical nodes run along the course of the internal jugular vein from the skull base to the brachiocephalic junction. These include the upper (jugulodigastric), middle, and lower jugular group. Lymph nodes are found in the posterior triangle which is formed by the anterior edge of the trapezius muscle posteriorly, the posterior edge of the sternocleidomastoid muscle anteriorly, and the clavicle inferiorly. These include the supraclavicular nodes and nodes along the lower half of the spinal accessory nerve and transverse cervical artery.

The anterior compartment group involves those surrounding the trachea and esophagus which includes the paratracheal nodes. Efferent lymphatics from the deep nodes drain into the venous system at the jugulosubclavian angle. From a surgical and pathologic standpoint, the lymph nodes are classified into levels 1 through 6.

Waldeyer's ring is considered the primary immune barrier for ingested or inhaled antigens and forms a major group of extranodal lymphoid tissue within the head and neck, comprising the palatine, pharyngeal, tubal, and lingual tonsils. The palatine tonsil consists of abundant lymphoid follicles, covered by stratified squamous epithelium with deep crypts in the surface. It lies within the oropharynx between the palatoglossal and palatopharyngeal muscles on either side. The pharyngeal tonsil lies within the nasopharynx at the periphery of the pharyngeal bursa. It consists of lymphatic nodules covered by pseudostratified columnar epithelium with a series of intervening folds on the surface. The tubal tonsil (also called Gerlach's tonsil) is formed by an extension of the pharyngeal tonsil anteriorly in the lateral nasopharyngeal wall mucosa. The lingual tonsil occurs on the posterior third of the tongue and consists of crypts lined by stratified squamous epithelium. Lymphoid tissue is also found in the major and minor saliva glands, the thyroid gland, and the dermis.

CRITICAL ELEMENTS IN THE HISTORY AND PHYSICAL EXAMINATION

Specific points in the history that need to be considered include any risk of immunodeficiency syndromes, including HIV, with associated increased incidence of both HD and NHL. Patients with a history of autoimmune disease, including Sjögren's syndrome and post organ transplant patients, are at an increased risk.[23] The risk of a sibling of someone with HD or NHL developing either HD or NHL is higher than in the normal population.[24] Young people who have had infectious mononucleosis (due to EBV) are at a significantly higher risk of developing HD.[25]

Constitutional symptoms (B symptoms) occur in approximately 40% of patients with HD and 10 to 15% of patients with NHL. Specific symptoms that should be sought include fever higher than 38°C, night sweats, and loss of more than 10% of total body weight over 6 months. Both HD and NHL patients may complain of severe itching over the whole body and even a rash may develop. Patients with HD have alcohol intolerance and frequently have pain in the area of involvement with alcohol ingestion.

The history and physical examination should focus on the detection of lymphadenophathy in the cervical and other node bearing areas, considering that the most frequent cause of a unilateral neck mass in the 21 to 40 year old age group is lymphoma.[26] Although the average age of patients with HD is younger and the incidence less common than NHL, both malignancies frequently present with lymphadenopathy above the clavicle, specifically along the internal jugular chain. Other lymph node groups in the head and neck tend to be involved more often with NHL than HD which is more likely to have disease in the mediastinum with an occasionally associated cough. In NHL, nodes are more likely in the abdomen (mesenteric nodes) and multiple other sites.

NHL is more likely to occur in extranodal sites with Waldeyer's ring being the most common. They are frequently multicentric and usually manifest as a bulky mass in the area without bone destruction.[27] Symptoms and signs will depend on the specific extranodal site involved. Involvement of the tonsil will usually present with a smooth unilateral or bilateral enlargement with associated throat discomfort. Adjacent lymph node involvement frequently occurs in this situation.[28]

The tongue base is generally difficult to visualize and nonspecific throat symptoms, including dysphagia and voice changes, may occur. Palpation of this area will identify a smooth, firm mass. Adenoidal involvement may present with nasal obstruction and hearing loss due to otitis media secondary to eustachian tube obstruction. The nasal cavities and paranasal sinuses are the next most frequent sites of involvement. Symptoms suggestive of chronic or recurrent sinusitis with nasal obstruction, facial pressure, or pain and bloody nasal discharge may occur. Extension beyond the sinuses may involve the orbit, resulting in proptosis and infraorbital nerve involvement with hypoesthesia of the cheek. T-cell lymphoma may present with local destruction of the midfacial region, including the nose.

Lymphomas involving the thyroid gland typically occur in patients with a history of Hashimoto's thyroiditis.[29,30] The gland is usually diffusely enlarged and indurated. Although the clinical course is often indolent and similar to MALT lymphomas, it may be aggressive with rapid onset and airway compromise similar to anaplastic thyroid carcinoma. Lymphomas involving the salivary glands are usually MALT lymphomas.[31] Parotid gland involvement usually consisting of bilateral, multiple, or poorly circumscribed lesions is often associated with cervical lymphadenopathy.[32] Lymphomas involving the orbit may present with symptoms localized to the eye and include irritation, foreign body sensation, redness, and a palpable mass.

APPROPRIATE DIAGNOSTIC OFFICE-BASED PROCEDURES

All patients with NHL and HD should have confirmation of the histopathology by an experienced hematopathologist and have a comprehensive clinical workup to assess the extent of disease prior to starting treatment.

Fine needle aspiration (FNA) is useful in distinguishing lymphomas from other pathology in the head and neck region, specifically carcinoma. Cytogenetics and molecular studies can be obtained from the cytologic specimen.[33] Flow cytometry may also give information regarding the phenotype (B or T) of the lymphoma utilizing immunohistochemical studies. Unfortunately, however, there are limitations to cytology because the histologic pattern of the malignancy in the lymph node is important for classification of the lymphoma and diagnosis of HD. FNA may also suggest lymphoma with benign disease, such as infectious mononucleosis, or miss the diagnosis of lymphoma when reactive hyperplasia occurs in association with lymphoma. The procedure itself is easily performed in the office. The most accessible and representative lymph node is sampled using a 25-gauge needle with multiple aspirations and passes to obtain the most representative sample. It is important to keep in mind that FNA is not cost effective and may, in fact, misguide treatment.[34,35] If the preliminary diagnosis of lymphoma is made, an adequate piece of the tissue must be obtained to determine the architecture and submitted for special molecular and cytogenetic studies before initiating therapy.

A formal biopsy is the definitive procedure required to diagnose and classify lymphoma.[36] Lymphomas and HD usually manifest with lymphadenopathy in the head and neck region and the most representative and accessible lymph nodes should be removed. Although this may be done as an office procedure, a sterile environment with general anesthesia is preferred. This is particularly true in anatomic areas in close proximity to cranial nerves that are at risk of injury. Local anesthesia may temporarily paralyze these nerves during the biopsy with an increased risk of iatrogenic injury. The spinal accessory nerve which has a long and very superficial location in the posterior triangle of the neck is particularly at risk of injury. Injury to this nerve may be associated with significant morbidity and is a relatively common cause for litigation.[37] Ideally, the entire lymph node should be removed in one piece with its capsule intact. If this is not possible, particularly with matted nodes surrounding important structures, a representative biopsy including the capsule and cortex of the lymph node should be obtained.

With extranodal involvement, biopsies may be undertaken in the office using local anesthesia. This will, however, depend on the area involved and its accessibility. The nasal cavity and postnasal space may be accessible in the office with endoscopic assistance. Tonsil and tongue base involvement will most likely require a formal procedure under general anesthesia. Areas such as the parotid gland and thyroid may be more difficult to biopsy because of the increased risk of nerve injury. In this situation, other sites should be sought or a more formal procedure undertaken after the patient is informed of the associated risks.

Once the diagnosis of NHL or HD is made, bone marrow aspiration and core biopsy can be performed in the office as part of the clinical staging workup. This is important as the approach to therapy differs between patients with localized and disseminated disease. This procedure is usually performed by the patient's medical oncologist and involves the aspiration of a fluid suspension of bone marrow from the posterior iliac crest. At the same time, a bone marrow core biopsy is obtained to assess the overall cellularity and architecture of the marrow. Bilateral bone marrow biopsies may increase the diagnostic yield.[38]

Standard laboratory testing should include a complete blood count, differential, erythrocyte sedimentation rate, platelets, albumin, serum lactate dehydrogenase (LDH), and liver and renal function tests. In the highly aggressive lymphomas, such as Burkitt's lymphoma, a lumbar puncture should also be performed. Burkitt's lymphoma is frequently associated with HIV infection and an HIV serology should be obtained in these situations, as well as patients with risk factors for HIV or unusual presentations.[39]

Multiple myeloma patients have increased levels of immunoglobulins in the blood and/or light chains (Bence-Jones protein) in the urine, and the diagnosis is confirmed by a bone marrow aspiration and biopsy, revealing an increased number of abnormal plasma cells (>15%) that are responsible for the increased monoclonal proteins in the plasma and/or urine. Other important features of myeloma include lytic skeletal lesions, hypercalcemia, and renal failure.

RECOMMENDED IMAGING STUDIES

Imaging studies are necessary in the initial evaluation of a mass or tumor within the head and neck. Once a diagnosis of lymphoma is established, further studies will need to be performed to define the primary disease and complete the staging. In the head and neck these include CT scanning or MRI. Chest x-rays and chest, abdomen and pelvic CT scans are needed to define the extent of the disease and complete the staging.

Cervical lymphadenopathy is the most common presentation of both NHL and HD. CT findings of multiple, bilateral, non-necrotic nodes involving levels 2, 3, 4, and 5, as well as superficial nodes, are typical of NHL (Fig 25–1). CT scans reveal nodal density to be equal to or less than muscle. It is important to differentiate cervical lymphadenopathy due to metastatic squamous cell carcinoma (SCCA) from lymphomas. Whereas nodal metastasis from SCCA of the head and neck may show necrosis, this is less common with lymphoma. SCCA is more likely

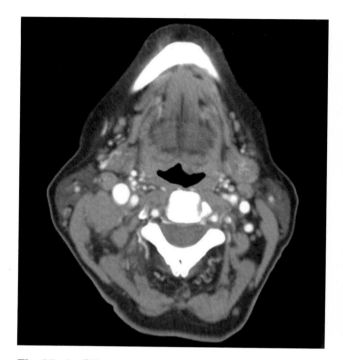

Fig 25–1. CT scan showing multiple, bilateral, non-necrotic lymph nodes with involvement of multiple levels typical of NHL.

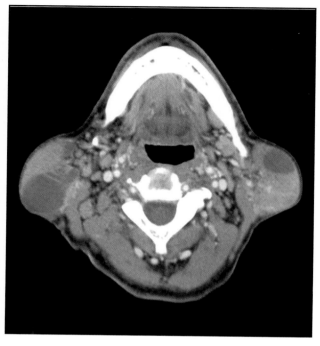

Fig 25–2. Bilateral parotid enlargement with multiple lesions in a patient with Sjögren's syndrome. Pathology revealed marginal zone B-cell lymphoma.

to show evidence of a primary tumor with necrotic and nonisodensity nodes, whereas NHL is more likely to have lymphadenopathy in levels 5 to 7.[40] If, however, necrosis with extranodal spread is noted, a more aggressive NHL is suggested.[41] Although CT scans cannot differentiate nodal disease of HD from NHL, involvement of extranodal sites such as Waldeyer's ring, nasopharynx, sinus, parotid, and thyroid is more suggestive of NHL. CT in these situations is helpful in evaluating the extent of the disease. In parotid gland involvement, bilateral, multiple, or poorly circumscribed parotid masses with cervical adenopathy are suggestive of lymphoma[32] (Fig 25–2). Although HD typically involves younger patients with neck and mediastinal lymphadenopathy, NHL involves older patients with extranodal site involvement, and an abdominal CT revealing mesenteric, high celiac nodes, and hepatic or splenic involvement. Multiple myeloma consists of multifocal, destructive bone tumors appearing radiologically as punched-out defects 1 to 4 cm in diameter.

In plasmacytoma, the bony lesions are solitary. With extraosseous lesions, presentation is often in the lungs, nasopharynx, or nasal sinuses.

MRI may be used together or instead of CT of the head and neck. On T1-weighted images, nodes are isointense to muscle and on T2-weighted images hyperintense to muscle.

Positron emission tomography (PET) scans, or more recently PET/CT, are not used routinely but are helpful in cases where the CT scan is equivocal. PET imaging has a high sensitivity compared to CT imaging.[42] In patients with localized disease, PET scans may be helpful in identifying occult disease or a recurrence.[43,44] The diagnostic specificity of the PET scans may be limited due to its sensitivity to inflammatory disease with increased false positivity.[45] This applies particularly to extranodal sites.[46] The newly developed PET/CT fusion appears to be more sensitive than PET alone.

Whereas lymphangiography may be helpful in staging HD to evaluate pelvic and periaortic lymph nodes, its application in staging has declined as the sensitivity of CT imaging and MRI have proven more useful.

EXAMPLES OF REPRESENTATIVE HISTOPATHOLOGY

Although lymphoid neoplasms may be suspected with clinical features, definitive histology of lymph nodes or other tissue is required. The majority (80–85%) of lymphoid neoplasms are of B-cell origin with the remainder being of T-cell and only rarely of NK origin. Neoplastic B and T cells lead to characteristic patterns of involvement. Follicular neoplasms will tend to proliferate in the B-cell area of the lymph node resulting in a nodular or follicular growth pattern whereas T-cell lymphomas grow in the paracortical T-cell zones.

Acute lymphoblastic leukemia/lymphoma is composed of immature lymphoblasts (precursor B or T lymphocytes). Histologically, normal tissue architecture is replaced by lymphoblasts that have scant cytoplasm and slightly larger nuclei.

CLL and small lymphocytic lymphoma may be morphologically, phenotypically, and genotypically indistinguishable. The lymph node architecture is diffusely effaced by small, fairly well-differentiated lymphocytes with slightly irregular nuclei and scant cytoplasm. There is widespread nodal disease and marrow involvement, and frequently the spleen is enlarged.

Follicular lymphoma closely resembles germinal center B-cells. There are two main cell types, small cells called centrocytes and larger cells called centroblasts.

Diffuse large B-cell lymphoma constitutes approximately 20% of all NHL. Morphologically, these tumors consist of a relatively large cell (4 to 5 times the diameter of a small lymphocyte) with a diffuse pattern of growth (Fig 25–3).

Burkitt's Lymphoma

Burkitt's lymphoma is aggressive and has a high mitotic index (Fig 25–4). Involved tissue is infiltrated

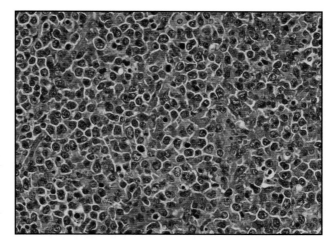

Fig 25–3. Diffuse large B-cell lymphoma (400×).

by intermediate-sized lymphoid cells. A characteristic "starry sky" pattern is formed by benign macrophages which ingest nuclear debris secondary to tumor cell death (Fig 25–5).

Mantle Cell Lymphoma

Mantle cell lymphoma closely resembles the normal mantle zone surrounding the germinal centers of a lymphoid follicle. It consists of a proliferation of homogeneous small B lymphocytes with round to irregular nuclear contours.

Marginal Zone Lymphoma

Marginal zone lymphoma includes a group of B-cell tumors that arise within the lymph nodes, spleen, or extranodal tissues. They have been referred to as MALT lymphomas because they occur at mucosal sites. Usually the predominant tumor cell resembles normal marginal zone B-cells (Fig 25–6).

Peripheral T-cell and NK-cell neoplasms include neoplasms that have phenotypes that resemble mature T cells or NK cells. Included in this group are the extranodal NK/T-cell lymphomas previously called lethal midline granuloma. These tumors consist of a mixture of small and large lymphoid cells or

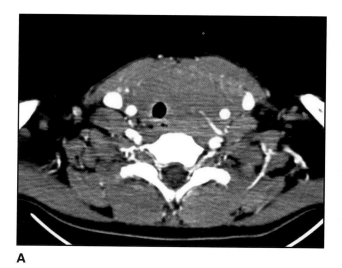

A

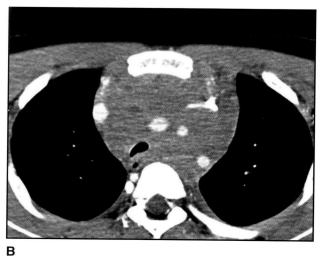

B

Fig 25–4. A. Burkitt's lymphoma (high-grade B cell type) presenting with shortness of breath and a midline neck mass in a 12-year-old male. **B.** Note the extensive mediastinal involvement.

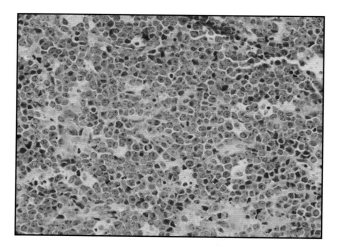

Fig 25–5. Burkitt's lymphoma. Note "starry sky" appearance and high mitotic rate (400×).

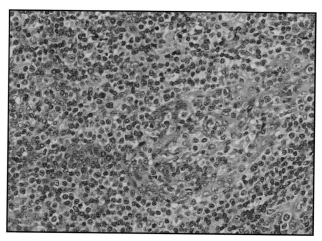

Fig 25–6. Marginal zone lymphoma of parotid gland. Lymphoepithelial lesion expands gland (400×).

predominantly large lymphoid cells that frequently invade blood vessels causing obstruction and extensive necrosis.

HD has diagnostic Reed-Sternberg cells which are large with multiple nuclei or a single nucleus with multiple nuclear lobes. Although these cells are needed for a diagnosis, there must be a background of non-neoplastic inflammatory cells (lymphocytes, plasma cells, and eosinophils) (Fig 25–7).

HD, nodular sclerosis subtype is characterized morphologically by a variant of the Reed-Sternberg cell called the lacunar cell. The lymphoid tissue is divided into circumscribed nodules by collagen bands. HD, mixed cellularity subtype, has abundant Reed-Sternberg cells with mononuclear variants. Small lymphocytes in the background are usually T cells. Lymphocyte depletion subtype is characterized by a relative abundance of Reed-Sternberg cells and a

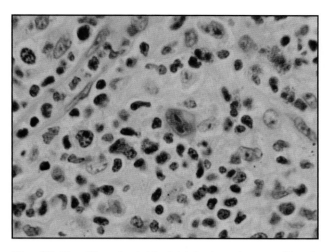

Fig 25–7. Classical Hodgkin's lymphoma. Reed-Sternberg cell in center along with eosinophils (1000×).

paucity of lymphocytes. The lymphocyte predominance subtype has few Reed-Sternberg cells and is characterized by an infiltrate of small lymphocytes mixed with the benign histiocytes.

AMERICAN JOINT COMMITTEE ON CANCER STAGING (AJCC) IN MALIGNANCY

Many different classification systems have been used to classify lymphoid neoplasms with much confusion. The working classification was simple consisting of 10 categories without requiring special studies such as immunophenotype or genetic studies. However, with continued refinement and the availability of newer methods and tests to more accurately identify neoplasms, the recognition of new categories and classification of the lymphoid neoplasms evolved. A new classification called the Revised European-American Classification of Lymphoid (REAL) neoplasms was introduced in 1994, incorporating new information such as immunophenotype and genetic features.

More recently, the World Health Organization (WHO) updated its classification of hematopoietic and lymphoid disease and adopted the REAL classification for lymphoid neoplasms. The REAL WHO classification is now the standard classification and includes HD, NHL, lymphoid leukemia, and plasma cell neoplasms, as well as several additional entities not recognized in the international working formulation. It includes immunophenotype and genetic information that characterize the variety of entities in this classification (Table 25-1).[47]

HD and plasma cell myeloma are recognized as B-cell lymphomas. The WHO classification divides HD into classical HD and nodular lymphocyte-predominant HD.[48] Classical HD includes nodular sclerosis, mixed cellularity, and lymphocyte-depleted and lymphocyte-rich HD.

The Ann Arbor classification system is the most widely used for staging lymphoma (Table 25-2).[49] The system was initially designed for HD which is a malignancy that spreads in a systematic pattern of anatomic continuity. Unlike HD, NHL does not follow this orderly anatomic pattern of spread, making it less useful in predicting prognosis. Despite the recognized limitations, the AJCC and the International Union Against Cancer (UICC) have adopted the Ann Arbor classification as the official system of staging HD and NHL. However, due to these limitations with NHL, prognostic factors for NHL have been evaluated, including tumor bulk, serum LDH, serum β-microglobulin level, and concomitant B symptoms. The International Prognostic Index is the most widely used today, particularly in patients with intermediate grade lymphoma. It includes age, Ann Arbor stage, serum LDH level, performance status, and number of extranodal sites.[50]

IDENTIFICATION OF CRITICAL DECISION POINTS

Lymphomas are a frequent cause of malignant lymphadenopathy in the head and neck. Although they are the most common nonepithelial tumors of the head and neck, recognizing the clinical presentation includes a detailed history and physical examination. Although cervical lymphadenopathy is the most common finding, extranodal involvement of various head and neck sites needs to be recognized.

Table 25–1. WHO Classification of Hematopoietic and Lymphoid Neoplasms

B-Cell Neoplasms	T-Cell and NK-Cell Neoplasms
Precursor B-cell neoplasm	Precursor T-cell neoplasm
Precursor B-lymphoblastic leukemia/lymphoma (precursor B-cell acute lymphoblastic leukemia)	Precursor T-lymphoblastic lymphoma/leukemia (precursor T-cell acute lymphoblastic leukemia)
Mature (peripheral) B-cell neoplasms[a]	Mature (peripheral) T-cell neoplasms
B-cell chronic lymphocytic leukemia/small lymphocytic lymphoma	T-cell prolymphocytic leukemia
B-cell prolymphocytic leukemia	T-cell granular lymphocytic leukemia
Lymphoplasmacytic lymphoma	Aggressive NK-cell leukemia
Splenic marginal zone B-cell lymphoma (± villous lymphocytes)	Adult T-cell lymphoma/leukemia (HTLV1+)[b]
	Extranodal NK/T-cell lymphoma, nasal type
Hairy cell leukemia	Enteropathy-type T-cell lymphoma
Plasma cell myeloma/plasmacytoma	Hepatosplenic gamma-delta T-cell lymphoma
Extranodal marginal zone B-cell lymphoma of MALT type	Subcutaneous panniculitis-like T-cell lymphoma
Nodal marginal zone B-cell lymphoma (± monocytoid B cells)	Mycosis fungoides/Sézary syndrome
	Anaplastic large-cell lymphoma, T/null cell, primary cutaneous type
Follicular lymphoma	Peripheral T-cell lymphoma, not otherwise characterized
Mantle cell lymphoma	
Diffuse large B-cell lymphoma	Angioimmunoblastic T-cell lymphoma
Mediastinal large B-cell lymphoma	Anaplastic large-cell lymphoma, T/null cell, primary systemic type
Primary effusion lymphoma	
Burkitt's lymphoma/Burkitt cell leukemia	

[a]B-cell and T-cell/NK-cell neoplasms are grouped according to major clinical presentations (predominantly disseminated/leukemic, primary extranodal, predominantly nodal).

[b]HTLV1+ indicates human T-cell leukemia virus; MALT, mucosa-associated lymphoid tissue; NK, natural killer.

With cervical lymphadenopathy in an adult, the decision to perform a biopsy should only be done once metastatic SCCA from the head and neck has been excluded. This may be obvious when a primary tumor site is identified. However, in situations when no obvious primary site is noted, SCCA may still need to be excluded. FNA is helpful in this situation and usually the cytologic report will suggest findings compatible with lymphoma with definitive biopsy recommended. Imaging with CT or MRI is usually suggestive of lymphoma, particularly when multiple nodes are noted involving levels 5 to 7. Sampling a representative node or an adequate part of the node involving the capsule and cortex is required. With extranodal NHL, an adequate tumor specimen should be obtained with a biopsy. Samples should be sent in normal saline avoiding formalin. Once a diagnosis is established, formal staging should be undertaken as previously described. Appropriate treatment is then based on the pathology and extent of disease.

ANALYSIS OF VARIOUS TREATMENT OPTIONS

Non-Hodgkin's Lymphoma

Treatment of lymphomas rarely requires surgery apart from the initial biopsy to establish a tissue diagnosis. Although radiation therapy and chemotherapy

Table 25–2. Ann Arbor Staging Classification for Hodgkin's Disease

Stage I	Involvement of a single lymph node region (I), or a single extralymphatic organ or site (I_E)
Stage II	Involvement of two or more lymph node regions on the same side of the diaphragm (II), or localized involvement of an extralymphatic organ or site (II_E)
Stage III	Involvement of lymph node regions on both sides of the diaphragm (III), or localized involvement of an extralymphatic organ or site (III_E) or spleen (III_S) or both ($IIIS_E$)
Stage IV	Diffuse or disseminated involvement of one or more extralymphatic organs with or without associated lymph node involvement
A	Asymptomatic
B	Fever, sweats, weight loss >10% of body weight

either alone or in combination form the mainstay of treatment, this is very dependent on the specific histology and tumor stage.

The National Comprehensive Cancer Network (NCCN) treatment guidelines for patients are developed for more common NHL histologic types. These include CLL/small lymphocyte lymphoma, follicular lymphoma, diffuse large B-cell lymphoma, marginal zone lymphoma, mantle cell lymphoma, and aggressive lymphoma subtypes, including Burkitt's, lymphoblastic lymphoma, and AIDS-related B-cell lymphomas. Although guidelines have not been developed for anaplastic and peripheral T-cell lymphomas, most are treated as aggressive diffuse large B-cell lymphomas.

CLL and small lymphocytic lymphoma are the same disease with different manifestations. Currently, CLL and small lymphocytic lymphoma are incurable with standard therapy. For localized disease locoregional radiotherapy or observation is recommended. With disease progression, patients who are symptomatic and have threatened end organ involvement or cytopenia, bulky disease, histologic transformation, or steady progression may be treated with chemotherapy. In all situations, the patient should

be enrolled in clinical trials, if indicated and appropriate. An appropriate choice for first-line therapy includes fludarabine with or without rituximab.[51,52]

Follicular lymphomas with nonbulky localized disease (Ann Arbor stage I-II) are candidates for curative radiotherapy, chemotherapy followed by radiotherapy, or extended field radiotherapy.[53] With localized bulky or stage III or IV disease, the decision to treat depends on symptoms, end organ threat, bulky disease, cytopenia, or progression of disease. Many treatment options are available in the absence of appropriate clinical trials, including locoregional radiotherapy and single agent or combination chemotherapy.

Marginal zone lymphomas are a heterogeneous group consisting of MALT lymphomas, nodal marginal zone lymphomas, and splenic marginal zone lymphomas. Nodal marginal zone lymphomas are treated like systemic indolent lymphomas. MALT lymphomas are divided into gastric versus nongastric due to the association of gastric MALT lymphomas with *Helicobacter pylori* infection.

In the head and neck, nongastric MALT lymphomas may arise from different sites including the skin, thyroid, salivary gland (parotid), and conjunctivae. For certain sites such as the parotid and thyroid, primary surgery may be appropriate.

Mantle cell lymphomas appear to be incurable with conventional chemotherapy. It has the worst characteristics of indolent and aggressive NHL.[54,55] Participation in clinical trials is encouraged, outside of which combined modality therapy or involved field radiotherapy is recommended.

Diffuse large B-cell lymphomas are the most common lymphoid malignancies in adults. In patients with localized (Ann Arbor stage I–II), nonbulky disease, treatment should be an abbreviated course (3 cycles) of rituximab, cyclophosphamide, doxorubicin, vincristine, and prednisone (R-CHOP) combined with involved field radiotherapy. Patients with bulky disease and local extranodal disease should be treated with a full course (6 to 8) cycles with involved field radiotherapy.[56-59]

Patients with advanced disease in the low or low-intermediate risk category (normal LDH level and performance status) should be treated with full course anthracycline-based chemotherapy which would include 6 to 8 cycles of R-CHOP.[57,60] Patients with high-risk categories should be treated in the context of appropriate clinical trials. They have less than 50% chance of being cured with standard therapy.

Highly aggressive lymphomas and lymphoblastic lymphomas are derived from precursor B-cells and usually involve extranodal sites. The majority of lymphoblastic lymphomas are derived from precursor T-cells and occur more frequently in younger aged patients, that is, children and adolescents and usually present as a large mediastinal mass. Treatment of Burkitt's lymphoma with intensive short-course chemotherapy has been successful in recent years. Induction therapy consists of a combination chemotherapy regimen, including alkalizing agents, anthracycline, intrathecal chemotherapy, and high-dose methotrexate with or without rituximab.[61-65] Lymphoblastic lymphoma is generally treated with regimens appropriate for acute lymphoblastic leukemia, such as cyclophosphamide and anthracyclines.

Nasofacial NK/T-cell lymphoma is treated with combination radiation therapy and chemotherapy, although the results are worse than other extranodal head and neck lymphomas.[66]

Hodgkin's Disease

In early nonbulky disease, combined treatment (chemotherapy and limited radiotherapy) is recommended. For patients with bulky mediastinal stage II disease with intermediate prognosis, combined treatment is also recommended. With stage III and IV disease, systemic treatment with or without radiation is recommended. If radiotherapy alone is used, doses of 30 to 44 Gy to the involved sites should be given. With combined treatment, the dose of radiotherapy will depend on bulky versus nonbulky disease. In bulky disease, irrespective of the stage, a dose of 20 to 36 Gy is used. In patients without bulky disease, the dose can be decreased to 20 to 30 Gy.

Chemotherapy forms an integral part of treatment. For early stage nonbulky disease (stage I to IIa), combined radiotherapy and chemotherapy (usually 4 cycles of adriamycin, bleomycin, vinblastine, and dacarbazine [ABVD]) are given. In certain selected patients, radiotherapy or chemotherapy alone may be used. Patients with bulky disease require combined radiotherapy and chemotherapy.[67,68] NCCN recommends ABVD for 4 cycles or Stanford V (mechlorethamine, doxorubicin, etoposide, vincristine, vinblastine, bleomycin, and prednisone) for 8 weeks.[69] In early stage I to II patients with B symptoms, combined chemotherapy with radiotherapy to a nodal region is recommended. In stage III to IV disease, the primary treatment is chemotherapy alone (ABVD) or chemotherapy with radiation therapy. The patient should be restaged at defined intervals after initial treatment with the addition of further chemotherapy, even if the patient has a complete response. ABVD is the gold standard for treatment of HD. ABVD regimens are superior to mechlorethamine, oncovin, procarbazine, and prednisone (MOPP) alone.[70]

Unfavorable factors have been identified which may reduce survival rates by 7 to 8% per year.[71] These include age of 45 or older, male gender, stage IV disease, albumin below 4 g/dL, hemoglobin below 10.5 g/dL, white cell count above 15,000 mm³, and lymphocytopenia. These factors may help to predict prognosis and dictate options, including more aggressive chemotherapy.

Localized plasma cell tumors are divided into medullary and extramedullary types. The medullary plasmacytomas usually progress to multiple myeloma in more than 50% of patients. Multiple myeloma is treated with chemotherapy with alkylating agents. Remission is induced in 50 to 70% of patients but the median survival is still 3 years. Some younger patients receiving allogeneic bone marrow transplants have long-standing remissions.[72]

Extramedullary plasmacytoma occurs in the submucosa of the upper aerodigestive tract. In 75% of patients the nasopharynx and the paranasal sinuses are involved.[73] It is less likely to progress to multiple myeloma. It is very radiosensitive and radiation therapy is the recommended treatment. Disease-free survival of greater than 70% at 10 years is reported.[74]

COMPLICATIONS OF THERAPY

There is a 1% to 5% mortality rate from complications associated with chemotherapy. Side effects and complications of chemotherapeutic agents increase with dose and duration of treatment. The most common side effects include nausea and vomiting, diarrhea, hair and weight loss, and depression. These effects are usually temporary and resolve. More serious side effects include neutropenia with associated secondary infection, anemia, thrombocytopenia, liver and kidney damage, and allergic reactions.

Long-term complications, including fatigue with associated aches and pains, are common and may last for years. Secondary cancers are the most worrisome with both solid and hematologic malignancies occurring with an incidence of 5%.[75] Infertility, osteoporosis, and heart failure may occur.

Complications from radiotherapy generally are less severe with lymphomas and HD compared to nonlymphoid malignancies of the head and neck. Radiotherapy causes complications depending on the specific sites of the body treated. Specifically with regard to the head and neck, these include xerostomia, mucositis, and dental caries. There may be generalized fatigue and weight loss. More serious acute complications include radiation pneumonitis and pulmonary fibrosis. Late complications include coronary artery disease, hypothyroidism, infertility (usually worse in women than men), impaired bone growth in children and young adults, and secondary malignancies of which lung and breast tumors are the most common. In general, complications are more severe when radiotherapy and chemotherapy are combined.

SUMMARY

Lymphomas are a heterogeneous group of lymphocytic neoplasms consisting of two major groups: HD and NHL. NHL is more common than HD and the incidence appears to be increasing. Although the average age of HD is younger and the frequency less common than NHL, both frequently present with cervical lymphoadenopathy above the clavicle. Although this is the most common presentation, extranodal involvement may occur with pathology involving other areas, including Waldeyer's ring, salivary glands, thyroid, and eyes. Typical B symptoms, for example, night sweats and weight loss, need to be recognized because they are present in approxi-

mately 40% of patients with HD and 10 to 15% of patients with NHL. Whereas FNA cytology is helpful, definitive pathology is almost always required. Over the past 3 to 4 decades, the classification of these tumors has evolved due to new technology applied to differentiate the unique molecular and genetic features of these tumors. Treatment and prognosis are directly related to this pathologic classification and stage of the disease. The head and neck surgeon needs to recognize the clinical presentation and establish a firm diagnosis so that the appropriate treatment can be instituted.

REFERENCES

1. Harris NL. Hodgkin's lymphomas: classification, diagnosis, and grading. *Semin Hematol.* 1999;36:220-232.
2. Bragg DG. Radiology of the lymphomas. *Curr Probl Diagn Radiol.* 1987;16:177-206.
3. Palackdharry CS. The epidemiology of non-Hodgkin's lymphoma: why the increased incidence? *Oncology (Williston Park).* 1994;8:67-73.
4. Urba WJ, Longo DL. Hodgkin's disease. *N Engl J Med.* 1992;326:678-687.
5. Raber MN. Clinical applications of flow cytometry. *Oncology (Williston Park).* 1988;2:35-43, 47.
6. Cobleigh MA, Kennedy JL. Non-Hodgkin's lymphomas of the upper aerodigestive tract and salivary glands. *Otolaryngol Clin North Am.* 1986;19:685-710.
7. Weisenburger DD. Epidemiology of non-Hodgkin's lymphoma: recent findings regarding an emerging epidemic. *Ann Oncol.* 1994;5:19-24.
8. Powles T, Matthews G, Bower M. AIDS related systemic non-Hodgkin's lymphoma. *Sex Transm Infect.* 2000;76:335-341.
9. Kaplan LD. HIV-associated lymphoma. *AIDS Clin Rev.* 1993-1994;145-166.
10. Kaplan LD, Abrams DI, Feigal E, et al. AIDS-associated non-Hodgkin's lymphoma in San Francisco. *JAMA.* 1989;261:719-724.
11. Zapater E, Bagan JV, Campos A, Armengot M, Abril V, Basterra J. Non-Hodgkin's lymphoma of the head and neck in association with HIV infection. *Ann Otolaryngol Chir Cervicofac.* 1996;113:69-72.
12. Finn DG. Lymphoma of the head and neck and acquired immunodeficiency syndrome: clinical

investigation and immunohistological study. *Laryngoscope*. 1995;105:1–18.

13. Wotherspoon AC, Ortiz-Hidalgo C, Falzon MR, Isaacson PG. *Helicobacter pylori*-associated gastritis and primary B-cell gastric lymphoma. *Lancet*. 1991;338:1175–1176.

14. Ambrosetti A, Zanotti R, Pattaro C, et al. Most cases of primary salivary mucosa-associated lymphoid tissue lymphoma are associated either with Sjögren's syndrome or hepatitis C virus infection. *Br J Haematol*. 2004;126:43–49.

15. Stein RS. Textbooks of hematology. In: Lee GR, Foerster J, Lukens J, Paraskevas F, Greer JP, Rodgers GM, eds. *Wintrobe's Clinical Hematology*. 10th ed. Baltimore, Md: Williams & Wilkins;1999: 2538.

16. Brousset P, Vassallo J, Knecht H, Delsol G, Lamant L, Odermatt BF. Detection of Epstein-Barr virus in Hodgkin's disease. *Appl Immunohistochem*. 1993; 1:213–219.

17. Brousset P, Schlaifer D, Meggetto F, et al. Persistence of the same viral strain in early and late relapses of Epstein-Barr virus-associated Hodgkin's disease. *Blood*. 1994;84:2447–2451.

18. Niedobitek G, Pazolt D, Teichmann M, Devergne O. Frequent expression of the Epstein-Barr virus (EBV)-induced gene, EBI3, an IL-12 p40-related cytokine, in Hodgkin and Reed-Sternberg cells. *J Pathol*. 2002;198:310–316.

19. Kandil A, Bazarbashi S, Mourad WA. The correlation of Epstein-Barr virus expression and lymphocyte subsets with the clinical presentation of nodular sclerosing Hodgkin disease. *Cancer*. 2001;91: 1957–1963.

20. Glavina-Durdov M, Jakic-Razumovic J, Capkun V, Murray P. Assessment of the prognostic impact of the Epstein-Barr virus-encoded latent membrane protein-1 expression in Hodgkin's disease. *Br J Cancer*. 2001;84:1227–1234.

21. Kumar V, Fausto N, Abbas A, eds. *Robbins and Cotran's Pathologic Basis of Disease*. 6th ed. Philadelphia, Pa: W B Saunders; 2004:651–674.

22. SEER Cancer Statistics Review 1975–2003 Web site. Table I–11. Retrieved October 24, 2006 from http://seer.cancer.gov/csr/1975_2003/results_single/sect_01_table. 11_2pgs. pdf

23. Grulich AE, Vajdic CM. The epidemiology of non-Hodgkin lymphoma. *Pathology*. 2005;37:409–419.

24. Chatterjee N, Hartge P, Cerhan JR, et al. Risk of non-Hodgkin's lymphoma and family history of lymphatic, hematologic, and other cancers. *Cancer Epidemiol Biomarkers Prev*. 2004;13:1415–1421.

25. Hjalgrim H, Askling J, Rostgaard K, et al. Characteristics of Hodgkin's lymphoma after infectious mononucleosis. *N Engl J Med*. 2003;349:1324–1332.

26. Bergeron RT, Osborn AG, Som PM. *Head and Neck Imaging Excluding the Brain*. St. Louis, Mo: Mosby; 1984:515.

27. DePena CA, Van Tassel P, Lee YY. Lymphoma of the head and neck. *Radiol Clin North Am*. 1990;28: 723–743.

28. Bruneton JN, Kerboul P, Denis F. Lymphomas of the face and neck. In: Bruneton J-N, Schneider M, eds. *Radiology of Lymphomas*. Berlin: Springer-Verlag; 1986:31–39.

29. Hyjek E, Isaacson PG. Primary B cell lymphoma of the thyroid and its relationship to Hashimoto's thyroiditis. *Hum Pathol*. 1988;19:1315–1326.

30. Matsuzuka F, Miyauchi A, Katayama S, et al. Clinical aspects of primary thyroid lymphoma: diagnosis and treatment based on our experience of 119 cases. *Thyroid*. 1993;3:93–99.

31. Isaacson P, Wright DH. Extranodal malignant lymphoma arising from mucosa-associated lymphoid tissue. *Cancer*. 1984;53:2515–2524.

32. Loggins JP, Urquhart A. Preoperative distinction of parotid lymphomas. *J Am Coll Surg*. 2004;199: 58–61.

33. Ordonez NG. Application of immunocytochemistry in the diagnosis of poorly differentiated neoplasms and tumors of unknown origin. *Cancer Bull*. 1989; 41:142–151.

34. Hehn ST, Grogan TM, Miller TP. Utility of fine-needle aspiration as a diagnostic technique in lymphoma. *J Clin Oncol*. 2004;22:3046–3052.

35. Meda BA, Buss DH, Woodruff RD, et al. Diagnosis and subclassification of primary and recurrent lymphoma. The usefulness and limitations of combined fine-needle aspiration cytomorphology and flow cytometry. *Am J Clin Pathol*. 2000;113:688–699.

36. Sneige N, Dekmezian RH, Katz RL, et al. Morphologic and immunocytochemical evaluation of 220 fine needle aspirates of malignant lymphoma and lymphoid hyperplasia. *Acta Cytol*. 1990;34:311–322.

37. Kim DH, Cho YJ, Tiel RL, Kline DG. Surgical outcomes of 111 spinal accessory nerve injuries. *Neurosurgery*. 2003;53:1106–1112.

38. Juneja SK, Wolf MM, Cooper IA. Value of bilateral bone marrow biopsy specimens in non-Hodgkin's lymphoma. *J Clin Pathol*. 1990;43:630–632.

39. Knowles DM. Etiology and pathogenesis of AIDS-related non-Hodgkin's lymphoma. *Hematol Oncol Clin North Am*. 2003;17:785–820.

40. Urquhart AC, Hutchins LG, Berg RL. Distinguishing non-Hodgkin lymphoma from squamous cell carcinoma tumors of the head and neck by computed tomography parameters. *Laryngoscope.* 2002;112: 1079-1083.

41. Hasberger HR, Wiggins RH, Hudgins PA, Davidson HC. *Diagnostic Imaging: Head and Neck.* Philadelphia, Pa: Amirysys-Elsevier Saunders; 2005.

42. Naumann R, Beuthien-Baumann B, Reiss A, et al. Substantial impact of FDG PET imaging on the therapy decision in patients with early-stage Hodgkin's lymphoma. *Br J Cancer.* 2004;90:620-625.

43. Jerusalem GH, Beguin YP. Positron emission tomography in non-Hodgkin's lymphoma (NHL): relationship between tracer uptake and pathological findings, including preliminary experience in the staging of low-grade NHL. *Clin Lymphoma.* 2002;3:56-61.

44. Blum RH, Seymour JF, Wirth A, MacManus M, Hicks RJ. Frequent impact of [18F]fluorodeoxyglucose positron emission tomography on the staging and management of patients with indolent non-Hodgkin's lymphoma. *Clin Lymphoma.* 2003;4: 43-49.

45. Wiedmann E, Baican B, Hertel A, et al. Positron emission tomography (PET) for staging and evaluation of response to treatment in patients with Hodgkin's disease. *Leuk Lymphoma.* 1999;34: 545-551.

46. Weinblatt ME, Zanzi I, Belakhlef A, Babchyck B, Kochen J. False-positive FDG-PET imaging of the thymus of a child with Hodgkin's disease. *J Nucl Med.* 1997;38:888-890.

47. Harris NL, Jaffe ES, Diebold J, et al. The World Health Organization classification of neoplastic diseases of the hematopoietic and lymphoid tissues. Report of the Clinical Advisory Committee meeting, Airlie House, Virginia, November, 1997. *Ann Oncol.* 1999;10:1419-1432.

48. Jaffe ES, Harris NL, Stein H, Vardiman JW, eds. *Pathology and Genetics of Tumors of Haematopoietic and Lymphoid Tissues.* Lyon, France: IARC Press; 2001.

49. Carbone PP, Kaplan HS, Musshoff K, Smithers DW, Tubiana M. Report of the Committee on Hodgkin's Disease Staging Classification. *Cancer Res.* 1971; 31:1860-1861.

50. [No authors listed] A predictive model for aggressive non-Hodgkin's lymphoma. The International Non-Hodgkin's Lymphoma Prognostic Factors Project. *N Engl J Med.* 1993;329:987-994.

51. Rai KR, Peterson BL, Appelbaum FR, et al. Fludarabine compared with chlorambucil as primary therapy for chronic lymphocytic leukemia. *N Engl J Med.* 2000;343:1750-1757.

52. Byrd JC, Peterson BL, Morrison VA, et al. Randomized phase 2 study of fludarabine with concurrent versus sequential treatment with rituximab in symptomatic, untreated patients with B-cell chronic lymphocytic leukemia: results from Cancer and Leukemia Group B 9712 (CALGB 9712). *Blood.* 2003;101:6-14.

53. MacManus MP, Seymour JF. Management of localized low-grade follicular lymphomas. *Austral Radiol.* 2001;45:326-334.

54. Fisher RI, Dahlberg S, Nathwani BN, Banks PM, Miller TP, Grogan TM. A clinical analysis of two indolent lymphoma entities: mantle cell lymphoma and marginal zone lymphoma (including the mucosa-associated lymphoid tissue and monocytoid B-cell subcategories): a Southwest Oncology Group study. *Blood.* 1995;85:1075-1082.

55. Samaha H, Dumontet C, Ketterer N, et al. Mantle cell lymphoma: a retrospective study of 121 cases. *Leukemia.* 1998;12:1281-1287.

56. Wu HJ, Zhang QY, Chen DF, Guan XJ, Zhang BL, Ma J. Comparison of rituximab plus CHOP regimen and CHOP regimen alone for treatment of newly diagnosed patients with diffuse large B-cell lymphoma. *Ai Zheng.* 2005;24:1498-1502.

57. Coiffier B, Lepage E, Briere J, et al. CHOP chemotherapy plus rituximab compared with CHOP alone in elderly patients with diffuse large-B-cell lymphoma. *N Engl J Med.* 2002;346:235-242.

58. Sehn LH, Donaldson J, Chhanabhai M, et al. Introduction of combined CHOP plus rituximab therapy dramatically improved outcome of diffuse large B-cell lymphoma in British Columbia. *J Clin Oncol.* 2005;23:5027-5033.

59. Coiffier B. Treatment of diffuse large B-cell lymphoma. *Curr Hematol Rep.* 2005;4:7-14.

60. Habermann TM, Weller EA, Morrison VA, et al. Phase III trial of rituximab-CHOP (R-CHOP) vss CHOP with a second randomization to maintenance rituximab (MR) or observation in patients 60 years of age and older with diffuse large B-cell lymphoma (DLBCL [Abstract]). *Blood.* 2003;102:6a.

61. Schwenn MR, Blattner SR, Lynch E, Weinstein HJ. HiC-COM: a 2-month intensive chemotherapy regimen for children with stage III and IV Burkitt's lymphoma and B-cell acute lymphoblastic leukemia. *J Clin Oncol.* 1991;9:133-138.

62. Mead GM, Sydes MR, Walewski J, et al. UKLG LY06 collaborators. An international evaluation of CODOX-M and CODOX-M alternating with IVAC in adult Burkitt's lymphoma: results of United Kingdom Lymphoma Group LY06 study. *Ann Oncol.* 2002;13:1264–1274.

63. Magrath I, Adde M, Shad A, et al. Adults and children with small non-cleaved-cell lymphoma have a similar excellent outcome when treated with the same chemotherapy regimen. *J Clin Oncol.* 1996; 14:925–934.

64. Lee EJ, Petroni GR, Schiffer CA, et al. Brief-duration high-intensity chemotherapy for patients with small noncleaved-cell lymphoma or FAB L3 acute lymphocytic leukemia: results of cancer and leukemia group B study 9251. *J Clin Oncol.* 2001;19:4014–4022.

65. Lacasce A, Howard O, Lib S, et al. Modified magrath regimens for adults with Burkitt and Burkitt-like lymphomas: preserved efficacy with decreased toxicity. *Leuk Lymphoma.* 2004;45:761–767.

66. Ho FC, Choy D, Loke SL, et al. Polymorphic reticulosis and conventional lymphomas of the nose and upper aerodigestive tract: a clinicopathologic study of 70 cases, and immunophenotypic studies of 16 cases. *Hum Pathol.* 1990;21:1041–1050.

67. Longo DL, Russo A, Duffey PL, et al. Treatment of advanced-stage massive mediastinal Hodgkin's disease: the case for combined modality treatment. *J Clin Oncol.* 1991;9:227–235.

68. Behar RA, Horning SJ, Hoppe RT. Hodgkin's disease with bulky mediastinal involvement: effective management with combined modality therapy. *Int J Radiat Oncol Biol Phys.* 1993;25:771–776.

69. National Comprehensive Cancer Network (NCCN) Web site. *Hodgkin Disease/Lymphoma.* Retrieved October 11, 2006 from http://www.nccn.org/professionals/physician_gls/PDF/hodgkins.pdf .

70. Canellos GP, Anderson JR, Propert KJ, et al. Chemotherapy of advanced Hodgkin's disease with MOPP, ABVD, or MOPP alternating with ABVD. *N Engl J Med.* 1992;327:1478–1484.

71. Hasenclever D, Diehl V. A prognostic score for advanced Hodgkin's disease. International Prognostic Factors Project on Advanced Hodgkin's Disease. *N Engl J Med.* 1998;339:1506–1514.

72. Huff CA, Jones RJ. Bone marrow transplantation for multiple myeloma: where we are today. *Curr Opin Oncol.* 2002;14:147–151.

73. Abemayor E, Canalis RF, Greenberg P, Wortham DG, Rowland JP, Sun NC. Plasma cell tumors of the head and neck. *J Otolaryngol.* 1988;17:376–381.

74. Wax MK, Yun KJ, Omar RA. Extramedullary plasmacytomas of the head and neck. *Otolaryngol Head Neck Surg.* 1993;109:877–885.

75. Varady E, Deak B, Molnar ZS, et al. Second malignancies after treatment for Hodgkin's disease. *Leuk Lymphoma.* 2001;42:1275–1281.

26

Surgery Following Radiation or Chemoradiation

Kerstin M. Stenson

DEFINITIONS OF UNIQUE TERMS

The last 10 years have witnessed a dramatic shift in the care of patients with advanced head and neck cancer. Successful functional preservation coupled with improved survival is frequently achieved with multimodality therapy. Toxicities of treatment have diminished as hospitals and cancer teams have learned to further support acute and chronic complications of treatment.

This chapter focuses on surgical issues surrounding care of patients who have undergone initial nonoperative treatment for head and neck cancer. Planned surgery, salvage surgery, and surgery for complications of multimodality therapy are addressed.

Multimodality therapy: The use of more than one modality, typically chemotherapy and radiation therapy, to treat patients with advanced head and neck carcinoma. The dual goals of multimodality therapy strive for functional preservation of the upper aerodigestive tract structures and improved survival rates.

Organ preservation therapy: This term is often misused synonymously with

multimodality therapy. The preferred term is *function preservation therapy* which indicates that the operations of speech, swallowing, and breathing are unimpaired or functioning at an acceptable level.

HISTORY AND PATHOPHYSIOLOGY

Surgeons have been discussing the operative challenges of caring for the previously radiated patient for nearly 40 years. Radiation injury to tissues has been recognized for decades and can significantly influence the healing of a surgical wound.[1-11] Radiation affects all cell types within the treatment field and each tissue type, whether it be skin, mucosa, muscle, fascia, or bone, responds differently to the radiation injury. *Acute radiation injury* corresponds to the time during the actual exposure to ionizing radiation and several weeks thereafter.[11] Epithelial tissues, such as mucosa, salivary tissue, and taste buds, are most sensitive to the acute radiation damage due to their rapidly proliferative nature. On a cellular level, radiation damages the DNA during mitosis of rapidly dividing cells. These cellular changes during the acute radiation injury account for the common side effects of mucositis, dry mouth, and decreased taste sensation. *Chronic radiation injury* affects the more slowly proliferating cells of vascular and connective tissues. This late radiation injury occurs 4 to 6 months after radiation.[11] During this time, capillaries progressively decrease in number, dilate, and undergo the changes of obliterative endarteritis. Fibrous tissue deposition gradually increases in the submucosal and subcutaneous tissue planes. Unlike acute radiation injury, whose changes are somewhat if not completely reversible, the chronic radiation injury of avascularity and fibrosis are dose dependent, progressive, and permanent. Clinically, the late radiation damage is seen as skin atrophy, telangiectasias, trismus, muscle fibrosis, hypothyroidism, and lymphatic obstruction. Trauma (surgical or otherwise) or infection of the irradiated field can result in a major nonhealing wound.

Historically, there are many reports in the literature referencing increased surgical morbidity in patients receiving preoperative radiation therapy, particularly if surgery crosses a mucosal barrier.[1-7] These include wound dehiscence, fistula formation, and carotid rupture. Analysis of more recent reports reflect more acceptable/comparable complication rates.[8,9,12] Two phenomenon likely account for this improvement in postradiotherapy surgical complications: increased prevalence of three-dimensional radiotherapy planning (limiting radiation dose to noninvolved structures), and improved ability to protect and reconstruct radiated wounds via free tissue transfer techniques. In addition, it has been theorized that a "surgical window" exists between the resolution of the acute radiation injury and the onset of the chronic injury in which technically feasible surgery can be completed through relatively normal tissue planes.[13] This intuitive concept is supported by the work of Hopewell et al, who studied the cellular basis of vascular irradiation damage.[14] He found that initial changes in vessels 2 to 4 months after radiation was associated with a loss of endothelial cells, which resulted in an abnormal proliferation of viable cells. This proliferation resulted in decreased size of the capillary bed from small vessel occlusion, that is, a radiation obliterative endarteritis. Later changes in the vasculature were associated with a reduction of smooth muscle cells.

Thus, surgical trauma prior to capillary occlusion (2–4 months) may result in wounds that heal relatively normally.

CRITICAL ELEMENTS OF THE HISTORY AND PHYSICAL EXAM

History

Critical elements of the history include a detailed account and summary of prior treatment, documenting the last date of radiation or chemoradiation. Functions of breathing, particularly symptoms of obstructive sleep apnea, speaking/voicing, and swallowing function should be carefully assessed. The patient's current and past weight gives insight into nutritional status and should be noted. Intensity and location of pain is a critical detail in understanding important treatment goals. Although surgical resection may not render a cure, surgical palliation may represent a powerful method of pain relief.

Physical Exam

A thorough head and neck examination clearly is required for complete assessment of the patient. Important points to document through visual assessment, physical exam, and fiberoptic laryngoscopy include extent of tumor, status of the airway, cranial nerve and sympathetic chain function, evidence of bone exposure, degree (if any) of trismus, and ability to manage secretions. Juxtaposition of tumor to common, internal, and/or external carotid artery branches should be determined. This latter point in the physical exam is fundamental in deciding if patient's wound is "safe" and helps establish the urgency of operative intervention. Often, the patient's prior treatments preclude complete accuracy of gross tumor extent. Here the physical exam is complemented well by imaging studies that help delineate anatomic details. Elective versus obligatory gastrostomy tube placement is discussed after nutritional status and ability to maintain adequate intake during treatment is evaluated.

APPROPRIATE DIAGNOSTIC OFFICE-BASED PROCEDURES

Completion of the physical exam is certainly aided by use of flexible fiberoptic laryngoscopy. Assessment of the patient's airway and potential intubation difficulties (if tracheotomy is not in place) is crucial to document and communicate to our anesthesia colleagues during the preoperative evaluation. If carcinoma recurrence has not been verified, pathologic documentation is paramount. The physician may consider biopsy with local anesthesia of oral or oropharyngeal lesions or fine needle aspiration of neck masses to facilitate the diagnosis and further workup. Another important condition to consider is thyroid function. Many patients who have undergone radiation become physiologically or clinically hypothyroid.[15,16] Wound healing effects of hypothyroidism are well documented and the physician should supplement as soon as possible prior to any scheduled surgery.[17,18]

RECOMMENDED IMAGING STUDIES

Imaging studies are critical in the evaluation of patients with recurrent carcinoma. Routinely, CT scans of the head, neck and chest are completed to characterize anatomic details and to evaluate evidence of distant disease. Both CT and MRI scanning provide detailed structural and anatomic information about extent and/or depth of invasion of head and neck cancer. CT scanning is particularly helpful in assessing subclinical adenopathy, especially when patients have been previously radiated or are heavily muscled or obese. In addition, bone and/or cartilage invasion can be evaluated. MRI scanning is known for its enhanced ability to render soft tissue detail, and has been reported to be superior to CT scanning in evaluating depth of invasion into soft tissue, discriminating tumor from mucus and detecting bone marrow invasion.

Positron emission tomography (PET) scanning is a useful adjunct in workup for metastatic disease and/or second primary tumors. Increasingly, PET scanning is being utilized in the management of patients with N-positive neck disease after chemoradiotherapy. Some authors believe that PET-scanning completed 6 weeks postchemoradiation can dependably isolate residual cancer.[19,20] Other researchers rely on the high negative predictive value (91–100%) of post-therapeutic PET scans in order to defer neck dissection.[21,22] Considering the less than perfect positive predictive value (33–80%), clinical judgment must be applied in those patients who have a positive PET scan, or a negative PET scan with gross residual nodal bulk. PET scan has also found a role in helping to differentiate laryngeal radionecrosis from recurrent laryngeal cancer.[23]

IDENTIFICATION OF CRITICAL DECISION POINTS

Recognition of the key points will help the head and neck surgeon to strategize the care of the patient who has undergone prior therapy.

Key Point 1

Is surgery part of a *planned* sequence of multimodality therapy?

This key point typically means planned neck surgery after concurrent chemoradiotherapy. There is much controversy surrounding this issue.

Key Point 2

Is surgery required to salvage recurrent or persistent cancer at the primary site and/or neck?

Multidisciplinary assessment of treatment options is critical. It is imperative here to recognize clinical and radiologic evidence of tumor invasion into the carotid artery and potential for carotid rupture (Fig 26-1). In other words, *is the wound safe?*

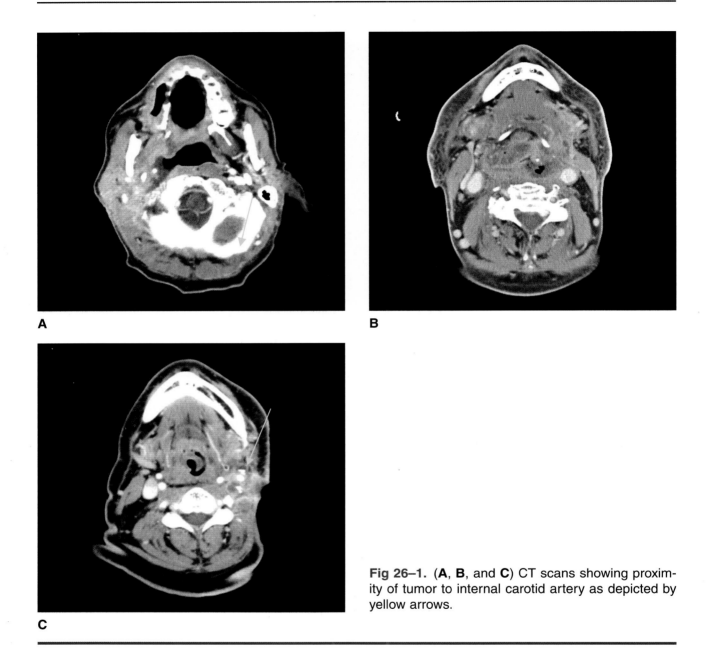

Fig 26–1. (**A**, **B**, and **C**) CT scans showing proximity of tumor to internal carotid artery as depicted by yellow arrows.

Key Point 3

Is surgery required for treatment of a patient with wound healing problems related to prior radiotherapy?

Diagnosis and management of bony, cartilaginous and soft tissue radionecrosis are addressed below.

Key Point 4

Is surgery required for definitive palliation?

Palliation of dysphagia related to fibrosis of the constrictor muscles/laryngeal apparatus or pain due to cancer ultimately can be accomplished with carefully planned surgery.

Thorough metastatic workup and preanesthesia testing is required when evaluating the feasibility of surgery in this group of patients. There are always competing and confounding clinical factors to consider when deciding when and if to operate. For example, would the head and neck surgeon perform carotid replacement and pectoralis flap in a patient with obvious lung metastases and imminent carotid rupture? Is an elective laryngectomy an acceptable option in a tracheotomy-dependent patient who cannot swallow?

Frequently the surgeon can decide whether or not to proceed with surgery if the following question can be answered in the affirmative: *If fit for general anesthesia, will surgery help the patient live better if not longer?* This thought process, along with the identification of the above key points, will facilitate the surgeon's dialogue with the patient and his or her family. Realistic expectations can be established through methodical and frank discussions. These in turn will improve the patient's understanding of their challenging situation, while facilitating the surgeon-patient relationship.[24]

KEY POINT 1: PLANNED SURGERY

The role of planned neck dissection (ND) in the context of concurrent chemoradiotherapy protocols remains controversial in that there is no clear consensus regarding which patients may obtain survival benefit from post-treatment ND. Surgeons have come to understand that residual post-treatment microscopic disease is not reliably predicted by CT scan imaging.[13,25-27] It is also understood that chemoradiotherapy is highly effective in sterilizing the neck in N0 (occult disease) and N1 neck stages and substantially decreases pathologically positive nodal disease and extracapsular spread in N-positive necks.[28] The possibility of post-therapeutic viable cancer in N-positive neck dissection specimens, has led many authors to recommend planned post-treatment ND in all patients with N2 or greater neck disease or those with residual clinical or radiographic disease, regardless of N-stage.[28-31] Others decide to perform ND for patients with pretreatment N3 neck disease[32] or if there is PET scan evidence of residual disease at 3 months post-treatment.[21,22,33] Still other authorities believe that the isolated neck recurrences are rare after attainment of a clinical and radiographic complete response and that the notion of planned neck dissection is obsolete.[34]

Technical Points

Prior to neck dissection, biopsy of the primary site and frozen section pathologic analysis must be performed. After pathologic documentation of complete response (ie, negative for carcinoma) at the primary site, planned neck dissection, at the same operative setting, can be considered. If a patient has positive pathology at the primary site, resection of the primary and neck would be required, usually at a separate operative setting so that informed consent can be obtained.

Most head and neck surgeons have learned that performing ND in patients who have undergone multimodality therapy is technically feasible with acceptable complication rates. CT scans are referred to regularly to aid in selection of neck dissection type. For example, if tissue planes between carotid sheath and sternocleidomastoid muscle (SCM) are discrete or if the jugular vein can be identified continuously from the thoracic inlet to the skull base, a selective neck dissection is planned (Fig 26–2).[13,35] If the jugular vein is not visualized, or if there is bulky residual disease that obliterates anatomic tissue planes, a more extensive neck dissection is planned. It is important to protect the carotid artery, typically with a pectoralis myofacial flap, if the SCM is sacrificed[36] (Fig 26–3). Again, preoperative counseling is paramount.

KEY POINT 2: SALVAGE SURGERY FOR PERSISTENT OR RECURRENT CANCER

Staging, Prognosis, and Costs

Several surgeons have studied the effectiveness of salvage surgery for patients with persistent or recurrent locoregional disease after chemo/radiotherapy.[37-42] In earlier studies, authors found prolonged survival

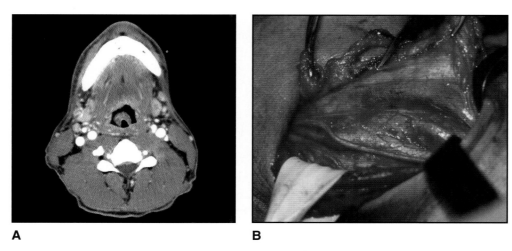

A   B

Fig 26–2. A. CT scan showing residual adenopathy at right level 2 with preserved tissue planes after concurrent chemoradiation. **B.** Anatomic surgical planes of selective neck dissection.

after salvage surgery ranging from approximately 19% to 53%. Despite these reasonable figures, many reported that salvage surgery provided limited survival benefit and was seldom feasible.

Recently Goodwin and others have shown that the restaging patients with recurrent cancer (ie, rT4, etc), independent of the initial stage, has clear prognostic power with respect to costs, survival, surgical complications, and quality of life (QOL).[37,42]. Goodwin performed a meta-analysis of 32 head and neck cancer surgical salvage reports in conjunction with a prospective observational study of 109 patients selecting salvage surgery.[37] He found that patients with stages I and II recurrent carcinoma had a 70% chance of living for at least 2 years after surgical salvage. This group also enjoyed a 60% to 85% chance of attaining successful QOL parameters. On the other hand, patients with stage III and IV recurrent head and neck cancer have a 23 to 33% chance of 2-year survival and only 30% to 40% chance of improved QOL—which may be only temporary—after salvage surgery. Likewise, these authors identified that economic costs, consisting of professional and hospital charges, were dramatically different between patients with early stage recurrences and late stage, that is, approximately $21,000 versus $47,000. The pro-

spective portion of the study showed no relationship between recurrence site and survival. These results, as well as our improved understanding of salvage surgery, help the surgeon and the multidisciplinary team to undertake a candid discussion with the patient. Thus informed, the patient is empowered to make the best possible decision with respect to recurrent cancer treatment.

Several institutions have realized that the majority of patients with postchemo/radiotherapy recurrences require more than salvage surgery for ultimate survival.[43-45] The largest trial studied 115 patients with recurrent locoregional carcinoma who underwent triple-agent chemotherapy (cisplatin, paclitaxel, and gemcytobine) and reirradiation with or without salvage surgery.[45] The overall survival and progression-free survival for the whole group was 22% and 33%, respectively. Forty-nine patients underwent salvage surgery prior to the chemotherapy and reirradiation. Three-year overall survival and progression-free survival was 39% and 51%, respectively, for these 49 patients, versus 11% and 19% for those 66 who did not undergo pretreatment cytoreductive surgery. Many patients had microscopic skip metastases or lymphovascular invasion despite efforts to achieve negative margins at the time of salvage

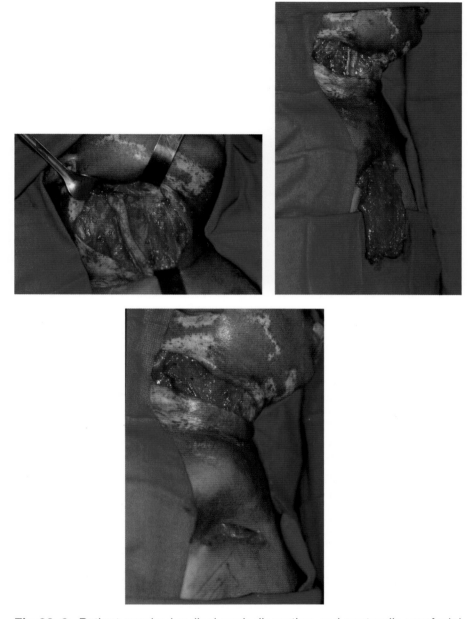

Fig 26–3. Patient required radical neck dissection and pectoralis myofacial flap after chemoradiation for large neck node.

surgery. Ultimately, margin status was not correlated with survival. Complications of osteoradionecrosis ($n = 13$) and carotid hemorrhage ($n = 6$; all in the nonoperated group) occurred, underscoring the potential risks and challenges of any retreatment protocols. Nonetheless, as Moscoso, Urken, and colleages stated more than a decade ago, "An expectation of increased post-operative morbidity should not interfere with the decision to proceed with multimodality salvage therapy . . ."[46]

Principles

Five main principles should be considered in patients who will undergo salvage surgery. The surgeon should:

1. *Carefully restage the disease at the time of recurrence, as the stage at recurrence most closely correlates with survival.*[37,47]
2. *Use vascularized tissue for reconstruction of mucosal defects or coverage of mucosal suture lines.*
3. *Use large-bore drains for management of potential fistulae.*[48]
4. *Have a thorough discussion with the patient and family regarding the risks and benefits of salvage surgery prior to resection.*
5. *Ultimately create a safe wound that will endure the ravages of poor nutrition and further treatment.*

Management of Recurrent Laryngeal Cancer

Early stage recurrences can be managed endoscopically or with open procedures.[49-53,54-59] The patient must have adequate pulmonary reserve which can be assessed via pulmonary function testing (FEV_1 >60% or FEV_1/FVC >50%), or by walking the patient up 1 to 2 flights of stairs (Ogura stair test).[60,61] Complete endoscopic visualization of the tumor is necessary for thorough removal. Frequent scheduled postoperative clinic visits are critical to document healing, assess nutrition and airway, and to evaluate for recurrence.

Late stage recurrences typically are managed with total laryngectomy[62-65] although Steiner and others have found modest success using endoscopic laser methods.[53] Following salvage total laryngectomy strong consideration should be given to prophylactic placement of a pectoralis myofascial flap over the neopharyngeal suture line to facilitate healing and prevent fistulae. If there is inadequate mucosa for primary closure of the neopharynx, the surgical team may inset a radial forearm free flap within the mucosal defect.[66] In all cases, the surgeon should provide the patient with a means to speak by performing a tracheoesophageal puncture (TEP) and voice prosthesis insertion during the primary resection. Voicing should begin via the TEP only after complete healing and risk of delayed fistulae is low, usually 2 to 3 weeks.

Management of Recurrent Oral Cavity, Oropharyngeal, and Hypopharyngeal Cancer

It is generally thought that increasing time to presalvage recurrence and salvage for nonlaryngeal sites poses significant challenges to survival.[42,47,67-71] This principle was not appreciated in either the prospective observational portion, nor the retrospective meta-analysis of Goodwin's 2000 study.[37] A more contemporary study of salvage surgery in nonlaryngeal sites reports an important intuitive concept: planned early *pathologic restaging* in patients with advanced carcinomas affords an opportunity for successful surgical salvage in patients for whom chemo/radiotherapy has failed.[72]

Vascularized tissue replacement via free flap reconstruction has been shown in many studies to be the most reliable method of reconstruction and wound protection.[73,74] Partial tongue, palate, or buccal defects are commonly repaired with fascial-cutaneous free flaps, such as the radial forearm free flap or the lateral thigh free flap.[75] For oral cavity and oropharyngeal recurrences that require a composite resection (including bone), the decision must be made whether or not to replace the bone. Certainly for anterior defects, oral competence and floor of mouth support is accomplished with structural support that is provided by vascularized bony replacement (Figs 26–4 and 26–5). However, lateral composite defects, particularly in patients who are edentulous or who cannot swallow, are more efficiently reconstructed with vascularized soft tissue only. Total glossectomy defects are usually managed with rectus myocutaneous free flap in order to replace the prerequisite mass. A flap with adequate bulk also permits use of a palatal-drop prosthesis, thus facilitating speech rehabilitation. Potential aspiration of secretions is managed with tracheotomy and enhanced pulmonary hygiene. Prophylactic laryngectomy is not routinely done to maximize speech potential (Fig 26–6).

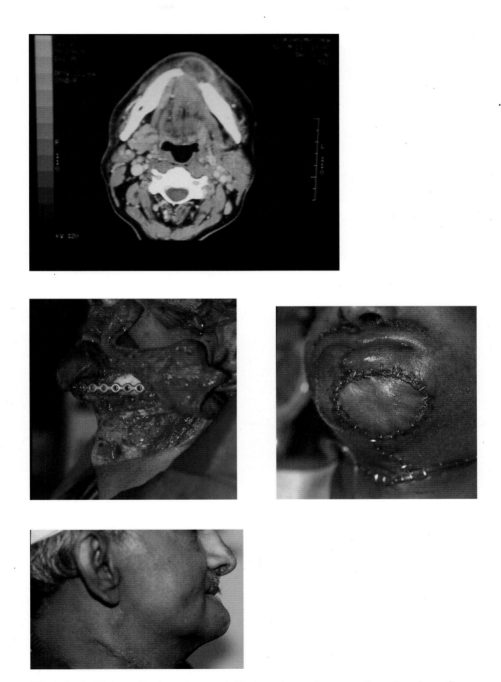

Fig 26–4. This patient underwent fibula osteocutaneous free flap for a floor-of-mouth recurrence that extended into the soft tissues. Note the preservation of the anterior mandibular contour.

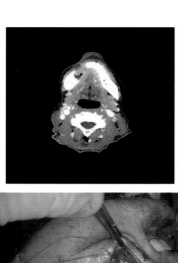
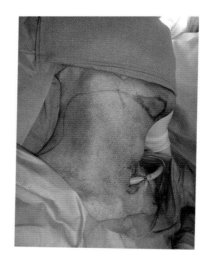
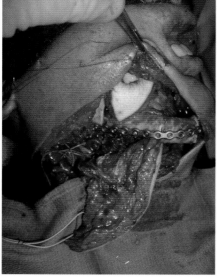
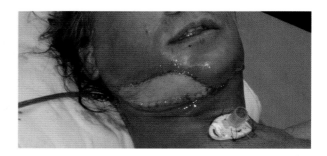
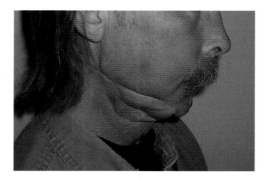

Fig 26–5. This patient had residual carcinoma within the soft tissues and mandible after concurrent chemoradiation

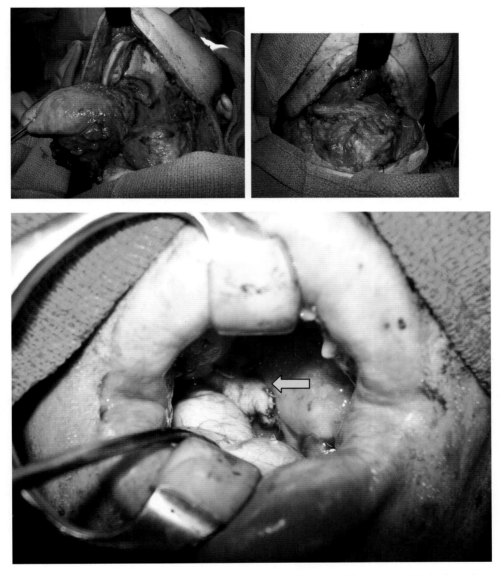

Fig 26–6. This patient required a total glossectomy with lateral thigh free-flap reconstruction. Note the small cutaneous extension used to reconstitute the soft palate.

For laryngopharyngectomy defects, surgeons may use a vascularized free jejunal segment.[76] Although this flap supplies visceral lining, experience has taught us that vascularized fasciocutaneous flaps provide less potential donor site morbidity and more functional speech, particularly when the lateral thigh free flap is utilized[77-79] (Fig 26–7). As in laryngectomy reconstructions, primary TEP should be performed. Voicing should not commence until full healing, usually 3 weeks postoperatively. Care must be taken if the inferior extent of the esophageal defect is well below the manubrium. In this situation, the proximal tracheal segment by necessity may become devascularized, a devastating complication. Here, the surgeon would choose a gastric pull-up (Fig 26–8).

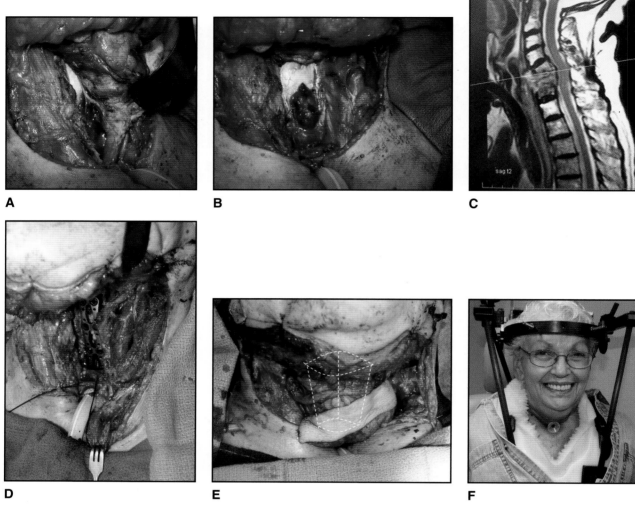

A   B   C

D   E   F

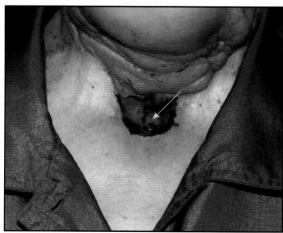

G

Fig 26–7. This patient suffered a recurrence of hypopharyngeal carcinoma after chemoradiotherapy. She had cervical bony destruction discovered postoperatively to be secondary to osteoradionecrosis. Arrow in (**A**) points to larynx with posterior pharyngeal defect. The arrow in (**B**) points to mass (found to be granulation tissue) on prevertebral fascia. (**C**) sagittal projection of the involved cervical spine. The patient was reconstructed with lateral thigh free-flap after cervical corpectomy, anterior spinal fusion with titanium cage, posterior spinal fusion, and Halo application (**F**). (**D**) anterior cervical hardware and (**E**) anterior skin paddle with radial forearm skin tube/neopharynx diagramed in overlay. (**G**) patient 2 weeks after completing chemotherapy and reirradiaiton. The arrow is pointing to the TEP (Provox™). She has been eating and speaking throughout treatment.

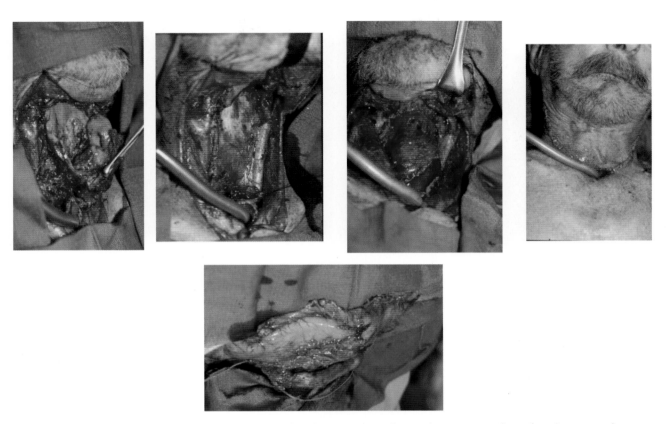

Fig 26–8. This patient required gastric pull-up for pharyngoesophageal reconstruction of a pharyngeal recurrence after chemoradiation.

Creativity and preoperative preparation by the head and neck reconstructive team is essential. A clear understanding of the three-dimensional aspects of the defect and potential location(s) of the recipient vessels is mandatory. Often, the same flap, either with different perforators or with de-epithelialized segments can be used to reconstruct mucosal defects as well as external neck skin defects[80,81] (Fig 26-9). The attentive surgeon will preserve potential recipient vessels such as external branches of the carotid artery and internal/external jugular veins if oncologically sound. Other potential recipient vessels include the transverse cervical vessels, thoracodorsal vessels, thoracoacromial system, or the subclavian artery/vein.[82-84] Use of the thoracoacromial system is facilitated by previous placement of a pectoralis flap, a common scenario in previously treated patients (Fig 26-10). Still, with use of careful technique and

loupe magnification, the thoracoacromial and subclavian systems can be dissected through an nonpedicled in situ pectoralis muscle.

Management of Nasopharyngeal Recurrences

Historically, recurrent disease in the nasopharynx has been viewed with some trepidation. Proximity of the tumor to the internal carotid artery as well as access to and clear exposure of the nasopharyngeal contents have posed particular challenges. Advances in surgical approaches, integration of skull base techniques, and control/protection of the carotid artery have made resection of selected nasopharyngeal recurrences feasible.[85-88] Long-term survival is better achieved for patients with early stage recurrences

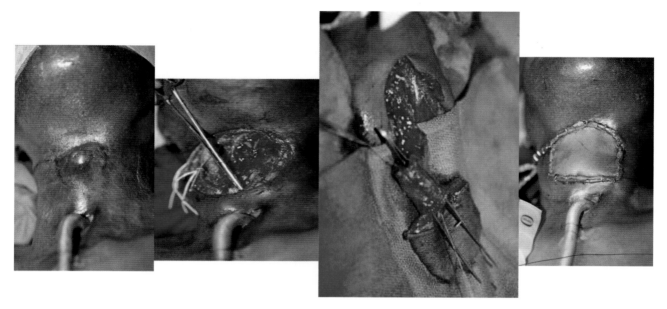

Fig 26–9. Patient wil neopharyngeal recurrence extending into skin. A radial forearm tubed "paddle flap" was used to reconstruct neopharynx and anterior skin.

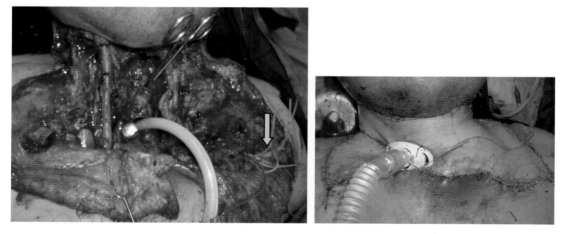

Fig 26–10. Patient with large pharyngocervical recurrence and previously placed pectoralis flap. Recipient vessels were (*arrow*) isolated at the thoracoacromial trunk for lateral thigh free-flap reconstruction.

and for those who undergo reirradiation. The facial translocation approach seems to provide the widest exposure. Other techniques, such as the cervicoparotid/transhyoid approach, may afford better protection of the facial nerve, improved internal carotid artery exposure, and more aesthetic incisions (Fig 26-11).[89]

Complications

Early reports of salvage surgery after organ preservation therapy revealed a high number of complications.[7,46] More recent analyses have shown modest major complications, such as fistulae, carotid rup-

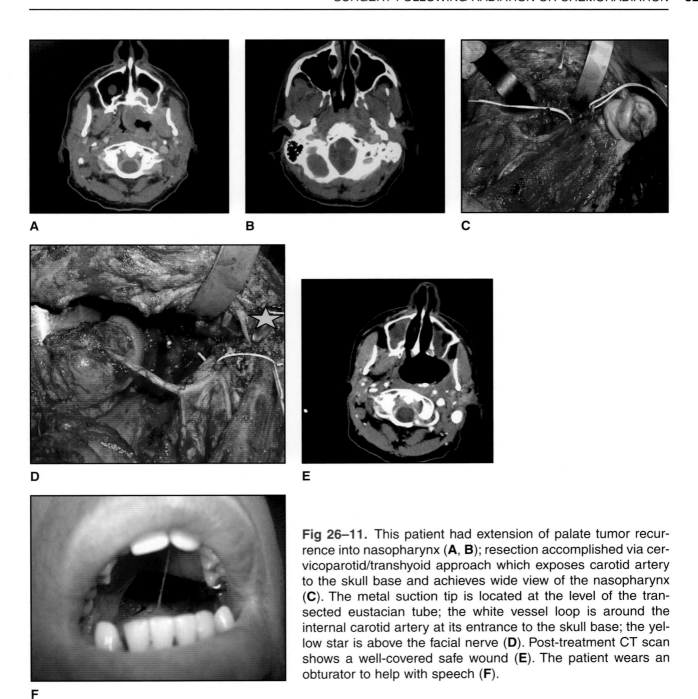

Fig 26–11. This patient had extension of palate tumor recurrence into nasopharynx (**A**, **B**); resection accomplished via cervicoparotid/transhyoid approach which exposes carotid artery to the skull base and achieves wide view of the nasopharynx (**C**). The metal suction tip is located at the level of the transected eustacian tube; the white vessel loop is around the internal carotid artery at its entrance to the skull base; the yellow star is above the facial nerve (**D**). Post-treatment CT scan shows a well-covered safe wound (**E**). The patient wears an obturator to help with speech (**F**).

ture, and other events requiring additional surgery, ranging from 10% to 28%.[47,62,71,90] This more acceptable level of complications likely reflects many factors, including increased use of free tissue for reconstruction, better nutrition during chemo/ radiotherapy, and decreased toxicity of radiation due to intensity modulated radiotherapy.

Potential fistulae are managed effectively in or out of the hospital with large-bore suction drains.[48] This method allows areas of salivary leakage to be diverted directly out the drainage tube. The skin flap and closure remain flat and intact. Wound care is much less burdensome with less time spent in the hospital. One can observe resolution of the fistula by observing the character of the exudate in the drainage tube as it changes from purulent to serous. This healing transformation takes from 2 to 5 weeks.

There are several potential complications that may occur principally in patients who require hypopharyngeal reconstruction.[91] Specifically, permanent hypocalcemia occurs in 45% of patients, either due to devascularization of the parathyroid glands or due to oncologic resection. This is even more problematic in patients who have a gastric pull-up due to problems with calcium absorption and metabolism.[92] In addition, there is approximately a 15% chance of stricture at the mucocutaneous anastamotic site. This can be managed through serial dilations and placement of mitomycin C to prevent restricture.[93]

Management of the Neck

The N0 Neck

Recent literature has shown that during primary site salvage surgery, there is little risk of node recurrence in a patient with a presalvage N0 neck.[94,95] Others reason that a selective neck dissection has little morbidity and should be completed, because an N0 neck may harbor microscopic disease.[96] In addition, recipient vessels must be meticulously preserved for free flap use during salvage surgery. A selective neck dissection simultaneously accomplishes oncologic removal of subclinical metastases and exposure of recipient vessels.

The N+ Neck: Carotid Artery Resection/Replacement

If tissue planes are preserved, as estimated from the preoperative CT scans, then a selective neck dissection usually can be accomplished for N+ neck with mobile nodes. If diseased nodes cannot easily be dissected away from the sternocleidomastoid muscle or jugular vein, modified radical or radical neck dissection is indicated. It is prudent to plan coverage of exposed vessels with the free-flap preparation or with a separate pectoralis myofascial flap.

Thorough review of the patient's physical examination and CT scans will help determine proximity of tumor to the carotid. Cranial nerve involvement and CT scan depiction of tumor that extends more than 180 degrees around the carotid artery predicts invasion.[97] The patient, family, and surgeon are ultimately faced with perhaps the most difficult dilemma in the field of head and neck oncology. The competing risks of disease progression with eventual carotid rupture and those of carotid resection and replacement must be systematically balanced and fully discussed with the patient.[98]

If the patient clearly has an unresectable recurrence, is not fit for surgery, or is at high risk for stroke, endovascular stent placement can provide palliation for imminent carotid blowout.[99-102] This is a temporizing measure only, as the stents are subject to contamination and displacement in an already fragile artery. Alternatively, if the patient is found to tolerate test balloon occlusion of the involved artery, he or she may undergo permanent occlusion.[103] Detachable balloons have generally fallen out of favor due to displacement (and resultant stroke) into the peripheral branches of the cerebral arteries. However, irretrievable coils can be utilized for permanent occlusion.

If the patient has resectable tumor and can be brought to surgery in a reasonable period of time, carotid resection and replacement should be strongly considered. There are important rationales that support this recommendation: (1) Intuitively, carotid replacement is the most physiologic means of repair and rehabilitation. (2) The risk of ischemic stroke and postoperative embolic stroke remains unpredictable during intraoperative carotid ligation.[39] (3) The contralateral carotid vessels are at risk for recurrent disease as well as the radiation-induced acceleration of atherosclerosis.[104,105] Most surgical teams utilize autogenous tissue, such as reverse saphenous vein graft or superficial femoral artery graft to replace the carotid.[108-110] Others advocate use of contralateral external carotid to middle cerebral artery bypass or stenting and exarterectomy.[111-113] Liberal use of a pectoralis myofascial flap or a vascularized perforator segment of a free flap is strongly advocated to protect the grafted artery from potential salivary contamination and to facilitate healing in the irradiated bed.[114] (Fig 26–12).

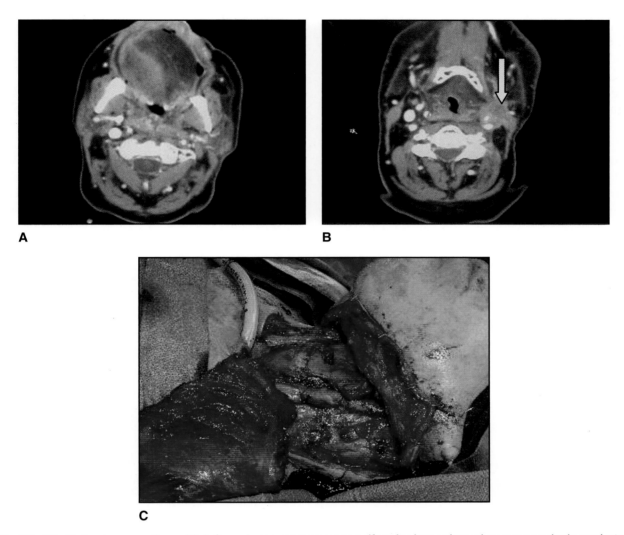

Fig 26–12. Patient presenting with left neck recurrence as manifest by hypoglossal nerve paralysis and atrophy of left tongue (**A**, **B**). In **C**, the carotid has been resected, replaced with saphenous vein, and is ready for pectoralis flap coverage.

KEY POINT 3: SURGERY FOR OSTEORADIONECROSIS (ORN) AND OTHER RADIATION-INDUCED WOUND HEALING PROBLEMS

Bone and soft tissue necrosis can be a painful and distressing complication of multimodality therapy. Nonoperative management is an option for some patients with limited wounds and minor complications such as mucosal ulceration, pain, fibrosis, or atrophic skin. Pentoxifylline has been shown to enhance healing as well as improve symptoms of pain and signs of fibrosis such as telangiectasias, edema, pain, and atrophy.[115-118] This effect of pentoxifylline works through increased deformity of erythrocytes, increased release of prostacyclin, and/or suppression of TNFα (tumor necrosis factor alpha). The outcome is increased oxygen delivery to the wound and decreased inflammatory products of radiation.

Most surgeons have learned to appreciate Marx's "3 H" principle: radiated tissue is hypoxic, hypocellular, and hypovascular and has limited ability to replace physiologic losses that occur during the composite tissue's normal cellular life span.[119] After collagen lysis and cellular death, the surrounding wound cannot provide enough other or basic requirements of tissue repair in order to heal.

It seems intuitive that if the wound hypoxia can be reversed, healing would be facilitated. To this end, Marx has explained how hyperbaric oxygen (HbO_2) can facilitate healing of radiated wounds.[120] During HbO_2 therapy sessions, the partial pressure of oxygen within the radiated tissue increases from 5 to 15 mm Hg to 1000 to 1300 mm Hg. This exposure stimulates fibroblasts to manufacture new collagen, which then forms the framework for endothelial proliferation from adjacent capillaries. This neovas-

cularization raises the local tissue oxygen levels to 20 to 35 mm Hg, thus promoting wound healing.

There is ongoing controversy over the benefits of HbO_2 as it relates to wound improvement in the head and neck population. There is literature to support its use alone, with sequestrectomy, and with vascularized and nonvascularized bone grafts.[121-124] The more compelling research has revealed that there is no benefit of HbO_2 for patients with overt ORN.[125] In addition, others reason that even in an adjuvant setting, HbO_2 cannot restore dead or impaired bone, is costly, and can delay definitive surgical treatment.[126] Hence, the surgical treatment of choice for nonhealing radiated wounds is to replace all necrotic and fibrotic bone, skin, and muscle with vascularized tissue[126-129] (Figs 26-13 through 26-17).

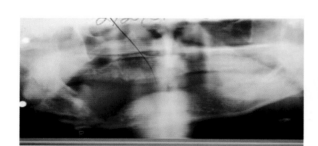

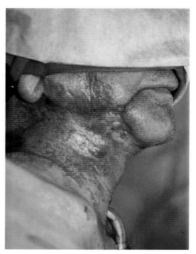

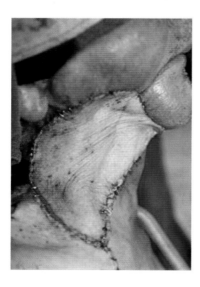

Fig 26–13. A patient with pathologic fracture due to ORN; patient is edentulous, unable to chew. He was reconstructed with radial forearm fasciacutaneous tissue.

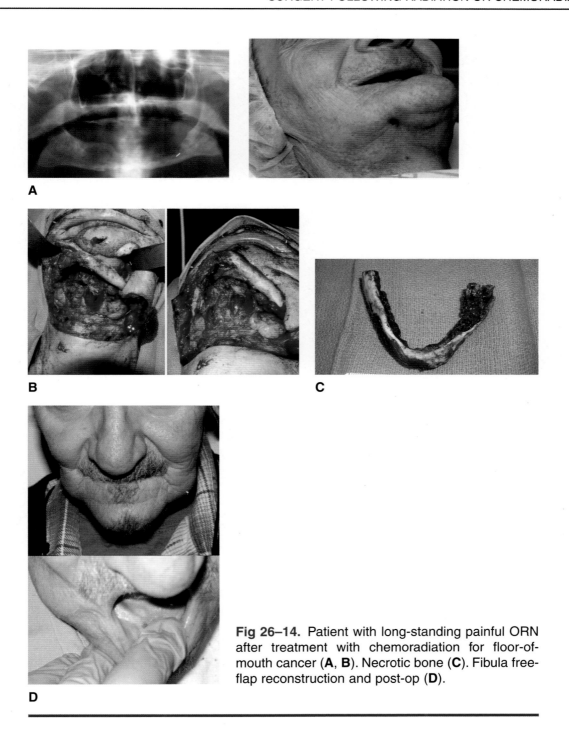

Fig 26–14. Patient with long-standing painful ORN after treatment with chemoradiation for floor-of-mouth cancer (**A**, **B**). Necrotic bone (**C**). Fibula free-flap reconstruction and post-op (**D**).

This fresh tissue likely offsets the need for perioperative HbO$_2$.

ORN of the mandible, maxilla, and other sites such as the skull base or cervical spine must be differentiated from residual carcinoma through thor-

ough biopsy. Management strategies for skull base ORN include endoscopic sequestrectomy, antibiotics, and HbO$_2$.[130,131] One may be unable to distinguish cervical spine ORN from invasive or metastatic cancer until the time of laryngopharynx resection

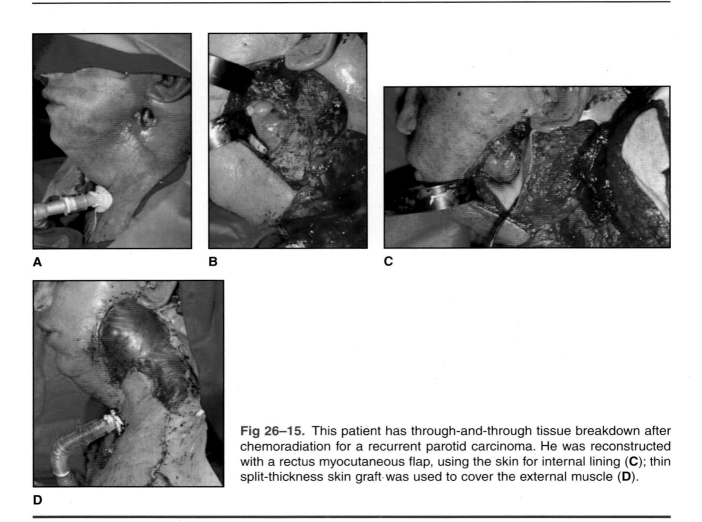

A

B

C

D

Fig 26–15. This patient has through-and-through tissue breakdown after chemoradiation for a recurrent parotid carcinoma. He was reconstructed with a rectus myocutaneous flap, using the skin for internal lining (**C**); thin split-thickness skin graft was used to cover the external muscle (**D**).

(see Fig 26–7). In either situation, the surgical team must be prepared for pharyngeal and cervical spine reconstruction which can be accomplished with vascularized osteocutaneous flaps.[132,133]

KEY POINT 4: SURGERY FOR PALLIATION OF PAIN OR DYSPHAGIA

Too often, adequate pain control is accompanied by lethargy or blunting of affect. The head and neck surgeon, along with the multidisciplinary team, should include surgical resection in their armamentarium of pain palliation. The patient and family can be made to understand that a surgery of this type may not increase survival as much as improve the quality of the patients remaining life (Fig 26–18).

In terms of dysphagia, the surgeon must work closely with speech and swallowing pathologists to determine the etiology. If there is a well-defined stricture and adequate function of the remaining constrictor muscles, antero- or retrograde dilation can be accomplished.[134,135] It is helpful to use fluoroscopy for accurate guide wire placement for

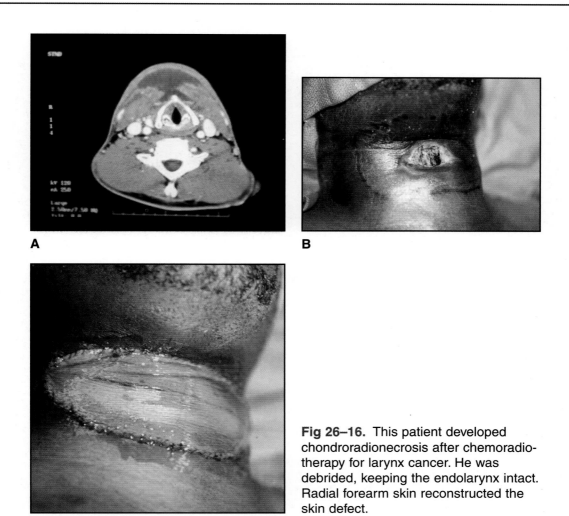

Fig 26–16. This patient developed chondroradionecrosis after chemoradiotherapy for larynx cancer. He was debrided, keeping the endolarynx intact. Radial forearm skin reconstructed the skin defect.

patients with small caliber or complete stenoses. Topical mitomycin C application may be helpful in preventing restricture in this population.

A clear understanding of the mechanism of dysphagia in a patient who has undergone chemo/radiotherapy must be ascertained prior to contemplation of ablative surgery. If the patient is tracheotomy dependent and cannot swallow secretions due to fibrosis of constrictor muscles, laryngectomy or laryngopharyngectomy may be considered. However, if the patient lacks sufficient tongue-base power to propel a food bolus down the neopharynx, a laryngectomy will *not* likely help the patient's situation.[136] Once again, thorough explanation with patient and family fosters understanding of this complex and challenging situation.

It must be made clear that due to extreme fibrosis and kyphosis of the neck, some patients are poor surgical candidates (Fig 26–19). These patients with woody induration of the soft tissues and neck contraction possess inadequate access for safe exposure of vessels, airway, and pharynx.

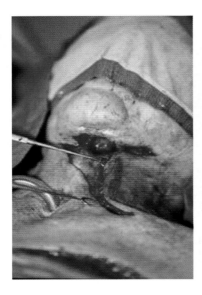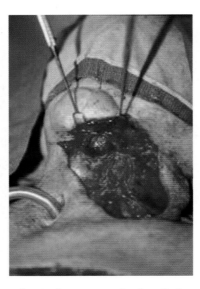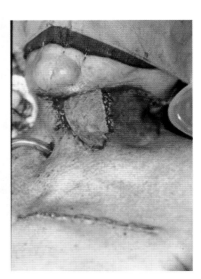

Fig 26–17. This patient underwent chemotherapy and reirradiation for a recurrent tongue cancer. He developed ORN of the hyoid bone which was debrided, and managed with pectoralis myofascial flap and long-term drain for fistulas prophylaxis.

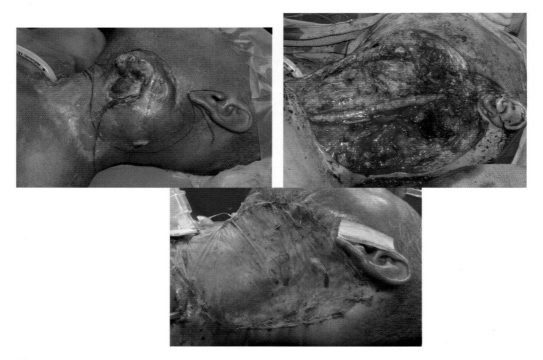

Fig 26–18. Patient with uncontrolled neck recurrence, potential for carotid rupture and distant metastatic disease. Radical neck surgery (with preservation of the carotid artery), alleviated pain, controlled odor, and eliminated risk of carotid rupture.

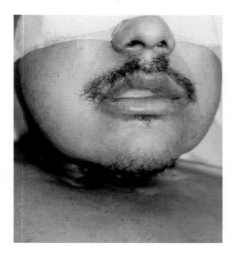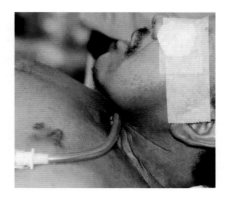

Fig 26–19. Patient after chemoradiation for a supraglottic cancer in approximately 1997. The patient displays severe soft tissue contraction and kyphosis. Laryngectomy for inability to swallow was aborted due to inadequate access for vessels control, airway, and pharyngeal access.

CONCLUSION

Overall, our patients are enjoying the improved survival and function preservation of contemporary chemoradiotherapy schema. Our steadfast role as anatomists, clinician/diagnosticians, and highly skilled and innovative technicians will not diminish.[137] The head and neck surgeon will continue to be the patient's strongest and often most effective advocate, through dedication to superior care and commitment to life-long learning.

Acknowledgments. The author gratefully acknowledges the Head and Neck Cancer Team at the University of Chicago including Dan Haraf, MD Everett Vokes, MD, Ezra Cohen, MD, Elizabeth Blair, MD, FACS, Louis Portugal, MD, FACS, Joe Salama, MD, Ellen MacCracken, MS, Allison Decker, RN, Roz Williams, and Eva Thomas, RN.

I am particularly indebted to Maureen Crowley, ANP, for her tireless dedication to our patients and to Larry Gottlieb, MD, FACS for his creativity, inspiration, and devotion to superior patient care.

Nicole Moran has earned special recognition for her exceptional help in preparing this chapter.

REFERENCES

1. Marchetta FC, Sako K, Maxwell W. Complications after radical head and neck surgery performed through previously irradiated tissues. *Am J Surg.* 1967;114:835–838.
2. Joseph D, Shumrick D. Risks of head and neck surgery in previously irradiated patients. *Arch Otolaryngol Head Neck Surg.* 1973;97:381–384.
3. Donald PJ. Complications of combined therapy in head and neck carcinomas. *Arch Otolaryngol Head Neck Surg.* 1978;104:329–332.
4. Marcial VA, Hanley JA, Ydrach A, et al. Tolerance of surgery after radical radiotherapy of carcinoma of the oropharynx. *Cancer.* 1980;46:1910–1912.
5. Corey JP, Caldarelli DD, Hutchinson JC, et al. Surgical complications in patients with head and neck cancer receiving chemotherapy. *Arch Otolaryngol Head Neck Surg.* 1986;112:437–439.
6. Panje WR, Namon AJ, Vokes E, et al. Surgical management of the head and neck cancer patient following concomitant multimodality therapy. *Laryngoscope.* 1995;105:97–101.
7. Sassler AM, Esclamado RM, Wolf GT. Surgery after organ preservation therapy: analysis of wound complications. *Arch Otolaryngol Head Neck Surg.* 1995;121(2):162–165.

8. Lavertu P, Bonafede JP, Adelstein DJ, et al. Comparison of surgical complications after organ-preservation therapy in patients with stage III or IV squamous cell head and neck cancer. *Arch Otolaryngol Head Neck Surg.* 1998;124:401–406.

9. Proctor E, Robbins KT, Vieira F, et al. Postoperative complications after chemoradiation for advanced head and neck cancer. *Head Neck.* 2004;26:272–277.

10. Hom DB, Adams GL, Monyak D. Irradiated soft tissue and its management. *Otolaryngol Clin North Am.* 1995;28(5):1003–1019.

11. Moore MJ. The effect of radiation on connective tissue. *Otolaryngol Clin North Am.* 1984;17(2):389–399.

12. Agra IM, Carvalho AL, Pontes E, et al. Postoperative complications after en bloc salvage surgery for head and neck cancer. *Arch Otolaryngol Head Neck Surg.* 2003;129:1317–1321.

13. Stenson KM, Haraf DJ, Pelzer H, et al. The role of cervical lymphadenectomy after aggressive concomitant chemoradiotherapy. *Arch Otolaryngol Head Neck Surg.* 2000;126:950–956.

14. Hopewell JW, Campling D, Calvo W, et al. Vascular irradiation damage: Its cellular basis and likely consequences. *Br J Cancer.* 1986;53 (suppl VII):181–191.

15. Colevas AD, Read R, Thornhill J, et al. Hypothyroidism incidence after multimodality treatment for stage III and IV squamous cell carcinomas of the head and neck. *Int J Radiat Oncol Biol Phys.* 2001;51(3):599–604.

16. Thorp MA, Levitt NS, Mortimore S, et al. Parathyroid and thyroid function five years after treatment of laryngeal and hypopharyngeal carcinoma. *Clin Otolaryngol.* 1999;24:104–108.

17. Cannon CR. Hypothyroidism in head and neck cancer patients: experimental and clinical observations. *Laryngoscope.* 1994;104(11 pt 2, suppl 66):1–21.

18. Talmi YP, Finkelstein Y, Zohar Y. Pharyngeal fistulas in postoperative hypothyroid patients. *Ann Otol Rhinol Laryngol.* 1989;98(4 pt 1): 267–268.

19. Goerres GW, Schmid DT, Bandhauer F, et al. Positron emission tomography in the early follow-up advanced head and neck cancer. *Arch Otolaryngol Head Neck Surg.* 2004;130:105–109.

20. Bailet JW, Sercarz JA, Abemayor E, et al. The use of positron emission tomography for early detection of recurrent head and neck squamous cell carcinoma in postradiotherapy patients. *Laryngoscope.* 1995;105:135–139.

21. Yao M, Graham MM, Hoffman HT, et al. The role of post-radiation therapy FDG PET in prediction of necessity for post-radiation therapy neck dissection in locally advanced head-and-neck squamous cell carcinoma. *Int J Radiat Oncol Biol Phys.* 2004;59(4):1001–1010.

22. Brkovich VS, Miller FR, Karnad AB, et al. The role of positron emission tomography scans in the management of the N-positive neck in head and neck squamous cell carcinoma after chemoradiotherapy. *Laryngoscope.* 2006;116(6):855–858.

23. McGuirt WF, Greven KM, Williams DW, et al. Laryngeal radionecrosis versus recurrent cancer: a clinical approach. *Ann Otol Rhinol Laryngol.* 1998;107:293–296.

24. Kern EB. The preoperative discussion as a prelude to managing a complication. *Arch Otolaryngol Head Neck Surg.* 2003;129:1163–1165.

25. Valazquez RA, McGruff HS, Sycamore DB, et al. The role of computed tomographic scans in the management of the N-positive neck in head and neck squamous cell carcinoma after chemoradiotherapy. *Arch Otolaryngol Head Neck Surg.* 2004;131(1):74–77.

26. Stenson KM, Dezheng H, Blair E, et al. Planned post-chemoradiation neck dissection: significance of radiation dose. *Laryngoscope.* 2006;116:33–36.

27. Frank DK, Hu KS, Culliney BE, et al. Planned neck dissection after concomitant radiochemotherapy for advanced head and neck cancer. *Laryngoscope.* 2005;115:1015–1020.

28. Moore MG, Bhattacharyya N. Effectiveness of chemotherapy and radiotherapy in sterilizing cervical nodal disease in squamous cell carcinoma of the head and neck. *Laryngoscope.* 2005;115:570–573.

29. McHam SA, Adelstein DJ, Rybicki LA, et al. Who merits a neck dissection after definitive chemoradiotherapy for N2-N3 squamous cell head and neck cancer? *Head Neck.* 2003;25:791–798.

30. Ampil FL, Mills GM, Caldito G, et al. Induction chemotherapy followed by concomitant chemoradiation-induced regression of advanced cervical lymphadenopathy in head and neck cancer as a predictor of outcome. *Otolaryngol Head Neck Surg.* 2002;126:602–606.

31. Strasser MD, Gleich LL, Miller MA, et al. Management implications of evaluating the N2 and N3 neck after organ preservation therapy. *Laryngoscope.* 1999;109:1776–1780.

32. Goguen LA, Posner MR, Tishler RB, et al. Examining the need for neck dissection in the era of

chemoradiation therapy for advanced head and neck cancer. *Arch Otolaryngol Head Neck Surg.* 2006;132:526-531.

33. Pellitteri PK, Ferlito A, Rinaldo A, et al. Planned neck dissection following chemoradiotherapy for advanced head and neck cancer: Is it necessary for all? *Head Neck.* 2006;28:166-175.

34. Corry J, Smith JG, Peters LJ. The concept of a planned neck dissection is obsolete. *Cancer.* 2001;7(6):472-474.

35. Robbins KT, Ferlito A, Suarez C, et al. Is there a role for selective neck dissection after chemoradiation for head and neck cancer? *J Am Coll Surg.* 2004;199(6):913-916.

36. Zbar RI, Funk GF, McCullough TM, et al. Pectoralis major myofascial flap: a valuable tool in contemporary head and neck reconstruction. *Head Neck.* 1997;19:412-418.

37. Goodwin WJ. Salvage surgery for patients with recurrent squamous cell carcinoma of the upper aerodigestive tract: when do the ends justify the means? *Laryngoscope.* 2000;110:1-18.

38. Taussky D, Dulguerov P, Abdelkarim SA. Salvage surgery after radical accelerated radiotherapy with concomitant boost technique for head and neck carcinomas. *Head Neck.* 2005;27:182-186.

39. Urken M, Biller H, Lawson W, et al. Salvage surgery for recurrent neck carcinoma after multimodality therapy. *Head Neck.* 1986;8:332-342.

40. Temam S, Pape E, Janot F, et al. Salvage surgery after failure of very accelerated radiotherapy in advanced head-and-neck squamous cell carcinoma. *Head Neck.* 2005;62(4):1078-1083.

41. Gleich LL, Ryzenman J, Gluckman JL, et al. Recurrent advanced (T3 or T4) head and neck squamous cell carcinoma. *Arch Otolaryngol Head Neck Surg.* 2004;130:35-38.

42. Agra IM, Carvalho AL, Samsonovski F, et al. Prognostic factors in salvage surgery for recurrent oral and oropharyngeal cancer. *Head Neck.* 2006;28:107-113.

43. Machtay M, Rosenthal DI, Chalial AA, et al. Pilot study of postoperative reirradiation, chemotherapy, and amifostine after surgical salvage for recurrent head-and-neck cancer. *Int J Radiat Oncol Biol Phys.* 2004;59(1):72-77.

44. Crevoisier RE, Domenge C, Wibault P, et al. Full dose reirradiation combined with chemotherapy after salvage surgery in head and neck carcinoma. *Cancer.* 2001;91:2071-2076.

45. Salama JK, Vokes EE, Chmura SJ, et al. Long-term outcome of concurrent chemotherapy and reirradiation for recurrent and second primary head-and-neck squamous cell carcinoma. *Head Neck.* 2006;64(2):382-391.

46. Moscoso JF, Urken ML, Dalton J, et al. Simultaneous interstitial radiotherapy with regional or free-flap reconstruction, following salvage surgery of recurrent head and neck carcinoma. *Otolaryngol Head Neck Surg.* 1994;120:965-972.

47. Davidson J, Keane T, Brown D, et al. Surgical salvage after radiotherapy for advanced laryngopharyngeal carcinoma. *Arch Otolaryngol Head Neck Surg.* 1997;123:420-424.

48. Bastian RW, Park AH. Suction drain management of salivary fistulas. *Laryngoscope.* 1995;105(12 pt 1):1337-1341.

49. Sewnaik A, Meeuwis CA, van der Kwast TH, et al. Partial laryngectomy for recurrent glottic carcinoma after radiotherapy. *Head Neck.* 2005;27:101-107.

50. Puxeddu R, Piazza C, Mensi MC, et al. Carbon dioxide laser salvage surgery after radiotherapy failure in T1 and T2 glottic carcinoma. *Otolaryngol Head Neck Surg.* 2004;130:84-88.

51. Quer M, Leon X, Orus C, et al. Endoscopic laser surgery in the treatment of radiation failure of early laryngeal carcinoma. *Head Neck.* 2000;22:520-523.

52. de Gier HH, Knegt PP, de Boer MF, et al. CO_2-laser treatment of recurrent glottic carcinoma. *Head Neck.* 2001;23:177-180.

53. Steiner W, Vogt P, Ambrosch P, et al. Transoral carbon dioxide laser microsurgery for recurrent glottic carcinoma after radiotherapy. *Head Neck.* 2004;26:477-484.

54. Rodriguez-Cuevas S, Labastida S, Gonzalez D, et al. Partial laryngectomy as salvage surgery for radiation failures in T1-T2 laryngeal cancer. *Head Neck.* 1998;20:630-633.

55. Spriano G, Pellini R, Romano G, et al. Supracricoid partial laryngectomy as salvage surgery after radiation failure. *Head Neck.* 2002;24:759-765.

56. McLaughlin MP, Parsons JT, Fein DA, et al. Salvage surgery after radiotherapy failure in T1-T2 squamous cell carcinoma of the glottic larynx. *Head Neck.* 1996;18:229-235.

57. Ganly I, Patel SG, Matsuo J, et al. Results of surgical salvage after failure of definitive radiation therapy for early-stage squamous cell carcinoma of the glottic larynx. *Arch Otolaryngol Head Neck Surg.* 2006;132:59-66.

58. DelGaudio JM, Fleming DJ, Esclamado RM, et al. Hemilaryngectomy for glottic carcinoma after

radiation therapy failure. *Arch Otolaryngol Head Neck Surg.* 1994;120:959-963.

59. Shaw HJ. Role of partial laryngectomy after irradiation in the treatment of laryngeal cancer: a view from the United Kingdom. *Ann Otol Rhinol Laryngol.* 1991;100:268-273.

60. Beckhardt RN, Murray JG, Ford CH, et al. Factors influencing functional outcome in supraglottic laryngectomy. *Head Neck.* 1994;16:232-239.

61. Hartig G, Truelson J, Weinstein G. Supraglottic cancer. *Head Neck.* 2000;22:426-434.

62. Weber RS, Berkey BA, Forastiere A, et al. Outcome of salvage total laryngectomy following organ preservation therapy: the radiation therapy oncology group trial 91-11. *Arch Otolaryngol Head Neck Surg.* 2003;129(1):44-49.

63. Parsons JT, Mendenhall WM, Stringer SP, et al. Salvage surgery following radiation failure in squamous cell carcinoma of the supraglottic larynx. *Int J Radiat Oncol Biol Phys.* 1995;32(3):605-609.

64. Leon X, Quer M, Orus C, et al. Results of salvage surgery for local or regional recurrence after larynx preservation with induction chemotherapy and radiotherapy. *Head Neck.* 2001;23:733-738.

65. Mercante G, Bacciu A, Banchini L, et al. Salvage surgery after radiation failure in squamous cell carcinoma of the larynx. *B-ENT.* 2005;1:107-111.

66. Teknos TN, Myers LL, Bradford CR, et al. Free tissue reconstruction of the hypopharynx after organ preservation therapy: analysis of wound complications. *Laryngoscope.* 2001;111:1192-1196.

67. Cherian T, Sebastian P, Ahamed MI, et al. Evaluation of salvage surgery in heavily irradiated cancer of the buccal mucosa. *Cancer.* 1991;68:295-299.

68. Gehanno P, Depondt J, Guedon C, et al. Primary and salvage surgery for cancer of the tonsillar region: a retrospective study of 120 patients. *Head Neck.* 1993;15:185-189.

69. Stoeckli SJ, Pawlik AB, Lipp M, et al. Salvage surgery after failure of nonsurgical therapy for carcinoma of the larynx and hypopharynx. *Arch Otolaryngol Head Neck Surg.* 2000;126:1473-1477.

70. Pacheco-Ojeda L, Marandas P, Julieron M, et al. Salvage surgery by composite resection for epidermoid carcinoma of the tonsillar region. *Arch Otolaryngol Head Neck Surg.* 1992;118:181-184.

71. Lin YC, Hsiao JR, Tsai ST. Salvage surgery as the primary treatment for recurrent oral squamous cell carcinoma. *Oral Oncol.* 2004;40:183-189.

72. Yom SS, Machtay M, Biel MA, et al. Survival impact of planned restaging and early surgical salvage following definitive chemoradiation for locally advanced squamous cell carcinomas of the oropharynx and hypopharynx. *Am J Clin Oncol.* 2005;28(4):385-392.

73. Chepeha DB, Annich G, Pynnonen M, et al. Pectoralis major myocutaneous flap vs revascularized free tissue transfer: complications, gastrostomy tube dependence, and hospitalization. *Arch Otolaryngol Head Neck Surg.* 2004;130(2):181-186.

74. Aitasalo K, Relander M, Virolainen E. Microvascular free tissue transfers after preoperative irradiation in head and neck reconstructions. *Acta Otolaryngol.* 1997; suppl 529: 247-250.

75. Hayden RE, Deschler DG. Lateral thigh free flap for head and neck reconstruction. *Laryngoscope.* 1999;109:1490-1494.

76. Disa JJ, Pusic AL, Hidalgo DA, et al. Microvascular reconstruction of the hypopharynx: defect classification, treatment algorithm, and functional outcome based on 165 consecutive cases. *Plast Reconstr Surg.* 2003;111:652-660.

77. Lewin JS, Barringer DA, May AH, et al. Functional outcomes after circumferential pharyngoesophageal reconstruction. *Laryngoscope.* 2005;115(7):1266-1271.

78. Lewin JA, Barringer DA, May AH, et al. Functional outcomes after laryngopharyngectomy with anterolateral thigh flap reconstruction. *Head Neck.* 2006;28(2):142-149.

79. Genden EM, Jacobson AS. The role of the anterolateral thigh flap for pharyngoesophageal reconstruction. *Arch Otolaryngol Head Neck Surg.* 2005;131(9):796-799.

80. Agarwal JP, Stenson KM, Gottlieb LJ. A simplified design of a dual insland fasciocutaneous free flap for simultaneous pharyngoesophageal and anterior neck reconstruction. *J Reconstr Microsurg.* 2006;22(2):105-112.

81. Taylor SM, Haughey BH. Combined pharyngoesophageal and cervical skin reconstruction using a single radial forearm flap. *Laryngoscope.* 2002;112:1315-1318.

82. Dolan R, Gooey J, Youngman JC, et al. Microvascular access in the multiply operated neck: thoracodorsal transposition. *Laryngoscope.* 1996;106:1436-1437.

83. Harris JR, Leug E, Genden E, et al. The thoracoacromial/cephalic vascular system for microvascular anastomoses in the vessel-depleted neck.

Arch Otolaryngol Head Neck Surg. 2002;128(3): 319-323.

84. Yu P. The transverse cervical vessels as recipient vessels for previously treated head and neck cancer patients. *Plast Reconstr Surg.* 2005;115: 1253-1258.

85. Chang KP, Hao SP, Tsang NM, et al. Salvage surgery for locally recurrent nasopharyngeal carcinoma-a 10-year experience. *Otolaryngol Head Neck Surg.* 2004;131:497-502.

86. Shu CH, Cheng H, Lirng JF, et al. Salvage surgery for recurrent nasopharyngeal carcinoma. *Laryngoscope.* 2000;110:1483-1488.

87. Hsu MM, Hong RL, Ting LL, et al. Factors affecting the overall survival after salvage surgery in patients with recurrent nasopharyngeal carcinoma at the primary site. *Arch Otolaryngol Head Neck Surg.* 2001;127:798-802.

88. Hao SP, Tsang NM, Chang CH. Salvage surgery for recurrent nasopharyngeal carcinoma. *Arch Otolaryngol Head Neck Surg.* 2002;128:63-67.

89. Biyani M, Stenson KM. *Cervical-parotid approach with transhyoid pharyngotomy: improved access to the nasopharynx and skull base* (Unpublished abstract). 2006.

90. Jorgensen K, Godballe C, Hansen O, Bastholt L. Cancer of the larynx: treatment results after primary radiotherapy with salvage surgery. *Acta Oncol.* 2002;41:69-76.

91. Clark J, Gilbert R, Irish J, et al. Morbidity after flap reconstruction of hypopharyngeal defects. *Laryngoscope.* 2006;166:173-181.

92. Price JC, Ridley MB. Hypocalcemia following pharyngoesophageal ablation and gastric pull-up reconstruction: pathophysiology and management. *Ann Otol Rhinol Laryngol.* 1988;97:521-526.

93. Annino DJ, Goguen LA. Mitomycin C for the treatment of pharyngoesophageal stricture after total laryngopharyngectomy and microvascular reconstruction. *Laryngoscope.* 2003;133:1499-1502.

94. Temam S, Koka V, Mamelle G, et al. treatment of the N0 neck during salvage surgery after radiotherapy of head and neck squamous cell carcinoma. *Head Neck.* 2005;27:653-658.

95. Farrag TY, Lin FR, Cummings CW, et al. Neck management in patients undergoing postradiotherapy salvage laryngeal surgery for recurrent/persistent laryngeal cancer. *Laryngoscope.* 2006;116: 1864-1866.

96. Wax MK, Touma J. Management of the N0 neck during salvage laryngectomy. *Laryngoscope.* 1999;109:4-7.

97. Yoo GH, Hocwald E, Korkmaz H, et al. Assessment of carotid artery invasion in patients with head and neck cancer. *Laryngoscope.* 2000;100: 386-390.

98. Freeman SB, Hamaker RC, Borrowdale RB, Huntly TC. Management of neck metastasis with carotid artery involvement. *Laryngoscope.* 2004;114:20-24.

99. Warren FM, Cohen JI, Nesbit GM, et al. Management of carotid blowout with endovascular stent grafts. *Laryngoscope.* 2002;112:428-433.

100. Levy EI, Horowitz MB, Koebbe C, Jungreis CC. Target-specific multimodality endovascular management of carotid artery blowout syndrome. *Ear Nose Throat.* 2002;81:115-118.

101. Desuter G, hammer F, Gardiner Q, et al. Carotid stenting for impending carotid blowout: suitable supportive care for head and neck cancer patients? *Palliative Med.* 2005;19:427-429.

102. Cohen J, Rad I. Contemporary management of carotid blowout. *Curr Opin Otolaryngol Head Neck Surg.* 2004;12:110-115.

103. Adams GL, Madison M, Remley K, Gapany M. Preoperative permanent balloon occlusion of internal carotid artery in patients with advanced head and neck squamous cell carcinoma. *Laryngoscope.* 1999;109:460-466.

104. Muzaffar K, Collins S, Labropoulos N, Baker WH. A prospective study of the effects of irradiation on the carotid artery. *Laryngoscope.* 2000;110: 1811-1814.

105. Hayes JC, Machtay M, Weber R, et al. Relative risk of stroke in head and neck carcinoma patients with external cervical radiation. *Laryngoscope.* 2002;112:1883-1887.

106. Katsuno S, Takemae T, Ishiyama T, Usami SI. Is carotid reconstruction for advanced cancer in the neck a safe procedure? *Otolaryngol Head Neck Surg.* 2001;124:222-224.

107. Mizra N, Gahtan V, Weber RS. Management of patients after elective carotid artery resection. *Am J Otolaryngol.* 1999;20:37-42.

108. Jacobs JR, Korkmaz H, Marks SC. One stage carotid artery resection: reconstruction in radiated head and neck carcinoma. *Am J Otolaryngol.* 2001;22:167-171.

109. Aslan I, Hafiz G, Baserer N, et al. management of carotid artery invasion in advanced malignancies

of the head and neck. *Ann Otol Rhinol Laryngol.* 2002;111:772-777.

110. Sessa CN, Morasch MD, Berguer R, et al. Carotid resection and replacement with autogenous arterial graft during operation for head and neck malignancy. *Ann Vasc Surg.* 1998;12:229-235.

111. Nussbaum ES, Levine SC, Hamlar D, Madison MT. Carotid stenting and exarterectomy in the management of head and neck cancer involving the internal carotid artery: technical case report. *Neurosurgery.* 2000;47:981-984.

112. Numata T, Konno A, Takeuch Y, et al. Contralateral external carotid-middle cerebral artery bypass for carotid artery resection. *Laryngoscope.* 1997; 107:665-667.

113. Chazono H, Okamoto Y, Matsizaki Z, et al. Extracranial-intracranial bypass for reconstruction of internal carotid artery in the management of head and neck cancer. *Ann Vasc Surg.* 2003; 17:260-265.

114. Okamoto Y, Inugami A, Matsuzaki Z, et al. Carotid resection for head and neck cancer. *Surgery.* 1996;120:54-59.

115. Futran ND, Trotti A, Gwede C. Pentoxifylline in the treatment of radiation-related soft tissue injury: preliminary observations. *Laryngoscope.* 1997;107:391-395.

116. Atgenc E, Celikkanat S, Kaymakci M, et al. Prophylactic effect of pentoxifylline on radiotherapy complications: a clinical study. *Otolaryngol Head Neck Surg.* 2004;130:351-356.

117. Delanian S, Depondt J, Lefaix JL. Major healing of refractory mandible osteoradionecrosis after treatment combing pentoxifylline and tocopherol: a phase II trial. *Head Neck.* 2005;27:114-123.

118. Okunieff P, Augustine E, Hicks J. Pentoxifylline in the treatment of radiation-induced fibrosis. *J Clin Oncol.* 2004;22:2207-2213.

119. Marx RE. Osteoradionecrosis: A new concept of its pathophysiology. *J Oral Maxillofac Surg.* 1983;41:283-288.

120. Marx RE, Ames JR. The use of hyperbaric oxygen therapy in bony reconstruction of the irradiated and tissue-deficient patient. *J Oral Maxillofac Surg.* 1982;40:412-420.

121. Hao SP, Chen HC, Wei FC, et al. Systematic management of osteoradionecrosis in the head and neck. *Laryngoscope.* 1999;109:1324-1328.

122. Notani KI, Yamzaki Y, Kitada H, et al. Management of mandibular osteoradionecrosis corresponding to the severity of osteoradionecrosis and the method of radiotherapy. *Head Neck.* 2003;25:181-186.

123. Narozny W, Sicko Z, Kot J, et al. Hyperbaric oxygen therapy in the treatment of complications of irradiation in head and neck area. *Undersea Hyperb Med.* 2005;32:103-110.

124. Peleg M, Lopez EA. The treatment of osteoradionecrosis of the mandible: the case for hyperbaric oxygen and bone graft reconstruction. *J Oral Maxillofac Surg.* 2006;64:956-960.

125. Annane D, Depondt J, Aubert P, et al. Hyperbaric oxygen therapy for radionecrosis of the jaw: a randomized, placebo-controlled, double-blind trial from the ORN96 study group. *J Clin Oncol.* 2004;22:4893-4900.

126. Gal TJ, Yueh B, Futran ND. Influence of prior hyperbaric oxygen therapy in complications following microvascular reconstruction for advanced osteoradionecrosis. *Arch Otolaryngol Head Neck Surg.* 2003;129:72-76.

127. Buchbinder D, Hilaire H. The use of free tissue transfer in advanced osteoradionecrosis of the mandible. *J Oral Maxillofac Surg.* 2006;64: 961-964.

128. Militsakh O, Wallace DI, Kriet JD, et al. The role of osteocutaneous radial forearm free flap in the treatment of mandibular osteoradionecrosis. *Otolaryngol Head Neck Surg.* 2005;133:80-83.

129. Coskunfirat OK, Wei FC, Huang WC, et al. Microvascular free tissue transfer for treatment of osteoradionecrosis of the maxilla. *Plast Reconstr Surg.* 2005;115:54-60.

130. Hunag XM, Zheng YQ, Zhang XM, et al. Diagnosis and management of skull base osteoradionecrosis after radiotherapy for nasopharyngeal carcinoma. *Laryngoscope.* 2006;116:1626-1631.

131. Chang KP, Tsang NM, Chen CY, et al. Endoscopic management of skull base osteoradionecrosis. *Laryngoscope.* 2000;110:1162-1165.

132. Ng RLH, Beahm E, Clayman GL, et al. Simultaneous reconstruction of the posterior pharyngeal wall and cervical spine with a free vascularized fibula osteocutaneous flap. *Plast Reconstr Surg.* 2002;109:1361-1365.

133. Donovan DJ, Huynh TV, Purdom EB, et al. Osteoradionecrosis of the cervical spine resulting from radiotherapy for primary head and neck malignancies: operative and non-operative management. *J Neurosurg: Spine.* 2005;3:159-164.

134. Lew RJ, Shah JN, Chalian A, et al. Technique of endoscopic retrograde puncture and dilation of

total esophageal stenosis in patients with radiation-induced strictures. *Head Neck*. 2004;26: 179-183.

135. Sullivan CA, Jaklitsch MT, Haddad R, et al. Endoscopic management of hypopharyngeal stenosis aftyer organ sparing therapy for head and neck cancer. *Laryngoscope*. 2004;114:1924-1931.

136. Lazarus C, Logeman JA, Shi G, et al. Does laryngectomy improve swallowing after chemoradiotherapy? *Arch Otolaryngol Head Neck Surg*. 2002;128:54-57.

137. Ridge JA. Head and neck surgeons still get to operate. *Am Soc Clin Oncol Proc/Abstr Book*. 2003;322-327.

27

Prosthetic and Implant Reconstruction of Treatment-Related Defects in the Head and Neck

John Beumer, III
Eleni D. Roumanas

Treatment of oral and facial cancers can result in severe oral dysfunction and facial disfigurement but today it is possible to restore many patients to near-normal form and function enabling them to continue to have useful and productive lives. In the late 1980s several technical improvements were made—for example, the development of osseointegrated dental implants and free vascularized flaps—but in recent times the most significant improvements have been the result of improved collaborations between medical and dental clinicians. In the leading cancer centers of the world, prosthodontists examine patients prior to their cancer treatment and work with their colleagues in surgical oncology, reconstructive surgery, and/or radiation oncology to minimize posttreatment morbidities and to develop plans to rehabilitate the patient. Our colleagues in surgery and radiation therapy have begun to realize that minor alterations in their surgical procedures or slight changes in the radiation fields or methods of radiation delivery can have a significant impact on the eventual posttreatment oral function and appearance of the patient. Presently, with a proper multidisciplinary approach to patient care, almost all patients, treated with surgical resection and/or radiation for oral or facial cancer can be very effectively rehabilitated, retaining their ability to speak, swallow, masticate, and control their saliva, enabling them to interact socially with family and friends.

An exception are those patients presenting with severe scarring, shrinkage, and immbolization of oral tissues secondary to chemoradiation. Substantial numbers of patients treated with chemoradiation are unable to swallow, and exhibit velopharyngeal incompetence and insufficiency. Severe post-therapy trismus makes maintenance of the dentitition and supporting periodontium extremely difficult if not impossible in many patients (Fig 27-1). To date, solutions have yet to be found for these very significant morbidities.

Head and neck cancer patients who require maxillofacial rehabilitation may be arbitrarily classified according to their post-treatment surgical defects and morbidity, which include maxillary, tongue-mandibular, and facial defects and the side effects of radiation treatments. This chapter concentrates primarily on the restoration of defects secondary to surgical ablation of head and neck tumors.

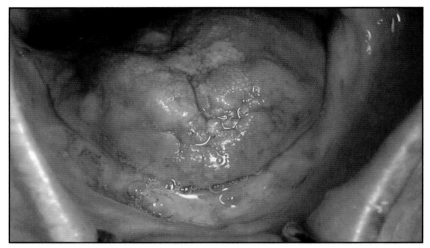

A

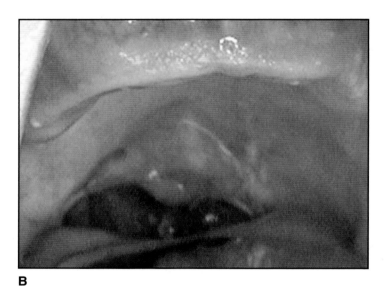

B

Fig 27–1. Tissue effects secondary to chemoradiation. **A.** Shrinkage and immobilization of the tongue compromise speech, swallowing, and mastication **B.** Shrinkage, scarring of velopharyngeal complex. Neither of these deficits is restorable with prosthodontic methods.

MAXILLARY DEFECTS

Disabilities

Most tumors of the paranasal sinus, palatal epithelium, or minor salivary glands require either a partial or radical maxillectomy. Defects of the hard or soft palate produce a variety of problems: hypernasality makes speech unintelligible; mastication efficiency is compromised, particularly for the edentulous patient; because teeth and denture-bearing tissue surfaces are lost and support, stability and retention of the maxillary prosthesis is compromised; swallowing is awkward, as food and liquids may be forced up into the nasal cavity and out the nose in an unrestored patient; nasal and sinus secretions collect in the defect area; and facial disfigurement can result from lack of midface bony support or resection of a branch of the facial nerve. In some cases, tumor invasion superiorly requires exenteration of the orbital contents.

Rehabilitation after resection of the hard or soft palate is best accomplished prosthodontically. Customarily, a temporary prosthesis, known as an immediate surgical obturator, is placed at the time of surgery. During the healing period, this prosthesis is relined periodically with temporary denture reliners to compensate for tissue changes secondary to organization and contracture of the tissues adjacent to the defect. When these tissues become well healed and dimensionally stable (usually 3 to 4 months after surgery), the definitive prosthesis is made.

Inadequate retention, stability, and support for the obturator prosthesis are the main problems associated with the use of an obturator prosthesis. The remaining teeth, therefore, become extremely valuable in providing support, retention, and stability for these restorations. The purpose of these prostheses is to restore the physical separation between the oral and nasal cavities, thereby restoring speech and swallowing to normal, and to provide support for the lip and cheek.

Prosthodontic Treatment

It is essential that the prosthodontist examine and consult with the patient before surgery. The sequence of treatment should be explained to the patient, and diagnostic casts and appropriate radiographs should be obtained. With this information, the prosthodontist is ready to consult with the surgeon about the design and fabrication of the surgical obturator. The surgeon can improve the prosthetic prognosis by considering the following modifications[1]:

1. A split-thickness skin graft should be used to line the raw cheek surface of the defect. The skin graft limits contracture of the cheek flap, provides a keratinized surface to support and stabilize the prosthesis, and forms a scar band at the junction of the skin graft and oral mucosa that can be engaged prosthodontically to improve

retention, stability, and support for the future obturator prosthesis (Fig 27–2).
2. If the surgeon can save some of the palatal mucosa normally included in the palatal resection and reflect this tissue during the bony resection of the palate, it can later be used to cover the medial cut margin of the palatal bone. If this palatal margin of the defect is covered with keratinized mucosa, the prosthesis may engage this surface more completely, thus improving its stability (resistance to lateral displacement during function).
3. An attempt should be made to save as much of the maxilla as possible, consistent with tumor control. The more the palatal-shelf area that remains, the more support (resistance to the vertical forces generated during mastication) will be provided for an obturator prosthesis. Retaining the premaxillary segment is particularly advantageous.
4. The transalveolar bony resection should be made as far from the tooth adjacent to the proposed defect as feasible. This practice leaves more bone around this tooth, improving its prognosis as a partial denture abutment.
5. If the soft palate does not retain the ability to effect velopharyngeal closure, it should be resected on the side of the tumor. If a posterior, nonfunctioning band of soft palate remains after surgery, it often prevents proper placement of the palatopharyngeal extension of the obturator prosthesis, compromising speech and swallowing (Fig 27–3).
6. In edentulous patients, the placement of osseointegrated implants into appropriate maxillary sites should be considered for patients not scheduled for postoperative radiation. These implants can be used later to facilitate the retention and stability of, and support for, the future obturator prosthesis (Fig 27–4).

Immediate Surgical Obturators

Immediate or early restoration of a palatal defect with an obturator will greatly ease and simplify the patient's postoperative course. The obturator provides a matrix upon which the surgical packing can

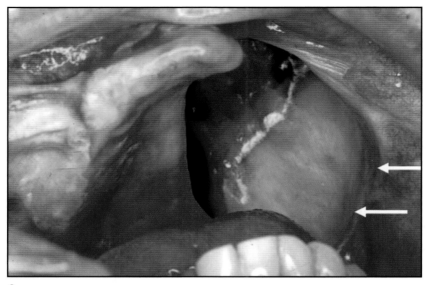

A

B

Fig 27–2. A split-thickness skin graft lining lateral wall of radical maxillectomy defect greatly enhances effectiveness of prosthetic rehabilitation. Note undercuts superior to the skin graft mucosal junction

be placed, minimizes contamination of the wound in the immediate postoperative period, and enables the patient to speak and swallow effectively immediately after surgery.

In order to fabricate the prosthesis, an irreversible hydrocolloid impression is obtained of the maxillary arch and the anterior portion of the soft palate, and the cast is retrieved. The obturator's size is determined by the surgical boundaries of the resection, as indicated by the surgeon. In the dentulous patient, teeth in the path of the surgical resection are removed from the cast (Fig 27–5). Care should be taken to extend the surgical obturator posteriorly past the proposed posterior soft palatal resection line to effectively seal off the defect. These prostheses are processed in autopolymerizing methyl

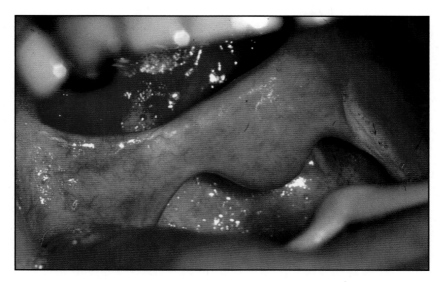

Fig 27–3. This nonfunctional posterior band of soft palate prevents optimal positioning of a pharyngeal obturator extension.

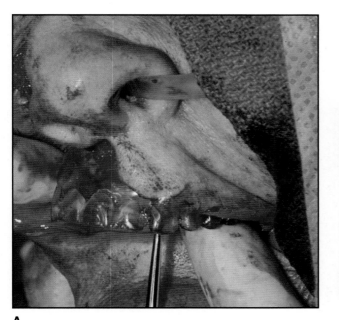

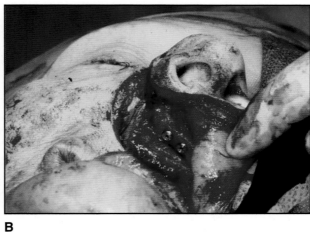

A

B

Fig 27–4. A and **B**. Implants are being placed immediately following completion of the maxillectomy.

methacrylate. They can be altered at surgery by trimming or by adding a temporary denture reliner. The prosthesis is wired to remaining teeth, alveolar ridge, or other available structures (eg, zygomatic arch, anterior nasal spine) or secured with lag screws (Fig 27-6).

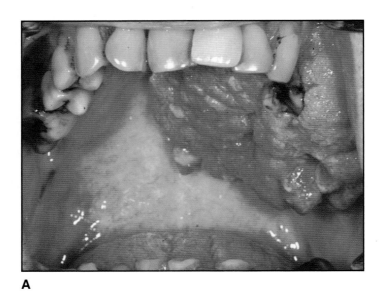

A

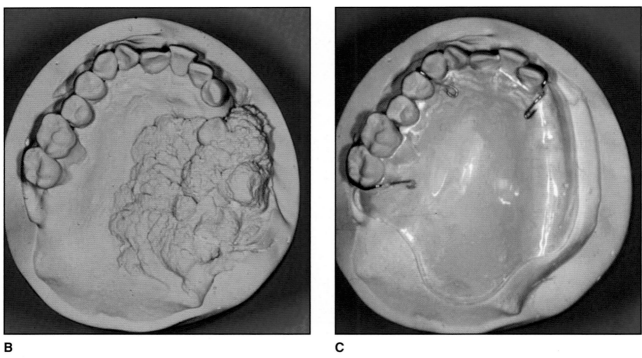

B   C

Fig 27–5. A and **B**. Tumor distorted palatal contours. **C**. After the cast is altered to remove teeth and restore palatal contours in the path of the resection, the immediate surgical obturator is completed on the cast.

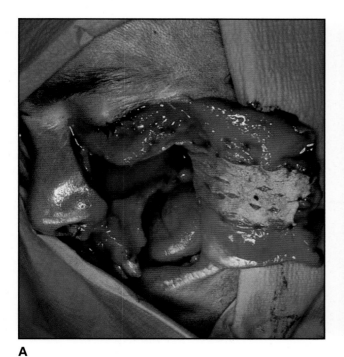

A

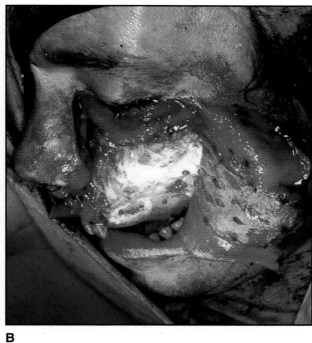

B

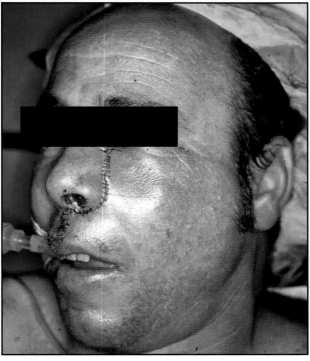

C

Fig 27–6. **A**. Radical maxillectomy defect. Note an external skin incision was used for surgical exposure. **B**. Prosthesis serves as a platform for placement of surgical packing. **C**. When wound is closed, facial contours are nearly normal.

After the surgical packing is removed (6 to 10 days after surgery), the prosthesis is relined with a temporary denture reliner. As healing progresses, the obturator is periodically relined and extended further into the defect, adaptation is improved, and anterior teeth are added as necessary. It is often desirable to add teeth to the prosthesis and reline it with autopolymerizing acrylic during this transitional stage (Fig 27–7). Three to 5 months after surgery, and after initial wound contracture is essentially complete, the definitive prosthesis is begun. Edentu-lous patients with maxillary defects often require a longer period of healing because the defect must be engaged more aggressively to maximize stability, support, and retention for the obturator prosthesis.

Definitive Obturator Prosthesis

Defects of the hard palate are restored most effectively with a prosthesis. Teeth greatly improve the retention and stability of the obturator prosthesis.

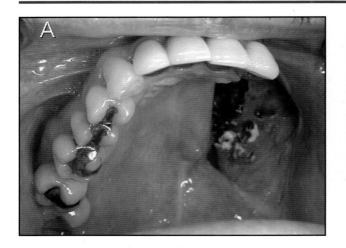
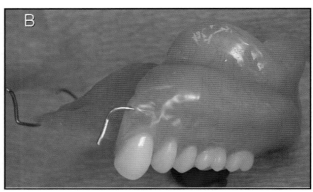
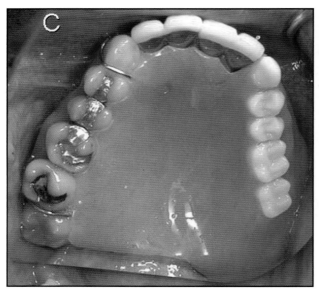
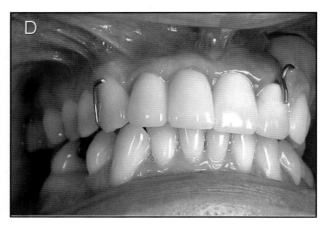

Fig 27–7. Interim obturator. Teeth have been added and the prosthesis relined with autopolymerizing acrylic resin. **A**. Partial maxillectomy defect 4-weeks post surgery. **B**. Interim obturator. **C** and **D**. Prosthesis in position.

Speech, swallowing, mastication, and facial contour can be restored with proper extensions and obturation. The obturator should extend maximally up the lateral wall of the defect (Fig 27–8). This high lateral extension increases retention and stability and helps recontour the lip and cheek. The movement of the medial side of the ramus into the distolateral area of the defect must be accounted for during impression procedures. The extension superiorly along the medial margin of the defect should not exceed the level of the repositioned palatal mucosa. Further superior extension will impede normal nasal airflow during speech and breathing and may result in unnecessary and painful ulceration of the respiratory mucosa lining the nasal septum. In some patients, extension across the nasal surface of the soft palate or into the nasal aperture may be necessary to provide acceptable retention.

Partial denture designs retaining the obturator prosthesis are complicated by: (1) multiple axis of rotation during function; (2) compromised support on the defect side; (3) lack of cross-arch stabilization because of the loss of dentition on the resected side; (4) extended length of the lever arms associated with the obturator prosthesis; and (5) the forces of gravity.

Teeth adjacent to the defect are subject to greater vertical and lateral forces and are more frequently lost than teeth in other positions because the defect offers little support and the long lever arms associated with the obturator prosthesis magnify the forces delivered to these teeth. If these abutment teeth are to be preserved, it is important they have positive rests so that occlusal forces can be directed along their long axis. If incisors are adjacent to the defect it is desirable to fit these teeth with porcelain fused to metal restorations with cingulum rests and to splint them together[2] (Fig 27–9).

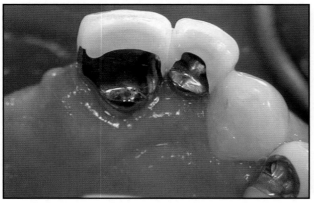

Fig 27–8. A diagrammatic frontal section of a radical maxillectomy with obturator prosthesis in position. Minimal medial extension enables normal airflow. Maximum lateral extension facilitates retention, stability, and support for the obturator prosthesis.

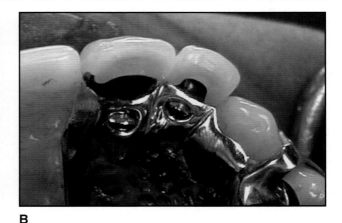

A   **B**

Fig 27–9. Abutments adjacent to defect are subject to more vertical and lateral forces and are more frequently lost than abutments in other positions. These incisors have been splinted with crowns and provided with cingulum rests.

The placement of osseointegrated implants dramatically improves function of the obturator prosthesis, particularly for edentulous patients.[3] The most desirable locations are the premaxillary segment and the maxillary tuberosity. The design concepts of tissue bars that are secured to the implants have much in common with the design concepts used for conventional edentulous patients. Implants are splinted together and the bar should be designed to direct occlusal loads along the long axis of the implants (Fig 27-10). Patients are advised to masticate on the unresected side. Forceful occlusion on the defect side will result in rapid wear of the attachments securing the obturator prosthesis to the tissue bar and may also result in bone loss around the implants, particularly the implant adjacent to the defect. When the prosthesis is completed (Fig 27-11), speech and swallowing are restored to normal limits. Most prostheses require relining within the first year because of slow but continuous changes of the tissues on the periphery of the surgical defect.

Surgical Reconstruction of Palatal Defects

It is possible to obturate hard and soft palate defects with free vascularized flaps. However, in almost all situations surgical reconstruction of such defects is

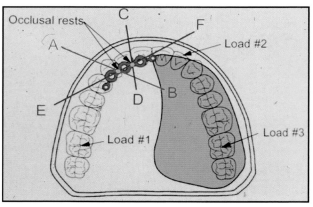

A

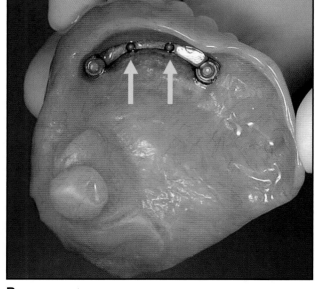

B

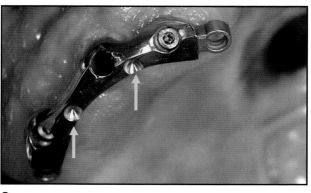

C

Fig 27–10. **A**. A diagrammatic representation of a patient in whom 3 implants have been placed in premaxilla. Resilient attachments have been connected to both ends of tissue bar. Note presence and location of occlusal rests, which control the axis of rotation when occlusal forces are delivered. **B** and **C**. A completed tissue bar and prosthesis. Note occlusal rests. These rests control axis of rotation and direct occlusal forces along long axis of implants.

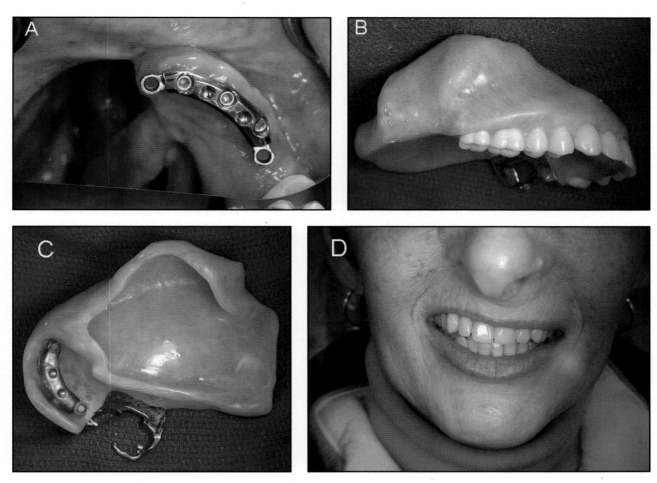

Fig 27–11. A. Maxillectomy defect with implant secured tissue bar. **B** and **C**. Obturator prosthesis. Note pharyngeal extension. **D**. Prosthesis inserted. Oral functions and esthetics are restored.

undesirable and actually impairs oral function. Restoration of unilateral defects of the hard palate with vascularized flaps is contraindicated in almost all instances. These flaps distort the palatal contours and compromise the tongue space (Fig 27-12). Bulky flaps preclude replacement of missing dentition in many patients and lack of tongue space further compromises speech articulation. In addition, secretions accumulate on the sinus side of the flaps, these secretions become crusted, and are subsequently colonized by microorganisms. These mucous crusts become odiferous and also cause local infections. Total palatal defects are the exception to this rule, however, and are best restored with a combination of surgical and prosthetic reconstruction. The fibula is preferred and subsequently implants

are placed and an implant-retained prosthesis is fabricated.

Definitive Soft Palate Prosthesis

Defects of the soft palate and velopharyngeal complex require different and more complex prosthetic treatment. Velopharyngeal closure normally occurs when the soft palate elevates and contacts the contracting lateral and posterior pharyngeal walls of the nasopharynx. The levator palati muscle is responsible for palate elevation and most lateral wall movement. When a portion of the soft palate or lateral pharyngeal wall is excised or when the soft palate is perforated, scarred, or neurologically impaired,

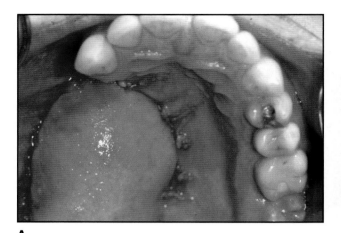
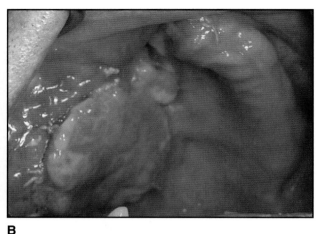

A   B

Fig 27–12. Flaps should not be used to reconstruct large unilateral defects such as these.

effective velopharyngeal closure cannot occur. Speech becomes hypernasal, and normal swallowing is not possible. With a properly extended and contoured pharyngeal obturator, the patient will be able to re-establish velopharyngeal closure if a residual portion of the velopharyngeal mechanism still exhibits some functional movement. The obturator must not interfere with breathing, impinge upon soft tissues during postural movements, or hamper the tongue during swallowing and speech.

In soft palate resections, if less than 30% to 40% of the soft palate is removed the defect can be successfully reconstructed with a free vascularized flap (Fig 27-13). However, if more is resected, the residual portion of the soft palate should be allowed to hang free and the defect obturated with a prosthesis. If the residual soft palate is tethered to the flap, the flap immobilizes the residual soft palate musculature and in most instances these types of defects are impossible to restore with an obturator prosthesis. The outcome will be hypernasal speech and leakage of bolus into the nasal cavities during swallowing (Fig 27-14).

The soft palate obturator remains in a fixed position in the nasopharynx and does not attempt to duplicate normal movements of the soft palate. The inferior surface of the obturator should be level with the hard palate contour, which in most patients is approximately the level of the anterior tubercle of the atlas. The inferior margin of the posterior surface of the obturator contacts Passavant's pad, if present, and extends approximately 10 mm superiorly into the nasopharynx. During breathing and the production of nasal speech sounds, the space around the obturator reflects the potential for muscular contraction. During swallowing and the production of other speech sounds, this sphincteric muscular network moves into contact with the stationary acrylic resin obturator, establishing velopharyngeal closure (Fig 27-15). A correctly constructed obturator will result in the return of normal speech and swallowing.

TONGUE-MANDIBLE DEFECTS

Disabilities

Disabilities resulting from tongue-mandibular resections include impaired speech articulation, difficulty swallowing, deviation of the mandible during functional movements, poor control of salivary secretions, and often cosmetic disfigurement. If the surgical wound is closed primarily (primary closure), the functional disabilities are compounded. Advanced tumors of the oral tongue and floor of the mouth often require extensive resection of soft tissue and adjacent mandible. The loss of large portions of the tongue prevents appropriate "valving" and/or inter-

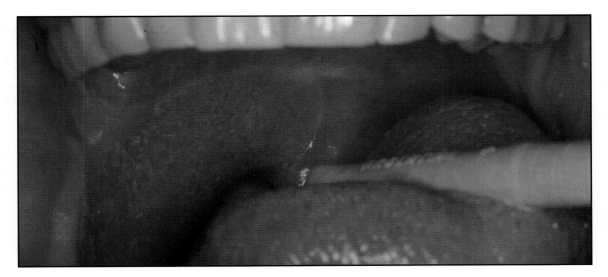

Fig 27–13. Tonsil-soft palate defect restored with a radial forearm flap. Sufficient mass of levator palati muscle remains to elevate the soft palate on the unresected side. Velopharyngeal closure is maintained.

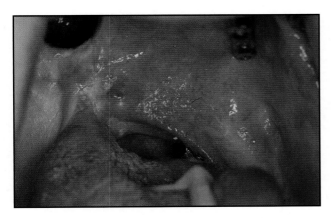

Fig 27–14. Following resection and reconstruction of this retromolar trigone lesion with a radial forearm flap, the soft palate was tethered to the flap. The result was velopharyngeal dysfunction and hypernasal speech.

action with other oral structures. This loss of bulk and mobility combined with the loss of motor and sensory innervation leads to misarticulation of most speech sounds. Deglutition is less impaired, and most patients learn to swallow fairly efficiently. Resections of the tongue and mandible also obliterate portions of the lingual and buccal sulci so that a means of collecting and channeling secretions pos-

teriorly no longer exists. In addition, the motor and sensory innervation of the lower lip on the resected side is often lost, further impairing speech, mastication, control of saliva, and dentures.

Tongue function is less affected if the resected portion is restored with free vascularized flaps. The myocutaneous flaps used in the 1980s restore bulk, prevent deviation of the mandible, and permit the reconstructed tongue to articulate more effectively with the palatal structures. However, myocutaneous flaps become scarred and immobile and limit the mobility of the reconstructed tongue. In contrast, tongues reconstructed with vascularized free flaps have the potential of supporting near-normal speech because they are less likely to become heavily scarred and immobile. Those with significant loss of soft tissue whose wounds are closed primarily suffer the greatest deviation.

If much of the mandible is removed and not reconstructed, the remaining functional mandibular segment will be retruded and deviated toward the surgical side. When the jaw is opened this deviation increases. These factors, combined with impaired tongue function, prevent effective mastication. The severity and permanence of mandibular deviation varies. However, some patients can attain reasonable occlusal relationships although some frontal

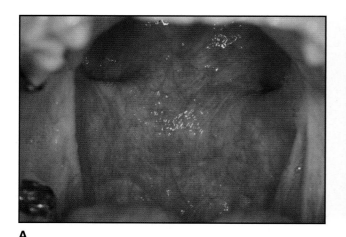

A

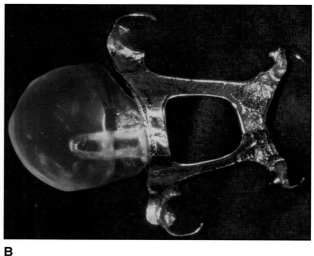

B

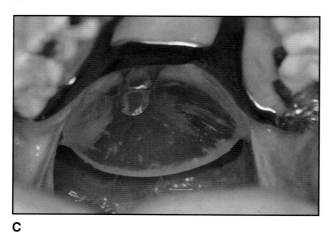

C

Fig 27–15. A. Soft palate defect after resection of an adenoidcystic carcinoma. **B.** Pharyngeal obturator extension attached to partial denture framework. **C.** Obturator in position. Note space around obturator. This space permits normal nasal breathing and production of nasal speech sounds. When muscles around obturator contract and closure is complete, swallowing and speech are restored without leakage of bolus or air into nasal cavity.

plane rotation will be observed (Fig 27–16). Therefore, it is highly desirable to reconstruct the mandible at the time of tumor ablation with a free vascularized flap.

When removal of tumors in the anterior floor of the mouth requires that the mandible be resected anteriorly, and when mandibular continuity is not restored, the two remaining posterior fragments are pulled medially by the residual mylohyoid muscles and superiorly by the muscles of mastication. Severe disfigurement and dysfunction result. Free flaps from the fibula can be used immediately to restore the lost hard and soft tissues, and most patients emerge with excellent function and acceptable appearance (Fig 27–17). The nature and degree of the disabili-

ties secondary to impaired tongue function after resection of lesions in the anterior floor of the mouth are proportional to the amount of tissue resected and to the nature of surgical closure. In most cases, motor control of the tongue is unimpaired and the functional deficits depend on the degree of tongue mobility.

Surgical Closure and Initial Reconstructive Steps

From the prosthodontic perspective the first priority, following surgical ablation of most lateral tongue-mandible defects, should be restoration of the soft

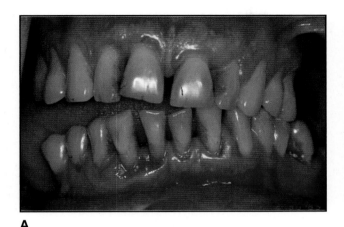

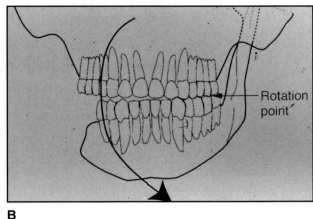

A **B**

Fig 27–16. Frontal plane rotation. **A**. As force of mandibular closure increases, mandible rotates around occlusal contacts on unresected side; **B**. remaining teeth on reseced side drop further out of occlusion.

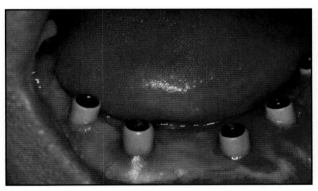

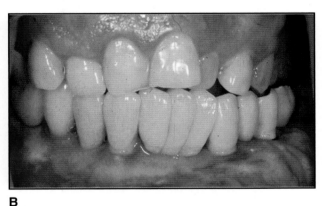

A **B**

Fig 27–17. Anterior mandible defect restored with fibula free flap and an implant supported porcelain fused to metal fixed partial denture. As the tongue was unaffected by the resection speech and mastication are near normal. **A**. Clinical view of the implants in place. **B**. Implant supported and retained prosthesis in position.

tissue deficit, particularly reconstruction of the tongue. With proper use of free flaps, tongue bulk can be restored and the mobility of the reconstructed tongue (Fig 27-18) results in acceptable speech, swallowing, and saliva control.[4] The advantage of free-tissue transfers (free flaps) over musculocutaneous flaps is the improved blood supply, enhancing wound healing and flap survival and the flexibility of the reconstructed tissues is enhanced. If large mandibular segments need to be restored, the fibula is the preferred donor site unless the soft tissue deficit is unusually large. The osteotomized fibula

provides sufficient length and bulk of bone and osseointegrated implants can be placed to retain and support a prosthesis (Fig 27-19).

Secondary Surgical Procedures

Vestibuloplasty, Tongue Release, and Skin Grafts

Vestibuloplasty and tongue release are of particular value when mandibular continuity has been main-

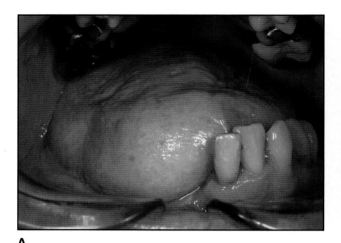
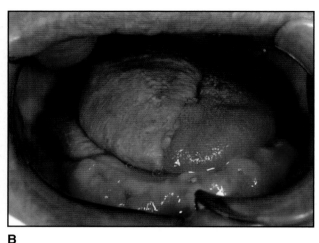

A   B

Fig 27–18. Free flaps were used to reconstruct these tongue defects

tained or restored. The creation of vestibules enables the patient to pool saliva more efficiently and allows for extension of denture flanges resulting in improved stability and retention (Fig 27–20). Creation of attached keratinized mucosa on the ridge surface with either a skin graft or a palatal graft provides additional stability for a partial or complete denture. The patient's appearance may also be improved because a prosthesis can now be molded to provide contour and support for the lower lip and cheek in the resected area. Improvement of speech is less noticeable in patients who lack tongue bulk and/or mobility.

Restoration of Mandibular Continuity

Surgically restoring mandibular discontinuity defects results in more normal mandibular movement patterns that enable the patient to exert force on both sides of the dental arch. This increases the stability of complete dentures. In dentulous patients, a properly reconstructed mandible restores dental occlusion to normal and will partially restore movement of the mandible to near normal.

Free Bone Grafts. Free grafts are rapidly being replaced by free flaps as a mean of restoring mandibular discontinuity defects, but are still being used by some clinicians. Reconstruction after extension resection of oral malignancies with free grafts is challenging because of the lack of sufficient soft tissues, compromised blood supply secondary to radiation therapy and/or radical neck dissection, and the difficulty in achieving proper fixation of the graft during the healing period. The primary goals are to restore facial form, mandibular continuity, and, in selected patients, appropriate volume and quality of bone should be provided for the placement of osseointegrated implants.

Autogenous graft sources include iliac crest, rib, and clavicle. Most commonly the defects are restored either with particulate autogenous marrow housed in a metal tray or with a block of bone, both usually obtained from the iliac crest (Fig 27–21). The use of myocutaneous flaps for closure of the initial wound facilitates free-bone grafting of continuity defects by enhancing the volume and vascularity of the recipient soft tissues.

Free Vascularized Flaps. A major advance in mandibular reconstruction has been the development of improved techniques in microvascular surgery, which allow for composite grafting of larger volumes of tissue. In microvascular free-tissue transfer (free flaps), bone, muscle, connective tissue, and skin can be autogenously grafted and remain viable. The grafting can be accomplished simultaneously with resection of the tumor, with excellent results.[4]

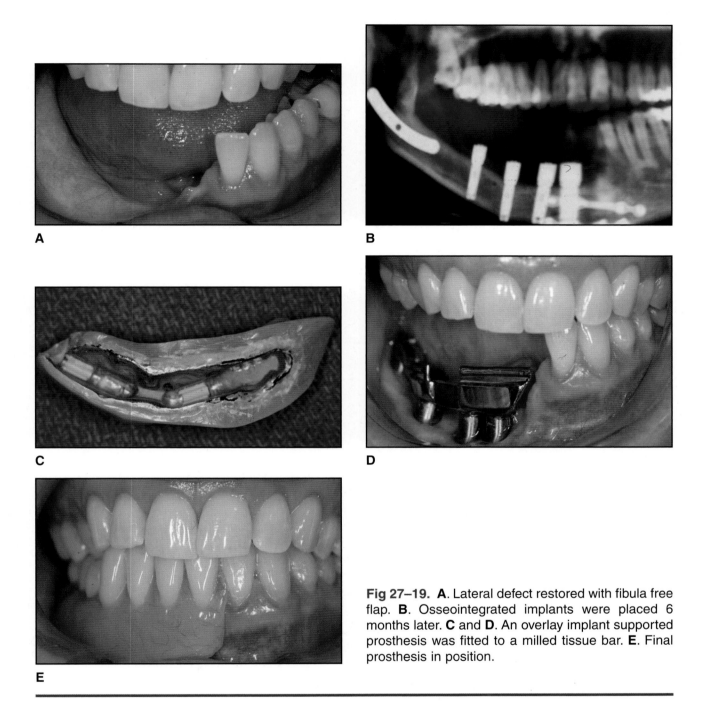

Fig 27–19. A. Lateral defect restored with fibula free flap. **B**. Osseointegrated implants were placed 6 months later. **C** and **D**. An overlay implant supported prosthesis was fitted to a milled tissue bar. **E**. Final prosthesis in position.

Numerous donor sites have been used. The radial forearm is favored for reconstruction of most extensive soft-tissue defects such as the tonsillar, partial-glossectomy, and floor-of-mouth defects (see Fig 27-13). The lateral thigh flap is an excellent choice to restore tongue bulk in a hemiglossectomy defect (see Fig 27-18). The composite fibula flap is the preferred donor site for most complex mandibular discontinuity defects (see Figs 27-17 and 27-19). Multiple osteotomies may be performed, without

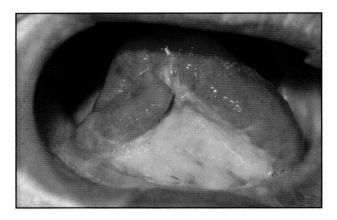

Fig 27–20. To overcome functional restrictions following surgery, tongue release and skin graft vestibuloplasty may improve tongue mobility, permit construction of dentures, and enable more effective control of saliva.

devascularizing the bone segments, to replicate the contour of the replaced mandible. Fibula thickness makes it an excellent recipient of osseointegrated implants.

Oral Function Following Tongue and Mandible Resection and Reconstruction

Even following successful reconstruction, functional deficits (deglutition, speech articulation, mastication efficiency) remain because of compromised motor and sensory control, inadequate tissue contour, and inadequate bulk of key tissues. Restoration of mastication efficiency is primarily dependent on the quality of tongue function. In addition, the plane of occlusion must be positioned so that the

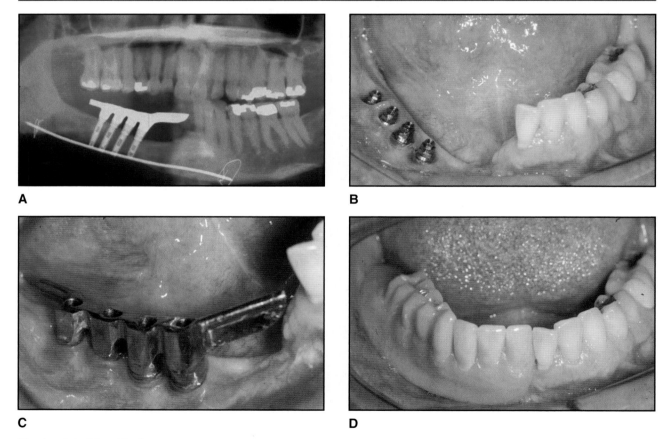

Fig 27–21. Mandibular discontinuity defect restored with free graft from iliac crest. **A** and **B**. Osseointegrated implants were placed several years later. **C** and **D**. Milled bar and overlay prosthesis in position.

tongue can effectively position the food bolus on the occlusal surfaces. Articulation of speech is also dependent on mobility and the presence of adequate bulk of the reconstructed tongue. Patients with reconstructed hemiglossectomy defects can learn to articulate, masticate, and swallow effectively, if they can elevate their reconstructed tongue to interact with the palatal vault, the maxillary dentition.[5-8]

Palatal Speech and Swallowing Aids

If the reconstructed tongue does not possess the ability to elevate sufficiently to interact with palatal structures, an acrylic resin template is made to engage the palatal contours and/or maxillary dentition (Fig 27-22). Their surfaces can be modified with modeling plastic or tissue-conditioning material (Fig 27-23) and eventually processed into acrylic resin. Guttural speech sounds, in particular, are enhanced with this type of aid.

Definitive Prosthetic Restoration

The functional outcomes of removable prostheses for patients with resections of the tongue and mandible primarily depend on the function of the residual tongue. In some patients with poor tongue function, only appearance and oral competence can be improved, whereas in others with good tongue function, mastication is a reasonable objective.[7,8] Partial denture designs should be consistent with the principles of design employed in normal patients with the exception that more bracing is employed to improve stability (resistance to lateral displacement) during mastication. After the partial denture casting has been fabricated, verified, and adjusted, an altered cast impression is obtained of the edentulous areas. Particular attention should be paid to the developing maximum lingual extension on the unresected side, especially the polished surfaces, which enhance retention and stability. Coverage of the buccal shelf on the unresected side is essential to maximize support. Centric relation

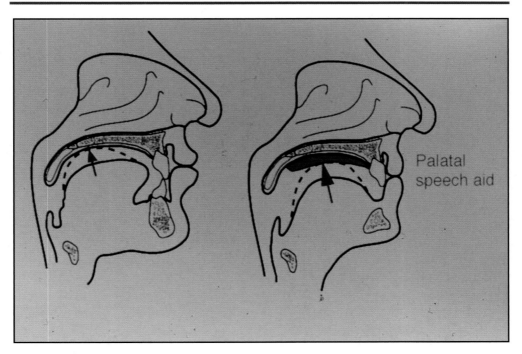

Fig 27–22. Insertion of palatal speech aid enables dorsum of reconstructed tongue to valve against prosthetic palate.

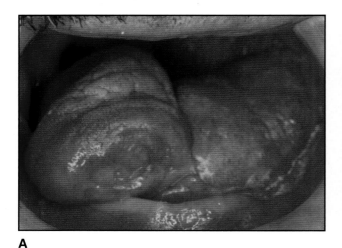

A

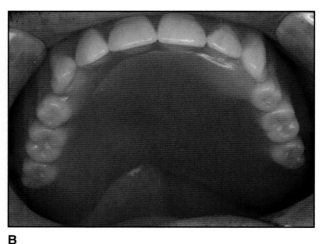

B

Fig 27–23. A. Hemiglossectomy defect repaired with myocutaneous flap. **B.** A thick layer of tissue conditioning material was used to fashion palatal speech aid.

records are made and occlusal schemes developed that are consistent with the unilateral mandibular movement patterns of mandibulectomy patients (Fig 27–24).

Resection Dentures

Dentures for edentulous patients with discontinuity defects of the mandible may provide esthetic improvement by replacing teeth and improving lip and cheek contours, but unless the reconstucted tongue has sufficient bulk, mobility, and control, mastication generally is not possible. A number of factors affect the patient's ability to function with resection dentures: (1) stability, support, and retention of the mandibular denture are compromised; (2) quality and quantity of saliva; (3) the angular pathway of mandibular closure, which induces lateral forces upon the dentures, tending to dislodge them; (4) abnormal maxillomandibular relationships that may prevent ideal placement of the denture teeth over their supporting structures; and (5) impairment of motor and/or sensory control of the tongue, lip, and cheek, limiting the patient's ability to control dentures during function. Implant-assisted resection dentures can overcome many of these difficulties, particularly those associated with compromised retention, stability, or support.

The status of the remaining tongue is probably the most important prognostic factor. If motor and/or sensory controls are not significantly impaired, and the tongue can be moved in several directions, resection denture stabilization and control of the food bolus during function become possible. Paradoxically, immobility of the tongue often permits a more aggressive extension of the lingual flange on the nonsurgical side, aiding stability and retention. Mandibular resections extending to the midline have a poor prosthetic prognosis without implant retention. If the resection is limited to the ramus-molar or even to the cuspid regions anteriorly, the prosthetic prognosis is more favorable. In some of these patients, remnants of the masseter or medial pterygoid muscle may remain attached to the mandible, enabling the development of bilaterally balanced occlusion. These patients demonstrate more-normal envelopes of motion, mandibular movement patterns, and near-normal ridge relationships, allowing for more favorable distribution of forces during mastication and swallowing.

Implant-Assisted Overlay Dentures

Patients with reasonable tongue bulk and mobility and with motor and sensory innervation intact on at least one side gain the most from implant-retained overlay dentures. The tongue is no longer required to

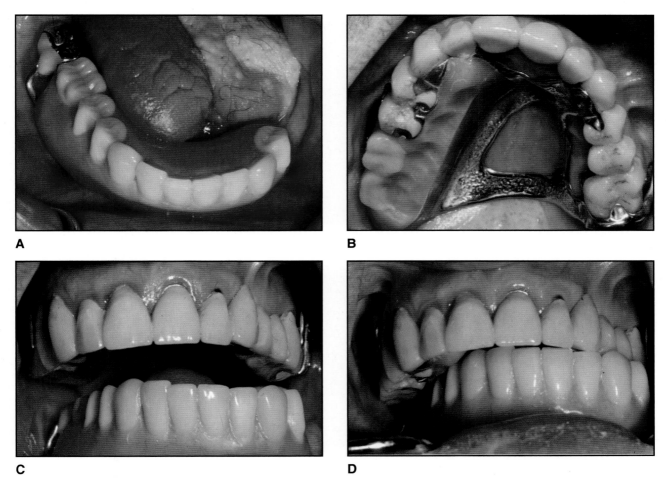

Fig 27–24. Patient with lateral tongue mandibular discontinuity defect. Left lateral tongue was reconstructed with a myocutaneous flap. **A**. Mandibular prosthesis in position. **B**. Maxillary prosthesis in position. Note functionally generated occlusal platform. **C** and **D**. Note angular path of closure.

control the denture, so it functions mainly to manipulate the food bolus during mastication and swallowing.

In mandibular resection patients, if implants are to be placed into the mandible to retain and support an overlay prosthesis, consideration should be given to placing implants in the opposing maxilla. The unilateral occlusal forces and increased lateral forces generated during the chewing cycle tend to dislodge the upper denture. In addition, xerostomia secondary to radiation therapy may compromise the peripheral seal. Therefore, implants should be considered if the retention and stability of a conventional maxillary denture is marginal (Fig 27-25).

In most patients, the only implant sites available in the edentulous resected mandible are located in

the symphyseal region. A minimum of two implants should be placed. However, more are desirable, if space allows. Tissue bar designs must take into account the axis of rotation of the overlay denture when occlusal forces are applied in the distal extension area on the nonresected side. A suitable design is shown in Figure 27-26.

Implant success rates in bone grafts used to restore mandibular continuity defects have been very good. Free bone grafts demonstrate a homogeneous calcification pattern that results in excellent bone anchorage (see Fig 27-21). Free flaps also provide sufficient quality and quantity of bone for excellent anchorage of implants, particularly with the fibula free flaps[9] (see Figs 27-17 and 27-19).

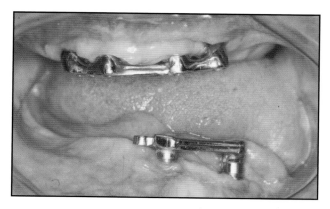

Fig 27–25. Implants have been placed in maxilla to counteract unilateral forces of occlusion. Note frontal plane rotation.

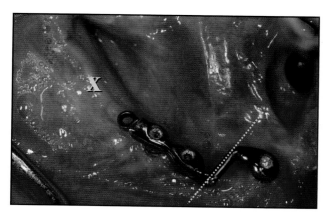

Fig 27–26. Typical tissue bar design for an edentulous lateral mandibular discontinuity defect. When occlusal load is applied in extension area (x) restoration rotates around "Hader" bar segment (*dotted line*).

FACIAL DEFECTS

Surgical Reconstruction Versus Prosthetic Restoration

Surgical reconstruction and prosthodontic restoration both have limitations. The surgeon is limited by the availability of tissue, damage to the local vascular bed, and the need for periodic visual inspection of an oncologic defect. The prosthodontist is limited by, movable tissue beds, and difficulties in retaining very large prostheses. The method of facial restoration should be considered before surgery and patients should participate in the decision-making process and have realistic expectations.

Surgical reconstruction of small facial defects is preferable. However, it is difficult for the surgeon to contour a facial component that is as effective in appearance as a well-made prosthesis. Osseointegrated implants in facial defects have changed patient perceptions about facial prostheses because of the retention achieved. Additionally, when a large resection is necessary and recurrence of tumor is probable, it is advantageous to be able to monitor the surgical site closely, which a prosthesis permits. Even when surgical reconstruction is deemed possible, most surgeons prefer to wait at least 1 year before surgical reconstruction. Also, surgical restoration of large defects is technically difficult and requires multiple procedures and hospitalizations, which may be further complicated if radiotherapy has been included.

Alterations at Surgery to Enhance the Prosthetic Prognosis

The key to fabricating esthetic facial prostheses are properly designed surgical defects. If surgical reconstruction of a facial defect following tumor ablation is not planned several factors need to be addressed. The key to an esthetic facial prosthesis is to create a defect with minimal distortion of adjacent facial structures. During nasal resections, the nasal bones should be resected and all raw tissues surfaces need to be lined with split-thickness skin grafts. Primary closure of skin to mucosal margins should be avoided, for this distorts nasolabial folds, and cheek and lip contours. In resections of the ear, total as opposed to partial resection is preferred. When possible, however, the tragus should be retained because this structure will hide the anterior margin of the prosthesis. During orbital exenteration the eyelids should be removed and the orbit lined with a skin graft. Covering a facial defect with free flaps precludes the fabrication of prosthetic restoration in almost all situations and should be avoided if possible.

Prosthetic Facial Restorations

The challenge to the prosthodontist is to fabricate an esthetically pleasing restoration (Fig 27-27). A conspicuous prosthesis may produce more anxiety and permit less social readjustment than a simple facial bandage or eye patch. The most critical period is the first 2 to 3 days after delivery. The patient must understand that a prosthesis has two different roles: for family, close friends, or business associates, it can only cosmetically replace the tissues excised; for the public at large, it generally provides enough concealment to render the reconstructed defect inconspicuous.

Materials and Methods of Retention for Facial Prostheses

Current materials all possess some undesirable characteristics.[10] The materials most often used are the silicone elastomers, which have achieved wide clinical acceptance. Adhesives can be used to retain facial prostheses but implant retention is preferred. Osseointegrated implants, results in extremely well-retained prostheses that permit vigorous physical activities. Patients favor implant retained facial prostheses over adhesive retained prostheses by a wide margin.[11]

Design Considerations

A presurgical moulage can be very helpful, especially if a total rhinectomy or total auriculectomy is anticipated. Impressions of the defect usually are obtained with elastic impression materials, taking care not to displace the tissues being recorded. The contours of the prostheses are sculpted in wax, both on the cast and on the patient. Surface characteristics, appropriate contour, coloration, and margin placement are equally important factors. Processing the materials is complicated and requires special instrumentation. Special flasks are necessary for processing large prostheses.

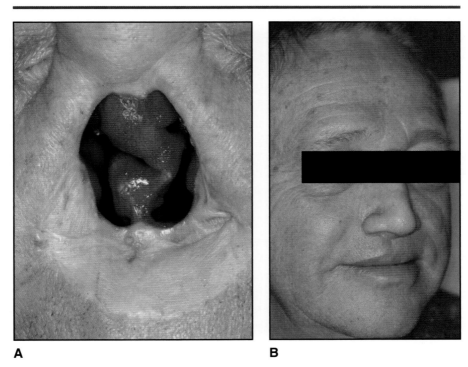

A   **B**

Fig 27–27. Prosthetic restoration of a nasal defect.

Coloration

Basic skin tones should be developed into a shade guide for each material. The base shade selected should be slightly lighter than the lightest skin tones of the patient, because as additional color is added extrinsically the prosthesis will darken.

Combined Oral and Facial Defects

When the integrity of the oral cavity has been destroyed, food and air escape during swallowing, speech is often unintelligible, and saliva control is difficult. Additionally, it is extremely difficult to adapt the margins of the prosthesis to maintain tissue contact during facial and mandibular movements. Retention of maxillary teeth or a portion of the hard palate improves the prosthetic prognosis. Placement of implants, as well as skin grafts to decrease tissue contraction and to create undercut areas for retention and stability, also improve the prosthetic prognosis.

Patients will experience less depression if as many functions as possible are restored immediately after surgery with a temporary prosthesis. These functions include swallowing food (thereby eliminating the need for a nasogastric tube or gastrostomy), controlling saliva, and speaking. The oral portion of the temporary prosthesis is constructed of acrylic resin and formed so that contact is established with healthy tissues adjacent to the defect. Functional contact with the remaining portions of the lips allows the patient to effectively seal the oral cavity. Tissue-bearing surfaces of the prosthesis are relined with temporary denture reliner at frequent intervals to accommodate tissue changes.

In constructing a definitive midface prosthesis, a custom tray is used for the master impression. Movable portions of the defect are recorded with a thermoplastic material. Record bases are fabricated, and centric relation records enable casts to be mounted on an articulator. Osseointegrated implants, eyeglass frames, adhesives, straps, teeth, and engagement of defect undercuts supply retention. The finished restoration usually provides the patient with acceptable appearance and function (Fig 27–28).

Craniofacial Implants

The use of osseointegrated implants has significantly improved patient acceptance of facial prostheses.[11] The retention provided by implants makes it possible to fabricate large prostheses and makes it possible to fabricate thinner margins, which enhance esthetics by blending and moving more effectively with adjacent mobile tissues. Other benefits include elimination of the occasional skin reaction to skin adhesives, ease and enhanced accuracy of prosthesis placement, improved patient comfort, and decreased daily maintenance, which also increases the life span of the facial prosthesis.

Treatment Planning

The implants must be positioned within the confines of the proposed facial prosthesis. In most patients, it is desirable to sculpt a wax replica of the future prosthesis and to use this replica to fabricate a surgical template. This template is sterilized and used as a guide during surgery to ensure proper implant position and angulation (Fig 27–29).

The number and arrangement of implants and possible bone sites are determined. In large extensive defects, CT scans and three-dimensional models are useful in evaluating potential bone sites and important adjacent structures. The health of skin and soft tissues circumscribing osseointegrated implants is easier to maintain if these tissues are thin (less then 5-mm thickness) and attached to underlying periosteum. If the skin contains hair follicles or scar tissue from past reconstructive procedures, these tissues should be removed and replaced with skin grafts.

Surgical Placement

Craniofacial implant fixtures are fabricated from pure titanium. They are available in either 3 or 4-mm lengths, with a 5-mm diameter flange. The short lengths are designed to permit placement in areas with limited available bone. The flange facilitates initial stabilization of the implant and prevents penetration into interior components. For ear defects, two or three implants are positioned pos-

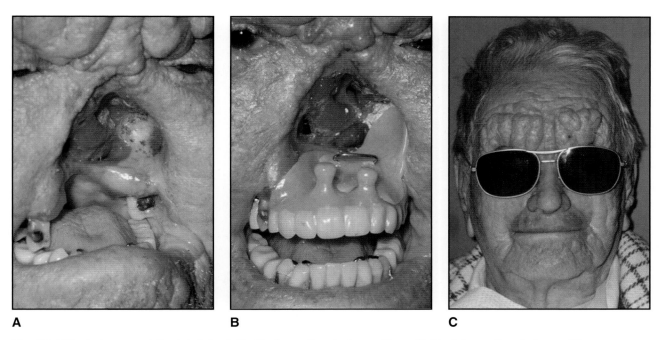

A   **B**   **C**

Fig 27–28. A. Large midfacial defect. **B.** Oral prosthesis in position. **C.** Facial prosthesis in position.

teriorly and superiorly to the ear canal (see Fig 27-29). For nasal defects, the preferred fixture location is the anterior portion of the floor of the nose (Fig 27-30). Care should be taken to avoid the roots of the teeth in the area. For orbital defects, the preferred location is the lateral portion of the superior orbital rim.

Several attachment systems have been used to connect the facial prosthesis to the implants, such as bar-clips, magnets, and O-ring types. For auricular and nasal or large midfacial prostheses we prefer the bar-clip systems because they provide superior retention (see Figs 27-30 and 27-31). We prefer magnetic retention for orbital prosthesis, because the ease of insertion of magnetically retained prostheses outweighs the possibilities of magnet corrosion and decreased retention over time. An acrylic resin substructure retaining the attachments is designed to fit within the contours of the silicone facial prosthesis. It should possess sufficient surface area so that the bond between the acrylic resin substructure and the silicone prosthesis will not fail during insertion or removal of the prosthesis.

Success rates for auricular sites have exceeded 90% in most studies and few complications have been encountered. Success rates of the floor-of-nose sites are around 80%. Success rates in the orbit have been less. Success rates are diminished if implant sites have been irradiated previously particularly in the orbit[12] (Tables 27-1 and 27-2).

IMPLANTS IN IRRADIATED TISSUES

Irradiation of head and neck tumors predispose to changes in bone, skin, and mucosa which affect the predictability of osseointegrated implants. Long-term function of osseointegrated implants is dependent on the presence of viable bone that is capable of remodeling and turnover as the implant is subjected to stresses associated with supporting, retaining, and stabilizing prosthetic restorations. The viability of irradiated bone may not be sufficient to ensure a long-term predictable result, particularly in anatomic sites such as the supraorbital rim and

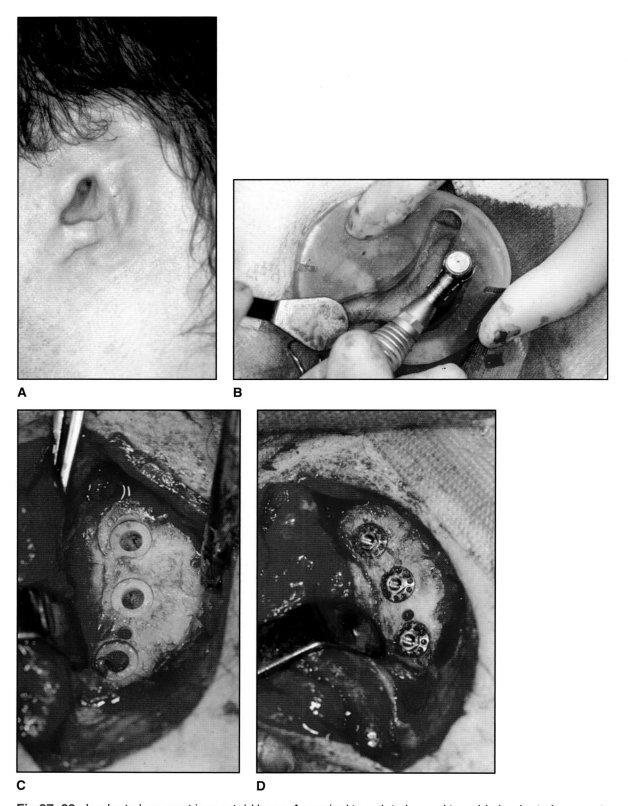

Fig 27–29. Implant placement in mastoid bone. A surgical template is used to guide implant placement.

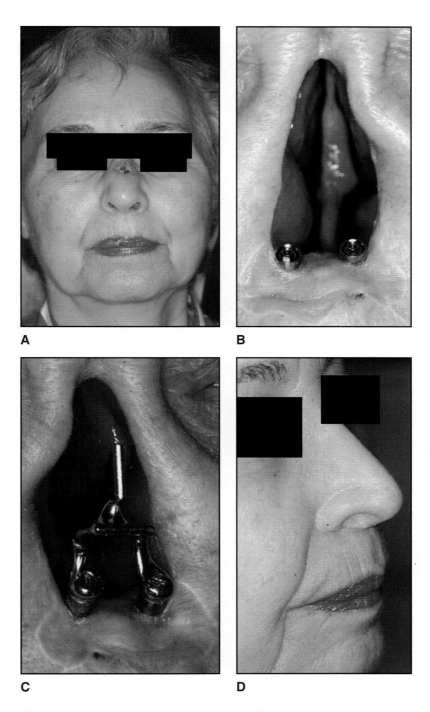

Fig 27–30. A. Patient presented with squamous carcinoma. **B**. Tissue bar for rhinectomy defect with "Hader" bar attachments arranged vertically and horizontally. **C**. Implants were placed at time of surgical resection. **D**. Prosthesis in position.

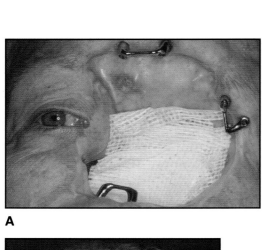

A

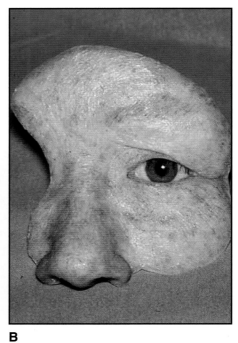

B

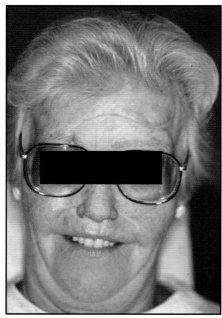

C

Fig 27–31. Large midfacial defect restored with implant retained prosthesis. **A**. Tissue bars in position. "Hader" bar retention system was used. **B**. Finished prosthesis. **C**. Prosthesis snaps in position.

the mandible. Even in the maxilla remodeling and turnover of bone subjected to high-dose radiotherapy (above 5000 cGy) may be adversely affected to the point where an implant subject to functional stresses cannot be sustained.

Predictability of Implants in Irradiated Bone

Preliminary reports and our own experience indicate that the success-failure rate of osseointegrated implants in irradiated bone appears to be dependent on the anatomic site selected, the dose to the site, and the use of hyperbaric oxygen. Animal experiments have shown that the quantity of the bone at the bone-implant interface is reduced. The early trends seen in recent clinical reports appear to substantiate the concerns raised in the animal studies; namely, a high percentage of implants in irradiated tissues demonstrate advanced bone loss at an early stage. Implants in irradiated tissues used to retain facial prostheses appear to have a significantly lower success rate than implants in nonirradiated tissues (see Tables 27–1 and 27–2).

Table 27–1. Nonirradiated Craniofacial Implants

Implant Sites	Patients Treated	Placed	Uncovered	Number of Implants Buried	Failed	Survival Rate
Auricular	35	111	97	8	5	94%
Nasal	16					
Piriform		27	25	0	5	80%
Glabella		6	6	0	4	33%
Orbital	9	28	25	2	7	70%
Overall	60	172	153	10	21	85%

Source: Data from Roumanas et al, 2002. Implant-retained prostheses for facial defects: An up to 14-year follow-up report on the survival rates of implants at UCLA.[12]

Table 27–2. Irradiated Craniofacial Implants

Implant Sites	Patients Treated	Placed	Uncovered	Number of Implants Buried	Failed	Survival Rate
Auricular	2	6	6	0	0	100%
Nasal	4					
Piriform		8	6	0	1	83%
Glabella		2	2	0	2	0%
Orbital	6	19	15	0	11	27%
Overall	12	35	29	0	14	52%

Source: Data from Roumanas et al, 2002. Implant-retained prostheses for facial defects: An up to 14-year follow-up report on the survival rates of implants at UCLA.[12]

In the maxilla as well, the implant failure rate in irradiated patients has been higher than in normal patients. Roumanas et al[3] reported on the results of 33 implants placed in the irradiated maxillae of 13 patients. All patients received at least 5000 cGY to the implant sites. Eleven of the 33 failed and were removed and 2 others were buried beneath the mucosa for a success rate of 60.6%. Many of the remaining implants demonstrated moderate to severe bone loss around the remaining implants (bone loss extending to at least the level of the fourth thread). Because of these results, some clinicians have attempted to improve the viability of bone with hyperbaric oxygen treatments prior to implant placement.

It seems clear from the current data that osseointegration is impaired in bone that has received doses in excess of 5000 cGy. Success rates, based on short-term clinical reports, are reduced as compared to nonirradiated sites, particularly in the orbit (Fig 27–32). The success rates are lower than in normal individuals even in the maxilla with an excellent blood supply. In addition, preliminary animal studies appear to indicate that the bone-implant interface may be significantly compromised making the implant less able to tolerate functional loads. Hyperbaric oxygen appears to help partially revitalize the bone, leading to improved success rates. Its high cost precludes its use in most patients.

Risk of Osteoradionecrosis

Risk of osteoradionecrosis in the mandible is probably best determined by an analysis of the bone necrosis rate seen following postradiation extractions. Based on these data, it should be relatively safe to place implants in irradiated mandibular sites if the dose is less than 5500 cGy. The risk would be quite high for doses above 6500 cGy (Fig 27–33). In such patients, if implants are necessary we recommend a course of hyperbaric oxygen. It should be noted that most patients with oral or pharyngeal tumors do not receive significant doses of radiation to the symphyseal region. Therefore, implants can be placed with a high degree of predictability in this region in most irradiated patients. In the maxilla the risk of bone necrosis is probably negligible. The use of hyperbaric oxygen can be justified only on the basis of improving success rates.

Irradiation of Existing Implants

Irradiation of titanium implants already in place results in backscatter and, therefore, the tissues on the radiation source side of the implants receive a higher dose than the other tissues in the field. The dose is increased about 15% to 20% up to 1 mm from the implant. Because of backscatter and the

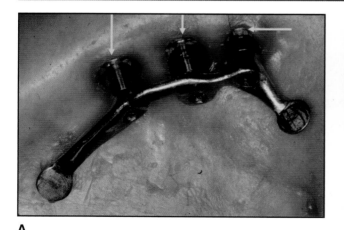
A

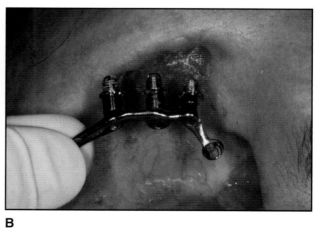
B

Fig 27–32. Implants in the irradiated orbit. **A.** Tissue bar retained by osseointegrated implants 2 years post-delivery. Note exposure of implant flanges. **B.** One year later, implants failed.

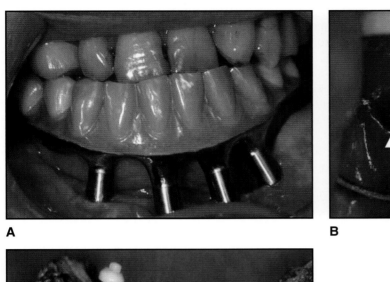

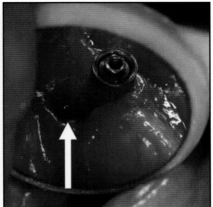

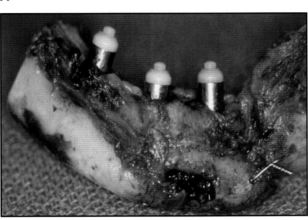

Fig 27–33. Osteoradionecrosis associated with osseointegrated implants. **A.** An implant support fixed prosthesis. **B.** Three years after implant placement the patient developed an infection associated with left posterior implant. **C.** Eventually, the mandible was resected.

increased numbers of elderly patients receiving implants, clinicians ask if osseointegrated implants should be removed in patients about to be irradiated for head and neck tumors. Available evidence suggests that when doses to the implant sites exceed 5000 cGy, all abutments and superstructures should be removed prior to radiation and skin and/or mucosa should be closed over the implant fixtures. When healing is complete, radiation therapy can begin.

REFERENCES

1. Beumer J, Curtis T, Marunick M, eds. *Maxillofacial Rehabilitation: Prosthodontic and Surgical Considerations.* St. Louis, Mo: Ishiyaku EuroAmerica, Inc; 1996.

2. Lyons KM, Beumer J, Caputo A. Abutment load transfer by removable partial denture obturator frameworks in different acquired maxillary defects. *J Prosthet Dent.* 2005;94:281–288.

3. Roumanas E, Nishimura R, Davis B, Beumer J, Clinical evaluation of implants retaining edentulous maxillary obturator prostheses. *J Prosthet Dent.* 1997(b); 77:184–190.

4. Urken ML, Weinberg H, Vickery C, et al. The combined sensate radial forearm and iliac crest free flaps for reconstruction of significant glossectomy-mandibulectomy defects. *Laryngoscope.* 1992;102: 543–558.

5. Curtis D, Sharma A, Finzen F, et al. Tongue and cheek function in the hemimandibulectomy patients. *J Dent Res.* 1994;73:187.

6. Marunick M, Mathog R. Mastication in patients treated for head and neck cancer. A pilot study. *J Prosthet Dent.* 1990;63:566–573.

7. Roumanas E, Garrett N, Blackwell K. Swallowing threshold performances with conventional and implant-supported prostheses post mandibular fibula free flap reconstruction. *J Prosth Dent.* 2006;960:289–297.

8. Garrett N, Roumanas E, Blackwell K, et al. Efficacy of conventional and implant-supported mandibular resection prostheses: study overview and treatment outcomes. *J Prosth Dent.* 2006;96:13–24.

9. Roumanas E, Markowitz B, Lorant J, et al. Reconstructed mandibular defects: fibula free flaps and osseointegrated implants. *Plast Reconstr Surg.* 1997(a);99:356–365.

10. Ma T, Clinical overview of materials for extraoral maxillofacial prosthetics. *Trans Acad Dent Mater.* 1992;5:9–23.

11. Chang TL, Garrett N, Roumanas E, Beumer J. Treatment satisfaction with facial prostheses. *J Prosthet Dent.* 2005;94:275–280.

12. Roumanas E, Freymiller E, Chang TL, Aghaloo T, Beumer J. Implant-retained prostheses for facial defects: an up to 14-year follow-up report on the survival rates of implants at UCLA. *Int J Prosthodont.* 2002;15(4):325-332.

28

Reconstruction of Head and Neck Defects

Brian B. Burkey
Jason P. Hunt
Chad A. Zender

INTRODUCTION AND THE HIERARCHY OF RECONSTRUCTION

Surgical defects following oncologic ablative procedures can have tremendous effects on a patient's function, cosmesis, and quality of life. The inability to reconstruct a defect can even serve as reason for a tumor to be labeled unresectable, leaving palliative care as the only option. Advances in reconstructive surgery, specifically with the development of free tissue transfer, have significantly increased the surgeon's armamentarium when attempting to maximize function and cosmesis as well as managing complications of oncologic treatments. Further advancements in biocompatibility of implants, prefabricated flaps, and tissue engineering will both tailor reconstructions and broaden the applications of reconstructive surgery.

Advances in reconstructive surgery are marked by developments of regional flaps as well as microvascular free tissue transfer. The deltopectoral fasciocutaneous flap was the first commonly used regional flap.[1] It paved the way for other regional flap developments such as the pectoralis major myocutaneous flap that was developed in the 1970s.[2] These served as the workhorses of head and neck reconstruction for several years. Even though the first report of a jejunum free flap was in 1959,[3] it was

not until the mid to late 1980s that free tissue transfer became a common technique in the reconstruction of head and neck defects.[4-6] This has improved our ability to restore structure and function to patients with massive defects of the head and neck.

Given the many tools of the reconstructive surgeon, the concepts of the reconstructive ladder and hierarchy of reconstruction must be remembered. This starts at the lowest rung of the ladder with primary closure of the defect. Ascending the ladder reveals the options of skin graft, local flap closure, regional flap closure, and free tissue transfer (Fig 28-1).

Reconstructive procedures should not be overly complex, as there is increased risk as one ascends the ladder. Choosing the correct reconstructive technique requires the analysis of the defect by looking at the location, size, and the number of tissues involved. Patient factors must also be considered as some patients are not suited for longer procedures because of comorbidities.

Defect Considerations

The location and composition are the first considerations for reconstruction of a particular defect. Assessment of the need for skin, soft tissue, and/or bone may indicate the defect may require two or more linings needed for different surfaces. The volume of

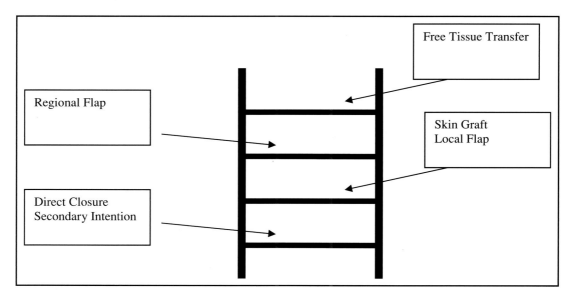

Fig 28–1. Reconstructive ladder.

the defect may direct the surgeon to one donor site over another. Also, the overall quality of tissue is a consideration in the reconstruction, that is, radiated tissue may require regional or distant transfer of tissue because of damage to local tissues.

Functional Considerations

One of the primary goals for the reconstructive surgeon is restoring function, not simply restoring form. This is not always easy to accomplish and requires a vast knowledge of the anatomy and physiology of the upper aerodigestive tract. Speech and swallowing are at the forefront of these considerations. An in-depth discussion of speech and swallowing is beyond the scope of this chapter; however, speech and swallowing must be balanced. It is important to know the wishes of the patient when planning reconstructive options. It may require maximizing speech or swallowing while sacrificing some degree of the other.

Patient Considerations

Although the goal of the reconstruction should be to restore the best function and cosmesis with the simplest measures, occasionally these objectives may have to be compromised because of patient factors. Head and neck cancer is commonly a disease of the elderly and often comes with significant co-morbidities. Postoperative complications are more often a result of medical factors than to surgical factors.[7,8] Thus, the overall medical status of the patient must be considered when choosing a method of reconstruction. This may necessitate the use of regional tissue to limit the length and complexity of surgery while accepting less, but still acceptable, functional recovery. At times, the reconstructive options may be equivalent in terms of function, but not in terms of cosmesis. The patient may choose to forgo the improved cosmesis of a more complex reconstruction with increased recovery time, for example, a composite free tissue transfer, for a quicker recovery from a less complex reconstruction with equivalent function, that is, a regional flap reconstruction (Fig 28-2).

RECONSTRUCTIVE APPROACH BY ANATOMIC SITE

Oral Cavity

Lip reconstruction is performed not only for cosmesis, but also to recreate oral competence. The goal of reconstruction is to preserve the dynamic nature

Defect Considerations	Tissue needed to be replaced (Bone, mucosa, skin, sensate tissue) Amount of bulk desired
Functional Considerations	Effect on Speech Effect on Swallowing Effect on Airway
Patient Considerations	Overall health of patient Body habitus Available recipient vessels Prior treatment (irradiation)

Fig 28–2. Reconstructive considerations.

of the lip complex and to avoid microstomia. Most defects less than one-half of the lip can be closed primarily allowing for good cosmesis and preservation of oral competence. The key to any closure of the lip is preservation of the vermilion line. Any inaccuracies in the alignment of the vermilion are noticeable to the eye and unsightly.

For defects larger than half the lip, primary closure typically is not the preferred method of closure. The lip-switch procedure, commonly referred to as the Abbe and Estlander flaps, are based on the sublabial artery. These flaps allow for preservation of oral competence, result in good cosmesis, and avoid microstomia. Their downsides are the necessity of two stages, numbness in the area of the transplanted lip, and a second scar from the harvest of the lip. The procedure involves taking a segment of normal lip from the uninvolved lip and switching it to the defect, leaving it pedicled by either the sublabial or superior labial artery. The Abbe flap is used for midline defects and requires a second stage to take down the pedicled labial artery, which is typically done after 2 to 3 weeks' delay. The Estlander flap is done for defects involving the oral commissure and can be done in one stage. The Karapandzic flap, which utilizes circumoral incisions and advances skin and orbicularis oris muscle for closure, can be used for defects larger than two-thirds of the lip. It does preserve neurovascular supply to the lip, but can result in microstomia. For even larger defects, the

Gilles or Webster procedures, or potentially free tissue transfer, can be utilized.

Restoring function of the oral cavity is a three-fold task. It requires that airway competence, mastication/swallowing, and speech be restored. The complexity of the oral cavity is evident when one looks at the results of improperly reconstructing a small floor of mouth cancer. If the reconstruction results in tethering of the tongue to the alveolus, both dysarthria and dysphagia may result. Another example is when an anterior mandibulectomy defect is created and the genial musculature is not resuspended to the reconstruction. This frequently results in glossoptosis and dysphagia, and compromises airway competence. These subtle yet complex relationships are vital for the reconstructive head and neck surgeon to recognize and restore.

Glossectomy defects can be separated based on size and what other structures are resected with the tongue. Most small glossectomy defects (less than one-quarter of the oral tongue) can be repaired with either primary closure, skin graft, or allowed to heal by secondary intention. The resulting articulation, swallowing, and airway competence is excellent. When the resection approaches one-half of the oral tongue (or more), and certainly when the floor of mouth is resected, more advanced reconstructive techniques are frequently utilized. When resection of the oral tongue reduces the bulk of the tongue, articulation may be impaired and the ability to move and propel the food bolus also can be hindered. Large glossectomy defects are rarely adequately reconstructed with primary closure, skin grafts, or pedicled flaps.

Floor of mouth defects must be reconstructed so that tongue mobility is preserved and separation of the oral cavity from the neck occurs. Small or superficial defects can be repaired by primary closure or left to heal by secondary intention. It must be remembered that healing by secondary intention does result in wound contracture and can result in tethering of the tongue. Reconstructing small to medium defects with split-thickness skin grafts can prevent or reduce a significant amount of tethering, but wound contracture and the lack of any bulk still limits this technique as a primary reconstructive option. Pedicled flaps such as the pectoralis frequently have too much bulk and as a result actually impair articulation and swallowing.

Microvascular surgery has revolutionized our ability to restore form and function in patients with glossectomy and floor of mouth defects. In subtotal defects, the radial forearm free flap has become invaluable because of its ease of harvest, soft pliable tissue, and limited bulk. It allows for tongue reconstruction while preserving mobility. The lateral arm free flap is another viable alternative in reconstructing glossectomy defects. Compared to the radial forearm flap, the lateral arm flap has more subcutaneous tissue in the proximal portions and tapers into a thinner flap over the distal aspects of the lateral arm. This is an excellent option when a little more bulk is required for tongue reconstruction, for example, in the tongue base, with the thin distal aspect of the flap reconstructing the floor of mouth. Both of these flaps have the potential for neural reconstruction, allowing for a sensate flap when the lingual nerve is resected. However, when a total oral glossectomy defect is reconstructed, it typically requires more bulk than what is obtained with a radial forearm or lateral arm free flap. The two workhorses of this reconstruction are the rectus free flap and the anterolateral thigh free flap. All total glossectomy reconstructions will result in immobile soft tissue and therefore bulk is necessary to allow for any significant amount of articulation and swallowing.

Buccal mucosa repair must preserve its soft tissue bulk to prevent the development of trismus.

Occasionally defects can be closed primarily, but frequently axial flaps like the nasolabial flap can be used and tunneled into the oral cavity if the resection permits. Larger defects and through-and-through defects often require free tissue reconstruction for acceptable form and function.

The maxillary alveolus and hard palate have a variety of reconstruction options available. Small defects can close by secondary intention or skin grafting, and occasionally a palatal island rotational flap can be used to close small oroantral connections. Larger defects can be relined with a skin graft and rehabilitated with an obturator. Obturators allow for excellent function and the ability to monitor the defect for recurrence very readily. The disadvantage is that they necessitate daily cleaning, some degree of manual dexterity, and may require several adjustments before they fit satisfactorily. Another option for reconstruction is free tissue transfer. This allows for one-stage repair and obviates the need for an obturator. It may also improve oral and nasal hygiene as compared to obturator use.

The method of reconstruction of mandibular defects depends on the location as well as the amount of bone resected. An isolated marginal mandibulectomy defect frequently can be covered with a split-thickness skin graft once the cortical bone is removed. This results in little morbidity and, if adequate bone height is maintained, implants may still be an option for dental rehabilitation. When a segmental defect is created, its location is one of the most important considerations. Traditionally, defects lateral to the mental foramen either were reconstructed with soft tissue only, that is, primary intraoral closure, or with a pectoralis flap, with or without a reconstruction bar. In select patients with significant comorbidities this is still a viable option; however, when the mandible is allowed to "swing" and dentition is present, significant malocclusion will develop. Patients will also develop significant volume loss due to bone removal and soft tissue atrophy. In lateral defects where a reconstruction plate is utilized, plate extrusion can develop in a delayed fashion, especially in the era of aggressive adjuvant therapy.

In select cases of mandibular reconstruction, avascular bone grafts are utilized. The initial procedure consists of the ablative surgery, restorative plating, and any soft tissue reconstruction. In the second "sterile" procedure, the avascular bone reconstruction would take place. This would be done through the neck because any form of contamination would result in graft loss. Cancellous bone is harvested (iliac crest) and "packaged" along the defect, medial to the plate, and held in place by cortical bone or a resorbable mesh. This can result in significant restoration of mandibular height even to the point of allowing dental implants. The lack of soft tissue, necessity of multiple procedures, and the increased use of chemoradiation postoperatively limit its utility.

Vascularized bone transfer has revolutionized the reconstruction of segmental mandibular defects. Microvascular surgery has allowed bone and soft tissue reconstruction at the time of the ablative procedure. Many sources of bone are available for reconstruction of the head and neck. Fibula, iliac crest, scapula, and radial bone are all potential donor sites. The fibula is probably the most frequently used site for mandibular reconstruction. It allows for reconstruction of the largest mandibular defects. The skin paddle is somewhat variable in terms of perforators, but several studies have proven that an osteocutaneous flap can be harvested reliably. The iliac crest and the scapula are viable alternatives when the fibula is not available. The scapula is particularly advantageous when both internal oral lining and external skin are needed. Some surgeons are also utilizing the radial bone for mandibular reconstruction. Only about one-third of the radius can be harvested, and it is usually necessary to plate the donor bone after harvest to avoid pathologic fracture. Because of the morbidity associated with its harvest, the limited bone stock available, and the other sites available, the use of radius bone is limited. A very important advantage of vascularized bone, in addition to single-stage reconstruction, is its resilience in the face of radiation. With the increasing use of adjuvant radiation and chemotherapy, and the subsequent hostile nature of the recipient tissue bed, the need for vascularized tissue has become very important.

Pharyngeal Reconstruction

Pharyngeal reconstruction is a difficult task. The pharyngeal phase of swallowing is dependent on many factors including the piston-like activity of the base of tongue, elevation of the soft palate, and the coordinated relaxation and contraction of pharyngeal musculature. Furthermore, the actions of the pharynx must be coordinated with the actions of the larynx to keep food and saliva out of the airway. The pharynx is also important in speech and airway competence. Resection of the soft palate will result in hypernasality and regurgitation of food boluses into the nasal cavity. Stenosis of the nasopharynx will result in hyponasal speech and significant rhinorrhea from a collection of nasal/nasopharyngeal secretions. If pharyngeal reconstruction does not preserve the vital relationships of the larynx to the pharynx, airway competence will be compromised and decannulation will be impossible.

When looking at palate reconstruction, the limitations of an adynamic reconstruction become evident. Complete soft palate resection is a very difficult defect to repair. Obturators fail because of their adynamic nature. Even free-tissue transfer reconstruction is difficult because of the inability to recreate the natural movement of the soft palate. The reconstruction goal should be to allow for a patent nasal airway during breathing and not allow too much air/food regurgitation during speech and swallowing. Partial defects that preserve some mobility of the palate can be reconstructed by suturing the adynamic portion of the palate reconstruction to the posterior pharyngeal wall. This decreases the size of the nasopharyngeal inlet and decreases the amount of work the dynamic segment must perform to create velopharyngeal competence.

Defects caused by the resection of smaller tumors involving the tonsil, palate, and pharyngeal wall can be allowed to granulate. Large areas of the base of tongue can be resected transorally and left to heal by secondary intention allowing for excellent function postoperatively. When transoral resection of tumors is not an option, or when such a resection will result in significant dysfunction in either speech or swallowing, reconstruction is warranted. Reconstruction of large tonsil and base of tongue defects has traditionally been done with pedicled flaps like the pectoralis flap, and it is still appropriate in select cases. The disadvantages of pedicled flap reconstruction in the repair of tonsil and tongue base defects are that the flap tends to pull away from surrounding soft tissue and can be too thick and bulky. The advent of free tissue transfer has allowed for thinner and more pliable flaps that are better suited for oropharyngeal reconstruction.

Hypopharyngeal and cervical esophageal reconstruction has always been challenging because of the complex relationship of the larynx to the upper digestive tract. Skin or dermal grafts can be used to reconstruct small areas of the hypopharynx, but isolated defects often can be left to granulate over the prevertebral fascia when resected transorally. When an open approach is needed or when the cervical esophagus is resected, complex flap coverage is necessary. Pedicled flaps have too much bulk when the larynx is preserved (eg, pectoralis), or are not reliable enough (eg, deltopectoral) for routine reconstruction. When a laryngectomy is performed with a partial pharyngectomy, especially in salvage surgery after failed radiation therapy, the pectoralis is a wonderful reconstructive option. In cases where a total pharyngectomy or cervical esophagectomy is performed, microvascular reconstruction has become the reconstructive method of choice. The tubed radial forearm or anterolateral thigh flaps, or the jejunal free tissue transfer, will all allow for the single-stage, satisfactory reconstruction of the hypopharynx or cervical esophagus.

Paranasal Sinus and Skull Base Reconstruction

When reconstructing the surgical defects of the paranasal sinuses and skull base, separation of the cranial vault from the skull base must be performed. Large resections of the paranasal sinuses alone, either open or endoscopic, do not necessarily need to be reconstructed. When the resection causes the loss of support of the eye, putting it at risk for enophthalmos, a superficial temporoparietal flap can be used to create a sling to resuspend the orbital contents. When reconstructing the anterior skull base, the pericranial flap based off the supraorbital vessels is used. It can be elevated separately from the bicoronal flap when performing an anterior craniofacial resection. If the supraorbital vessels have been compromised and the defect is small, sometimes small avascular grafts (eg, tensor fascia lata) can be used if the dura is repaired primarily. In larger defects, free tissue transfer is utilized to separate the cranial vault from the nasal cavity, and when necessary, to reconstruct soft tissue defects of the face. Few pedicled flaps are able to reach the skull base, but for lateral skull base defects (eg, lateral temporal bone resections) a pedicled trapezius or latissimus flap can be used.

RECONSTRUCTIVE METHODS

Primary Closure

Primary closure is the most direct way to reconstruct a defect and should be used when possible. Neck or facial incisions should be located along relaxed skin tension lines and take into account surrounding structures, as well as future contracture as scars mature. However, the ability to close a wound primarily is not the indication to close a wound primarily. This may leave distortion of surrounding structures, poor function, broadening of scars, and wound complications if undue tension exists around the wound. Undermining may allow less tension and improve closure results.

Glossectomy defects may be closed primarily in many situations without impact on swallowing or speech. However, defects involving a significant portion of the floor of mouth often require graft or flap reconstruction to prevent tethering of the tongue and speech difficulties. The principal application of primary closure exists with limited skin defects of the neck and face. Grafting and flap techniques often are required for other head and neck defects.

Grafts

Grafts include skin, dermis, fat, and alloplastic materials. Skin grafts can be harvested as split thickness or full thickness. Split-thickness skin grafts are used for defects of the skin and oral cavity, and may be meshed to allow increased coverage of nonmucosal surfaces. The goal of the skin graft is to cover open areas and limit contracture of surfaces. Appropriate surfaces to graft on include periosteum, perichondrium, paratenon, dermis, muscle, and granulation tissue. Contracture of 10% or more is expected. Oral cavity resurfacing is an ideal indication for this technique. It can provide quicker healing and minimize tethering of the tongue. The skin grafts must be securely bolstered to the tissue while vascular ingrowth occurs. The graft survives by plasmatic imbibition during the first 2 to 3 days before vascular ingrowth occurs. Five to 7 days is considered adequate bolstering. Skin grafting over muscle flaps or underlying muscle of the neck is appropriate in patients of significant morbidities in which a lengthy surgery is to be avoided. The thigh is a common donor site and grafts of 0.0012 to 0.0020 inches can be used. Thicker grafts allow less contracture, and have lesser survival due to less inflow from the recipient bed. Caution should be used when the recipient bed is irradiated or infected.

Full-thickness skin grafts are most commonly utilized for small defects of the nose. These full-thickness grafts are commonly harvested from skin near a supraclavicular, preauricular, or postauricular crease. Dermal grafting and fascial grafting has also been utilized in situations to prevent Frey's syndrome from parotidectomy defects. Fascia lata can be harvested from the thigh for static facial slings for facial paralysis.

Alloplastic materials are available for use as well. Cadaveric skin in the form of acellular dermis was first used in burn defects for skin coverage. It has been used for parotidectomy defects to provide bulk and prevent Frey's syndrome.[9] Dural defects can also be closed with the use of acellular dermis.[10]

Local Flap Reconstruction

Local flap reconstruction is commonly applied to cutaneous defects of the face, as these flaps have superior color match, contour, and texture. Mastery of local flaps will aid the surgeon in reliably and cosmetically reconstructing defects particularly of the nose, cheeks, and forehead. Common flap techniques include advancement, rotation, and transposition. A full description of each local flap is beyond the scope of this chapter.

Considerations in designing a local flap include reducing tension, hiding scars, and avoiding distortion of nearby structures. Advancing tissue should utilize nearby mobile tissue. Scars can be camouflaged in creases, shadows of the face, and/or hairlines when possible. Length-to-width ratio should not exceed 3:1 when depending on a random subdermal plexus blood supply; but, when patterned on an axial blood supply, the ratio can be larger. The melolabial flap is the only commonly used local flap considered to have an axial blood supply, based on the angular artery (Fig 28–3). The tension of the closure should be minimized to improve survival and reduce scarring. Also, factors such as cigarette smoking and infection will increase complications of the flap and one should be more conservative in these situations.

Regional Flap Reconstruction

Regional flaps have been revolutionary in head and neck reconstruction. They involve the transfer of tissue from a nearby location, though not immediately

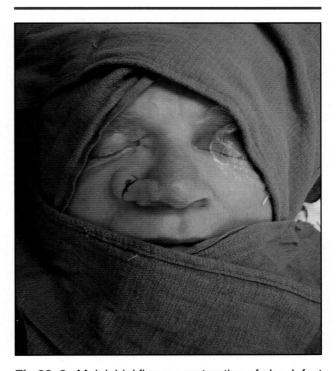

Fig 28–3. Melolabial flap reconstruction of alar defect in a delayed fashion. Flap previously transferred and currently undergoing division and inset.

adjacent to the defect. The flap types include muscle only, myofascial, myocutaneous, fasciocutaneous, and cutaneous flaps based on an axial blood supply. The ability to utilize an axial blood supply allows the reconstruction of defects that are relatively far from the donor site. The axial blood supply also allows a relatively vascular tissue to be utilized for the reconstruction. This is very important for wounds that are contaminated. The first design was the deltopectoral flap in the 1960s.[1] This allowed readily available tissue to reconstruct external skin defects and defects of the lining of the aerodigestive tract. Since that time, other flaps have become more prevalent for use in the reconstruction of head and neck defects.

Pectoralis Major Flap

The pectoralis major flap has been the regional workhorse flap in the reconstruction of head and neck defects for the past two and a half decades. It was originally described in the late 1970s by Ariyan[2] and can be transferred as a muscle-only flap, myofascial flap, or myocutaneous flap. It has even been transferred with chondral cartilage and rib, though this was found to have a high rate of cartilage/bone resorption.[11,12] It is based on the pectoral branch of the thoracoacromial artery, that is located approximately two-thirds of the distance from the sternoclavicular joint to the acromium. It does not prevent the use of a deltopectoral flap as long as it is raised in a subfascial plane and the second through fourth intercostal perforators are preserved. The applications of the pectoralis major flap include carotid coverage after radical neck dissection in irradiated patients, glossectomy defects, oropharyngeal defects, and laryngopharyngeal defects. The flap can variably reach the nasopharynx, but distal flap loss may occur if too much tension exists. Overall, the flap is very reliable and easily harvested, but may be too bulky for some applications, depending on body habitus.

Deltopectoral

The deltopectoral flap is a fasciocutaneous regional flap. The skin is supplied by the second, third, and fourth intercostal perforators to an area of skin from the sternum extending to the overlying skin of the deltoid. This flap can reach defects of the face and lateral skull in addition to providing external coverage of the neck and internal lining of the pharynx. When harvesting the flap, care must be taken to raise the flap in a subfascial plane. Also, previous pectoralis flap harvest may prevent the use of the deltopectoral flap if the perforators are damaged or if the pectoralis muscle is raised with the fascia required on the undersurface of the deltopectoral flap. The flap's use has significantly decreased with the advancement of other regional flaps as well as free tissue transfer. However, its use should be considered when other options are not available or are contraindicated, for example, in patients with a history of previous flap failure.

Latissimus Flap

This is a very versatile flap that was originally described in 1896,[13] and its use in the head and neck was developed by Quillen in 1979.[14] It is a myocutaneous flap based on the thoracodorsal artery from the subscapular system, and it can be utilized as a regional flap or as a microvascular transfer. We limit the discussion in this section to its regional flap applications. The flap is harvested utilizing the latissimus muscle with overlying skin. The skin does become less reliable as it extends beyond the muscle. The skin harvested can be extended onto the iliac crest of the hip. The skin paddle can be designed in an oval pattern but better as an otter-tail design extending from the axilla to the iliac crest. The harvest can occur simultaneously with the patient in a partial lateral decubitus position, with the ipsilateral arm prepped into the operative field. A muscle-only flap can also be rotated with or without a skin graft for muscle coverage. The donor site can be closed primarily in most situations and has very tolerable morbidities. Seromas are common but usually resolve with conservative measures. The applications of this flap include skin coverage of the neck and lateral skull base, intraoral lining of glossectomy and palatal defects, and lining of pharyngeal defects.

Trapezius Flap

The trapezius system is a versatile group of tissues with three distinct muscular or myocutaneous flaps available for harvest: superior, lateral, and lower island. As early as 1842, Mutter[15] described a method that involved using the skin based on the midline back that allowed release of scar contracture of the neck. Conley[16] used this skin with the underlying trapezius muscle and even transferred a segment of vascularized clavicle. The flap was later popularized by Ariyan[17] and McCraw and Dibbell[18] in what is now known as the superior island trapezius flap. This is a very reliable flap, but is limited by a short arc of rotation. This tissue can also be laterally based on the transverse cervical artery which increases its arc of rotation, but is contraindicated in cases of neck dissections where the transverse cervical artery has been ligated.[19,20]

The lower island trapezius flap was introduced by Baek et al in 1980 and advanced by Netterville[21] and is based on the dorsal scapular artery. It has a large arc of rotation and the donor site has limited morbidity. Applications include reconstruction of the skin of the neck and scalp, but it is particularly useful for reconstruction of lateral skull base defects, especially when the ablative procedure can be performed in the lateral decubitus position as well. The proximal portion of the flap can be de-epithelialized and buried under the skin of the upper back so that only the island needed for the defect is exposed. Skin grafts can be utilized, but primary closure is possible in most situations. The disadvantages include the need to reposition the patient intraoperatively. The patient must be positioned with a pillow under the back during the first several days postoperatively to avoid compression of the pedicle. Complications of the trapezius flap include hematoma and prolonged seromas.

Other Regional Flaps

There are several other regional flaps available for reconstruction of the head and neck: sternocleidomastoid, temporalis, temporoparietal fascial flap, submental flap, platysma flap, and so forth. These are based on axial blood supply and one must ensure the vascular pedicle is not damaged prior to transfer or during the transfer. The application is usually limited by the ability of the flap to reach the defect, based on its arc of rotation. They can be utilized with a skin graft in some instances.

Free-Flap Reconstruction

Sitting on the top rung of the reconstructive ladder, free tissue transfer allows customized reconstruction of head and neck extirpative and traumatic tissue defects. Regional flaps rely on the tissues near the defect, whereas free tissue transfer allows the reconstructive surgeon to utilize many different locations and tissue types in the body, both close to and distant from the defect. The tissue can be chosen based on its composition of tissue types, (eg, bone, muscle, fascia, skin), pedicle length, donor morbidity, and patient factors; instead of, simply its ability to reach the defect.

Cutaneous and Myocutaneous

Radial Forearm Flap. This flap is the workhorse flap for reconstruction of oral cavity defects. The radial forearm free flap (RFFF) was initially described by Yang in 1981[22] in the Chinese literature and it offers a thin, pliable fasciocutaneous skin paddle that can encompass nearly the entire forearm excepting a thin strip of skin on the ulnar aspect. The pedicle length can be as much as 20 cm, with large caliber pedicle vessels at 2.0 to 2.5 cm in size. This fasciocutaneous flap is ideal for oral cavity reconstruction, easily adapting to the contours of the oral cavity including the floor of the mouth, gingivolabial sulci, and so forth. Pharyngeal and upper esophageal defects, as well as partial palatectomy defects, are reconstructed well with the RFFF. It allows sensate capabilities using the lateral antebrachial cutaneous nerve.[23] It is based on the radial artery with its venae comitantes as the deep venous system. The superficial venous system of the cephalic vein is commonly utilized for venous drainage. The cephalic vein and venae comitantes are connected by bridging veins near the antecubital fossa, so that a single vein can be harvested in most situations that encompasses both the superficial and deep venous systems. Up to 12 cm of length and 40% of the circumference of the radius bone can be harvested as well as part of an osteocutaneous flap. Harvesting the palmaris longus tendon with the flap allows for reconstruction of the entire lower lip with suspension of the flap to the modiolus or zygoma[24] and this can also be useful for midface reconstruction.

The skin paddle can be folded on itself, and a portion can be de-epithelialized to allow reconstruction of through-and-through defects such as a buccal carcinoma eroding through the external skin. Other applications include skin replacement of the head and neck, and reconstruction of defects of the maxilla and palate that require an osteocutaneous flap (Fig 28–4). This is discussed further in the section on osteocutaneous flaps later in the chapter.

The disadvantages include a donor site that can be cosmetically displeasing due to the need for a skin graft on the forearm. There is the possibility of decreased range of motion at the wrist; therefore, we use the nondominant hand whenever possible. Numbness to the thumb and dorsal hand are possible risks at the donor site. The risk of ischemia to the hand is low if the superficial and deep palmar arches are intact as evident by a positive Allen's test. If there is any question of the Allen's test, further vascular Doppler studies can be utilized.

Lateral Arm Flap. The lateral arm flap was first reported by Song in 1982[25] and Katsaros et al published the first comprehensive study of the flap in 1984[26] which provides an alternative to the RFFF (Fig 28–5). The primary difference in comparison to the RFFF is the ability to have two distinct tissue types that include the relatively thicker skin of the lateral upper arm and the very thin skin over the lateral epicondyle.[27] This is particularly useful for reconstructing tongue defects extending onto the soft palate or pharynx. Up to one-third of the circumference of the arm can be harvested with primary closure. It is based on the profunda brachii artery terminating as the posterior radial collateral artery, which is not essential for vascularity to the distal arm. The pedicle length is relatively short at 8 cm with smaller caliber vessels that average 1.5 mm. It rarely is transferred with up to 10 cm of the humerus for an osteocutaneous flap. There

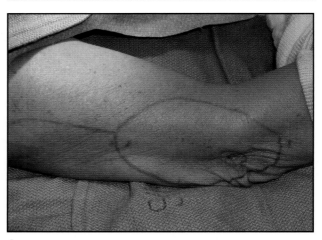

A

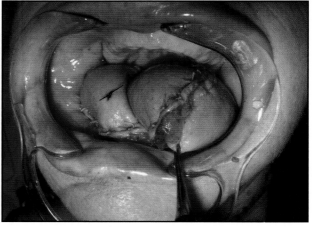

B

Fig 28–5. Lateral arm flap reconstruction. **A.** Flap design on lateral arm. **B.** Immediate postoperative reconstruction of tongue-soft palate defect.

Fig 28–4. Radial forearm free-flap reconstruction of infrastructure maxillectomy defect.

are two nerves originating proximally from the radial nerve that provide sensory input to the flap. The lower lateral cutaneous nerve to the arm (posterior cutaneous nerve to the arm) provides the major sensory input,[28] with secondary input arising from the posterior cutaneous nerve to the forearm. The donor site can be closed primarily in most cases with acceptable cosmetic result. This dissection must be performed with care as the pedicle runs in close proximity to the radial nerve. Applications are similar to that of the radial forearm free flap.

Rectus Abdominus Flap. The rectus free flap can be harvested as a muscular or musculocutaneous free flap and usually provides a significantly bulky soft tissue transfer. It was described by Brown et al[29] in 1975 with the transfer of skin based on the periumbilical perforators. Drever[30] later described the transfer of abdominal skin with the underlying rectus muscle. The variability of the flap is derived from the varying amounts of skin and muscle that can be transferred as well as the various orientations of the skin paddle. A large portion of the rectus muscle can be transferred with skin from the abdomen and lower chest. The skin island can be oriented vertically as a vertical rectus abdominus muscle flap (VRAM), transversely as a transverse rectus abdominus flap (TRAM), or obliquely. The skin perforators can be dissected through the rectus muscle in a muscle-sparing technique which allows a cutaneous perforator flap. All flaps are based on the deep inferior epigastric vessels that are large caliber at 3 to 4 mm in size. The pedicle length is sufficient to reach defects of the scalp (8 to 10 cm). Sensate capabilities are possible based on the lower six intercostal nerves, but rarely utilized.

A thorough understanding of the anatomy of the abdominal wall is a prerequisite to harvesting the rectus flap. Above the arcuate line, there is an anterior and posterior rectus sheath and when the anterior sheath is harvested, one relies on the posterior rectus sheath to prevent herniation, or augments the sheath with mesh. There is considerable debate regarding the need for mesh augmentation of the anterior rectus sheath, and there is also an anterior rectus sheath-sparing technique in the harvest of the flap.[31] Below the arcuate line, there is

no posterior sheath and the anterior rectus sheath must be preserved and reapproximated.

Applications for use of the rectus flap include lateral skull base defects requiring bulk, maxillectomy and orbitomaxillectomy defects, and total glossectomy defects.[32-34] Of note, the muscle component will atrophy over time requiring overcorrection of the defect at the time of tissue transfer.

Anterolateral Thigh Flap. The anterolateral thigh flap has become a very important tool in head and neck reconstruction (Fig 28-6 and Fig 28-7). It is a fasciocutaneous flap that can support underlying vastus lateralis muscle and the tensor fascia lata. It can be a primary flap for head and neck reconstruction, though it is often utilized as an alternative to the radial forearm free flap. It allows transfer of a large skin paddle with up to 12 cm of the width of the thigh being transferred while still closing the donor site primarily. Alternatively, a skin graft can be used for donor site closure when larger skin paddles are transferred. The lack of donor site morbidity makes this flap an attractive choice for many soft tissue applications, though the vascularity and tissue thickness can be variable.[35] It may be thinned primarily at the time of reconstruction, but this should be performed with caution.[36] It is pedicled on the descending branch of the lateral circumflex femoral artery and venae comitantes, which may provide a length of 10 to 12 cm. There is sensate capability via the lateral femoral cutaneous nerve. The soft tissue applications include partial or total glossectomy defects, lateral skull base defects, soft tissue defects of the midface, laryngopharyngeal defects, as well as defects of the external skin of the head and neck. There is little donor site morbidity, although there is potential for denervation of the vastus lateralis and a low risk of ischemia of the rectus femoris muscles.

Latissimus Dorsi Flap. The latissumus flap previously described as a regional flap may also be transferred as a free flap. The microvascular transfer of this musculocutanous flap was first described in 1979 by Watson et al.[37] It is based on the thoracodorsal artery which has an average diameter of 2.7 mm and provides a length of up to 16 cm.[38] Its applications are similar to the anterolateral thigh flap. One unique application is for large scalp defects,[39] where it can

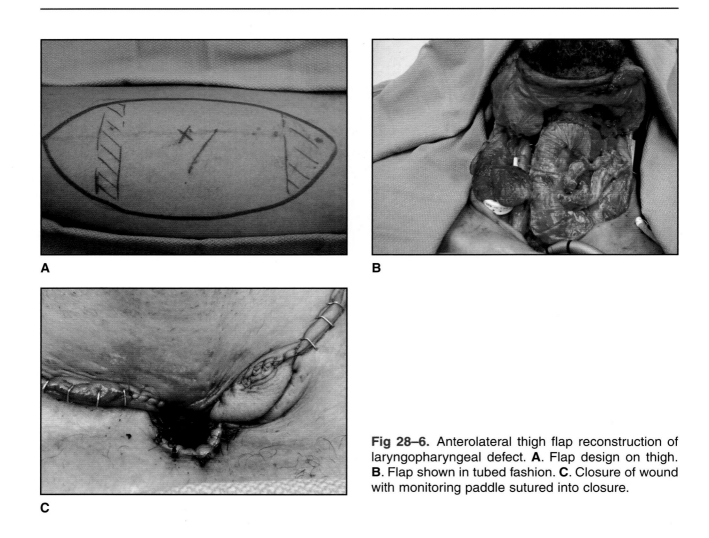

Fig 28–6. Anterolateral thigh flap reconstruction of laryngopharyngeal defect. **A**. Flap design on thigh. **B**. Flap shown in tubed fashion. **C**. Closure of wound with monitoring paddle sutured into closure.

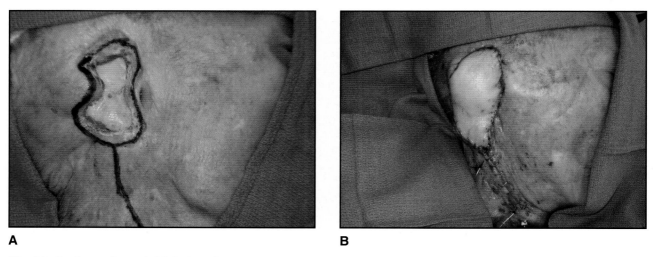

Fig 28–7. Anterolateral thigh free-flap reconstruction of lateral temporal bone defect that failed an advancement flap closure. **A**. Preoperative defect of the lateral skull base. **B**. Postoperative reconstruction results.

be transferred as a thin, broad, muscle-only flap with a split-thickness skin graft (Fig 28–8). Due to the difficulty of simultaneously harvesting the flap from the back, it often serves as an alternative to other soft tissue flaps. Donor site morbidity is minor and includes a mild decrease in shoulder stability and seroma formation.

Osseous and Osteocutaneous Flaps

Fibular Osteocutaneous Free Flap. The advancement of the fibular free flap has revolutionized the ability to restore function and cosmesis for composite oromandibular defects. Taylor first described the flap in 1975 for reconstruction of an open fracture of the lower extremity.[40] Extremity reconstruction remained the primary application until Hidalgo adapted the flap for complex head and neck defects in 1989.[41] It is now the standard for reconstruction of segmental mandibulectomy defects. The fibula is a long, thin, nonweight-bearing bone. Bone stock is good and 22 to 25 cm of bone can be harvested while preserving 5 to 7 cm at the knee and ankle for joint stability. It can be harvested as an osseous or osteocutaneous flap, and the perforator to the skin is reliable and can support a skin island of up to 10 × 22 cm.[42] Transfer of muscle (flexor hallucis longus or soleus) can provide bulk for larger defects. The

vascular pedicle is based on the peroneal vessels and can reach lengths of 12 to 15 cm depending on the length of bone needed. Wedge-shaped closing ostectomies are required for contouring the fibula for mandible reconstruction. The blood supply is provided by the periosteum and must be maintained when performing ostectomies. The bone stock is good and usually adequate to support osseointegrated implants,[43] although this is an expensive endeavor that most patients do not pursue. Using the lateral sural cutaneous nerve, a sensate flap can be utilized. The donor site is acceptable, but almost always requires a skin graft if a skin paddle is used. Long-term difficulty with the extremity or gait is uncommon.

The donor site can be closed primarily with skin paddles less than 4 cm. Although there may be some anesthesia to the lateral leg and foot and minor stiffness at the ankle, there is usually no significant long-term donor site morbidity.[44] Although the primary application in the head and neck is for mandibular reconstruction, the fibular free flap provides good reconstruction for composite defects of the midface as well (Fig 28–9).

Scapular Flaps. The scapular flap can be harvested as a fasciocutaneous flap or an osteocutaneous flap. A relatively large skin paddle can be harvested with

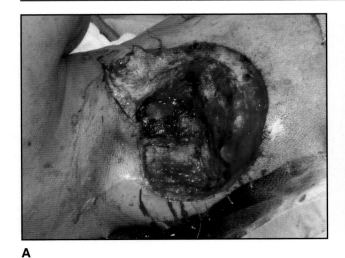
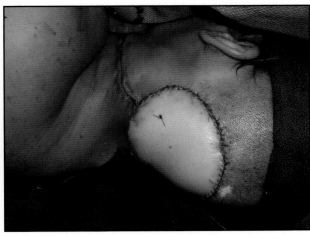

A   **B**

Fig 28–8. Latissimus dorsi free-flap reconstruction of posterior scalp defect. **A.** Defect after tumor extirpation. **B.** Immediate postoperative result.

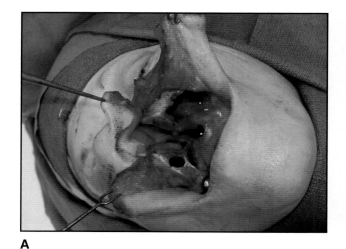

A

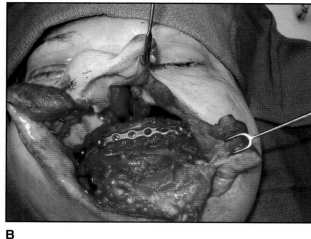

B

C

Fig 28–9. Fibular free-flap reconstruction of maxillary defect. **A.** Intraoperative defect after anterior palatectomy. **B.** Closure of defect with plated fibula and associated skin paddle. **C.** Immediate postoperative result showing skin closure of lip and palate.

primary closure. The pedicle is based on the circumflex scapular artery and vein that are large-caliber vessels. The advantage of this flap is the separation of the skin paddle and bone segments that allows freedom for insetting in challenging three-dimensional defects. The length of bone that can be harvested from the lateral scapular border ranges from 10 to 14 cm. Applications include reconstruction of oromandibular defects, mid-face defects, as well as soft tissue defects not easily restored with other soft tissue transfers.

Iliac Crest-Internal Oblique Osteocutaneous Flap.
The iliac crest flap is an osteocutaneous flap that serves as an alternative to the fibula flap for oro-

mandibular reconstruction. In the early 1980s, it was the workhorse of mandible reconstruction. As the fibula became more popular, its use is now very limited. It is based on the deep circumflex iliac artery system (DCIA). This composite flap may include skin, iliac bone, and the internal oblique muscle. The bone stock is very good and well suited for osseointegrated implants. However, the bone does not have segmental perforators like the fibula which increases the risk of devitalizing bone when creating osteotomies. The soft tissue that accompanies the bone is often too bulky for oromandibular reconstruction. There are no sensate capabilities. In general, its use is reserved for cases where the fibula and scapula are not available.

Other Composite Flaps. In addition to the above osteocutaneous flaps, it should be mentioned that the radial forearm and lateral arm flaps also can be utilized with bone from the radius and humerus, respectively. The radial forearm osteocutaneous flap can be harvested with up to 12 cm of the radius utilizing up to 40% of the circumference. This has been utilized for oromandibular reconstruction. The bone stock is not suitable for osteointegrated implants as compared to the fibula and there is the risk of pathologic fracture of the radius. However, this bone is ideal for midface reconstruction where a thin pliable skin paddle can be utilized for reconstruction of the palate. The lateral arm flap with humerus is also available for utilization, but its use is rare.

Jejunum

Pharyngoesophageal and upper cervical esophageal defects are well-suited for reconstruction by the jejunum flap. This free tissue transfer is based on the mesenteric arcade vessels. It is usually harvested from the second loop of jejunum that is based on the superior mesenteric artery and vein. During reconstruction, the bowel must be placed in an isoperistaltic direction. The diameter approximates that of the upper esophagus, but proximally, the jejunum must be bivalved to create an appropriate size match to the pharynx. A segment of flap usually is externalized for monitoring for the first week postoperatively. This serves as an alternative to tubed radial forearm or anterolateral thigh flaps or a gastric transposition. The advantage over the gastric transposition is the ability to reconstruct at any level in the pharynx, whereas the stomach has difficulty reaching above the tongue base.[45] The potential disadvantage is the need for a laparotomy, although endoscopic harvest is possible. Also, tracheoesophageal puncture after this flap reconstruction creates a wet voice.

SUMMARY

Restoration of acceptable form and function following resection of head and neck tumors is a critical element of comprehensive cancer care. The contemporary head and neck reconstructive surgeon should have the creativity and flexibility to correctly apply techniques from all levels of the reconstructive "ladder." They should have a working knowledge of biomaterials and understand the principles of rigid fixation and prosthetic reconstruction of head and neck defects. She or he also should have expertise in several alternative techniques for each defect encountered, including a plan to salvage a failed reconstruction. Patients requiring extensive head and neck resections and reconstructions should have a careful preoperative evaluation and assessment of comorbidities which aids in the correct selection of individuals able to tolerate extended surgical procedures. Close collaboration and communication between ablative and reconstructive surgical teams is necessary to reduce operative time and facilitate harvest and inset of distant flaps. Meticulous postoperative care and flap monitoring can result in early detection of impending flap failure and prompt early intervention and increase the likelihood of flap rescue. Finally, we must prospectively study and collect objective data on the quality of life and functional outcomes of patients undergoing these resource-intensive reconstructive procedures.

REFERENCES

1. Bakamjian VY. Total reconstruction of the pharynx with a medially based deltopectoral skin flap. *NY State J Med.* 1968;1:2771-2778.
2. Ariyan S. The pectoralis major myocutaneous flap. a versatile flap for reconstruction in the head and neck. *Plast Reconstr Surg.* 1979;63:73-81.
3. Seidenberg B, Rosenak SS, Hurwitt ES, et al. Immediate reconstruction of the cervical esophagus by a revascularized isolated jejunum segment. *Ann Surg.* 1959;149:162-171.
4. Coleman JJ, Searles JM, Hester TR, et al. Ten-year experience with free jejunal autograft. *Am J Surg.* 1987;154:394-398.
5. Soutar DS, McGregor IA. The radial forearm flap in intraoral reconstruction: the experience of 60 consecutive cases. *Plast Reconstr Surg.* 1986;78:1-8.
6. Hidalgo D. Fibula free flap: a new method of mandible reconstruction. *Plast Reconstr Surgery* 1989;84:71-79.

7. Ferrier MB, Spuesens EB, Le Cessie S, et al. Comorbidity as a major risk factor for mortality and complications in head and neck surgery. *Arch Otolaryngol Head Neck Surg.* 2005;131:27-32.

8. Suh JD, Sercarz JA, Abemayor E, et al. Analysis of outcome and complications in 400 cases of microvascular head and neck reconstruction. *Arch Otolaryngol Head Neck Surg.* 2004;130:962-966.

9. Govindaraj S, Cohen M, Genden EM, et al. The use of acellular dermis in the prevention of Frey's syndrome. *Laryngoscope.* 2001;111:1993-1998.

10. Warren WL, Medary MB, Dureza CD, et al. Dural repair using acellular human dermis: experience with 200 cases: technique assessment. *Neurosurgery.* 2000;46:1391-1396.

11. Cuono C, Ariyan S. Immediate reconstruction of a composite mandibular defect with a regional osteomusculocutaneous flap. *Plast Reconstr Surg.* 1980;65:477-484.

12. Lam K, Wei W, Sui K. The pectoralis major costomyocutaneous flap for mandible reconstruction. *Plast Reconstr Surg.* 1984;73:904-910.

13. Tansini I. Spora il mio nuovo processo di amputazione della mammaella per cancre. *Riforma Med* (Palerma, Napoli). 1896;12:3-5.

14. Quillen C. Latissimus dorsi myocutaneous flaps in head and neck reconstruction. *Plast Reconstr Surg.* 1979;63:664-670.

15. Mutter J. Cases of deformities of burns, relieved by operation. *Am J Med Sci.* 1842;4:66-70.

16. Conley J. Use of composite flaps containing bone for major repairs in the head and neck. *Plast Reconstr Surg.* 1972;49:522-526.

17. Ariyan S. One-stage repair of a cervical esophagostome with two myocutaneous flaps from the neck and shoulder. *Plast Reconstr Surg.* 1979;63:426-249.

18. McCraw JB, Dibbell DG. Experimental definition of independent myocutaneous vascular territories. *Plast Reconstr Surgery.* 1977;60:212-220.

19. Demergasso F. *The lateral trapezius flap.* Presented at the Third International Symposium of Plastic and Reconstructive Surgery, New Orleans, La; April 29-May 4,1979.

20. Panje WR. *The island (lateral) trapezius flap.* Presented at the Third International Symposium of Plastic and Reconstructive Surgery, New Orleans, La; April 29-May 4,1979.

21. Netterville JL, Wood D. The lower trapezius flap: vascular anatomy and surgical technique. *Arch Otolaryngol Head Neck Surg.* 1991;117:73-76.

22. Yang G, Chen B, Gao Y, et al. Forearm free skin flap transposition. *Natl Med J China.* 1981;61:139-141.

23. Boyd B, Mulholland S, Gullane P, etc. Reinnervated lateral antebrachial cutaneous neurosome flaps in oral reconstruction: are we making sense? *Plast Reconstr Surg.* 1994;93(7):1360-1362.

24. Sadove R, Luce E, McGrath P. Reconstruction of the lower lip with a composite radial forearm-palmaris longus free flap. *Plast Reconstr Surg.* 1991;88:209-214.

25. Song R, Song Y, Yu Y, Song Y. The upper arm free flap. *Clin Plat Surg.* 1982;9:27-35.

26. Katsaros J, Schusterman M, Beppu M, Banis JC, et al. The lateral upper arm flap: anatomy and clinical applications. *Ann Plast Surg.* 1984;12:489-500.

27. Vico PG, Coessens BC. The distally based lateral arm flap for intra-oral soft tissue reconstruction. *Head Neck.* 1997;19:33-36.

28. Matloub HS, Sanger JR, Godina M. The lateral arm flap. In: A neurosensory free flap. Williams HB, ed. *Transactions of the VIII International Congress of Plastic Surgery.* Montreal IPRS; June 1993:125.

29. Brown R, Vasconez L, Jurkiewics M. Transverse abdominal flaps and the deep epigastric arcade. *Plast Reconstr Surg.* 1975;55:416-419.

30. Drever J: The epigastric island flap. *Plast Reconstr Surg.* 1977;59:343-346.

31. Erni D, Harder YD. The dissection of the rectus abdominus myocutaneous flap with complete preservation of the anterior rectus sheath. *Br J Plast Surg.* 2003;56:395-400.

32. Cordeiro PG, Santamaria E, Krause DH, et al. Reconstruction of total maxillectomy defects with preservation of the orbital contents. *Plast Reconstr Surg.* 1998;102:1874-1884.

33. Jones N, Sekhar L, Schramm V. Free rectus abdominus muscle flap reconstruction of the middle and posterior cranial fossa. *Plast Reconstr Surg.* 1986;78:471-479.

34. Lyos AT, Evans GR, Perez D, et al. Tongue reconstruction: outcomes with the rectus abdominus flap. *Plast Reconstr Surg.* 1999;103:442-447.

35. Kimata Y, Uchiyama K, Ebihara S, et al. Anatomic variations and technical problems of the anterolateral thigh flap: a report of 74 cases. *Plast Reconstr Surgery.* 1998;102:1517-1523.

36. Ross GL, Dunn R, Kirkpatrick J, et al. To thin or not to thin: the use of the anterolateral thigh flap in the reconstruction of intraoral defects. *Br J Plast Surg.* 2003;56:409-413.

37. Watson JS, Craig R, Orton C. The free latissimus dorsi myocutaneous flap. *Plast Reconstr Surg.* 1979;64:299-305.

38. Bartlett SP, May JW, Taremchuck MJ. The latissimus dorsi muscle. A fresh cadaver study of the primary neurovascular pedicle. *Plast Reconstr Surg.* 1981;67:631-636.

39. Pennington D, Stern H, Lee K. Free flap reconstruction of large defects of the scalp and calvarium. *Plast Reconstr Surg.* 1989;83:655-661.

40. Taylor GI, Miller GD, Ham FJ. The free vascularized bone graft. A clinical extension of microvascular techniques. *Plast Reconstr Surg.* 1975;55:533-544.

41. Hidalgo DA. Fibular flap: a new method of mandibular reconstruction. *Plast Reconstr Surg.* 1989;84:71-79.

42. Wei FC, Seah CS, Tsai YC, et al. Fibula osteoseptocutaneous flap for reconstruction of composite mandible defects. *Plast Reconstr Surg.* 1994;93:294-304.

43. Frodel JL, Funk GF, Capper DT, et al. Osseointegrated implants: a comparative study of bone thickness in four vascularized bone flaps. *Plast Reconstr Surg.* 1993;92:449-455.

44. Cordeiro PG, Disa JJ, Hidalgo DA, et al. Reconstruction of the mandible with osseous free flaps: a ten year experience with 150 consecutive patients. *Plast Reconstr Surg.* 1999;104:1314-1320.

45. Spiro RH. Gastric transposition for head and neck cancer: a critical update. *Am J Surg.* 1991;162:348-352.

29

Rehabilitation of Swallowing and Speech Following Treatment of Head and Neck Malignancies

Donna S. Lundy
Paula A. Sullivan
Michelle G. Bernstein

Adequate control of the lips, tongue, and palate are vital for both swallowing and speech function. Any impairment in the strength, range of motion, and/or flexibility of these dynamic structures may affect both swallowing and speech. Efficient swallowing and clear, intelligible speech are highly integrated processes involving intact structures and coordinated sequences of intricate motor and sensory events. Swallowing and speech function may be affected directly by the disease process, surgical treatment of cancer involving the structures of the head and neck, as well as the nature and type of reconstruction. These functions also may be impaired due to the complications or side effects from organ preservation protocols involving chemo- and radiation therapy. In addition, damage to the neurologic innervation of the muscles involved with swallowing and speech may occur directly from oncologic interventions and adversely impact critical function.

This chapter first focuses on the definitions of the involved processes of swallowing and speech. Appropriate evaluative procedures are then presented for both swallowing and speech/voice function. Next, typical deficits that may arise from cancer treatment to specific head and neck regions are discussed as they impact swallowing and speech abilities. Finally, rehabilitation measures are addressed.

DEFINITIONS OF UNIQUE TERMS

Swallowing

The act of swallowing, or deglutition, is a highly coordinated process involving four phases (oral preparatory, oral, pharyngeal, and esophageal). In the normal swallow, these phases interact in a rapid, dynamic, and integrated manner.[1] The coordinated sequence of intricate motor and sensory events within these phases enables liquid and solid boluses to pass without incident from the oral cavity to the stomach.[2,3] Normal adults swallow an average of 1000 times each day with the majority being an involuntary response to salivation.[4] Saliva is produced at a rate of about 0.5 ml/min resulting in a swallowing rate of one swallow per minute in alert states[5] and less frequently while asleep. The functions of saliva are to assist in the formation of a moist, cohesive bolus and to keep the oral mucosa moist, which facilitates transit through the upper aerodigestive tract and aids in deglutition.

The word dysphagia originates from the Greek *dys*, meaning difficulty and *phagia* meaning to eat.[6] Dysphagia is typically defined as "a difficulty in swallowing, commonly linked to blockage or motor disorders of the esophagus," according to the *Signet Mosby Medical Dictionary*.[7] This definition, although accurate, simplifies the many factors and considerations associated with swallowing disorders.

Swallowing Phases

The preliminary swallowing phase is the oral preparatory stage where the bolus (food ready to be swallowed) is introduced into the oral cavity. It is mixed with saliva, shaped, and positioned on the tongue in a cohesive form in preparation for swallowing. Oral propulsion involves voluntary control and coordination of lip closure, jaw motion, buccal tone, and tongue motion.[8] In addition, the tongue base contacts the uvula to prevent posterior spillage of the bolus.[5] Chewing motion is needed to manipulate more solidlike boluses and involves rotary and lateral motion of the tongue and mandible.[9] During food preparation, the bolus is held between the tongue and the palate or anterior floor of mouth. Thus, the most important components of the oral preparatory phase are adequate tongue mobility to manipulate the bolus and to access the recesses in the oral cavity, and a competent palatoglossal sphincter to prevent premature bolus loss over the base of the tongue.[10]

The oral or oral propulsive stage of swallowing follows the oral preparatory phase and allows for propulsion of the bolus from the oral cavity into the oropharynx. The oral phase is also under voluntary control. This phase is initiated by the onset of the leading bolus and involves a complex act of closely related events including the onset of tongue tip movement, tongue base movement, and vertical hyoid motion.[11] In a more detailed description, Dodds and colleagues[5] explain the involvement of the base of tongue as it descends in synchrony with the palatoglossal sphincter opening. The uvula and soft palate, then, elevate to facilitate passageway into the oropharynx. As the bolus continues in its passage, the tongue pumps it into the oropharynx through sequential contractions along the palate. Oral transit time usually takes less than 1 second.[9]

The pharyngeal stage includes a series of involuntary, highly coordinated neuromuscular events that draw the pharyngeal wall upward over the bolus and propel the bolus through the hypopharynx for entry into the esophagus. This phase is considered to be the most complex and critical. Typically, the pharyngeal phase is initiated as the bolus head reaches the ramus of the mandible at the junction of the tongue base and is controlled by velopharyngeal, laryngeal, and cricopharyngeal valving actions. The velopharyngeal valving assists in swallowing coordination and prevents nasal regurgitation. Laryngeal valving prevents penetration and/or aspiration into the airway. Cricopharyngeal valving permits bolus entry into the esophagus.

Pharyngeal transit occurs in two phases. The first phase or initial thrust occurs as the bolus thrust propels most of the bolus into the esophagus by lingual pressure, laryngeal elevation, and gravity.[10] The epiglottis then inverts to cover the larynx and the vocal folds adduct to prevent aspiration.[12] It is important to recognize that the most critical level of laryngeal closure does not occur at the level of the vocal folds but rather is dependent on the anterior tilting of the larynx that permits the arytenoids to abut the laryngeal surface of the epiglottis.[8] Following this, the hyolaryngeal complex moves anteriorly and posteriorly to generate adequate bolus pressure to provide anterior traction to stimulate the cricopharyngeus muscle to relax and open the upper esophageal sphincter (UES). The second phase, or mucosal clearance stage, occurs in a sequential manner as the pharynx, due to its close contact between the anterior and posterior mucosal surfaces, squeezes the tongue base and initiates pharyngeal peristalsis. At the same time, the larynx lowers due to contact with the hypopharyngeal peristaltic wave.[10] As the bolus approaches the upper esophageal sphincter, the cricopharyngeus muscle remains in tonic contraction but relaxes to allow bolus transport into the esophagus.[13] Average pharyngeal transit time is within 1 second.[9]

The final phase is the esophageal stage. The upper esophageal sphincter (UES), at the superior end of the esophagus, remains contracted until signaled by the cricopharyngeal muscle to relax for bolus passage. This process, along with peristaltic contractions in the esophagus, assists in transporting the bolus to the lower esophageal sphincter (LES), and ultimately into the stomach.[14] The combined time for bolus transit from the oral phase through entry into the stomach takes less than 20 seconds.[12]

Speech

Speech clarity is dependent on adequate articulation, oral-nasal resonance, and voice quality. Articulation is highly reliant on brisk movements of the oral structures to move from one placement to the next in a rapid sequence within connected speech. Impairments due to surgical resection and its reconstruction and/or scarring may interfere with clear production of individual speech sounds. In addition, a dysarthria, or speech disorder resulting in impairment to any of the speech subsystems including respiration, articulation, and phonation, may result when neurointegrity to the involved muscles is compromised either directly from tumor involvement or surgical resection or indirectly due to scarring or compression along the course of the nerve. Trismus, or limited opening of the oral aperture, may decrease the size of the resonating oral cavity adversely affecting vocal quality. When trismus is severe with limited oral cavity opening, articulation may be compromised. Xerostomia may affect vocal resonance as the lack of lubrication to the vocal tract and the larynx itself may produce varying degrees of hoarseness.

Velopharyngeal function is another area that may be involved following treatment for head and neck cancer. The primary purpose of the soft palate is to provide separation between the oral and nasal cavities both during swallowing to prevent nasal regurgitation and to aerate and equalize pressures in the middle ear. Secondarily, the soft palate serves to prevent excessive nasality during speech by blocking nasal airflow for all speech sounds with the exception of the nasal consonants (/m, n, -ng/). Velopharyngeal incompetence (VPI) may result from surgical resection of lesions extending to the palate with inadequate remaining tissues available to make closure. VPI also may arise due to scarring of the palate causing inadequate tissue mobility or neurological denervation of cranial nerves IX and X either temporarily or permanently.

EVALUATIVE PROCEDURES

Swallowing

The purpose of a swallowing evaluation is to determine the safety and efficiency of an individual's ability to tolerate food and liquids by mouth. The detection of aspiration, material entering the airway below the level of the true vocal folds, and deep penetration, entry of material into the laryngeal vestibule but above the level of the true vocal folds, should be considered a symptom of underlying abnormal physiologic response rather than a diagnosis. Evaluation of dysphagia is most frequently approached in a multidisciplinary fashion as swallowing difficulties in head and neck cancer patients are complex and typically result from multiple causes and in a combination of systems. Commonly, dysphagia assessment may include assistance from speech-language pathology, otolaryngology, gastroenterology, nutrition services, and/or neurology along with primary care physicians, dentistry, and many other professionals whose role may influence dysphagia diagnostics. The following presents an overview of the various means of assessing swallowing function.

Clinical Examination/Bedside Assessment

The initial phase of swallowing assessment is to obtain a complete clinical examination/bedside assessment. Goals of the clinical assessment of swallowing are to screen for the presence of dysphagia, determine risk of aspiration, ascertain the need for nonoral nutrition, and determine the need for additional assessment procedures. The clinical examination is composed of patient history including subjective symptoms, health history, surgical history, and documentation of other pertinent factors like mental, pulmonary, and/or respiratory status. It is important to understand the description of the swallowing problem, onset and progression of the symptoms, as well as the frequency, duration, intermittent versus constant presentation, and/or exacerbating versus alleviating factors associated with the swallowing difficulty.[15] Quality of life measures, weight loss factors, and other descriptions are of further importance with consideration for the clinical assessment. Following careful history taking, a bedside or clinical swallowing evaluation is performed incorporating an oropharyngeal examination including food and liquid swallows using graduated bolus amounts while monitoring laryngeal elevation, voice quality, and patient reaction, such as coughing (Fig 29–1).[16]

The gag reflex and laryngopharyngeal sensation also are commonly assessed. However, the bedside evaluation is considered "subjective in nature and is not sensitive to silent aspiration," according to Hoppers and Holm.[17] Lim and colleagues[18] compared the accuracy of bedside clinical methods and found that the oxygen desaturation test combined with the 50-mL water swallow test were reasonable screening tests to identify risk of aspiration in acute stroke patients.[18] The water swallow test alone either at 3-oz or 50-mL, however, were not found to be good tools for silent aspiration.[19-18] Nevertheless, this would be a useful screening tool to identify patients at bedside who are found to be at low risk for aspirating and may be safe to return to oral feeding.[18]

Videofluoroscopic Swallowing Study (VFSS)/Modified Barium Swallow (MBS)

The most widely accepted tool for assessment of swallowing function is the videofluoroscopic swallow study (VFSS), also known as the modified barium swallow study (MBS). This method involves a comprehensive radiographic visualization of all structures during each swallowing phase for analysis of the oral preparation, oral, pharyngeal, and esophageal phases of the swallow.[17] The MBS is designed to identify swallowing anatomy and physiology, as well as to define effectiveness of interventions to improve swallow safety and efficiency. Optimally, a VFSS should be performed on all patients prior to any treatment as studies have demonstrated that many patients exhibit pretreatment swallowing disorders.[20] Knowledge of these pretreatment disorders is helpful in predicting and ultimately managing post-treatment swallowing disorders.

During the MBS, the patient is placed in lateral and anteroposterior positions while consuming different consistencies of barium within radiology projections.[16] The bolus amount can be modified during the test. Swallowing treatment techniques should be introduced and their effectiveness on swallowing safety and efficiency evaluated (Fig 29–2). Treatment techniques include postural change procedures for heightening sensory input, and voluntary swallow maneuvers which can further assist in treatment strategies and the potential for successful diet modification. As well, the procedure itself can be modified to clinician/patient needs and preferences.

The etiology of aspiration is visualized during the modified barium swallow study, which further assists the clinician in dysphagia assessment. For instance, aspiration occurring before, during, or after the swallow can suggest differences in oropharyngeal control. Aspiration before the swallow typically indicates poor tongue control and delayed or absent swallowing response. Aspiration during the swallow implies incomplete laryngeal closure and/or epiglottal dysfunction. Aspiration after the swallow suggests reduced pharyngeal peristalsis, reduced laryngeal

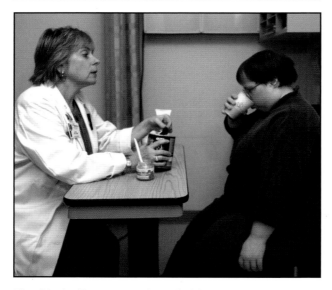

Fig 29–1. Demonstration of chin down posture during clinical examination of swallowing.

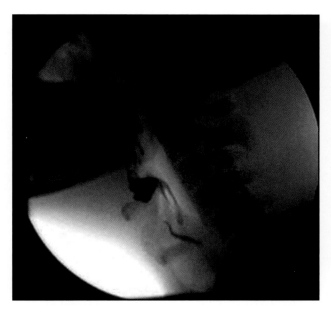

Fig 29–2. Lateral radiograph of a patient s/p base of tongue resection with vallecular pooling.

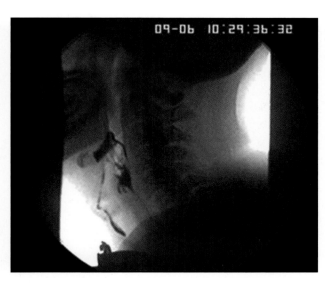

Fig 29–3. Lateral radiograph of a patient s/p base of tongue resection with aspiration postswallow due to pooled vallecular material spilling into unprotected airway.

elevation, unilateral pharyngeal weakness, or crico-pharyngeal dysfunction (Fig 29-3).

Swallowing maneuvers and techniques can be implemented during the study depending on the aspiration etiology and assess the benefit of treatment strategies in eliminating or reducing aspiration.

Advantages of the MBS include aspiration detection and effectiveness of swallowing maneuvers and techniques. Disadvantages include patient mobility to radiology, lack of direct anatomic visualization, and financial expense.[17]

It should also be noted that the MBS is designed primarily to evaluate oropharyngeal physiology. Screening of the esophagus frequently is done during an MBS but does not replace the need for a formal and complete barium esophagram as it does not provide enough barium to fill the esophagus and delineate the walls for better evaluation.

Flexible Fiberoptic Endoscopic Examination of Swallowing (FEES)

Flexible endoscopic examination of swallowing (FEES) is designed to identify swallowing anatomy of the hypopharynx and larynx; determine adequacy of pharyngeal swallow, sensory components of swallow, and presence of gross aspiration through direct visualization (Fig 29-4).

The advantage of performing FEES is the visualization of structures, especially laryngeal anatomy including voice deficit assessment.[17] Also, this method of assessment can be performed with portable equipment. Disadvantages of FEES include the "whiteout" phase where the muscles during pharyngeal contraction block visualization during the actual swallow. Thus, interpretation of the etiology of aspiration is based on inference after the fact.

Fiberoptic Endoscopic Evaluation of Swallowing with Sensory Testing (FEESST)

Fiberoptic endoscopic evaluation of swallowing with sensory testing (FEESST) combines the FEES test with delivering air pulse stimuli to the mucosa innervated by the superior laryngeal nerve to determine laryngopharyngeal sensory discrimination.[21] This is a more recent development in dysphagia assessment designed to test both the motor and sensory components of swallowing while offering a comprehensive assessment as the initial swallowing

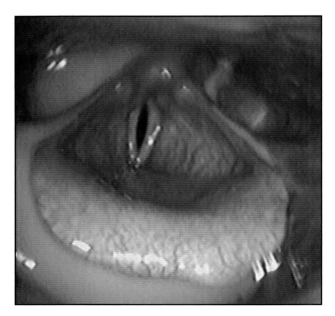

Fig 29–4. Still shot during FEES exam of same patient s/p base of tongue resection showing green-dyed bolus in valleculae.

evaluation.[21] Furthermore, a subsequent study reported by Aviv et al[22] concluded that FEESST is a safe method of evaluating dysphagia. No cases of airway compromise, no significant heart rate changes, 81% reported none to mild discomfort, and only 3 instances of self-limited epistaxis were reported with administration of FEESST to 155 patients of varying underlying diagnoses.[22]

Although findings to date indicate that patients with an absent laryngeal adductor reflex (LAR) are at a statistically significant increased risk for penetration and aspiration, a disadvantage of the FEEST is that it does not provide any information necessary to guide swallowing intervention.

Transnasal Esophagoscopy (TNE)

Transnasal esophagoscopy more recently has been introduced as a relatively easy and safe tool that can be performed without sedation in the clinic setting[23-25] to evaluate the status of the esophagus. It also has been suggested that TNE can be used to facilitate in office unsedated dilation therapy for esophageal strictures.[25-26] In general, studies have

shown that TNE is better tolerated than conventional oral esophagoscopy with conscious sedation.[27] TNE is most commonly utilized as a screening procedure to evaluate for precancerous or cancerous lesions of the esophagus in patients with symptomatic dysphagia.[23] It also has been used for unsedated esophageal dilation to treat symptomatic esophageal narrowing.[25,26] One retrospective review[28] of 1,100 consecutive patients who underwent TNE for a variety of reasons revealed that 93.9% of patients were able to tolerate the procedure with minimal discomfort. Greater than 90% of patients who had previous oral esophagoscopy with conscious sedation stated they preferred TNE. It should be noted that although TNE has been shown to be a satisfactory method of screening the esophagus in the clinic setting, it does not replace a MBS or FEES examination that assess the oropharyngeal aspects of swallowing function.

Manometry

Oropharyngeal manometry can be used for dysphagia assessment with transnasal insertion of a manometric catheter into the oropharynx, which can measure oropharyngeal pressures and/or timing of oropharyngeal events during the swallow from attached sensors on the catheter.[29] This method of diagnostics remains controversial due to difficulty with interpretation limited by asymmetric configuration of the upper esophageal sphincter and rapid events in the pharynx; however, newer manometric systems with improved pressure measurements may improve diagnostic benefit in the future.[6] Furthermore, normative data are not yet available for interpretation of dysphagia with manometry, and may be more indicative for use during swallowing rehabilitation.[29]

Esophageal manometry is designed to assess esophageal motility disorders and may be implicated if VFSS, FEES, and/or other assessments have suggested unremarkable results with no obvious source of oropharyngeal dysphagia.[6] In these cases, esophageal manometry may be considered to evaluate the presence of a motility disorder, such as achalasia or esophageal spasm.[6] Of further note, many of these techniques have similar indications for esophageal assessments, which would be referred for gastroenterological services.

Scintigraphy

Scintigraphy can be used as a method for evaluating the oropharyngeal swallowing. This method allows for precise quantification of actual percentages of the bolus aspirated or percentages of residue in the mouth or pharynx.[30] The scintigraphic technique includes usage of a gamma camera along with radioactive skin markers delineating oral and pharyngeal regions of interest. The images are then acquired during swallowing of varied water bolus swallows following which, time-activity curves are generated and residual counts are obtained using a scintigraphic computer.[31]

Oropharyngoesophageal scintigraphy was found to be useful as a preliminary examination in outpatients with possible laryngopharyngeal reflux (LPR) separating LPR from gastroesophageal reflux (GERD) prior to determining the need for more invasive instrumental examinations.[32] Additionally, Logemann et al[31] found that oropharyngeal scintigraphy is the only instrumental diagnostic procedure for measuring residue in the oral cavity or pharynx; however, this method is not widely available and VFSS is the most common technique for the disordered pharyngeal swallow. Furthermore, Argon et al[33] found correlating data between findings of scintigraphic and electrophysiologic measures of oropharyngeal dysphagia in patients with signs of airway aspiration.[33]

Electromyography (EMG)

Different muscle groups can be examined with usage of EMG guidance. In cases of oropharyngeal EMG examination for dysphagia, surface electrodes are placed on the submental muscle groups such as the mylohyoid, geniohyoid, and infrahyoid muscle groups.[34] Water swallows are administered as well as monitoring of saliva swallows while muscle activity is measured and recorded by the EMG system. EMG evaluates the timing and muscular effort of each swallowing event.[35]

Vaiman et al[34] have found surface EMGs to be a simple and reliable method for screening evaluation of swallowing with regard to muscle activity especially considering the availability of normative data for diagnostic purposes, objectification of complaints, localization of pathologic process, and comparison

purposes in preoperative, postoperative, and in EMG monitoring during otolaryngologic treatments. Furthermore, surface EMG has been found useful as biofeedback during dysphagia therapy.[36]

Ultrasonography

In this method, a linear array probe may be positioned around the laryngopharyngeal musculature to visualize the contour and acoustic shadows of bones/cartilage associated with swallowing control. For example, Kuhl et al[37] had positioned the probe above the larynx with visualization of the hyoid bone and the thyroid cartilage to measure laryngeal elevation during water and saliva swallows with comparison between hyoid and thyroid cartilage at rest and during the swallow.[37]

Kuhl and colleagues[37] have found ultrasound sonographic techniques to be a viable and noninvasive, repeatable method before and after swallowing therapy using the investigation of laryngeal excursion during swallowing. As decreased laryngeal elevation and adduction are found to be a major mechanism in dysphagia and aspiration risk,[38] ultrasonography can be used as a dysphagia tool as it can show the distinction in decreased laryngeal motion.

Limitations of ultrasonography include the lacking correlation of hyoid and larynx movements to the bolus positions as the imaging only allows for anatomic distances without timing aspects.[39] Although the use of ultrasound is not common practice in dysphagia assessment, it has proven useful in many medical facets and may prove to be more useful for dysphagia in the future.

Speech/Voice

Evaluation of speech and voice parameters following head and neck cancer treatment is guided by the perceptual assessment of the disorder. Disordered articulation, whether a true dysarthria is present or impaired due to structural changes, may either be evaluated with subjective means or more objectively with standardized tests of articulation and intelligibility such as the Fisher Logemann Test of Articulation Competence[40] and the Assessment of Dysarthric Speech.[41] Evaluation of voice and resonance problems requires visualization of the structures involved both at rest and during function.

Structural assessment of the vocal folds may be done with a variety of visualization techniques including flexible fiberoptic laryngoscopy and strobolaryngoscopy. Radiologic evaluation of the vocal folds is rarely needed as the structures are readily seen in the clinical setting with the above tools. Voice evaluation is typically a team approach with otolaryngologists and speech-language pathologists (SLP) working together to assess both structure and physiology. The ultimate medical diagnosis of laryngeal status is made by the physician whereas the SLP may render assessment of vocal fold physiology through performance and interpretation of stroboscopic images. Additional measures of vocal function including acoustic and aerodynamic data may be performed to document the status of an individual patient. These measures may then be repeated over time for comparative purposes.

Velopharyngeal insufficiency (VPI) is best assessed by videonasendoscopy where dynamic images of the nasopharynx during production of specific speech tasks are viewed. In individuals where videonasendoscopy is not possible, videofluoroscopy can be performed. To adequately view the valving action of the nasopharynx, barium is injected through the nasal cavities to coat the nasopharynx prior to fluoroscopy. The individual is then stimulated to produce various speech tasks. Images obtained either from nasendoscopy or fluoroscopy help not only to determine the presence of VPI but also the direction of treatment. Static radiographic images are not helpful in assessing the adequacy of velopharyngeal closure as they cannot capture the dynamic nature of the sphincteric closure.

TYPICAL DEFICITS FOLLOWING SURGICAL TREATMENT FOR HEAD AND NECK CANCER

Oral Cavity

Expected deficits from cancers arising in the oral cavity are dependent on the amount of residual tissue, range of motion, flexibility, and scarring. Both swallowing and speech difficulties can arise from surgical resection and chemoradiation therapy.

From a swallowing perspective, oral cavity lesions reconstructed with a variety of techniques from primary closure to microvascular free flaps have been reported to result in increased oral transit times, increased oral residue post-swallow, and worse function with thicker materials.[42-44] Swallowing function is best preserved in anterior tongue lesions with minimal effect on pharyngeal phase function or aspiration.[42,45] McConnel and colleagues[46] studied individuals with oral tongue lesions and their incidence of dysphagia and found that those that underwent primary closure had the lowest incidence of swallowing dysfunction. They further found that there was no significant difference between individuals reconstructed with local versus free flaps.

Speech also may be altered following treatment for oral cavity lesions. The nature of the deficit is related to difficulties making necessary articulatory contacts in a precise enough manner and with adequate speed to accommodate connected speech. McConnel et al[46] reported that individuals that underwent split-thickness skin grafts for anterior floor of mouth lesions had better speech outcome than those closed with hemitongue flaps. Speech intelligibility is dependent on the mobility of the residual tongue more than its volume.[47] In addition, speech may be compromised by the effect of the reconstructed area on adjacent structure's functions.[48] Bulkier pedicle flaps have been shown to interfere with the critical range, rate, and coordination of articulatory movements that are needed for intelligible speech.[42] In a retrospective study of 23 individuals with tongue lesions reconstructed with radial forearm free flap versus lateral upper arm free flap, no significant difference were found between the two groups with both experiencing similar decreased tongue mobility.[49] Hsiao and colleagues[50] found that the reconstructed flap remained adynamic but provided bulk to allow the remaining tongue to achieve necessary movements assisting in speech intelligibility.

Oropharynx

Oropharyngeal lesions, especially those involving the base of tongue, have the potential for worse effects on swallowing as the tongue base is critical to bolus propulsion and upper esophageal sphincter opening. Composite resections may further impair velopharyngeal valving and adversely affect laryngeal motion and cricopharyngeal relaxation.

Managing swallowing difficulties following treatment for oropharyngeal lesions is more challenging as the tongue base and/or pharyngeal wall are often affected. Fujimoto and colleagues[51] looked at the amount of base of tongue that was resected and the presence of aspiration and found that when more than 50% was removed, dysphagia severity significantly increased. Pauloski and colleagues[20] prospectively investigated 144 individuals with oral or oropharyngeal lesions. They found that the extent of base of tongue resection was more related to the presence of dysphagia than the nature of reconstruction. Conversely, Seikaly and colleagues[52] prospectively investigated individuals that underwent radial forearm free-flap reconstructions for oropharyngeal cancers and found that 94% resumed a normal or soft diet and 6% aspirated. They further reported that the amount of base of tongue resected was not related to swallow function. However, it should be noted that comparison with other reconstructive options was not made.

Speech problems following treatment for oropharyngeal cancer resections relate to alterations in resonance and difficulties with velar consonant production (/k, g/). The degree of difficulty is related to the amount of tissue resected and pliability/flexibility of both remaining and reconstructed areas. Base of tongue resections frequently result in altered resonance as the upper vocal tract is altered. Involvement of the nasopharynx may result in velopharyngeal insufficiency (VPI) and perceived hypernasality.

Larynx

Treatment for early glottic carcinoma typically is accomplished with either radiation therapy or surgical excision with equivalent 5-year cure rates of 85% to 90%.[53] In general, swallowing difficulties do not arise from treatment for early T1 glottic cancers; however, dysphonia is a more frequent occurrence. Some studies have suggested better voice outcome following radiation therapy as the linearity of the vocal fold vibratory edge is not affected.[54] Orlikoff and Krauss[55] have shown that dysphonia may result from the tumor bulk and tissue invasion leading to vocal folds that are mismatched structurally and biomechanically. However, dysphonia may also result from radiation therapy. Scar formation following resolution of the original tumor may lead to stiffening of the mucosal lining.[56] Additionally, xerostomia following radiation may decrease the necessary lubrication of the vocal tract and may cause the patient to use great phonatory effort.[57]

Minimally invasive surgical procedures for laryngeal cancer have become increasingly more popular. As the surgeries are less invasive, it is anticipated that the effects on swallowing function might be less pervasive; however, the actual impact is not completely known. Bernal-Sprekelsen et al[58] retrospectively assessed 210 consecutive individuals treated with laser excision for glottic cancer, not including T1 lesions. They found that the nasogastric tube (NG) was required in 23% with small tumors for 2 to 8 days and 63% with more advanced tumors for 14 to 23 days. Aspiration pneumonia developed in 12 individuals. A tracheostomy was needed in 8 due to severe dysphagia and 13 individuals underwent conversion from an NG to a PEG tube for a prolonged period of time with 5 remaining NPO permanently.

In addition, newer surgical advances have resulted in preservation of a portion of the larynx in individuals with more advanced disease who might otherwise have needed a total laryngectomy. The obvious advantage is maintenance of their sound source. However, Dworkin and colleagues[59] retrospectively compared 10 individuals each who had undergone either supracricoid versus total laryngectomy. They found that the supracricoid group had significantly increased residue post-swallow, intermittent aspiration during respiration, and prolonged use of feeding tubes as their primary means of nutrition. Total laryngectomy, on the other hand, does not remove the potential for dysphagia. McConnel et al[60] looked at the impact of removing the larynx on swallowing function and found that increased resistance to flow was present due to loss of superior and anterior laryngeal movement reducing UES opening with average pharyngeal transit times doubling. Ackerstaff and colleagues[61] also looked at dysphagia following total laryngectomy and found that

50% experienced difficulties with solids resulting in a diet change in 25%. Mendelsohn[64] found that total laryngectomy resulted in prolonged mealtimes in 74%. Dysphagia following laryngectomy significantly increases when there is concomitant loss of base of tongue.[60] Later, McConnel[63] reported the presence of hypopharyngeal stenosis in 70%.

Dysphonia following laryngeal conservation procedures is relative to the amount of preserved vocal folds and their mobility. In general, some degree of hoarseness is expected due to lack of complete glottal closure with resultant air loss.

TYPICAL DEFICITS FOLLOWING ORGAN PRESERVATION TREATMENT

In the last 5 years, organ preservation strategies using chemoradiation therapy (chemotherapy given concurrently with radiation) have evolved as available treatment alternatives. Multiple trails have identified that anatomic laryngeal preservation can be accomplished without increase in local regional recurrences or reduced survival. However, organ sparing treatment often negatively impacts oral and pharyngeal motility for swallow.

Both external beam radiotherapy and chemotherapy cause significant morbidities and diminished quality of life. The most common side effects that affect swallowing and speech function are xerostomia, fibrosis, mucositis, edema, odynophagia, and altered sense of taste. Changes in swallow physiology occur with reduction of structural movement for these critical functions. Swallowing deficits worsen over time as tissues become more fibrotic. Sluggish movements of oral and pharyngeal structures as well as reduction in range of motion of the tongue base, pharyngeal wall, hyolaryngeal complex, and upper esophageal segment opening result. A reduction in tongue strength also is common.[64] Although adequate lubrication is vital to swallowing function to allow solids to be mixed in the oral preparatory phase and ease transit through the oral through esophageal phases, the critical amounts are not known. Logemann and colleagues[65] prospectively studied 30 patients who had undergone chemo- and radia-

tion therapy for oropharyngeal cancers and compared the amount of saliva from pretreatment to 3-, 6-, and 12-months post-completion. They found that saliva was significantly reduced following treatment as expected. However, they also found that despite the diminished amount of saliva, it did not significantly interfere with bolus transit as evident via videofluoroscopic swallow studies. Logemann concluded that the perception of dry mouth was worse than its actual effect on the swallow process.

Woo[66] retrospectively studied 31 symptomatic patients following radiation therapy alone for nasopharyngeal cancer with a FEES examination and found that 94% had pharyngeal retention, 87% had delayed or absent swallow response, 81% had reduced pharyngeal constriction, 58% had VPI, and 41% had silent aspiration. In another study, Smith and colleagues[67] prospectively investigated 29 patients with advanced oropharyngeal or hypopharyngeal cancer treated with chemo- and radiation therapy to determine if dysphagia was related to overall radiation dosage. They found that odynophagia was significantly worse with higher dosages of radiation, 60 versus 74 Gy. They also found that at 12 months postcompletion of treatment, 78% of those who received the higher dosage (74 Gy) were PEG dependent versus 18% at the lower dosage (60 Gy). Newer types of delivery of radiotherapy such as Intensity Modulated Radiation Therapy (IMRT) are being used to shape the focus and intensity of the radiation beam to reduce the damage to the critical structures involved in swallowing. To date, studies have not shown a significant difference in the severity of dysphagia if present.[68,69] Eisbruch and colleagues[70] prospectively evaluated 29 patients with unresectable stage IV head and neck cancer who were treated with chemo- and radiation therapy. They found that aspiration was present in 3 patients prior to treatment, 13 in the early post-treatment period, and 8 in the late-treatment period. In addition, 6 patients developed aspiration pneumonia and 1 resulted in death. Finally, swallowing problems are not confined to the immediate treatment and post-treatment period. Lazarus[71] looked at individuals who were more than 10 years postradiation therapy for head and neck cancer and found significantly decreased base of tongue contact with the pharyngeal wall, decreased laryngeal elevation, decreased vocal fold closure, and a high incidence of aspiration after the swallow. These findings were irrespective of the original site of lesion.

SPEECH AND SWALLOWING REHABILITATION CONSIDERATIONS

As some degree of communication and swallowing deficits develop in nearly all patients following treatment of head and neck malignancies, it is important that patients and their families are educated about the likelihood of these deficits and the need for post-treatment rehabilitation. Pretreatment counseling by all members of the interdisciplinary team including the surgeon, speech-language pathologist, nurse, social worker, dietitian, and physical therapist is essential to prepare the patient and family for their cancer treatment and rehabilitation. Information obtained will assist team members in assessing patients' ability to actively comply and participate in their treatment as well as identify possible barriers to head and neck oncologic intervention.

Swallowing

Treatment of dysphagia is driven by the symptoms present and based on the results of a comprehensive and thorough evaluation as detailed above. It is important to recognize that aspiration is not a diagnosis but rather a symptom of underlying abnormal physiologic and/or structural impairment in the individual's ability to protect their airway during swallowing. The goal of the evaluation is to determine the exact physiologic abnormalities that result in material either entering the airway (aspiration) and/or remaining in the pharynx after the swallow placing the individual at risk for aspiration after the swallow has been completed. Specific strategies and maneuvers are normally presented during the evaluation to determine their potential effect on the swallow as detailed in the above section. Swallowing management is then based on this information (Fig 29–5).

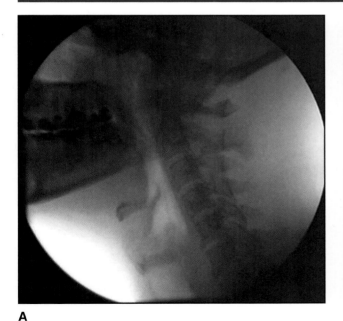

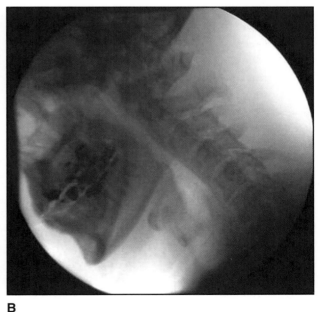

A   **B**

Fig 29–5. A. Lateral radiograph of normal. **B**. Lateral radiograph of normal with chin down posture demonstrating increased vallecular space and closer approximation of base of tongue to pharyngeal wall.

The first decision to be made when treating an individual with dysphagia is whether they can continue to take nutrition orally or will need an alternate means of feeding. Silent aspiration does not preclude oral intake if the patient is able to respond to strategies and/or maneuvers to protect the airway. In general, patients who aspirate may continue to eat orally if they can completely clear the material from their airway either spontaneously, or respond successfully to maneuvers, strategies, and/or dietary modifications, and are cognitively and physically able to comply with the needed recommendations.

In addition, the amount of time and energy required to maintain an oral diet is a consideration. Patients who require more than 10 seconds to swallow a single bolus will benefit from alternative nutritional intake due to the lengthy time needed that may result in fatigue and inadequate nutritional intake. As well, individuals that are unable to swallow any consistency of food with less than 10% aspiration or more than 10% of all boluses regardless of their response to strategies and maneuvers will benefit from tube feeding.

The decision of what type of alternative means of nutrition to consider is dependent on the patient's underlying medical condition, estimated length of time tube feeding may be needed, and both patient and treating clinicians' preferences. Park and colleagues[72] have shown that both nasogastric tube (NG) and percutaneous gastrostomy tubes (PEG) have similar rates of complications and aspiration pneumonia. However, they found that PEG tubes are more efficacious in providing nutritional needs. It should also be remembered that patients may continue to take oral nutrition with a feeding tube in place as long as it is deemed safe. Weaning from a feeding tube typically is a gradual process with increasing amounts of oral intake being ingested while decreasing tube feeding until patients can maintain their nutritional needs via the mouth alone.

Dietary modifications are frequently recommended when an individual is able to preferentially tolerate specific consistencies without aspirating better than others. Diet modification may include thickening liquids for individuals who aspirate on thinner consistencies. The degree of thickening is again determined by the assessment as various consistencies (thin liquid, nectar, honey, pudding, cookie coated, and barium tablets of calibrated diameters) typically are presented during the swallowing assessment. Other patients may experience difficulty with particulate materials such as crackers or other foods that are crumbly and may break apart and collect in the recesses in the oropharynx. Individuals with esophageal strictures may find more solidlike foods difficult but may benefit from alternating liquid and solid swallows. Alternating solid and liquid boluses or washing down solid boluses with liquids also is beneficial for individuals who have significant xerostomia following radiation treatment. Saliva is needed to mix with drier, more solid foods to form a cohesive bolus. Bolus volume and method of feeding are other important dietary concerns. Some patients do better with larger boluses that they are better able to sense in their oral cavity whereas others do better with smaller boluses. Additionally, cup drinking has been shown to assist the maintenance of laryngeal elevation and thus is beneficial for some patients with poor laryngeal coordination or impaired suprahyoid muscle function. Others may find drinking through a straw beneficial. Regardless of the recommended dietary modification, it is imperative that the patient have the ability to comply or have others present who can take on that responsibility during feedings (Fig 29–6).

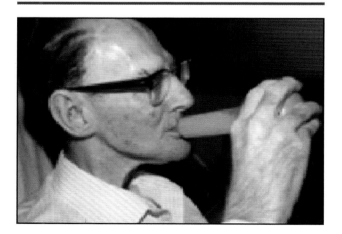

Fig 29–6. Patient s/p glossectomy using syringe to inject bolus to posterior oral cavity for swallowing.

Directed swallowing therapy is indicated when specific physiologic abnormalities are detected on the swallowing study. The timing of therapy usually is determined by the patient's underlying medical condition; that is, adequate healing following surgical intervention. In addition, other factors including adequate mental status to follow directions are considered. Oral facilitative exercises typically are prescribed for patients with difficulties manipulating a bolus due to altered and/or weakened range of motion (ROM) and strength of the tongue, lips, palate, and pharynx (Fig 29-7).

Logemann and colleagues[73] have found that ROM exercises in patients following surgical treatment for head and neck cancer result in significant improvement in both speech and swallowing. Specific devices have been designed to facilitate tongue exercises including the Tongue transducer,[74] Tongue Array with pressure transducers (Kay Elemetrics, Lincoln Park, NJ), Iowa Oral Performance Instru-

ment (IOPI),[75] and the Madison Oral Strengthening Therapeutic Device (MOST)[76] (Fig 29-8).

Both the IOPI and the MOST have undergone therapeutic trials and demonstrated efficacy in improving tongue strength that has translated to improvement in swallowing function.[77-78] Lazarus and colleagues[64] further have reported that tongue strength correlates with the ability to propel a bolus through the oral cavity whereas reduced tongue strength results in increased transit times and the amount of residue remaining after the swallow.

Trismus can be helped with therapeutic exercise aimed at gradually stretching the oromandibular joints. This is frequently accomplished by gradually increasing the number of tongue depressors inserted between the upper and lower teeth. In addition, Therabite Jaw Motion Rehabilitation System[79] has been successfully used for trismus and provides the patient the ability to gradually control resistance along with increased oral aperture.

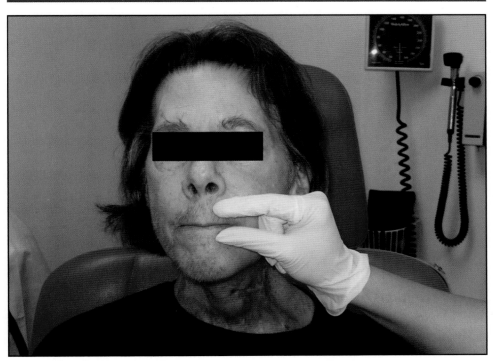

A

Fig 29–7. A. Lip resistance exercises: active closure against finger pressure to open. *continues*

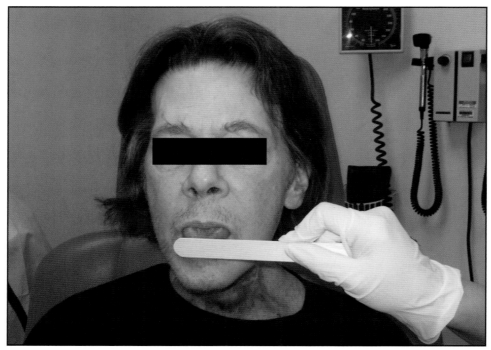

B

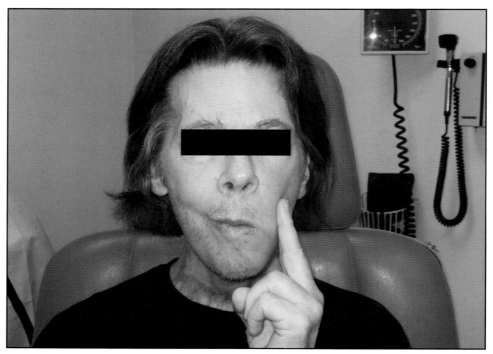

C

Fig 29–7. *continued* **B.** Tongue resistance exercises: active protrusion against tongue depressor. **C.** Tongue resistance exercises: active lateralization against cheek and digital pressure.

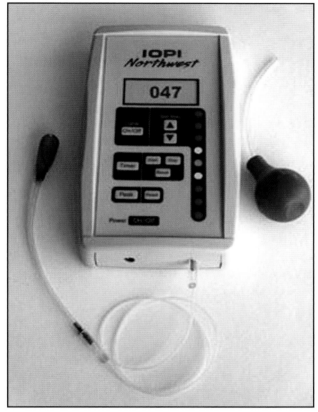

A

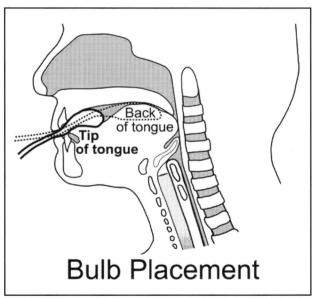

B

Fig 29–8. A. IOPI instrument. **B**. Schemata of tongue bulb in place.

Additional exercises can be performed for specific swallowing difficulties. Delayed triggering of the swallow response typically results in premature spillage of the bolus over the base of the tongue into the valleculae prior to the initiation of swallowing. Liquids are usually worse as they travel quicker. Thermal-tactile stimulation is aimed at improving the initiation of the pharyngeal swallow.[80] An iced laryngeal mirror (size 00) is applied to the anterior faucial arches with gentle but firm pressure in a stroking fashion to stimulate the swallow. This technique has been shown to alert the central nervous system to the presence of a bolus and the need to swallow, thus improving triggering of the swallow.[81]

Tongue base retraction to the posterior pharyngeal wall is critical to propel the bolus and assist initiation of cricopharyngeal relaxation and open the upper esophageal sphincter (UES). The Masako maneuver is designed to improve tongue base retraction and is practiced by having patients swallow with the tip of their tongue between their front teeth.[82]

Laryngeal elevation also is critical to airway protection during the swallow and may be restricted for a variety of underlying medical conditions including the presence of a tracheostomy tube, radiation fibrosis, or postsurgical scarring. Exercises to improve laryngeal motion are necessary to facilitate the anterior and superior movement that allows for separation of the airway from the pharynx. The Mendelsohn maneuver was developed to improve this function and involves voluntary laryngeal elevation and also has been shown to improve UES opening.[83] This exercise is accomplished by elevating the larynx as typically done at the beginning of a swallow and maintaining the contraction for a few seconds. In addition, vocal exercises including sliding glissandos, and sustaining a tone in a falsetto pitch level improve glottal closure, laryngeal elevation, and pharyngeal contraction.

Incomplete cricopharyngeal relaxation or cricopharyngeal dysfunction (CPD) results in pooling following the swallow. CPD may be a primary problem with the UES or a reaction to inadequate laryngeal motion and/or tongue base retraction. For primary causes of CPD, the Shaker exercises have been shown to improve laryngeal motion and UES relaxation.[84] This exercise is performed with the patient supine without pillow support under the head. The patient then elevates the head only, keeping the shoulders and upper body flat, to look toward their feet. For patients with secondary causes of CPD, exercises aimed at improving laryngeal elevation and tongue base retraction are recommended. In addition, both medical and surgical options have been tried to relax the cricopharyngeus and facilitate improved UES opening. Cricopharyngeal myotomy frequently is performed as part of a total laryngectomy and may be utilized secondarily in individuals with dysphagia related to CPD. However, efficacy of the procedure is questionable. Jacobs and colleagues[85] prospectively studied individuals undergoing supraglottic laryngectomy and/or tonsil with base of tongue resection and randomized them to myotomy or not.[85] They failed to find a significant difference between the two groups. Chemical denervation with botox injections also has been attempted with CPD. Although no randomized prospective clinical trials have been reported, subjective improvement in swallowing function with decreased pooling in the hypopharynx has been reported following botox injection into the cricopharyngeus muscle[86] (Fig 29-9).

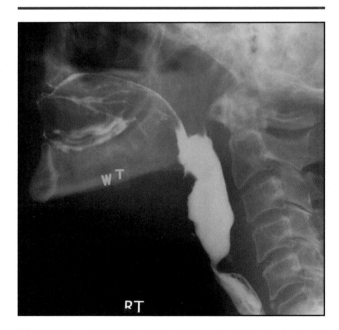

Fig 29-9. Lateral radiograph of patient s/p total laryngectomy with cricopharyngeal bar (posterior indentation).

Velopharyngeal incompetence (VPI) may result in nasal regurgitation and further impact swallowing function. Frequently, nasal regurgitation is more pronounced with thinner liquids as compared with other consistencies.

If VPI is due to a palatal defect following surgery or trauma, an obturator may be indicated to recreate the separation between the oral and nasal cavities. Palatal obturators have been shown to prevent nasal regurgitation as well as improving hypernasality[87] (Fig 29-10).

For individuals with VPI due to neurologic weakness of the soft palate, a palatal lift device can be made to hold the palate in an elevated position reducing the nasal regurgitation and improving speech. Surgical management for VPI also is an option and has been found to work better for structural versus neurologic deficits.

It should be noted that other techniques have been proposed for swallowing intervention including electrical stimulation (e-stim) but have not been adequately assessed and efficacy data are missing. Therapy for swallowing and/or speech following treatment for oral cavity lesions is specific to the deficits present.

Finally, the timing of swallowing intervention is an important factor. Currently, clinical trials are underway to evaluate the efficacy and timing of specific therapeutic techniques on swallow function. Timing of swallowing intervention varies depending on the oncologic treatment given to treat the head and neck cancer. Treatment after surgical resection ideally is initiated once the surgeon indicates that the patient has healed adequately, usually 3 to 10 days postsurgery. Delaying rehabilitation after surgical resection and prior to initiating postoperative radiotherapy can affect outcome. Rademaker at al[88] found that the recovery of partial laryngectomy patients who were relearning to swallow was delayed in those who had not reestablished oral intake prior to the initiation of postoperative radiotherapy. Treatment is usually performed while patients are undergoing chemoradiotherapy. However, treatment may be modified or delayed and swallowing function may be significantly compromised as the treatment often causes changes to oral and pharyngeal mucosa and structures. Patients should be encouraged to continue swallowing exercises on a daily basis long

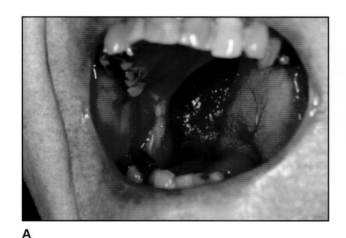

A

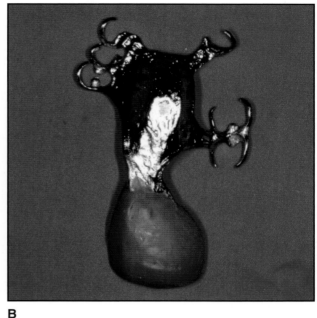

B

C

Fig 29–10. A. s/p composite resection with palatal defect. **B**. Palatal obturator. **C**. Placement of obturator into palatal defect.

after treatment, ideally for the rest of their lives, as the effects of chemoradiation therapy can occur years after treatment is completed. Head and neck cancer patients also should be educated to inform their physician of any negative decline in swallowing function as this can be indicative of disease recurrence or progression of tissue changes related to their cancer treatment(s). In general, speech-language pathologists do not perform aggressive swallowing therapy while patients are undergoing treatment but may guide the patient through exer-

cises to maintain as much function as possible. More aggressive therapy typically begins after the acute side effects of treatment have subsided.

Speech

Speech and voice therapy following treatment for head and neck cancer is aimed at restoring maximal, realistic function in the quickest amount of time. Rehabilitation of articulatory deficits that are related to decreased range of motion, strength, and flexibility of the dynamic articulators are treated similarly to the same deficits as they affect swallowing. Thus, oral facilitative exercises are also effective for speech/articulatory problems as detailed above.

Management of VPI is based on the nature and degree of insufficiency. In general, prosthetic options (obturators and palatal lifts) are made by the prosthodontists with information from the speech-language pathologist with regard to the area that needs augmenting to maximize oral/nasal resonance balance. Individuals with neurologic-based VPI do better with palatal lifts than surgical procedures whereas surgical defects can be managed either surgically or with an appliance. Speech therapy may be helpful to retrain the individual in obtaining the best benefit from either prosthetic or surgical management.

Dysphonia that results from either surgical and/or chemo- and radiation therapy may frequently be multifactorial. Xerostomia reduces lubrication to the vocal tract and when present alone may adversely affect vocal quality. Laryngopharyngeal reflux is common in the head and neck cancer population and its presence may further compound dysphonia. In addition, any scarring or reduced mobility that affects glottal closure or mucosal wave resolution may further impair vocal quality. Management of these problems is challenging. Patients usually are placed on a vocal hygiene program including increasing hydration, minimizing products that dehydrate the vocal tract (caffeine, tobacco, alcohol), anti-reflux precautions, and vocal conservation measures. Directed voice therapy to improve the technical aspects of voice usage also is indicated when the patient is hyperfunctioning their mechanism. It should be noted that the presence of vocal hyperfunction in these patients may represent a compensatory mechanism as otherwise vocal output would be even worse. Thus, therapy needs to take into account the nature of the difficulty to best plan the strategy. Traditional therapy aimed at improving breath management, tone focus, and minimizing hard glottal attacks all have been found to be useful.[55] Fex and Henricksson[89] found that concurrent voice therapy and instruction on vocal hygiene can significantly reduce the extent of tissue damage associated with radiation therapy.

Therapy following total laryngectomy has evolved over the years particularly after the advent of the tracheoesophageal puncture (TEP) that was introduced by Drs Blom and Singer.[90] The more traditional approaches focusing on the development of esophageal speech and/or use of an electrolarynx are not as widely used. However, the benefits and disadvantages of each method need to be taken into consideration with the individual patient's needs when determining the most appropriate method of alaryngeal speech rehabilitation. Although most studies demonstrate the superiority of the TEP in terms of voice outcome, it is important to recognize that not all patients are candidates for surgical voice restoration. There are physical and behavioral prerequisites that need to be met to increase likelihood of success with this method. Additionally, it is important to consider the patient's preference.

CONCLUSIONS

Evaluation and management of speech and swallowing disorders in head and neck cancer patients requires a thorough knowledge of the nature of the patient's oncologic treatment in order to design efficient and effective assessment and treatment strategies. Enhanced functional outcomes are best achieved via early intervention designed to improve nutritional status, normalize oral intake, and improve communication abilities.

REFERENCES

1. Robbins J, Hamilton J, Lof G, Kempster G. Oropharyngeal swallowing in normal adults of different ages. *Gastroenterology.* 1992;103:823–829.
2. Dodds WJ. The physiology of swallowing. *Dysphagia.* 1989;3:171–178.
3. Miller A. Neurophysiological basis of swallowing. *Dysphagia.* 1986;1:91–100.
4. Gleeson DC. Oropharyngeal swallowing and aging: a review. *J Comm Disord.* 1999;32:373–395.
5. Dodds WJ, Stewart ET, Logemann JA. Physiology and radiology of the normal oral and pharyngeal phases of swallowing. *Am J Roentgenol.* 1990; 158:953–963.

6. Mujica VR, Conklin J. When it's hard to swallow. What to look for in patients with dysphagia. *Postgrad Med.* 1999;105:141-142.

7. Glanze WD, Anderson KN, Anderson LE, eds. *The Signet Mosby Medical Dictionary.* Rev ed. New York, NY: Penguin Books, USA Inc; 1996:272-273.

8. Logemann JA. Swallowing physiology and pathophysiology. *Otolaryngol Clin North Am.* 1988;21:613-623.

9. Logemann JA. The dysphagia diagnostic procedure as a treatment efficacy trial. *Clin Comm Disor.* 1993;3:1-10.

10. Mendelsohn MS. New concepts in dysphagia management. *J Otolaryngol.* 1993;22(suppl 1):1-24.

11. Cook IJ, Dodds WJ, Dantas RO, et al. Timing of videofluoroscopic, manometric events, and bolus transit during the oral and pharyngeal phases of swallowing. *Dysphagia.* 1989;4:8-15.

12. Gaziano JE. Evaluation and management of oropharyngeal dysphagia in head and neck cancer. *Cancer Control.* 2002;9:400-409.

13. Robbins JG, Levin RL. Swallowing after unilateral stroke of the cerebral cortex: preliminary experience. *Dysphagia.* 1988;3:11-17.

14. Miller A, Bieger D, Conklin JL. Functional controls of deglutition. In: Perlman AL, Schulze-Delrieu, K eds. *Deglutition and Its Disorders.* San Diego, Calif: Singular; 1997:43-97.

15. Miller RM. Clinical examination for dysphagia. In: Groher ME, ed. *Dysphagia: Diagnosis and Management.* 3rd ed. Newton, Mass: Butterworth-Heinemann; 1997:169-189.

16. Ramsey DJC, Smithard, DG, Kalra, L. Early assessments of dysphagia and aspiration risk in acute stroke patients. *Stroke.* 2003;34:1252-1257.

17. Hoppers P, Holm SE. The role of fiberoptic endoscopy in dysphagia rehabilitation. *J Head Trauma Rehab.* 1999;14:475-485.

18. Lim SHB, Lieu PK, Phua SY, et al. Accuracy of bedside clinical methods compared with fiberoptic examination of swallowing (FEES) in determining the risk of aspiration in acute stroke patients. *Dysphagia.* 2001;16:1-6.

19. Mari F, Matei M, Ceravolo MG, Pisani A, Montesi A, Provinciali, L. Predictive value of clinical indices in detecting aspiration in patients with neurological disorders. *J Neurol Neurosurg Psych.* 1997;63:456-460.

20. Pauloski BR, Rademaker AW, Logemann JA, et al. Pre-treatment swallowing function in patients with head and neck cancer. *Head Neck.* 2000;22:474-482.

21. Aviv JE, Kim T, Sacco RL, et al. FEESST: a new bedside endoscopic test of the motor and sensory components of swallowing. *Ann Otolaryngol Rhinol Laryngol.* 1998;107:378-387.

22. Aviv JE, Kaplan ST, Thomson JE, Spitzer J, Diamond B, Close LG. The safety of flexible endoscopic evaluation of swallowing with sensory testing (FEESST): an analysis of 500 consecutive evaluations. *Dysphagia.* 2000;15;39-44.

23. Aviv JE, Takoudes TG, Ma G, Close L. Office-based esophagoscopy: a preliminary report. *Otolaryngol Head Neck Surg.* 2001;125:170-175.

24. Belafsky, PC. Office endoscopy for the laryngologist/bronchoesophagologist. *Curr Opin Otolaryngol Head Neck Surg.* 2002;10:467-470.

25. Postma GN, Bach KK, Belafsky PC, Koufman JA. The role of transnasal esophagoscopy in head and neck oncology. *Laryngoscope.* 2002;112:2242-2243.

26. Belafsky PC, Postma GN, Daniel E, Koufman JA. Transnasal esophagoscopy. *Otolaryngol Head Neck Surg.* 2001;125:588-589.

27. Dean R, Dua K, Massey B, Berger W, Hogan WJ, Shaker R. A comparative study of unsedated transnasal esophagogastroduodenoscopy and convention EGD. *Gastrointest Endoscopy.* 1996;44:422-424.

28. Dumortier J, Napoleon B, Hedelius F, et al. Unsedated transnasal EGD in daily practice: results with 1100 consecutive patients. *Gastrointest Endoscopy.* 2003;57(2):198-204.

29. Hiss SG, Huckabee, ML. Timing of pharyngeal and upper esophageal sphincter pressures as a function of normal and effortful swallowing in young healthy adults. *Dysphagia.* 2005;20:149-156.

30. Hamlet S, Choi J, Zormweier M, et al. Normal adult swallowing of liquid, viscous material: scintigraphic data on bolus transit and oropharyngeal residues. *Dysphagia.* 1996;11:41-47.

31. Logemann JA, Williams RB, Rademaker A, Pauloski BR, Lazarus CL, Cook I. The relationship between observations and measures of oral and pharyngeal residue from videofluorography and scintigraphy. *Dysphagia.* 2005;20:226-231.

32. Galli J, Volante M, Parrilla C, Rigante M, Valenza V. Oropharyngeal scintigraphy in the diagnostic algorithm of laryngopharyngeal reflux diseases: a useful exam? *Otolaryngol Head Neck Surg.* 2005;132:717-721.

33. Argon M, Secil Y, Duygun U, et al. The value of scintigraphy in the evaluation of oropharyngeal dysphagia. *Eur J Nucl Med Molec Imag.* 2004;31:94-98.

34. Vaiman M, Eviatar E, Segal S. Surface electromyographic studies of swallowing in normal subjects:

a review of 440 adults. Report 1. Quantitative data: timing measures. *Otolaryngol Head Neck Surg.* 2004;131:548-555.

35. Carnaby-Mann GD, Crary MA. Pill swallowing by adults with dysphagia. *Arch Otolaryngol Head Neck Surg.* 2005;131:970-975.

36. Crary MA, Carnaby-Mann GD, Groher ME, Helseth E. Functional benefits of dysphagia therapy using adjunctive sEMG biofeedback. *Dysphagia.* 2004; 19:160-164.

37. Kuhl V, Eicke BM, Dieterich M, Urban PP. Sonographic analysis of laryngeal elevation during swallowing. *J Neurol.* 2003;250:333-337.

38. Logemann JA. *Evaluation and Treatment of Swallowing Disorders.* San Diego, Calif: College-Hill Press; 1983.

39. Casas MJ, Seo AH, Keny DJ. Sonographic examination of the oral phase of swallowing: bolus image enhancement. *J Clin Ultrasound.* 2002;30:83-87.

40. Fisher, HB, Logemann, JA. *The Fisher-Logemann Test of Articulation.* Austin, Tex: Competence. Pro-Ed;1971.

41. Yorkston KM, Beukelman DR, Traynor CD. Articulatory adequacy in dysarthric speakers: a comparison of judging formats. *J Comm Disord.* 1988;21: 351-361.

42. Pauloski, BR, Logemann, JA, Rademaker, AW, et al. Speech and swallowing function after anterior tongue and floor of mouth resection with distal flap reconstruction. *J Med Speech-Lang Pathol.* 1993;2:191-210.

43. Hamlet S, Faull J, Klein B, et al. Mastication and swallowing in patients with postirradiation xerostomia. *Int J Radiat Oncol Biol Phys.* 1997;37: 789-796.

44. Jacobson MC, Franssen E, Fliss DM, Birt BD, Gilbert RW. Free forearm flap in oral reconstruction. Functional outcome. *Arch Otolaryngol Head Neck Surg.* 1995;121:959-964.

45. Logemann JA, Bytell DA. Swallowing disorders in three types of head and neck surgical patients. *Cancer.* 1979;44:1095-1105.

46. McConnel F, Teichgraeber J, Adler R. A comparison of three methods of oral reconstruction. *Arch Otolaryngol Head Neck Surg.* 1987;113:495-500.

47. Imai S, Michi K. Articulatory function after resection of the tongue and floor of the mouth: Palatometric and perceptual evaluation. *J Speech Hear Res.* 1992;35:68-78.

48. Leonard R, Goodrich S, McMenamin P, Donald P. Differentiation of speakers with glossectomies by acoustic and perceptual measures. *Am J Speech-Lang Pathol.* 1992;1:56-63.

49. Hara I, Gellrich NC, Duker J, et al. Swallowing and speech function after intraoral soft tissue reconstruction with lateral upper arm free flap and radial forearm free flap. *Br J Oral Maxillofac Surg.* 2003;41:161-169.

50. Hsiao SF, Wu YT, Wu HD, Wang TG. Comparison of effectiveness of pressure threshold and targeted resistance devices for inspiratory muscle training in patients with chronic obstructive pulmonary disease. *J Formosan Med Associ.* 2003;102: 240-245.

51. Fujimoto Y, Hasegawa Y, Nakayama B, Matsuura H. Usefulness and limitation of cricopharyngeal myotomy and laryngeal suspension after wide resection of the tongue or oropharynx. *Nippon Jibiinkoka Gakkai Kaiho (Jap).* 1998;101:307-311.

52. Seikaly H, Rieger J, Wolfaardt J, Moysa G, Harris J, Jha N. Functional outcomes after primary oropharyngeal cancer resection and reconstruction with the radial forearm free flap. *Laryngoscope.* 2003; 113:897-904.

53. Zeitels SM. Phonomicrosurgical treatment of early glottic cancer and carcinoma in situ. *Am J Surg.* 1996;172:704-709.

54. Zeitels SM. Premalignant epithelium and microinvasive cancer of the vocal fold. The evolution of phonomicrosurgical management. *Laryngoscope.* 1995;67(suppl 1):1-5.

55. Orlikoff RF, Krauss DH. Dysphonia following nonsurgical management of advance laryngeal carcinoma. *Am J Speech Lang Pathol.* 1996;5:47-52.

56. Harrison LB, Solomon B, Miller S, Fass DE, Armstrong J, Sessions RB. Prospective computer-assisted voice analysis for patients with early stage glottic cancer: a preliminary report of the functional result of laryngeal irradiation. *Int J Radiat Oncol Biol Phys.* 1990;19:123-127.

57. Verdolini K, Titze IR, Fennell A. Dependence of phonatory effort on hydration level. *J Speech Hear Res.* 1994;37:1001-1007.

58. Bernal-Sprekelson M, Vilaseca-Gonzalez I, Blanch-Alejandro JL. Predictive values for aspiration after endoscopic laser resections of malignant tumors of the hypopharynx and larynx. *Head Neck.* 2004;26:103-110.

59. Dworkin JP, Meleca RJ, Zacharek MA, et al. Voice and deglutition functions after the supracricoid and total laryngectomy procedures for advanced stage laryngeal carcinoma. *Otolaryngol Head Neck Surg.* 2003;129:311-320.

60. McConnel FM, Mendelsohn MS, Logemann JA. Examination of swallowing after total laryngectomy using manofluorography. *Head Neck Surg.* 1986; 9:3-12.
61. Ackerstaff AH, Hilgers FJM, Aaronson NK, Balm AJM. Communication, functional disorders and lifestyle changes after total laryngectomy. *Clin Otolaryngol.* 1994;19:295-300.
62. Mendelsohn MS. The Modified Barium Swallow database. *Dysphagia.* 1994;9:47-53.
63. McConnel FM, Hester TR, Mendelsohn MS, Logemann JA. Manoflorography of deglutition after total laryngectomy. *Plast Reconstr Surg.* 1988;81: 346-351.
64. Lazarus CL, Logemann JA, Pauloski BR, et al. Swallowing and tongue function following treatment for oral and oropharyngeal cancer. *J Speech Lang Hear Res.* 2000;43:1011-1023.
65. Logemann JA, Pauloski BR, Rademaker AW, et al. Xerostomia: 12-month changes in saliva production and its relationship to perception and performance of swallow function, oral intake, and diet after chemoradiation. *Head Neck.* 2003;25:1082.
66. Woo P. Arytenoid adduction and medialization laryngoplasty. *Otolaryngol Clin North Am.* 2000; 33:817-840.
67. Smith RV, Goldman SY, Beitler JJ, Wadler SS. Decreased short- and long-term swallowing problems with altered radiotherapy dosing used in an organ-sparing protocol for advanced pharyngeal carcinoma. *Arch Otolaryngol Head Neck Surg.* 2004;130:831-836.
68. Milano MT, Vokes EE, Kao J, et al. Intensity-modulated radiation therapy in advanced head and neck patients treated with intensive chemotherapy: preliminary experience and future directions. *Int J Oncol.* 2006;28:1141-1151.
69. Garden AS, Forster K, Wong PF, Morrison WH, Schechter NR, Ang KK. Results of radiotherapy for T2N0 glottic carcinoma: does the "2" stand for twice-daily treatment? *Int J Radiat Oncol Biol Phys.* 2003;55:322-328.
70. Eisbruch A, Lyden T, Bradford CR, et al. Objective assessment of swallowing dysfunction and aspiration after radiation concurrent with chemotherapy for head-and-neck cancer. *Int J Radiat Oncol Biol Phys.* 2002;53:4-5.
71. Lazarus CL. Effects of radiation therapy and voluntary maneuvers on swallow functioning in head and neck cancer patients. *Clin Comm Disord.* 1993;3:11-20.
72. Park RH, Allison MC, Lang J, et al. Randomized comparison of percutaneous endoscopic gastrostomy and nasogastric tube feeding in patients with persisting neurological dysphagia. *Br Med J.* 1992;304:1406-1409.
73. Logemann JA, Pauloski BR, Rademaker AW, Colangelo LA. Speech and swallowing rehabilitation for head and neck cancer patients. *Oncology.* 1997; 11:651-656.
74. Barlow SW, Abbs JH. Force transducers for the evaluation of labial, lingual, and mandibular motor impairments. *J Speech Hear Res.* 1983;26:616-621.
75. Robin DA, Somodi LB, Luschei ES. Measurement of tongue strength and endurance in normal and articulation disordered participants. In: Moore CA, Yorkston KM, Beukelman DR, eds. *Dysarthria and Apraxia of Speech: Perspectives on Management.* Baltimore, Md. Brookes; 1991:173-184.
76. Robbins J. Oral strengthening and swallowing outcomes. *Perspec Swallow Swallow Disord.* SID 13. 2003;12:16-19.
77. Sullivan P, Hind JA, Robbins J. Lingual exercise protocol for head and neck cancer: a case study. *Dysphagia.* 2001;16:154.
78. Lazarus CL, Logemann JA, Huang CF, Rademaker AW. Effects of two types of tongue strengthening exercises in young normals. *Folia Phoniatr Logoped.* 2003;55:199-205.
79. Rodriguez B. *Management of trismus in head and neck practice.* Presented at Society of Otorhinotolaryngology and Head and Neck Nurses 19th Annual Congress. New Orleans, La; 1995.
80. Bisch EM, Logemann JA, Rademaker AW, Kahrilas PJ, Lazarus CL. Pharyngeal effects of bolus volume, viscosity, and temperature in patients with dysphagia resulting from neurologic impairment and in normal subjects. *J Speech Hear Res.* 1994;37: 1041-1059.
81. Lazzara G, Lazarus C, Logemann JA. Impact of thermal stimulation on the triggering of the swallowing reflex. *Dysphagia.*1986;1:73-77.
82. Fujiu M, Logemann JA. Effect of a tongue-holding maneuver on posterior pharyngeal wall movement during deglutition. *Am J Speech Lang Pathol.* 1996;5:23-30.
83. Kahrilas PJ, Dodds WJ, Dent J, Logemann JA, Shaker R. Upper esophageal sphincter function during deglutition. *Gastroenterology.* 1988;95:52-62.
84. Shaker R, Kern M, Bardan E, et al. Augmentation of deglutitive upper esophageal sphincter opening

in the elderly by exercise. *Am J Physiol.* 1997;272:
1518-1522.

85. Jacobs JR, Logemann J, Pajak TF, et al. Failure of
cricopharyngeal myotomy to improve dysphagia
following head and neck cancer surgery. *Arch Otolaryngol Head Neck Surg.* 1999;126:804-805.

86. Blitzer A, Brin MF. Use of botulinum toxin for diagnosis and management of cricopharyngeal achalasia.
Otolaryngol Head Neck Surg. 1997;116:328-330.

87. DaBreo EL, Ghalichebaf M. Provisional restoration
for a patient with cleft lip and palate: a clinical
report. *J Prosth Dent.* 1990;63:119-121.

88. Rademaker AW, Logemann JA, Pauloski BR, et al.
Recovery of postoperative swallowing in patients
undergoing partial laryngectomy. *Head Neck.*
1993;15:325-334.

89. Fex S, Henriksson B. Phoniatric treatment combined with radiotherapy of laryngeal cancer for the
avoidance of radiation damage. *Acta Otolaryngol.*
1970;263:128-129.

90. Singer MI, Blom ED. An endoscopic technique for
restoration of voice after laryngectomy. *Ann Otol
Rhinol Laryngol.* 1980;89:529-533.

30

Interpreting and Reporting Results of Head and Neck Cancer Treatment

Kristen B. Pytynia

INTRODUCTION

Head and neck cancer affects 40,000 people each year in the United States.[1] Globally, head and neck cancer, specifically squamous cell carcinoma (SCC), has reached epidemic proportions, affecting over 600,000 people annually.[2] Head and neck cancer is the most common cancer in India due to high rates of use of tobacco and other orally active carcinogenic compounds.[3] Despite advances in surgical and radiation techniques as well as new chemotherapy compounds and concurrent chemoradiation protocols, the survival from head and neck cancer has not increased significantly over the past 6 decades. These statistics underscore the importance of clinical trials directed at improving the survival and function of those afflicted with this cancer.

Head and neck cancer can be particularly difficult to treat due to the complex functions that are innate to this region, particularly those related to speech, swallowing, and breathing. These systems can be affected by both tumor and subsequent therapy. Furthermore, patients can also suffer severe cosmetic deformities. Quality of life studies have shown that patients place great importance on social activities, such as eating in public, speaking on the phone, or having visible deformities.[4,5] Clinical trials are paramount to the advancement of quality of life outcomes in patients with head and neck cancer. The wide range of possible cancer or treatment related side effects, along with the rarity of head and neck cancer when compared to other sites (breast, prostate, lung) dictate that head and neck cancer patients, particularly those with advanced stage, should be treated by an experienced medical team.

Quality of life and survival issues combine to make the multidisciplinary approach essential for patients with head and neck cancer. The multidisciplinary approach involves medical personnel of many different specialties in the patient's treatment plan. The head and neck cancer treatment team should include head and neck oncologic surgeons, medical oncologists, radiation oncologists, dental oncologists, oral and maxillofacial surgeons, prosthedontists, speech therapists, audiologists, physical therapists, and others. The multidisciplinary approach allows all aspects of a patient's care to be considered prior to receiving initial therapy, with a combined goal of improving both survival and functional outcomes. Over the past 3 decades, this has radically changed the medical approach to head and neck cancer. Patients that in the past would have been treated with morbid surgical excisions may now be successfully treated with chemotherapy, radiation therapy, and less extensive surgery. One particular example is tonsil squamous cell carcinoma. Tonsil SCC has been found to be particularly sensitive to radiation alone or chemoradiation for extensive disease, allowing patients to avoid radical surgical excisions while maintaining survival rates and improving speech and swallowing function. Radiation with or without chemotherapy has now become the recommended therapy for locoregionally advanced tonsil cancer in the United States.[6]

It is the use of the multidisciplinary approach that has stimulated clinical trials in head and neck cancer. Trials are conducted with the aims of improving survival and quality of life. One of the first large scale trials was the Department of Veterans Affairs laryngeal cancer study, which examined the use of radiation and chemotherapy for advanced squamous cell carcinoma of the larynx, with the main outcome measure being laryngeal preservation. This study showed that organ sparing chemoradiation can be a viable alternative to total laryngectomy in certain patients with squamous cell carcinoma.[7] A subsequent Intergroup 91-11 study showed that laryngeal preservation ranged from 69% to 84% with chemoradiation.[8,9] Quality of life studies have shown a mild improvement in quality of life in patients with chemoradiation, though other studies suggest this may not be due to organ preservation.[4,10]

Clinical trials allow multiple institutions to cooperate and better determine what treatments are best for each subset of head and neck cancer patients. Cooperation among multiple institutions allows for enrollment of a larger number of patients than single institution trials. Oncologists at smaller institutions may then benefit from information gathered from larger clinical trials in order to determine the best treatment options for their patient population. This chapter arms the clinician with the skills necessary to properly assess the validity of a clinical trial, and possible applications for clinical trials data in their head and neck cancer population.

INTERPRETATION OF TRIALS

Clinical trials are classified according to the Food and Drug Administration. Phase I trials are designed to assess the safety of a new treatment on human patients after laboratory studies show promise. For pharmaceutical trials, phase I trials may use escalating doses of the new therapy in order to determine the safety profile. Endpoints of phase I studies are related to toxicity only, not disease status, as the goal is to evaluate safety only and these studies do not claim to report efficacy of the agent(s) studied. Phase II trials are initiated after phase I trials have proven that a therapy is safe. Phase II trials are used to determine the efficacy of the therapy, that is, to show if the new therapy has the desired effect, usually prolonging disease-free survival or preventing known treatment related side effects. Phase II trials often include dose escalation to determine the proper dosing of the new therapeutic drug. Phase II trials consist of a small number of people (20-100 depending on the prevalence of the disease), and often the patients enrolled in Phase II studies have no other alternative treatments. Therefore, poor outcomes in a phase II trial may not be indicative of a treatments efficacy, but rather the patient population studied. Phase III trials expand upon phase II trials by enrolling a larger number of patients, typically greater than 100, who are randomly placed into control or experimental groups to compare endpoints between these groups. Phase III trials must report outcome endpoints, including overall survival, disease-specific survival, and disease-free survival, as well as toxicity. Trials may be closed early if unexpected toxicity or deaths are found, or if preliminary results show significant improvement in survival in the experimental group.[11]

The largest and best known organizations running clinical trials for head and neck cancer patients in the United States are the Radiation Therapy Oncology Group (RTOG), the Eastern Clinical Oncology Group (ECOG), the National Cancer Institute, and the Southwest Clinical Oncology Group (SWOG). The American College of Surgeon's Oncology Group (ACOSOG) focuses on trials involving surgical management of oncology patients. These groups are dedicated to discovering treatment techniques to maximize the quality of life and survival of oncology patients. Trials initiated by these groups are particularly useful in uncommon disease states. The larger number of patients that can be recruited by cooperative groups enable enough patients to be enrolled in studies on uncommon diseases to potentially reach statistically significant results. Institutions that participate in the trials are members of the groups, but the oncology groups themselves act independently, without influence from the institutions' political or financial interests. In these trials, patient inclusion criteria, medication doses, and adverse outcomes are strictly monitored. This allows patients to be treated safely with experimental medications to possibly improve the treatment of patients with head and neck cancer. Strict guidelines for patient care, and inclusion criteria, and the ability to recruit patients from multiple institutions (thereby increasing the power of the study) make the outcomes of the various oncology groups some of the most compelling. Patients with advanced disease or those undergoing new treatments should be treated on a national or regional protocol. This not only ensures the quality of their care but also adds to the depth of knowledge about head and neck cancer.

Trials also may be conducted within a single institution. All institutions that conduct clinical trials have an internal regulatory committee which governs clinical trials, called the Institutional Review Board (IRB). The goal of the IRB is to ensure the safety of the patients as well as the scientific merit of each trial. Protocols must be reviewed for safety and merit, and approved by each institution prior to commencing the study. Committees are composed of medical personnel from multiple disciplines, ethicists, and legal professionals. Often they will suggest changes that must be made to ensure patient safety. Protocols that do not meet the minimum standard of care are rejected. All trials must have IRB approval prior to subject recruitment, and are monitored throughout the trial. Furthermore, most journals require that a trial has IRB approval before they will consider publishing results. All of these controls are designed to ensure patient safety scientific validity and integrity.

Patients often worry that participation in clinical trials means that they are receiving experimental therapy. This is most often not the case. Clinical trials, particularly phase III trials, may use agents that have been well studied in other patients but not yet studied in the head and neck cancer population, or not yet studied in combination with other agents. The trial may be designed to determine the right dose of a chemotherapy agent or timing of radiation therapy. Clinical trials should not automatically be interpreted as experimental therapy, but rather as an attempt to provide a specific dose or combination of therapies under strictly regulated conditions. Patients, particularly those with advanced disease, should be encouraged to have treatment under pro-

tocol-based clinical trials in an attempt to improve evidenced based medicine for patients with head and neck cancer.

Clinical trials include strict criteria for inclusion and exclusion. One common area of exclusion is a patient's performance status. Patients who are too ill to undergo the stress of the treatment are often excluded from the trials. The ECOG performance status (range from 0 to 5) is one commonly used measure the performance (Table 30-1). There are also strict controls over which events must be reported. If the patient has a treatment related toxicity or death, this must be reported in a timely manner to the IRB or group monitoring the study. Toxicities related to treatment include hematologic, gastrointestinal, neurologic, cardiac, pulmonary, or infectious events.

Statistics

In order to understand clinical trials, one must first understand the outcome measures reported by these

Table 30–1. ECOG Performance Status*

Grade	ECOG
0	Fully active, able to carry on all predisease performance without restriction
1	Restricted in physically strenuous activity but ambulatory and able to carry out work of a light or sedentary nature (eg, light housework, office work)
2	Ambulatory and capable of all self-care but unable to carry out any work activities. Up and about more than 50% of waking hours
3	Capable of only limited self-care, confined to bed or chair more than 50% of waking hours
4	Completely disabled. Cannot carry on any self-care. Totally confined to bed or chair
5	Dead

From Eastern Cooperative Oncology Group, Robert Comis MD, Group Chair.[12]

Source: Oken, Creech, Tormey, et al. *Am J Clin Oncol.* 1982;5: 649–655.[12]

studies. Survival is an important endpoint of oncologic clinical trials. Survival analysis allows the reader to determine if the study protocol increases the lifetime of patients who receive therapy. The study protocol can be a new surgical technique, a new or different dose of chemotherapy, a new radiation technique, or even a nonchemotherapy drug that may reduce fatal side effects. The survival improvement should be statistically significant, meaning that the improvement was not random chance, but has been shown mathematically to be related to the introduction of the new treatment. It is mathematically impossible to irrefutably prove that a new treatment improves survival; therefore, mathematicians, and clinicians accept the 95% level as acceptable, meaning that a study is significant if there is a 95% likelihood that the survival difference is due to the new treatment rather than by chance alone. The p value indicates the chance that the results of the study are due to chance, and therefore a p value of less than 0.05 (corresponding to 5%) is an acceptable level to determine relevance of the study. Therefore, when analyzing survival studies, the study should include the time that each group survived, as well as the p value associated with this difference in survival times.

The survival time is reported as the mean survival time. This is the average time that all patients in the group survived, calculated by adding each patient's survival time and dividing by the number of patients in the study. As studies are limited by the amount of time each patient is followed, the maximum amount of survival will be the longest time that a patient survived. Note that this often is limited by the duration of the study, in that some patients will still be surviving at the time the study is reported, and therefore their survival time is from when they enrolled until the study ended. The mean is not equivalent to the median, which is the middle survival value if all survival times are placed in a numerically ascending row. The astute reader will note that a study can report biased results if they report a mean and do not include a median. For example, in a study with 5 patients (pts), pt 1 survived 1 day, pt 2 survived 2 days, pt 3 survived 3 days pt survived 4 days, and pt 5 survived 500 days. There is quite a difference in survival between pts 1 to 4 and pt 5. The mean survival is 102 days, whereas the median survival is 3 days. In this case, the median is more reflective of the actual survival among the group rather than the mean. Large differences between the mean and the median can alert the reader to a possible bias, and both mean and median values should be reported. The 95% confidence interval (CI) of the mean also should be reported. The 95% CI is calculated by the examining the difference of each value within the series from the calculated mean, squaring the difference, multiplying the sum of squares by $1/n$ where n is the number of subjects in the set, and taking the square root of that entire value. Although it sounds complex, the importance of the 95% CI is that it is a range of values in which 95% of the actual numbers will lie. If the 95% CI is similar to the mean, this tells the reader that most of the specific values of survival were close to the mean. If the 95% CI is a wide range, this alerts the readers that there was a large range of actual survival values, and that the study must be interpreted with a little more caution. Again, a strong study will report the mean, the median, and the 95% CI so that readers may determine for themselves how reliable the reported mean may actually be.

The three most common survival outcome measures are overall survival, disease-specific survival, and recurrence-free or disease-free survival. Overall survival measures the time interval from the completion of treatment to death by any cause whether it is disease related or due to an unrelated cause. If a patient has a heart attack, or a motor vehicle accident, or dies from recurrent disease, these events are all considered an endpoint for overall survival. When patients die, they are said to have experienced an event, or outcome. Each event is specific to the type of analysis being conducted. In overall survival analyses, the event is the death of the patient. Other analyses examine more specific events. Disease-specific survival relates to deaths due to a particular disease only, and only patients who die of that disease will be considered to have an event. If the patient dies of another cause, he or she will not be included as having an event. Only those who die due to their disease are included in this analysis. Recurrence-free (or disease-free) survival analysis analyzes the time to disease recurrence. If a patient develops a recurrence, he is considered to have an event, and is no longer followed for that particular outcome, as it has already occurred. In this case, unlike overall survival or disease-specific survival, the event is recurrence, not death. Whether the patient survives the recurrence is irrelevant; this analysis only considers recurrence. The specific definition of outcome measures and each event becomes important during the upcoming discussion of Kaplan Meier survival values. The most effective study protocols will produce an improvement in not only overall survival, but also disease-free and recurrence-free survival.

Relative Risk

The statistical terms used to convey the risk associated with exposure to a possible causative factor is termed a relative risk. Similar though not mathematically equal terms are odds ratio, or hazard ratio, depending on whether the study is prospective or retrospective, and whether survival is the particular measurement of analysis. Relative risk (RR) is defined as the ratio of the incidence of an event in one group given an exposure (experimental group) compared to the incidence of an event in another group given no exposure (control group). For example, we would like to know the effect of postoperative chemotherapy in addition to radiation compared to radiation alone in high-risk patients, and we will use the data published by Bernier et al.[13] For this type of analysis, it is important to define the experimental and control groups. In the current case, the experimental exposure is the postoperative concurrent administration of chemotherapy with radiation and the experimental group is that group of patients who received postoperative chemoradiation. The control group is the group of patients who do not undergo postoperative chemoradiation but undergo radiation alone. The event is death at 5 years. The RR is the incidence of death in the experimental group compared to the incidence of death in the control group. A RR greater than one means that the exposed group (chemoradiation group) is more likely to die at 5 years compared to the nonexposed group(radiation only group). A RR is calculated by a 2 × 2 table. The 2 × 2 table is critical to understand relative risk. We will now construct a 2 × 2 table (Table 30–2). Remember that we include in our analysis only those that have been followed up for 5 years, or died by

Table 30–2. 2 × 2 Table to Calculate Relative Risk

	Dead	Alive	Total
Experimental Postoperative chemoradiation	A 45	B 47	A + B 92
Control Postoperative radiation	C 71	D 31	C + D 102
	A + C 116	B + D 78	A + B + C + D 194

5 years. Patients who are alive but have not been followed for 5 years are not included, as we cannot predict what will happen to them. The experimental and control group are the columns, and dead and alive are the rows.

The incidence of death at 5 years given postoperative chemoradiation (experimental group) is the number of people who have died after chemoradiation over the total number of people who have received chemoradiation, A/ (A+B) = 45/92 = 0.48.

The incidence of death at 5 years given postoperative radiation only (control group) is the number of people who have died after postoperative radiation only over the total number of people who have received postoperative radiation only, C/ (C+D) = 71/102 = 0.69.

The RR is the ratio of those incidences.

$$RR = \frac{A/ (A+B)}{C/ (C+D)} = \frac{45/92}{71/102} = 0.70$$

Note that any RR (not just survival) can be determined by filling out the appropriate 2 × 2 table. As long as the exposure and the event are defined, the RR can be calculated. For example, the risk of developing SCCHN after exposure to a chemical spill could be determined easily. In this example, cases would have SCCHN, controls would not, and the exposure would take the palce of the dead or alive columns as above. The new 2 × 2 table would look like Table 30–3.

The same formula $RR = \frac{A/ (A+B)}{C/ (C+D)}$ could be used to determine RR.

Table 30–3. Example of Determining RR Using Exposure and Event Data

	Exposed	Not Exposed	Total
Case: SCHHN	A	B	A + B
Control: No SCCHN	C	D	C + D
	A + C	B + D	A + B + C + D

Odds ratio (OR), hazard ratio (HR), and risk ratio are all terms similar to Relative Risk, but not equivalent. These terms all differ based on the timing of the study, but are all related as they are all ratios of events in exposed versus nonexposed persons. Retrospective studies start with cases and controls, then look back to examine differences in events that may have influenced some patients to become cases and others to remain controls. The OR is the measure used in retrospective cases. For example, in studying the effect of smoking on the development of SCCHN, cases and controls would be questioned about smoking history. The OR associated would be the chance of developing SCCHN in those exposed to smoking compared to the chance of developing SCCHN in those not exposed to smoking, which easily could be determined by filling out the above 2 × 2 table and again determining the ratio. Note that this differs from RR in that we started with a select group of cases and controls and looked back to see whether or not exposure had happened, rather than monitoring and controlling the exposure. The word risk cannot be used in retrospective studies, as exposure was not controlled. The hazards ratio is similar to a RR, except that it is used exclusively in survival analysis and employs a mathematical analysis that accounts for change in risk over time. This is especially important in studies in which the risk of death may change over time. For example, we know that patients with SCCHN are more likely to die within the first 2 years of diagnosis, and therefore the risk of death changes over time. A strong study will report the hazards ratio, but a relative risk can be very similar if large enough subjects are analyzed and the timing of the study is only a few years.

When conducting clinical research, it is standard to express the goals of the study as the null hypothesis and the alternative hypothesis. The null hypothesis is that there is no difference in the risk of death of patients who receive postoperative chemoradiation compared to those who receive postoperative radiation only: RR = 1. The alternative hypothesis is that there is a change in the risk of death of patients who receive postoperative chemoradiation compared to those who receive postoperative radiation only. If RR >1, then there is a greater chance of death among the experimental group, or a greater chance of death in those who received postoperative chemoradiation therapy. If RR <1, then there is a smaller chance of death among the experimental group. Here, because our RR = 0.70, we accept the alternative hypothesis that there is a smaller chance of death (0.7 times smaller) after postoperative chemoradiation compared to those with postoperative radiation alone because.

It is very difficult to prove with 100% accuracy that the null hypothesis is invalid, therefore, scientific research has accepted that a 5% error rate is an acceptable error rate. This is referred to as the p value. A p value of 0.05 means that there is a 5% chance of wrongly rejecting the null hypothesis. A p value of 0.001 means that there is a 0.1% chance of incorrectly rejecting the null hypothesis. The 95% confidence interval (95% CI) is a range of values of the relative risk. This is mathematically determined in such a way that there a 95% likelihood that the real value is within that range. If the 95% CI contains the value of the null hypothesis, then the results of the study are not significant. This means that there is a greater than 5% chance that the null hypothesis is valid. Looking at it mathematically, this means that the actual ratio may be <1, 1, or >1, as all of these are included within the 95% CI. For example, a RR = 1.2 {95% CI [0.6–2.0]} means that the calculated relative risk was 1.2 and the 95% confidence interval for the relative risk ranges from 0.6 to 2.0. If the relative risk is 1, then there is no increased risk with exposure, if the relative risk is <1 then there is a decreased risk with exposure and if the relative risk is >1, then there is an increased risk with exposure. You can see in the current example that all of these possibilities are within the 95% confidence interval and, thus, you cannot tell whether there is any increased risk with the exposure. This example shows that the value of the relative risk is often not as important as the 95% CI. Substituting the data for postoperative chemoradiation example, the RR = 0.70, and the 95% CI is 0.55 to 0.90. The p value is <0.01. Note that all of the possible values of the RR in the 95% CI (0.55-0.9) are less than 1. We can therefore accept the alternative hypothesis and say that there is a 0.7 times decreased risk of death with postoperative chemoradiation therapy compared to postoperative radiation only. We are 95% confident of this because the p value is less than 0.05, and the 95% CI does not contain the value 1.

Kaplan Meier Survival Curve

The Kaplan Meier survival curve is a graphic representation of the outcomes reported by clinical trials and other studies. The Kaplan Meier survival curves allow the reader to quickly and easily understand the data presented with the variable or outcome studied defined for each curve. Most often, curves look at survival, either overall survival, disease-related survival, or recurrence-free survival. The curve is created by graphing the percentage of people surviving on the y-axis versus the length of time the patient survived on the x-axis. Each patient has a point on the curve. In clinical trials, all patients are not followed until their death. Some continue to survive past the length of time on the graph, and others are considered to be "censored" out. A patient will be censored out when they no longer have any follow-up. This can occur for multiple reasons. A patient can be censored because they were lost to follow-up, or because the follow-up time for that patient is limited. These patients have not died, and, therefore, cannot be considered to have had an event. After a patient is censored that patient is not counted as an event, rather the patient is mathematically removed from the study. For example, if a study of 100 people shows 2 deaths in the first year and 2 censored patients, the survival without the consideration of the 2 censored patients would be 98 survivors out of 100 patients still alive in the study, 98/100 = 98%. In a Kaplan Meier calculation, the 2 censored patients are mathematically removed from the patient pool as if they were not a part of the study from that point on. In this case, the calcu-

lation would be performed as if the patient pool contained 98 patients rather than 100. The survival calculation would be 96 survivors out of 98 patients still in the study, or 96/98 = 97.96%. If 2 more patients are censored out in the next time interval, and 2 more die, the survival for that time period is 92/96 = 95.83%. This is multiplied by the previous survival rate (97.96 * 95.83 = 93.87%) to come up with an overall survival rate of 93.87%. If we had not accounted for the censored patients, our survival rate at the end of the second time interval would be 94/100 = 94%. As you can see, there is little impact on the results if the number of censored patients is relatively small. As the number of censored patients reaches more than 10% of the study population the impact of the censoring becomes important. In a typical Kaplan Meier graph, as you move to the right along the x-axis, more and more patients are censored. This can make the right side of the graph less accurate than the left. In patients with head and neck cancer, the majority of patients will recur within the first 2 years, and almost all recurrences will occur before 5 years. Therefore, any survival curve that does not have a mean follow-up time of 2 years should be suspect. Those patients with short follow-ups will be censored and, thus, the right side of the graph will represent significantly fewer patients and be less accurate. The Kaplan Meier survival curve can be applied to overall death from any cause, to death due to disease, or even time to recurrence, as long as the event is defined.

Quality of Life

Quality of life (QOL) issues also are important, particularly in patients with head and neck cancer, and measures should be reported in clinical trials. The complex relationship between function and form in the head and neck impacts all aspects of social and emotional health. Patients find that communication, swallowing, and decreased pain are important QOL measures. A well-designed trial should report on the patients' QOL, for example, eating habits, tracheostomy dependence, feeding tube dependence, and other side effects of therapy. Many have criticized the VA laryngeal trial for not including in the original report information on speech and swallowing function after chemoradiation of the larynges. Subsequent reports on long-term survivors of the VA laryngeal trial have shown that the organ preservation group scored significantly better on many QOL domains, but not necessarily on speech.[4]

Types of Reported Studies

In order to understand clinical trials, we must further understand the types of studies that are reported and several types are found in the clinical literature: case reports, case series, retrospective reviews, case control studies, and prospective clinical trials. Case reports and case series can illustrate interesting examples of treatment options, but they do not provide evidence. The information gleaned from case reports and case series often fuel prospective clinical trials. Retrospective studies are studies that analyze existing data and report the outcome of that data. Retrospective studies cannot manipulate any of the data within the study. Treatment has already been given prior to the beginning of the study; therefore, data from retrospective analyses reflect the outcomes from that treatment. Furthermore, treatment likely is not standardized across the entire study population. Retrospective studies vary in quality according to their inclusion criteria as well as the information gathered. A prospective study begins with no patients, and recruits patients into the study as they are diagnosed. The treatment is dictated according to strict guidelines. Clinical trials are, by definition, all prospective. Patients are recruited by strict criteria, and treated according to a well-defined treatment plan. The prospective recruitment of patients limits the variability of both patient variables by only recruiting a strict subset of patients as well as treatment variability by assigning patients to strict treatment protocols. The studies that provide the strongest evidence and hence have the greatest clinical impact are randomized, prospective clinical trials. The term randomized refers to patients being assigned an arm of treatment (control or experimental) based on change, with the patient having no input as to the type of treatment. Randomization is usually done with a computer program, assigning patients to the control or experimental arm. Prospective studies also may be nonrandomized, with the patient picking the type of treatment they receive, either experimental or control treatment. If patients are not randomized, this may introduce inequalities between the two groups. For example, if head and neck cancer patients who are being recruited are stage 3 and 4, and, for some reason, the stage 3 patients think they have less disease, they may all opt for the control therapy. A failure of the experimental arm in this case may be due to the placement of patients with more advanced disease in the experimental arm rather than a failure of therapy.

All studies are subject to errors introduced by bias, or unequal factors that may affect the results of the study. There are many types of bias. Patients themselves introduce bias (patient selection bias) when they refuse to enter a trial because they do not want to be randomized. Bias can also be introduced by physicians recruiting for clinical trials, creating physician selection bias. Physicians may be reluctant to recommend treatment within a trial setting if they do not believe the treatment is beneficial, or may only recommend enrollment to certain patients. In some situations, nonrandomized studies may not include a control arm, but rather use historical controls as the control arm. This may introduce further selection bias as the historical controls may not have undergone the exact treatment. For example, in a chemoradiation trial, the historical controls may have outdated techniques of radiation therapy, and therefore not be comparable to a control arm with contemporary radiation techniques. Other types of bias can be introduced by the methods of the study. If patients are classified into stage or diagnosis is made by methods other than the gold standard, misclassification may introduce further bias. Improper statistical analysis may introduce analysis bias. An exhaustive review of the many types of bias is beyond the scope of this chapter, although reviews on bias are available.[14] A strong study should attempt to reduce bias or, at the very least, explain where bias may have occurred.

Meta-Analysis

Meta-analysis is a statistical method of pooling the results of multiple studies in an attempt to strengthen the power of those studies by increasing patient numbers. Because different studies do not necessarily employ the same methods, each meta-analysis has strict criteria as to which studies can be included. Meta-analysis is an excellent method of reviewing recent trials and ensuring that the results of the trial are reproducible and stand the test of time. A meta-analysis differs from a review because the meta-analysis systematically reviews all published studies that meet the criteria. The meta-analysis may not exclude qualifying studies, thus reducing biased viewpoints sometimes seen in invited review articles. The actual data are acquired from the original authors, and the pooled data are analyzed. An excellent review of the techniques and pitfalls of meta-analysis was authored by Rosenfeld.[15] Meta-analysis has gained popularity over the past few decades as the importance of evidence-based medicine has been recognized. The Cochrane Review is one organization dedicated to improving the quality of evidence-based medicine, and they have a number of head and neck related meta-analyses available.[16]

Evidence-Based Medicine

In order to make the research validity of clinical trials easily understandable to readers, a number of high-quality journals now include recommendations as to the quality of the study at the end of each abstract. The most commonly used recommendation system is the Strength of Recommendation Taxonomy. In the SORT classification, studies are graded as A, B, or C. Studies earning a grade A recommendation have consistent high-quality evidence. High-quality evidence is designated as level 1, and these are usually from prospective randomized trials. Grade B studies have poor or inconsistent evidence, designated as level 2. This may be from randomized clinical trails in which a significant proportion of the patients do not complete the treatment as recommended, or the recommended treatment does not meet the standard of care. Grade C studies are not recommended as they have no direct evidence. They include level 3 evidence that may be from case reports, retrospective studies, or case series.[17]

When analyzing a clinical trial, there are a number of factors that should be examined in determining if the study is valid. The study should explicitly state both its research question and the methods used to answer that question. The research methods should be detailed enough to replicate the study, including surgical techniques, pharmaceutical doses and scheduling, radiation timing and fractionation, and patient recruiting methods. The statistical methods used to analyze the data should be listed. The study should also explicitly state the clinical characteristics and demographics of the two groups. The two groups should be equal in the stage of disease, performance status, age, and gender. Any difference between the two groups could introduce bias.

Intergroup 0099: Nasopharyngeal Cancer

Armed with a fundamental understanding of the many factors related to outcome measures, we will examine a clinical trial in depth. This discussion will point out that there is much more to a good study than just statistics. Intergroup 0099 examined the effect of concomitant chemoradiation and adjuvant chemotherapy compared to standard radiation therapy in patients with previously untreated stage 3 and stage 4 nasopharyngeal carcinoma. This was a landmark trial that has permanently changed the way that nasopharyngeal cancer is treated. However, this study was not without its critics, and the controversy surrounding this trial is a good example of some of the difficulties with clinical trials.

Intergroup 0099 was a randomized prospective trial sponsored jointly by SWOG, ECOG, and RTOG. Previously untreated stage 3 and 4A patients with nasopharyngeal carcinoma and a performance status of 0 to 2 were recruited. Patients were randomized to the control group, which consisted of daily radiation of 1.8 to 2.0 Gy to a total dose of 70 Gy to the primary site and 50 to 70 Gy to the neck depending on the bulk of vocal disease. The experimental group received the same radiation as well as chemotherapy, concurrent cisplatin 100 mg/m² on days 1, 22, and 43 during radiation therapy followed by 3 courses of adjuvant cisplatin 80 mg/m² and 5FU every 4 weeks. The endpoints of the study were progression-free survival and overall survival.

There were 193 patients initially enrolled in Intergroup 0099; however, 38 were excluded for noncompliance or incomplete follow-up information. The clinical characteristics of the patients in the experimental and control groups were similar.

The vast majority of patients in each arm were stage 4. The average age was similar, 50 compared to 52. There were similar percentages of males and females in each group. The majority of patients in each group were classified as World Health Organization (WHO) type 2 or 3 (nonkeratinizing or undifferentiated carcinoma). The chemoradiation group had statistically significant improved progression-free survival (radiation 24% 3-yr versus chemoradiation 69% 3-yr survival, p <0.001) and overall survival (radiation 47% 3-yr versus chemoradiation 78% 3-yr survival, p = 0.005). The study actually was closed early due to the large difference in survival at interim analysis. These statistics show that the 3-year progression-free survival was 24% for the radiation group and 69% for the chemoradiation group. Twenty-four percent seems to be much less than 69%, but without the p value, the significance could not be determined. In this case, the p value was less than 0.001. That means that there is a less than 0.1% chance that the 3-year progression-free survival for radiation is not different for those treated with chemoradiation. This is a strong result. Similarly, the overall survival was 47% with radiation and 78% with chemoradiation with a less than 0.5% chance that these values are really the same. Overall, this means that chemoradiation improves progression-free survival and overall survival compared to radiation therapy alone.

Of note, the majority of patients in the chemotherapy arm did not complete the chemotherapy as outlined in the protocol: 63% of patients completed all 3 concurrent treatments and 55% of patients completed all 3 adjuvant treatments; 33% of patients did not have any adjuvant chemotherapy at all. Reasons for not completing chemotherapy include treatment toxicity and patient preference.

Although Intergroup 0099 showed a significant improvement in survival in patients with advanced nasopharyngeal cancer who received chemoradiation compared to radiation alone, there were a number of critiques. The survival of patients in the radiation arm in Intergroup 0099 was worse than historical controls. Of 193 patients initially enrolled, 38 were excluded, most for incomplete evaluations or paperwork. The Intergroup 0099 trial closed early due to a significant survival advantage in the interim analysis. This introduced bias and may overestimate the actual benefit. There was a higher percentage of WHO type I compared to what would be expected in endemic areas (Asia, Northern Africa).[18] Subsequent studies have shown chemoradiation is useful in endemic areas.[19] Others cited the low number of patients able to finish the protocol as outlined, and wondered if less chemotherapy could be used.[20] Investigation into the exact timing most appropriate for chemotherapy continues today. Despite the valid critiques, Intergroup 0099 was an excellent clinical trial that changed the way nasopharyngeal cancer is treated and has benefited many patients.[21]

This evaluation of Intergroup 0099 illustrates some of the inherent difficulties of clinical trials. Patient and physician compliance, treatment-related side effects, and trial methods all can introduce variability and possible bias into a clinical trial. We cannot discount all trials that have any source of bias, as there are no perfect trials when dealing with human subjects. However, being aware of the possible sources of bias may help the clinician determine if his or her patient might benefit from participation in a clinical trial.

CONCLUSION

Clinical trials are a useful means of demonstrating the likely effect of an experimental therapy. The ideal clinical trial will have sufficient power to show a difference between treatments, will be repeatable at other institutions, will contain quality of life measures such as speech and swallowing outcomes, and will have minimal toxicity compared to the control group. A strong word of caution must be issued in examining the results of clinical trials. Clinical trials are most often conducted at large institutions, and often enroll multiple institutions, with extra resources devoted to the care of patients participating in the trial. These results cannot necessarily be extended to community hospitals. The excellent outcomes of patients on some clinical trials are due not only to close patient observation but also to experience of the clinicians. There are, and always will be, factors that are not explicitly stated in the protocol, but rather are due to physician experience. Patients' long-term survival and quality of life outcomes are best served by treatment at a large institution with experience treating patients with head and neck cancer.

REFERENCES

1. Jemal A, Siegel R, Ward E, et al. Cancer statistics, 2006. *CA Cancer J Clin.* 2006;56:106-130.

2. Parkin DM, Bray F, Ferlay J, Pisani P. Global cancer statistics, 2002. *CA Cancer J Clin.* 2005;55:74-108.

3. Sen U, Sankaranarayanan R, Mandal S, Ramanakumar AV, Parkin DM, Siddiqi M. Cancer patterns in eastern India: the first report of the Kolkata Cancer Registry. *Int J Cancer.* 2002;100:86-91.

4. Terrell JE, Ronis DL, Fowler KE, et al. Clinical predictors of quality of life in patients with head and neck cancer. *Arch Otolaryngol Head Neck Surg.* 2004;130:401-408.

5. Hanna E, Sherman A, Cash D, et al. Quality of life for patients following total laryngectomy vs chemoradiation for laryngeal preservation. *Arch Otolaryngol Head Neck Surg.* 2004;130:875-879.

6. Parsons JT, Mendenhall WM, Stringer SP, et al. Squamous cell carcinoma of the oropharynx: surgery, radiation therapy, or both. *Cancer.* 2002;94:2967-2980.

7. Induction chemotherapy plus radiation compared with surgery plus radiation in patients with advanced laryngeal cancer. The Department of Veterans Affairs Laryngeal Cancer Study Group. *N Engl J Med.* 1991;324:1685-1690.

8. Weber RS, Berkey BA, Forastiere A, et al. Outcome of salvage total laryngectomy following organ preservation therapy: the radiation therapy oncology group trial 91-11. *Arch Otolaryngol Head Neck Surg.* 2003;129:44-49.

9. Forastiere AA, Goepfert H, Maor M, et al. Concurrent chemotherapy and radiotherapy for organ preservation in advanced laryngeal cancer. *N Engl J Med.* 2003;349:2091-2098.

10. Hillman RE, Walsh MJ, Wolf GT, Fisher SG, Hong WK. Functional outcomes following treatment for advanced laryngeal cancer. Part I—voice preservation in advanced laryngeal cancer. Part II—laryngectomy rehabilitation: the state of the art in the VA system. research speech–language pathologists. Department of Veterans Affairs Laryngeal Cancer Study Group. *Ann Otol Rhinol Laryngol Suppl.* 1998;172:1-27.

11. Code of federal regulations.

12. Oken MM, Creech RH, Tormey DC, et al. Toxicity and response criteria of the Eastern Cooperative Oncology Group. *Am J Clin Oncol.* 1982;5:649-655.

13. Bernier J, Domenge C, Ozsahin M, et al. Postoperative irradiation with or without concomitant chemotherapy for locally advanced head and neck cancer. *N Engl J Med.* 2004;350:1945-1952.

14. Hartman JM, Forsen JW Jr, Wallace MS, Neely JG. Tutorials in clinical research: Part IV: recognizing and controlling bias. *Laryngoscope.* 2002;112:23-31.

15. Rosenfeld RM. Meta-analysis. *ORL J Otorhinolaryngol Relat Spec.* 2004;66:186-195.

16. The Cochrane Library. Retrieved October 12 from www.thecochranelibrary.com

17. Ebell MH, Siwek J, Weiss BD, et al. Strength of recommendation taxonomy (SORT): a patient-centered approach to grading evidence in the medical literature. *Am Fam Physician.* 2004;69:548-556.

18. Rischin D, Peters LJ. The local-regionally advanced nasopharyngeal carcinoma jigsaw puzzle: where does the chemotherapy piece fit? *J Clin Oncol.* 2002;20:1968-1970.

19. Lin JC, Jan JS, Hsu CY, Liang WM, Jiang RS, Wang WY. Phase III study of concurrent chemoradiotherapy versus radiotherapy alone for advanced nasopharyngeal carcinoma: positive effect on overall and progression-free survival. *J Clin Oncol.* 2003;21:631-637.

20. Faivre S, Janot F, Armand JP. Optimal management of nasopharyngeal carcinoma. *Curr Opin Oncol.* 2004;16:231-235.

21. Baujat B, Audry H, Bourhis J, et al. Chemotherapy in locally advanced nasopharyngeal carcinoma: an individual patient data meta-analysis of eight randomized trials and 1753 patients. *Int J Radiat Oncol Biol Phys.* 2006;64:47-56.

Index